Pediatric Cardiology

THE REQUISITES IN PEDIATRICS

Victoria L. Vetter, M.D.
Professor of Pediatrics
University of Pennsylvania School of Medicine
Chief, Division of Pediatric Cardiology
The Children's Hospital of Philadelphia
Philadelphia, Pennsylvania

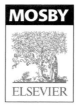

MOSBY

ELSEVIER

MOSBY
ELSEVIER

1600 John F. Kennedy Boulevard
Suite 1800
Philadelphia, PA 19103-2899

THE REQUISITES ™
THE REQUISITES
THE REQUISITES
THE REQUISITES
THE REQUISITES

THE REQUISITES is a proprietary trademark
of Mosby, Inc.

PEDIATRIC CARDIOLOGY: THE REQUISITES IN PEDIATRICS

ISBN-13: 978-0-323-02367-2
ISBN-10: 0-323-02367-3

Notice

Knowledge and best practice in this field are constantly changing. As new research and experience broaden our knowledge, changes in practice, treatment and drug therapy may become necessary or appropriate. Readers are advised to check the most current information provided (i) on procedures featured or (ii) by the manufacturer of each product to be administered, to verify the recommended dose or formula, the method and duration of administration, and contraindications. It is the responsibility of the practitioner, relying on his or her own experience and knowledge of the patient, to make diagnoses, to determine dosages and the best treatment for each individual patient, and to take all appropriate safety precautions. To the fullest extent of the law, neither the Publisher nor the Editor assumes any liability for any injury and/or damage to persons or property arising out or related to any use of the material contained in this book.

Library of Congress Cataloging-in-Publication Data

Vetter, Victoria L.
  Pediatric cardiology / Victoria L. Vetter.
    p. ; cm. – (The requisites in pediatrics)
  Includes index.
  ISBN-13: 978-0-323-02367-2
  ISBN-10: 0-323-02367-3
   1. Pediatric cardiology. I. Title. II. Series.
  [DNLM: 1. Cardiovascular Diseases–Child. WS 290 V591p 2006]
RJ421. V48 2006
618.92'12–dc22   2005056227

Acquisitions Editor: Joanne Husovski
Development Editor: Patrick M.N. Stone
Senior Project Manager: Cecelia Bayruns
Design Direction: Steven Stave

Printed in the United States of America

Last digit is the print number: 9 8 7 6 5 4 3 2 1

Dedication

I would like to dedicate this book to these special individuals.

To my mentors at CHOP,
Sidney Friedman
and
William J. Rashkind

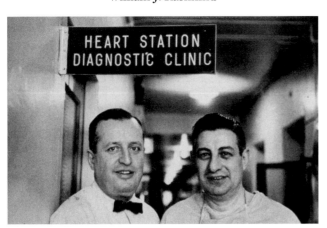

To my parents,
Albert E. Vetter, Jr.,
and
Mildred Irene Vetter

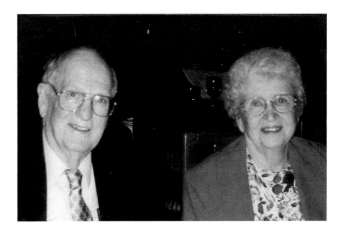

To my husband,
Anthony S. Jennings

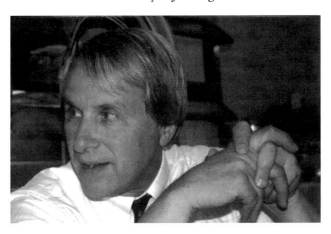

To my children,

Jason   Jennifer   Jonathan

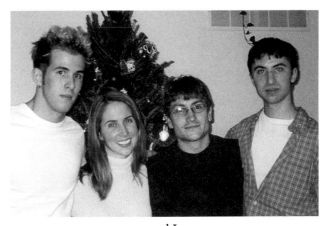

and Jason, my
son-in-law

Contributors

Maryanne R.K. Chrisant, M.D.
Assistant Professor of Pediatrics
The University of Pennsylvania School of Medicine
Medical Director, Pediatric Heart Failure and Heart
  Transplant Programs
The Children's Hospital of Philadelphia
Philadelphia, Pennsylvania

Bernard J. Clark III, M.D.
Associate Chief Executive of the Practice
Nemours Children's Clinic
A.I. duPont Hospital for Children
Wilmington, Delaware
Formerly, Professor of Pediatrics
The University of Pennsylvania School of Medicine
Medical Director
Division of Cardiology
The Children's Hospital of Philadelphia
Philadelphia, Pennsylvania

Meryl S. Cohen, M.D.
Assistant Professor of Pediatrics
The University of Pennsylvania School of Medicine
Interim Director, Non-Invasive Cardiovascular Laboratory
The Children's Hospital of Philadelphia
Philadelphia, Pennsylvania

Richard M. Donner, M.D.
Clinical Professor of Pediatrics
The University of Pennsylvania School of Medicine
Associate Cardiologist
The Children's Hospital of Philadelphia
Philadelphia, Pennsylvania

Matthew J. Gillespie, M.D.
Assistant Professor of Pediatrics
The University of Pennsylvania School of Medicine
Assistant Cardiologist, Division of Cardiology
The Children's Hospital of Philadelphia
Philadelphia, Pennsylvania

Marie M. Gleason, M.D., FACC, FAAP
Clinical Professor of Pediatrics
The University of Pennsylvania School of Medicine
Director, Outpatient and Community Cardiology
The Children's Hospital of Philadelphia
Philadelphia, Pennsylvania

Elizabeth Goldmuntz, M.D.
Associate Professor of Pediatrics
The University of Pennsylvania School of Medicine
Associate Cardiologist
Division of Cardiology
The Children's Hospital of Philadelphia
Philadelphia, Pennsylvania

Alexa N. Hogarty, M.D.
Clinical Associate in Pediatrics
The University of Pennsylvania School of Medicine
Attending Cardiologist
Division of Cardiology, Department of Pediatrics
The Children's Hospital of Philadelphia
Philadelphia, Pennsylvania

Fraz Ahmed Ismat, M.D.
Instructor in Pediatrics
University of Pennsylvania School of Medicine
Attending Cardiologist
The Children's Hospital of Philadelphia
Philadelphia, Pennsylvania

Vijaya M. Joshi, M.D.
Assistant Professor of Pediatrics
The University of Tennessee School of Medicine
Director of Echocardiography
Le Bonheur Children's Medical Center
Memphis, Tennessee
Formerly, Clinical Instructor
The University of Pennsylvania School of Medicine
Clinical Assistant Professor of Pediatrics
The Children's Hospital of Philadelphia
Philadelphia, Pennsylvania

Jonathan R. Kaltman, M.D.
Assistant Professor of Pediatrics
The University of Pennsylvania School of Medicine
Assistant Cardiologist, Division of Cardiology
The Children's Hospital of Philadelphia
Philadelphia, Pennsylvania

Jacqueline Kreutzer, M.D., FACC
Assistant Professor of Pediatrics
Director, Cardiac Catheterization Laboratory
Children's Hospital of Pittsburgh
Pittsburgh, Pennsylvania
Assistant Cardiologist, Division of Cardiology
The Children's Hospital of Philadelphia
Philadelphia, Pennsylvania

P. Nelson Le, M.D.
Fellow, Division of Cardiology
The Children's Hospital of Philadelphia
Clinical Instructor
The University of Pennsylvania School of Medicine
Philadelphia, Pennsylvania

Mark D. Levin, M.D.
Research Fellow
Division of Cardiology
The Children's Hospital of Philadelphia
Philadelphia, Pennsylvania

Nandini Madan, M.D.
Staff Cardiologist
Heart Center for Children
St. Christopher's Hospital for Children
Philadelphia, Pennsylvania
Formerly, Electrophysiology Fellow
Division of Cardiology
The Children's Hospital of Philadelphia
Instructor in Pediatrics
The University of Pennsylvania School of Medicine
Philadelphia, Pennsylvania

Bradley S. Marino, M.D., MPP, MFCE
Assistant Professor of Anesthesia and Pediatrics
The University of Pennsylvania School of Medicine
Divisions of Critical Care Medicine and Cardiology
The Children's Hospital of Philadelphia
Philadelphia, Pennsylvania

Jondavid Menteer, M.D.
Assistant Professor of Clinical Pediatrics
Keck School of Medicine
University of Southern California
Transplant Cardiologist
Children's Hospital Los Angeles
Los Angeles, California
Formerly, Instructor in Pediatrics
The University of Pennsylvania School of Medicine
Fellow, Division of Cardiology
The Children's Hospital of Philadelphia
Philadelphia, Pennsylvania

Adam M. Ostrow, M.D.
Formerly, Instructor in Pediatrics
The University of Pennsylvania School of Medicine
Fellow, Division of Cardiology
The Children's Hospital of Philadelphia
Philadelphia, Pennsylvania

Stephen Paridon, M.D.
Associate Professor of Pediatrics
University of Pennsylvania School of Medicine
Director, Cardiovascular Exercise Laboratory
The Children's Hospital of Philadelphia
Philadelphia, Pennsylvania

Larry A. Rhodes, M.D.
Professor of Pediatrics
West Virginia University School of Medicine
Section Chief, Pediatric Cardiology
West Virginia University Hospital
Morgantown, West Virginia
Formerly, Associate Professor of Pediatrics
The University of Pennsylvania School of Medicine
Director of Electrophysiology, Division of Cardiology
The Children's Hospital of Philadelphia
Philadelphia, Pennsylvania

Jonathan Rome, M.D.
Associate Professor of Pediatrics
The University of Pennsylvania School of Medicine
Director, Cardiac Catheterization Laboratory
The Children's Hospital of Philadelphia
Philadelphia, Pennsylvania

Jack Rychik, M.D.
Associate Professor of Pediatrics
The University of Pennsylvania School of Medicine
Director, Fetal Heart Program
Cardiac Center at The Children's Hospital of Philadelphia
Philadelphia, Pennsylvania

Heike E. Schneider, M.D.
Pediatric Cardiology and Intensive Care Medicine
Georg-August-Universität Göttingen
Göttingen, Germany
Formerly, Interventional Cardiology Fellow, Division of
    Cardiology
The Children's Hospital of Philadelphia
Philadelphia, Pennsylvania

Amy H. Schultz, M.D.
Assistant Professor of Pediatrics
University of Washington School of Medicine
Attending Physician, Division of Cardiology
Children's Hospital and Regional Medical Center
Seattle, Washington
Formerly, Instructor in Pediatrics
University of Pennsylvania School of Medicine
Assistant Cardiologist, Division of Cardiology
The Children's Hospital of Philadelphia
Philadelphia, Pennsylvania

Sepehr Sekhavat, M.D.
Assistant Professor of Pediatrics
Boston University School of Medicine
Boston, Massachusetts
Formerly, Instructor in Pediatrics
The University of Pennsylvania School of Medicine
Fellow, Division of Cardiology
The Children's Hospital of Philadelphia
Philadelphia, Pennsylvania

V. Ben Sivarajan, M.D., FRCP, FAAP
Senior Registrar in Critical Care Medicine
Royal Children's Hospital
Melbourne, Australia
Formerly, Clinical Instructor
The University of Pennsylvania School of Medicine
Fellow, Division of Cardiology
The Children's Hospital of Philadelphia
Philadelphia, Pennsylvania

Sarah Tabbutt, M.D., Ph.D.
Assistant Professor of Cardiology and Critical Care
    Medicine
The University of Pennsylvania School of Medicine
Interim Medical Director, Cardiac Intensive Care
The Children's Hospital of Philadelphia
Philadelphia, Pennsylvania

Ronn E. Tanel, M.D.
Assistant Professor of Pediatrics
The University of Pennsylvania School of Medicine
Attending Cardiologist
Division of Cardiology
The Children's Hospital of Philadelphia
Philadelphia, Pennsylvania

Victoria L. Vetter, M.D.
Professor of Pediatrics
University of Pennsylvania School of Medicine
Chief, Division of Pediatric Cardiology
The Children's Hospital of Philadelphia
Philadelphia, Pennsylvania

Ilana Zeltser, M.D.
Assistant Professor of Pediatrics/Cardiology
University of Texas Southwestern Medical School
Children's Medical Center at Dallas
Dallas, Texas
Formerly, Instructor in Pediatrics
The University of Pennsylvania School of Medicine
Fellow, Division of Cardiology
The Children's Hospital of Philadelphia
Philadelphia, Pennsylvania

Foreword

For much of the early history of medicine, the heart was considered to be the most sacred and mystical of all human organs. As a General Pediatrician, I tend to expect that the children I care for will have strong, properly functioning hearts. However, in situations where the heart is congenitally malformed or affected by inflammation or myopathy, it is reassuring and important to have a pediatric cardiologist and cardiac surgeon at my side to help me with decisions about further diagnostic testing and imaging, instituting medical therapy, and assessing the need for surgical intervention.

It is with that image of partnership in mind that the fifth volume of **The Requisites in Pediatrics**, *Pediatric Cardiology*, is offered. This carefully edited book by Dr. Vetter meets the goal of the series. The editors and authors were asked to discuss the common pediatric conditions within their specialty and to include practical information that would guide primary care providers, resident physicians, nurse practitioners, and students in the care of their patients. Therefore, the information in this volume is intended to be an adjunct to all care providers, to strengthen our understanding and improve treatment of heart disease in infants, children, and young adults.

The book, containing sixteen chapters, begins with an excellent review of the heart exam in the pediatric patient. It is filled with pearls of wisdom from the experienced authors. Chapter 6, by Dr. Paridon, begins with an outstanding review of the infection endocarditis, ranging from the changing epidemiology over the last 50 years to evidence-based discussion of diagnosis and treatment.

Chapter 11 is unique in my experience, beginning with the "goals of this chapter" for the reader. Drs. Gillespie, Schneider, and Rome give the reader a detailed review and explanation of cardiac catheterization in pediatrics. The discussion of the indications for balloon dilations, balloon septostomy, and endovascular stent deployment is excellent. Chapter 15, by Dr. Clark, is very helpful for the general pediatrician in outpatient and inpatient care. It contains practical information about the management of children and young adults with heart disease, including advice on anticipatory guidance for families about safe travel and exercise. Dr. Clark discusses medications to avoid in patients with arrhythmias and the implications of pregnancy in young women with heart disease.

I extend my deep appreciation to Dr. Vetter and the authors for providing an outstanding volume that offers detailed and practical information on pediatric cardiology. We hope you will enjoy this fifth volume in **The Requisites in Pediatrics.**

Louis M. Bell, M.D.
Patrick S. Pasquariello, Jr. Chair in General Pediatrics
Professor of Pediatrics
University of Pennsylvania School of Medicine
Chief, Division of General Pediatrics
Attending Physician, General Pediatrics
and Infectious Diseases
The Children's Hospital of Philadelphia
Philadelphia, Pennsylvania

Preface

Although congenital heart defects were described in pathological specimens in the seventeenth century, pediatric cardiology began as a specialty in 1930 with Helen Taussig's Cardiac Clinic at The Harriet Lane Home of the Johns Hopkins Hospital. Rheumatic heart disease was the major "treatable" heart disease of children at that time, as congenital heart disease remained largely descriptive. In 1938, Robert Gross successfully ligated the patent ductus arteriosus of a 7-year-old girl and congenital heart disease began its journey to the present era. The field of pediatric cardiology began the current era only slightly over 60 years ago with the incredibly courageous actions of a surgical team, cardiologists, family members, and a patient at the Johns Hopkins Hospital in 1944 with the first Blalock-Taussig shunt. Ten years later, in 1954, a similar team at the University of Minnesota performed the first open heart surgery on a congenital heart disease patient using cross circulation; this was quickly followed by the use of mechanical cardiopulmonary bypass by John Kirklin in 1955. Six years later, in 1961, pediatric cardiology became the first Subboard of Pediatrics to be formed. Over the ensuing years, the field has developed and expanded into the broad expanse that is called Pediatric Cardiology with treatment available for essentially all congenital heart defects. It continues as a vibrant and constantly changing specialty, and thus writing a book with the "requisites in pediatric cardiology"—necessary or essential information—has been challenging.

Heart disease in pediatrics spans a wide range of ages, from the fetus to the young adult, and includes congenital heart disease—the most common birth defect known, occurring in 8 of 1000 live births—and acquired heart disease. The etiologies of both of these categories are complex with the genetic and molecular implications just beginning to be understood.

Congenital heart disease includes structural intracardiac abnormalities, extracardiac vascular abnormalities, and coronary artery anomalies. The genetic association is borne out by the presence of congenital heart disease in association with genetic syndromes, as well as the identification of specific genes associated with distinct types of congenital heart defects. Additionally, heart disease may be acquired in childhood by association with inflammatory or infectious etiologies, or systemic disease. Atherosclerotic heart disease, the number one health problem of adults, has its origins in childhood. Abnormal cardiac function, or congestive heart failure, may be seen in association with congenital heart defects, cardiomyopathies, or inflammation of the heart such as myocarditis, pericarditis, or endocarditis. Abnormal heart rates and rhythms are seen in children with known structural heart disease and in those with normal hearts.

A variety of signs and symptoms may concern or alert the parent or pediatrician to seek a cardiac evaluation. These include heart murmurs; abnormally low, high, or irregular heart rates or palpitations; dizziness; near fainting or syncope; fatigue or exercise intolerance; and chest pain.

Treatment of heart disease may include pharmacologic agents, cardiac catheterization including therapeutic or interventional catheterization technologies, electrophysiologic diagnostic and therapeutic techniques including catheter ablation and pacing devices, and cardiothoracic surgery.

Knowledge of preventive cardiology should be applied to the pediatric population in an effort to affect the development of cardiovascular disease in adults.

This book is written for the practitioners who treat children with concerns involving the heart or who care for children or adults with congenital heart disease across all age ranges. To care for the fetus with heart disease, one must know the in utero effects of the heart disease, as well as the subsequent treatment of the disease in the neonate. To care for the pediatric patient with heart disease, one must understand the disease, how to diagnose it, how to treat it, and, of increasing importance, how to identify and treat the sequelae of pediatric heart disease. Fortunately, in the current era, most of these children with heart disease grow into adulthood. To care for the adult who has had heart disease since birth or childhood, knowledge of these requisites in pediatric cardiology is truly essential, for one must understand the background of the patient to understand the present condition and prepare for the future sequelae. As knowledge regarding prevention of cardiac disease beginning or presenting in childhood is acquired, this will become an important component of pediatric cardiology.

We are all students, just at different points in time. Thus, this book is meant to provide useful information to medical students, pediatric residents, pediatric nurses, pediatricians, pediatric cardiology fellows, pediatric cardiologists, our pediatric cardiac surgical and cardiac anesthesia and critical care colleagues, and all others involved in the care of pediatric cardiology patients. This book can be used to provide basic or more extensive information determined by the need of the reader. The initial emphasis on the history and physical exam should be recognized as an indicator that the individual patient and the information derived from that patient informs all future interactions with the patient. A thorough history and physical exam of the cardiac patient and an understanding of the implications will direct future diagnostic tests, interventional procedures, and treatments described in the fetal diagnosis, catheterization, pharmacology, and surgical chapters. A broad base of knowledge exists about pediatric cardiology, but taken in logical and compact portions as is the case in this book, this important knowledge can be readily applied to the patient. The text of each chapter is meant to provide the necessary information for all types of students. The Major Points in each chapter describe the most important concepts, and the References point to additional information for those interested in a more in-depth exploration of the topics.

Today pediatric cardiology truly is a multidisciplinary field. The care of the cardiac patient involves the family and the pediatric cardiologist, often including those with many different subspecialty skills. Additionally, cardiothoracic surgeons, cardiac anesthesiologists, cardiac nurses, and other support staff are essential to the care of these very special and unique patients.

Victoria L. Vetter, M.D.

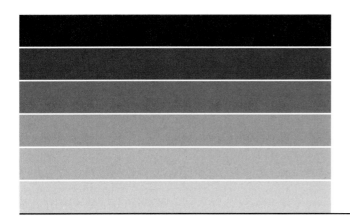

Acknowledgments

I would like to thank a number of individuals for their assistance in this project.

The first is Paullette Shamwell-Briggs, my administrative assistant, who has been invaluable in coordinating, organizing, and generally shepherding this project from start to finish. Without her assistance, the book would not have been completed.

All of the chapter authors, fellows and faculty, are owed a debt of gratitude. The time and effort spent in this type of project is often taken from one's personal time, and that fact is recognized and acknowledged. You are all incredible doctors and people and deserve recognition for being the best in your field. The knowledge you share in these pages and each day has an impact far beyond your day-to-day care of patients.

Over 30 years of exposure to the best that pediatric cardiology has to offer has led me to be the editor of this book. I would like to acknowledge and thank those who have been my teachers. This includes Jacqueline A. Noonan at the University of Kentucky, who provided my first exposure to pediatric cardiology and quickly incorporated her enthusiasm for the field into my psyche. The next stop on the path was at Johns Hopkins Hospital, where I encountered Helen Taussig, Catherine Neil, Richard Rowe, and Robert Freedom. With no question left as to the most exciting field in pediatrics, my education was furthered by Thomas P. Graham at Vanderbilt University. The final step in my "formal educa-

tion" in pediatric cardiology came from William J. Rashkind and Sidney Friedman at the Children's Hospital of Philadelphia, from whom I learned different but equally important aspects of the field. Additionally, at CHOP, Henry Wagner and Charles Causo were important in shaping my early pediatric cardiology education. My area of subspecialty, electrophysiology, is a result of the guidance and friendship of Leonard Horowitz of the Cardiology Division of the University of Pennsylvania School of Medicine and Mark Josephson, who allowed a pediatric cardiology fellow into his clinical laboratory and to read the drafts of the chapter of his first book as they were written. The early research experience that taught me so much about critical thinking is a result of research done in the laboratories of Neil Moore and Joseph Spear of the School of Veterinary Medicine of the University of Pennsylvania. Scores of others, including students, residents, fellows, and colleagues, have taught me over the years, and all are acknowledged here.

Importantly, I would like to thank my very special patients and their families, from whom I have learned more than any textbook or formal education could provide.

Finally, I would like to thank and acknowledge the many Elsevier staff who have assisted our group of authors with this project. Your patience and assistance have been invaluable.

Contents

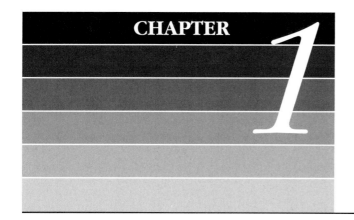

CHAPTER 1

Pediatric Evaluation of the Cardiac Patient

Exam, Murmurs, Exercise Intolerance, Chest Pain, Palpitations, and Syncope

V. BEN SIVARAJAN

VICTORIA L. VETTER

MARIE M. GLEASON

CARDIAC EXAMINATION

Background

The role of the primary care provider in assessing the status of the cardiovascular system is extremely important. It is through the careful evaluation of neonates, children, and adolescents by a primary care provider that congenital and acquired heart problems are discovered; referral can then be made to a pediatric cardiologist for further evaluation and treatment. Once these patients are identified, primary care providers function as the remote eyes of the pediatric cardiologist. Their assessments of the cardiovascular system at well and sick visits determine whether additional evaluation by the sub-specialist is indicated.

The success of a good physician lies in the ability to obtain an accurate history and to perform an excellent physical examination. These skills provide the basis for appropriate referral and management of children with congenital or acquired heart disease and, in some instances, can be lifesaving. As such, it is important to review the components of the history and the physical examination that are critical in assessing the cardiovascular system.[1-3]

History

The history should start with the chief complaint and a relatively rapid determination of how sick the child might be. What have the parents observed and what have they been told by others, including other physicians, caretakers, and teachers? If the child can speak for himself, he should be allowed to provide as much history as possible before the clinician hears the parents' account.

The age of the child at the onset of symptoms is critically important in pointing the clinician in the appropriate direction. Any cardiac or respiratory symptoms in a newborn must be considered serious.

The type and onset of symptoms, their duration and intensity, interference with normal childhood activities, and associated findings should be ascertained. If the symptom is one of cyanosis or duskiness, questioning should determine whether the cyanosis is central (i.e., seen in mucous membranes such as blue tongue and lips, indicating desaturation), or peripheral (indicating a response to cold temperatures). Circumoral cyanosis associated with increased venous pressure or crying is not a central form of cyanosis, and pulse oximetry will be normal.

Symptoms of respiratory distress must be evaluated for severity, onset, and association with fever, feeding, or other activity. Differentiating between an infection and heart failure may be difficult because a respiratory infection may increase the symptoms of congestive heart failure. Poor feeding with diaphoresis would be more suggestive of congestive heart failure exacerbated by a respiratory infection. Other respiratory symptoms, such as stridor or dysphagia, might point to a vascular ring or sling.

The growth and feeding history of the child are important. The parent can generally relate whether the infant or child is too tired to eat or is uninterested in food. In a child who is several months to several years of age, the growth chart is essential in following the general state of growth and nutrition. With congestive heart failure, weight is more affected than height or head circumference. The major symptoms of congestive heart failure in the infant are poor feeding, diaphoresis, increased or labored respirations, growth failure, and frequent respiratory infections.

A complete review of systems can reveal information about the cardiac system. A decrease in urinary output might signal congestive heart failure. A careful review of the exercise tolerance of the child and changes in activity level may reveal limitations imposed by cardiac physiology. Feeding is the major activity of the infant, and "exercise intolerance" is marked by tiring during feeding, by increased respiratory effort, or by failure to continue eating shortly after beginning, even though the baby still seems to be hungry. Frequent respiratory infections are seen in children with left-to-right shunts through large ventricular septal defects (VSDs).

History of abnormalities in the central nervous system or delayed development, especially in the presence of a syndrome or other congenital defects, may point to an associated congenital heart defect. This is commonly seen with trisomy 21, and DiGeorge, Williams, and Noonan's syndromes. A history of abnormalities in the musculoskeletal system could point to various types of acquired heart disease, including cardiomyopathies, rheumatic fever, and Lyme disease.

The family history is extremely important, because there are many genetic causes of congenital heart disease and predispositions to acquired heart disease. Prenatal and maternal history may reveal important information such as maternal infection or medication exposure that could have affected the fetus. Maternal conditions such as lupus or diabetes mellitus are associated with an increased incidence of heart problems in the child.

Observation and Inspection

With time and experience, a health care provider develops a sense of when a patient is well or unwell. This same instinctive global assessment is a very important component of the examination of the patient with known or suspected heart disease. The overall appearance of the child helps the clinician determine the urgency associated with the particular patient. The following are several specific features that should be evaluated prior to touching the patient:

1. Does the patient show signs of distress (e.g., tachypnea, shortness of breath, clamminess, or diaphoresis)?
2. Is the child responsive, interactive, happy, or irritable?
3. Is there any change in color (e.g., pallor or cyanosis)?
4. Are there any dysmorphic features?
5. Are there any obvious skeletal abnormalities of the chest, back, or extremities? Is there a precordial bulge or asymmetry of the chest?
6. Is the patient age-appropriate for height and weight?
7. Is the patient developmentally delayed in motor skills, speech, or cognition?

Vital Signs

Whenever possible, vital signs should be recorded and available to the practitioner at the start of the examination. Temperature should be documented because fever can significantly impact other vital signs. Fever history (length and degree of fever and response to antipyretics) is important in assessing the patient for acquired heart disease. Height and weight should be plotted on appropriate growth charts (normal, trisomy 21, or premature). In the absence of specific genetic conditions, head circumference and length are generally spared in children with clinically significant heart disease. Utilization of calories for weight gain is adversely affected by increased cardiac work, making serial assessment of weight gain velocity an important indicator of cardiac well-being in the pediatric population. Heart rate and respiratory rate should be documented and interpreted in light of the patient's general state at the time (e.g., quiet and cooperative, febrile, or crying). The effort or work of breathing, as well as its precise rate, should be noted. Nasal flaring and suprasternal, subcostal, and intercostal retractions should be reported.

Documentation of blood pressure is essential when assessing the cardiovascular system. Blood pressure measurements should be obtained in primary care offices from infancy, recognizing that patient cooperation will vary in younger patients and that automated blood pressure machines with multiple-size pediatric cuffs will be needed, especially for infants. Upper extremity hypertension can be an important first sign of coarctation of the aorta but is often missed in children younger than 3 years if blood pressures are not obtained. In order to maximize yield on blood pressure screening for hypertension, the right arm is the preferred site for recording serial measurements. If elevated blood pressure is noted in the right arm, a left arm and a leg blood pressure should be obtained. In the primary care office, documentation of systemic oxygen saturation with pulse oximetry is generally reserved for patients with active respiratory issues or known cyanotic heart disease.[4] Additionally, measurement

of pulse oximetry is helpful in children with cardiac murmurs, especially those younger than 1 month of age.

Many cyanotic cardiac patients have decreased pulmonary blood flow (e.g., tetralogy of Fallot [TOF]), but there is a subgroup of patients with cyanotic heart disease who have adequate pulmonary blood flow but abnormal intracardiac mixing of desaturated and saturated blood. Although the oxygen saturation needs to be less than 88–90% to produce visible cyanosis, a pulse oximetry reading of less than 94% in a quiet infant or child should be considered abnormal. The appearance of cyanosis is influenced by anemia and hyperpigmentation of the patient. Documentation of oxygen saturation of less than 94% in the lower extremity would alert the practitioner either to cyanotic congenital heart disease or to any condition in which there is right-to-left shunting through the patent ductus arteriosus (PDA) into the descending aorta. This differential cyanosis is seen in left heart obstructive lesions such as coarctation of the aorta, interrupted aortic arch, hypoplastic left heart syndrome, critical aortic stenosis, or pulmonary hypertension with an open PDA (Table 1-1).

Palpation

Beginning the cardiac examination with gentle palpation of the precordium using the palm rather than the fingertips, instead of immediate auscultation of the heart sounds, can be beneficial in several ways. In younger children, it is a nonthreatening, soothing gesture, which may allay the fear of painful procedures. From a physician's perspective, there is important information to be obtained regarding the heart, including:

1. Is the chest hyperdynamic or asymmetric, or is a bony deformity present?
2. Is there a heave?
3. Is there a thrill?
4. Is the cardiac impulse displaced?

Thrills are best felt with the palm of the hand at the lower sternal border (where they are more likely to be associated with VSDs than mitral or tricuspid regurgitation), or the right upper sternal border (RUSB) or suprasternal notch (where they are most likely to be associated with severe aortic stenosis). The point of maximal impulse should be within the midclavicular line in the fourth (through 4 years of age) or fifth left intercostal space. The suprasternal notch should be palpated for thrills generated by turbulent blood flow in the ascending aorta. Vigorous aortic pulsations (seen in aortic insufficiency), or jugular venous distention (seen in congestive heart failure), should be noted. Palpation of the abdomen for the size and location of the liver and spleen is important. All extremities should be examined for the presence of palpable pulses of equal intensity and timing. In small patients with a large patent ductus arteriosus or in any

Table 1-1   Signs and Symptoms in Heart Disease

Feature	Abnormality	Possible Cardiac Implications
Temperature	Fever	Tachycardia Peripheral vasoconstriction
Height	> 95%ile < 5%ile	Marfan syndrome, mitral valve prolapse Genetic syndrome
Weight	> 95%ile < 5%ile	Exercise intolerance Hypertension
Pulse oximetry (lower extremity)	< 93%	Cyanotic heart disease / mixing lesions Persistent pulmonary hypertension Parenchymal lung disease

Heart rate	Bradycardia	Third-degree atrioventricular block
		    Congenital complete heart block
		    Acquired (carditis, Lyme)

	Tachycardia	Sinus tachycardia
		    Carditis, congestive heart failure (CHF)
		    Effusions (pleural, pericardial)
		Supraventricular tachycardia
		Ventricular tachycardia

	Irregular	Sinus arrhythmia Premature atrial or ventricular contractions PACs, PVCs Second-degree atrioventricular block
Respirations	Tachypnea	CHF Effusions (pericardial, pleural) Metabolic acidosis
Blood pressure	Hypotension	Septic shock, metabolic acidosis Critical left heart obstruction
	Hypertension	Coarctation of the aorta Syndromes: Williams, Turner's Essential/familial

patient with severe aortic valve regurgitation, the pulses will be "full" or "bounding" because of the wide pulse pressure. The neck should be palpated for thyroid abnormalities; hyperthyroidism with goiter formation can have significant cardiac implications such as tachycardia, hypertension, ectopy, exercise intolerance, or high-output congestive heart failure (seen in thyroid storm).

Auscultation

Heart Sounds

The heart sounds should be assessed in both the right and left chests, including auscultation anteriorly, posteriorly, and in both axillae. A practitioner may diagnose dextrocardia when the heart sounds are louder in the right chest even though they are audible in the left chest. The precordium should be interrogated in a stepwise fashion, encompassing the five important areas: (1) right upper sternal border (RUSB), (2) left upper sternal border (LUSB), (3) left mid-sternal border (LMSB), (4) left lower sternal border (LLSB), and (5) left-sided apical region (LVap).

Any irregularity of the heart rate should be noted, with particular attention to variation with breathing (sinus arrhythmia). If the patient is old enough to hold his or her breath, irregularity secondary to sinus arrhythmia should disappear with a breath hold. Auscultation of the neck, skull, and liver areas may identify arteriovenous malformations in these areas or carotid bruits and venous hums.

Much information is obtained from the heart sounds. The first heart sound (S_1) represents closure of the tricuspid and mitral valves at the onset of systole and is best heard at the apex. The component parts may be appreciated separately (called splitting of a heart sound) at the LLSB in older children and adolescents with slower heart rates, with the mitral component normally first. On occasion, the splitting will be very noticeable, and sometimes the sound is mistakenly interpreted as a click. S_1 will be single in patients with an atretic atrioventricular (AV) valve or tachycardia. A loud S_1 occurs with increased flow across the mitral valve from large left-to-right shunts, such as a large VSD or patent ductus arteriosus, or moderate to severe mitral regurgitation, and is best heard at the apex. When there is increased flow across the tricuspid valve, as in a large atrial septal defect (ASD) or tricuspid regurgitation, the accentuated first sound is best heard at the LLSB. Accentuation of the S_1 occurs with marked mitral or tricuspid stenosis. With a short PR interval, as in Wolff-Parkinson-White (WPW) syndrome, and with increased cardiac output, the S_1 is increased. A soft first heart sound is present in congestive heart failure or with prolonged atrioventricular (AV) conduction.

The second heart sounds are best heard in the second and third left intercostal spaces. The second heart sound (S_2) represents closure of the aortic (A_2) and pulmonary (P_2) valves at the end of systole, in that order. An accurate assessment of the quality of this heart sound is critical in a thorough cardiac examination. Under normal circumstances, systemic vascular resistance (SVR) is higher than pulmonary vascular resistance (PVR), allowing slightly longer systolic ejection time into the pulmonary bed. As a result, the aortic valve closes before the pulmonary valve (A_2P_2). This splitting of S_2 also varies with the respiratory cycle. During inspiration, increased central venous return to the right heart takes longer to cross the right ventricular outflow tract. Closure of the pulmonary valve is delayed compared to the ejection time in expiration; thus, the aortic and pulmonic components of S_2 are more readily separated from each other in inspiration. This variability in the timing of A_2 and P_2 with the respiratory cycle is termed physiologic splitting. If this variability is not appreciated beyond infancy or at slower heart rates, an abnormality of the cardiopulmonary system must be suspected.

The intensity of the components of the second heart sound reflects not only the pressure in the respective vessels, but also their position within the thorax and the thickness of the chest wall. In D-transposition of the great arteries (D-TGA), for example, the second heart sound is "single" because the posterior pulmonic component cannot be heard. Likewise, in TOF, the soft pulmonic component from a stenotic valve may not be audible. A loud pulmonic component or an apparent single S_2 may signal the presence of pulmonary artery hypertension if heard beyond the neonatal period when pulmonary resistance may normally be elevated (Table 1-2).

Physiologic splitting of S_2 occurs only when PVR is normal, so any abnormality of PVR will alter this physiologic effect. The higher the PVR caused by a large left-to-right shunt or pulmonary vascular disease, the shorter the pulmonary ejection time. P_2 will occur closer to A_2 and, although they are still separate from each other, the splitting is termed narrow. When PVR is equal to or greater than SVR, closure of A_2 and P_2 will be nearly simultaneous, resulting in an audible "single" S_2. This is a sign of severe pulmonary hypertension. Alternatively, the splitting of S_2 will be accentuated ("widened") under certain circumstances. When the right heart is volume-loaded from a left-to-right shunt at the atrial level, the physiologic variation between A_2 and P_2 is lost as the stroke volume is increased, both in inspiration and expiration. Another situation in which S_2 shows "fixed splitting" is in the presence of a complete right bundle branch block. This intraventricular conduction delay causes a slight prolongation of right ventricular ejection time, so P_2 is always delayed compared to normal.

A third heart sound (S_3) may normally be present in infants because it occurs at the peak of ventricular inflow into a compliant ventricle. As the ventricle ages, the velocity of ventricular filling diminishes and S_3 cannot be heard. S_3 is best heard at the cardiac apex or the LLSB. It becomes more prominent when there is increased volume of ventricular inflow (as is seen in lesions with left-to-right shunts causing increased pulmonary blood flow), valvar regurgitation, and high cardiac output (as is seen with anemia). The physiologic low-pitched S_3 sound that can occur in well children and adolescents takes on the intonation of "Kentucky." Referring to an S_3 as a *gallop* generally connotes other findings consistent with congestive heart failure. A gallop is a lower-pitched sound that occurs in diastole, during the ventricular filling phase, and is best heard with the bell of the stethoscope.

A fourth heart sound (S_4) occurs during atrial contraction and is associated with a limitation of ventricular distensibility. It has been associated with cardiomyopathy and hypertension and is more common in adults, again heard best at the apex or the LLSB. In the adult population, S_4 gallops are pathologic and signify the presence of a noncompliant ventricle, occurring immediately before S_1. Occasionally, in children with congestive heart failure, the same situation applies.

Other heart sounds may be present. *Clicks* are sounds made by the opening of abnormal valves. The most common clicks occur in systole and are related to abnormalities of the aortic, pulmonic, and mitral valves. Ejection clicks

Table 1-2 Clinical Clues from the S_2			
Normal physiologic splitting			Normal; related to increased preload of right ventricle (delays P_2)
expiration	A_2_____P_2		
inspiration	A_2_____P_2		
Widely split			Seen in right heart dilation with normal pulmonary artery pressure (left to right shunts: atrial septal defect [ASD], partial anomalous pulmonary venous return) or with right bundle branch block
expiration	A_2_____P_2		
inspiration	A_2_____P_2		
Narrowly split	A_2____P_2		May be normal variant
"Single S_2"	A_2-P_2		In congenital heart disease where the aorta is anteriorly positioned, or a single semilunar valve is present
Narrow spilt with accentuated P_2	A_2-P_2		Seen in significant pulmonary arterial hypertension

occur early in systole, immediately after S_1, and represent the opening of a structurally abnormal aortic or pulmonary valve, which is usually bicuspid. Pulmonic ejection clicks are best heard at the LUSB and aortic clicks at the LLSB. Clicks with onset midway between S_1 and S_2 occur in mitral valve prolapse as the closed, myxomatous valve billows backwards toward the left atrium in mid to late systole. Tricuspid valve abnormalities occur less commonly, but additional heart sounds may be heard in Ebstein's anomaly of the tricuspid valve, probably due to motion of the redundant leaflets and to atrial hypertension.

Extracardiac Sounds

The most common of these sounds is the pericardial friction rub heard in association with pericarditis. This can best be described as a rough, scratchy sound with a sandpaper quality, present in systole, diastole, or both. Rubs are usually best heard along the left sternal border and apex, often with better results with the patient in the sitting position, leaning forward. Rubs may be intermittent and may disappear as the pericardial effusion become larger.

Cardiac Murmurs

The primary reason for referral of a pediatric patient to a cardiologist is the presence of a cardiac murmur. A cardiac murmur is an additional sound heard in systole or diastole, caused by turbulence of blood flow or by vibrations within the heart or major cardiac vessels. Cardiac murmurs are very common during childhood and adolescence. As many as four out of five normal children will have a cardiac murmur, referred to as a functional, benign, physiologic, or innocent murmur, noted sometime during their life.[5,6] The primary care provider may become quite comfortable in assessing functional murmurs, and that is appropriate. Referral to a pediatric cardiologist is indicated if a cardiac murmur has characteristics that suggest pathology, if there is a history of heart disease in the family, or if a clinical symptom suggesting a cardiac abnormality exists in the child.[7,8]

Etiology

Heart murmurs are sounds from the heart that can be auscultated with the stethoscope and are not normally present. They are generated by fluid vibrations or turbulence and relate to the speed with which blood is traveling through the heart and across the great vessels. There are two major categories of murmurs:

1. Innocent, functional, or physiologic, with no underlying structural heart disease
2. Pathologic, indicating a structural abnormality of the heart resulting in an abnormal pattern or turbulence of blood flow

Fortunately, most murmurs heard in childhood are innocent, but they can be quite variable in their intensity, location, and quality. Congenital heart disease occurs in approximately 8 out of 1000 live births and is the most common form of birth defect seen by all primary care providers. Murmurs can be accentuated by intercurrent illnesses and fever, which increase heart rate, cardiac output, or both. It may be difficult to distinguish between innocent and pathologic murmurs, especially if a new health care provider is hearing the murmur for the first time or if it is heard during an illness or febrile episode.

Evaluation

In order to characterize a murmur accurately, objective information needs to be obtained. Murmurs are classified according to at least five characteristics, including (1) timing in the cardiac cycle, (2) location and radiation, (3) loudness and pitch, (4) characteristics or qualities, and (5) duration. The age of appearance provides important information to the examiner. A combination of these criteria can often lead to a specific diagnosis.[9]

Age at Appearance   Murmurs that are audible within the first few hours of life are often due to structural heart disease, particularly outflow tract obstruction and valvular heart disease, because their flow characteristics are independent of pulmonary vascular resistance changes. These murmurs are often related to tricuspid valve regurgitation but can also represent either aortic or pulmonary valve stenosis, or else subvalvar aortic or subvalvar pulmonary stenosis. Often these murmurs are associated with complex congenital heart diseases such as TOF or tricuspid atresia. In cases of pulmonary atresia, as pulmonary resistance falls, blood flows to the lungs through a PDA or collaterals and produces a murmur that can be heard early. PVR drops in the first few days after birth in a variable manner and continues to decrease during the first few months of life. During that time frame, congenital shunt lesions, such as VSD, AV canal (endocardial cushion) defect, PDA, and atrial septal defect, all become audible. Occasionally, these murmurs are heard shortly after birth.

Of importance, too, are the circumstances under which a murmur is detected. Innocent murmurs are very common between the ages of 2 and 6 years and again in adolescence, and are frequently heard at well-child checkups or sports physicals. Innocent murmurs are more easily detected at times of illness, especially with fever. Flow murmurs related to physiologic anemia may be heard in the first few months of life.

Timing in the Cardiac Cycle   Timing is described as systolic, diastolic, or continuous. Most innocent cardiac murmurs in children and adolescents occur in systole, during ventricular contraction. Pathologic murmurs commonly occur in systole and include those resulting from turbulent flow across a ventricular outflow tract (pulmonic or aortic), or regurgitation across an AV valve. In addition, the murmur of a VSD occurs in systole.

Systolic murmurs are further classified as pan- or holosystolic murmurs, systolic ejection murmurs, and late systolic murmurs. Holosystolic murmurs begin with the first heart sound and extend through systole, but they do not need to encompass all of systole. This type of murmur is typical for a VSD or AV valve regurgitation. Ejection murmurs occur after S_1 during the ejection period of systole and represent flow disturbance from stenosis in the right or left ventricular outflow tracts (RVOT or LVOT). The murmurs may be referred to as crescendo-decrescendo murmurs. Late systolic murmurs often occur after a mid-systolic ejection click and represent mitral regurgitation through a prolapsing mitral valve.

Murmurs that occur during cardiac relaxation, in diastole, are less common and generally should be considered pathologic. Diastolic murmurs that occur early, during the isovolumetric period, represent aortic or pulmonary valve regurgitation. Mid-diastolic murmurs occur during the transition from rapid to slow filling of the ventricle and represent the flow associated with large left-to-right shunts across the fixed orifice of the tricuspid valve (with ASD), or the mitral valve (with VSD) and are referred to as *rumbles*. They may occur with moderate to severe AV valve regurgitation. Late, protodiastolic, or presystolic murmurs often represent accentuation of mid-diastolic murmurs associated with AV valve stenosis. In the current era, this accentuation can result from acquired rheumatic mitral stenosis. Diastolic murmurs at the base of the heart generally represent leakage through a semilunar valve: aortic, pulmonic, or truncal. Aortic and truncal valve regurgitant murmurs have a higher pitch than those of pulmonary regurgitation, unless pulmonary hypertension exists. Aortic regurgitation is best heard along the LUSB while upright, and pulmonary regurgitation is accentuated in the supine position, due to increased central venous return.

Continuous murmurs persist past S_2 and are generated by uninterrupted flow through a blood vessel or channel, both in systole and diastole, without cessation at S_2. With the one exception of the venous hum, continuous murmurs are pathologic. Continuous murmurs do not necessarily fill all of diastole. Also, continuous murmurs may be louder in systole, suggesting a connection between the arterial and venous systems, including PDA, bronchial collateral, and arteriovenous malformations. Depending on the loudness of the murmur, S_2 may be difficult to appreciate. Most continuous murmurs are audible best at the base of the heart and the back.

One unusual situation is a high-pitched, "whirring," continuous murmur at the LMSB or LLSB, which represents continuous flow through a rarely found coronary-cameral fistula. In this condition, either the right or left coronary artery has one or more connections to a cardiac chamber, usually the right ventricle (RV) or right atrium (RA) or to a blood vessel, particularly the main pulmonary artery. In children, these are usually congenital in nature, but they can develop after myocardial biopsy.

Continuous murmurs louder in diastole are most commonly the benign venous hum but can occur with cerebral or hepatic AV malformation, which are heard in their respective anatomic locations.

Location and Radiation Cardiac murmurs may be localized or widespread, especially in small or thin children. It is important to listen in all regions of the chest, including the five precordial areas (RUSB, LUSB, LMSB, LLSB, and apex), as well as both axillae, the posterior chest, and the neck. One should determine where the murmur is loudest and from where it radiates, as this information can help categorize the origin of the murmur. In less complex defects, murmurs heard at the RUSB are from the aortic area, LUSB from the pulmonic area, LMSB or right lower midsternal border (RLSB) murmurs are from the tricuspid area or are caused by a VSD, and LLSB and apex murmurs are from the mitral valve.

Pathologic murmurs generally have a wider area of radiation that indicates direction of the turbulent flow. If a murmur is audible in the back and the child is outside of the age group for physiologic peripheral pulmonary stenosis, a pathologic cause should be suspected. Murmurs from the LVOT typically radiate to the right posterior chest and neck, especially the right carotid area. Those from the RVOT radiate to the left posterior chest. VSD murmurs typically radiate to the RLSB and LV apical areas, and mitral regurgitant murmurs radiate to the left axilla and lower left posterior chest. Importantly, when possible, the patient should be examined in both the upright and supine positions because the intensity of murmurs can be altered by position. Asking an older, cooperative patient to perform a Valsalva maneuver (bearing down or pushing the abdomen outward) can help identify certain murmurs that are altered by systemic vascular resistance, particularly those from mitral valve prolapse or hypertrophic obstructive cardiomyopathy.

Loudness and Pitch In an effort to be objective, all murmurs are categorized on a scale of 1 to 6, although some use only a maximal number of 4 for diastolic murmurs (Table 1-3). Any murmur of grade 4 or above has an associated thrill. The designation of grade 2 and 3 status is variable, depending upon the examiners and their

Table 1-3 Loudness Grading of Murmurs	
Type	**Description**
Grade 1	Soft, must listen carefully to hear
Grade 2	Soft but easily heard
Grade 3	Moderately loud but no thrill
Grade 4	Loud with a thrill present
Grade 5	Loud, heard with part of stethoscope off chest wall
Grade 6	Loud, heard with all of stethoscope off chest wall

interpretations of "soft but easily heard" (grade 2) vs. "moderately loud" (grade 3). Most innocent murmurs fall in the range of grades 1–3.

Intensity of a murmur is subject to change depending on other physiologic factors such as fever, anemia, and tachycardia. Generally, loud murmurs reflect increasing pathology, with the exception of the VSD. A restrictive VSD will have a significant pressure gradient across the defect and will produce a loud murmur. Conversely, some large defects have a lower pressure gradient between the ventricles with a less turbulent flow, producing a softer murmur. Similarly, a murmur may be diminished in the setting of poor cardiac contractility (e.g., critical aortic stenosis with congestive heart failure), so the loudness of the murmur may not correlate directly to the level of severity of the lesion. With regard to stenotic lesions, tighter stenosis produces a higher-pitched murmur. Likewise, higher-pitched murmurs occur when the pressure difference is greater; for example, aortic or mitral regurgitant murmurs are high-pitched, compared with tricuspid or pulmonary regurgitation with normal pulmonary vascular resistance. When pulmonary artery hypertension is present, pulmonary regurgitation becomes a high-pitched murmur. Diastolic murmurs across AV valves are generally low-pitched.

High-pitched murmurs are better appreciated with the diaphragm of the stethoscope and low-pitched murmurs with the bell.

Characteristics or Quality Murmurs are characterized as harsh or blowing, to-and-fro, flow, musical, vibratory, twangy, squeaky, or scratchy, in addition to the other previously discussed descriptors such as ejection, regurgitant, and holosystolic. These additional qualifiers become somewhat individualized. "Harsh" is a good descriptor for the quality of a VSD or outflow tract murmur, and "blowing" refers to a regurgitant murmur of AV valve insufficiency. "To-and-fro" murmurs refer to systolic and diastolic murmurs such as those produced by pulmonary stenosis (PS) and pulmonary insufficiency (PI) especially in the setting of tetralogy of Fallot with absent pulmonic valve leaflets. They are not equivalent to a continuous murmur. The "musical," "vibratory," "twangy," and "flow" are generally reserved for describing functional or innocent murmurs, and the other qualities refer to pathologic murmurs. Using the above descriptors, one can identify the classical characteristics of a variety of cardiac lesions (Table 1-4).

Innocent Murmurs
There are several types of functional or innocent murmurs, and these are more common in the general pediatric population than pathologic murmurs. Functional murmurs should have no associated symptoms or abnormal cardiac tests; in addition, the heart sounds are normal, they are less than grade 4 in intensity, and they generally are systolic and short (Table 1-5).

Innocent murmurs may represent flow across the pulmonic valve or peripheral pulmonic vessels (heard in the first few months of life related to the relative "stenosis" of the peripheral pulmonic vessels due to lack of pulmonary blood flow in utero). Increased cardiac output from exercise, anemia, or a febrile state will increase the intensity of any flow murmur. Pulmonic flow murmurs should be distinguished from true pulmonary valve stenosis, a small ASD or PDA, or pathologic peripheral pulmonary artery stenosis.

A venous hum from flow in the jugular venous system is frequently heard as a continuous murmur in the upper anterior chest and is more accentuated in diastole. The intensity is altered by position. When the patient is supine with the head turned to one side and pressure is placed over the neck vessels, venous return into the superior vena cava is decreased and the murmur is absent or markedly diminished. The murmur is heard best with the patient sitting and is less audible in the supine position.

This murmur should be distinguished from the pathologic causes of continuous murmurs, especially PDA. Listening over the clavicles and manipulating the arms may alter supraclavicular functional murmurs. Carotid bruits are also heard in the neck but do not have an associated aortic stenosis murmur over the precordium. Still's functional murmurs, also referred to as vibratory, musical, or twangy systolic murmurs, are heard from the LLSB to the apex and are loudest in the supine position, often becoming softer or disappearing with sitting. These common murmurs need to be distinguished from VSD and are generally much more pleasant sounds.

Patients with functional murmurs often require no further testing. However, if the pediatrician or family physician cannot determine whether the murmur is functional or not, the next step should be referral to a pediatric cardiologist. An echocardiogram should not be used to determine the presence of cardiac disease without first consulting a pediatric cardiologist. In many instances, an echocardiogram is not necessary; with most patients, an experienced pediatric cardiologist can determine the presence of a functional murmur by listening. Likewise, a normal electrocardiogram (ECG) does not rule out organic heart disease. The remainder of the physical examination should address the presence or absence of findings that can indirectly or directly relate to the cardiovascular system.

REMAINDER OF THE PHYSICAL EXAM

Pulmonary and Back Exams

One should look for the presence of skeletal abnormalities such as pectus excavatum, pectus carinatum, and scoliosis and also for the presence of thoracotomy

Table 1-4   Characteristic Descriptors of Cardiac Lesions

Lesion	Timing	Location	Radiation	Loudness	Pitch	Quality	Duration
ASD (Large)	Systolic	LUSB	Back, axillae	1-3	Mid	Crescendo-decrescendo ejection	Mid
	+ Diastolic	LLSB	None	1-3	Low	Rumble	Short
VSD (Large)	Systolic	LLSB	RLSB, apex	1-6	High	Harsh	Holosystolic
	+ Diastolic	Apex	Back	1-6	Low	Rumble	Short
PDA	Continuous	LUSB Below left clavicle	Back	1-6	High-mid	Machinery	Dependent on PVR
CAVC	Systolic	LUSB LLSB	Back	1-6	High (VSD) High (MR/TR)	Harsh Blowing	Holosystolic
	+ Diastolic	LLSB		2-3	Low	Rumble	Short
PS	Systolic	LUSB + Click at LMSB	Back, axillae	1-6	Mid	Crescendo-decresendo ejection	Starts after S_1
PR	Early diastolic	LUSB		2-3	Low		Mid
AS	Systolic	RUSB + Click at apex	Carotids, right posterior chest LUSB, LMSB	1-6	High	Harsh ejection	Starts after S_1
AR	Early diastolic	RUSB	LUSB, LMSB	2-4	High-mid	Blowing	Mid
MR	Systolic	Apex	LLSB, Left axilla, left posterior chest	1-6	High	Blowing	Holosystolic
MS	Presystolic (diastole)	Apex		1-3	Low	Crescendo	Short
TR	Systolic	RLSB	LLSB	1-6	High	Blowing	Holosystolic
TS	Mid diastolic	RLSB	LLSB	1-3	Low	Rumble	Short

ASD, Atrial septal defect; *AR*, aortic regurgitation; *AS*, aortic stenosis; *CAVC*, common atrioventricular canal; *MR*, mitral regurgitation; *MS*, mitral stenosis; *PDA*, patent ductus arteriosus; *PR*, pulmonic regurgitation; *PS*, pulmonic stenosis; *PVR*, pulmonary vascular resistance; *TR*, tricuspid regurgitation; *TS*, tricuspid stenosis; *VSD*, ventricular septal defect; *LLSB*, left lower sternal border; *LUSB*, left upper sternal border; *RUSB*, right upper sternal border; *RLSB*, right lower sternal border.

Table 1-5 Innocent Murmurs		
Murmur	Location	Timing
Still's, vibratory, musical, twangy	LLSB to apex	Systolic
Pulmonic flow	LUSB	Systolic
Venous hum	Upper precordium, neck	Continuous
Carotid bruit	Neck	Continuous
Supraclavicular	Above clavicles	Systolic or continuous

and sternotomy scars. During auscultation, one should assess the adequacy of breath sounds because diminished breath sounds in some areas can represent the presence of pleural effusion, pneumothorax, or cardiac enlargement. The presence of rales, indicative of pulmonary edema, or wheezing, related to left atrial dilation and bronchial compression, should also be noted.

Abdominal Exam

On inspection, the clinician should assess for distention, indicating possible ascites. On palpation, one should assess for hepatic congestion and enlargement, which are seen in congestive heart failure or pulmonary hypertension. Splenomegaly may be seen in endocarditis or portal venous hypertension. Prominent superficial venous collateral vessels are seen with obstruction to deep veins, such as the inferior vena cava. In addition, the presence of a fluid wave, indicating ascites, should be determined.

Extremity Exam

On inspection, the extremities should be evaluated for signs of Marfan syndrome, including an increased arm span, a reduced upper-to-lower segment ratio, a reduced extension at the elbows, and pes planus. Patients may also have arachnodactyly, manifested by a wrist or thumb sign. A "wrist sign" is positive if being that the patient can encircle the left wrist with the thumb and fifth finger of the right hand; a "thumb sign" is positive if the patient can flatten the thumb along the palm of the hand, wrap the fingers over the thumb, and see the tip of the thumb at or beyond the fifth finger. It is important to ask about hyperextensibility of joints because some patients with connective tissue disorders may not have typical skeletal findings.

The examiner should look for the presence of extremity cyanosis and should determine whether it is true cyanosis, associated with central desaturation of mucous membranes, or acrocyanosis, associated with normal central saturation. Pulse oximetry can define whether true desaturation exists. Long-term cyanosis leads to clubbing of the fingertips and toes but is relatively rare on a cardiac basis in the current medical era.

Finally, assessment for edema is important. In the pediatric population, this is most often seen in the face and sacral areas in babies and in the lower extremities in ambulatory children. It can occur in right heart failure with pulmonary hypertension, in patients with hypoproteinemia (e.g., protein-losing enteropathy or proteinuria related to nephrotic syndrome) or in conditions associated with fluid retention (e.g., renal insufficiency). The timing of capillary refill is an indication of the circulation time representing cardiac output from the heart. When the toe is squeezed, a delayed capillary refill of greater than 3 seconds suggests decreased cardiac output or congestive heart failure. Likewise, cool extremities in a warm environment may indicate decreased cardiac output.

CARDIAC TESTING

When a cardiac murmur is appreciated and the quality, location, radiation, and intensity are determined, the practitioner must assess this in the context of the patient's current medical status, past medical history, and family history and then must determine whether cardiac testing is indicated.[10]

In a well child, there is a strong likelihood that a cardiac murmur is innocent or else represents a mild form of congenital heart disease such as a small VSD, ASD, or PDA or mild aortic or pulmonary stenosis. From a surveillance perspective, differentiating among these is important with regard to follow-up and the necessity for antibiotic prophylaxis against endocarditis. On the other hand, well-appearing children may have clinically significant congenital heart diseases that merit intervention, even in the absence of clinical symptoms. These conditions include moderate to large secundum or primum ASDs, partial anomalous pulmonary venous return with right ventricular volume overload, small ventricular septal defects with aortic regurgitation or significant RVOT/LVOT obstruction, subaortic stenosis (membranous or hypertrophic obstructive cardiomyopathy), and coarctation of the aorta.

A normal baseline ECG never rules out structural heart disease; an abnormal ECG not only necessitates referral to a cardiologist but also implies that a structural or functional abnormality of the heart may exist. The ECG also supplies information regarding electrical conduction abnormalities (e.g., AV block, delta waves of WPW, bundle branch block, and prolongation of the corrected QT interval) that would not otherwise be appreciated on auscultation. Normal ECG standards vary with age and heart rate. The ECG should be assessed for a variety of measurements, which will indicate heart rate, conduction intervals, and the presence of atrial or ventricular hypertrophy, as well as abnormalities suggesting myocardial stress or ischemia (Table 1-6). The origin of the rhythm, sinus or other, can be determined from the electrocardiogram (Fig. 1-1).

A chest radiograph should be performed in any child with desaturation, respiratory symptoms or distress, dysmorphic features, or failure to thrive. Heart size is evaluated, arch sidedness and abdominal situs are documented, the pulmonary vasculature is assessed, and bony abnormalities (e.g., abnormal or missing ribs or scoliosis) may be detected (Fig. 1-2). Echocardiography is an extremely useful noninvasive tool in the assessment of children and adults with suspected cardiac problems. However, in most well children with innocent murmurs, it is unnecessary if the murmur is typical and the ECG is normal, and also is expensive and potentially emotionally traumatic. A cardiac consultation by a pediatric cardiologist should precede the performance of an echocardiogram.

EXERCISE INTOLERANCE

Background

Some medical conditions can exist insidiously, without the patient's or parents' knowledge, if there is no impact on day-to-day activities. Once physical or mental performance becomes impaired, there is some urgency in determining the cause and assessing whether any therapy is available. Fortunately, most pediatric patients are quite energetic, so any deviation from that expected level of activity brings them to medical attention rather quickly. Although several medical conditions can be implicated in patients who have exercise intolerance, limited physical capabilities, or both, a cardiac cause should be considered.

Before proceeding further, one must understand the normal physiology of exercise. The function of the circulation is to provide oxygen, glucose, and fatty acids to the body organs and muscle cells in order for the skeletal muscle to repetitively contract. As work increases, there is a progressive rise in heart rate, cardiac output, and systolic blood pressure. Systemic vascular resistance drops,

allowing increased delivery of blood to muscles and other tissues. There is also a rise in pulmonary artery pressure and a slight drop in pulmonary vascular resistance. In addition, the waste products of exercise, carbon dioxide and lactate, must be removed from the tissues. Finally, pulmonary work increases, both to provide additional oxygen and to expel carbon dioxide. If there is any deficiency or inefficiency, including abnormalities at the muscle cell level, abnormal pulmonary function, skeletal deformity of the chest affecting respiratory reserve, or a cardiac condition that limits cardiac output, exercise intolerance will occur.

Etiology

It is incumbent on the consulting cardiologist to rule out a cardiac source of exercise intolerance, although this may not be the most likely cause. Other factors responsible for exercise intolerance include the sequelae of systemic illnesses, including a postviral condition or mononucleosis; neuromuscular, metabolic, mitochondrial, or endocrine conditions (i.e., diabetes or thyroid dysfunction); pulmonary conditions with exercise-induced asthma or reactive airway disease; and anemia.

There are multiple cardiac causes of exercise intolerance in children. These include lesions that limit cardiac output because of abnormal cardiac muscle function, such as dilated cardiomyopathy, which may be idiopathic or acquired through an inflammatory process such as myocarditis or rheumatic fever, caused by anthracycline therapy in oncology patients; restrictive cardiomyopathy; ischemia related to coronary insufficiency, caused by Kawasaki disease, a congenital coronary anomaly, or following congenital heart surgery that involved coronary manipulation such as an arterial switch for D-transposition of the great vessels; and reimplantation or baffle surgery for an anomalous left coronary artery from the pulmonary artery (ALCAPA) or after a Ross procedure.

In addition, exercise intolerance can result from lesions that limit cardiac output because of outflow tract obstruction, including multiple forms of aortic stenosis (valvar, subvalvar, or supravalvar stenosis), hypertrophic cardiomyopathy, coarctation of the aorta, and severe pulmonary valve stenosis.

Other etiologies of cardiac-induced exercise intolerance include lesions that limit cardiac output because of valve leakage, such as (1) severe aortic valve regurgitation, which can be congenital or acquired from endocarditis or rheumatic fever; (2) severe mitral valve regurgitation, which can be congenital from cleft mitral valve or from mitral valve prolapse, or else acquired from endocarditis or rheumatic fever; (3) severe pulmonary regurgitation following surgery for TOF, surgery for pulmonary valve atresia, or critical pulmonic stenosis; (4) severe tricuspid

Table 1-6 Normal ECG Values for Age

Age	Heart Rate Min–Max	Mean Frontal Plane QRS Axis	P-R Interval	QRS Duration	R in V_1	S in V_1	R:S Ratio in V_1	R in V_6	S in V_6	R:S Ratio in V_6
0–1 mo	100–180 (120)	+75 to +180 (+120)	0.08–0.12 (.10)	0.04–0.08 (.06)	4–25 (15)	1–20 (10)	0.5–∞ (1.5)	1–21 (6)	0–12 (4)	0.1–∞ (2)
2–3 mo	110–180 (120)	+35 to +135 (+100)	0.08–0.12 (.10)	0.04–0.08 (.06)	2–20 (11)	1–18 (7)	0.3–10 (1.5)	3–20 (10)	0–6 (2)	1.5–∞ (4)
4–12 mo	100–180 (150)	+30 to +135 (+60)	0.09–0.13 (.12)	0.04–0.08 (.06)	3–20 (10)	1–16 (8)	0.3–4.0 (1.2)	6–20 (13)	0–4 (2)	2.0–∞ (6)
1–3 yr	100–180 (130)	0 to +110 (+60)	0.10–0.14 (.12)	0.04–0.08 (.06)	1–18 (9)	1–27 (13)	0.5–1.5 (0.8)	3–24 (12)	0–4 (2)	3.0–∞ (20)
4–5 yr	60–150 (100)	0 to +110 (+60)	0.11–0.15 (.13)	0.05–0.09 (.07)	1–18 (7)	1–30 (14)	0.1–1.5 (0.7)	4–24 (13)	0–4 (2)	2.0–∞ (20)
6–8 yr	60–130 (100)	−15 to +110 (+60)	0.12–0.16 (.14)	0.05–0.09 (.07)	1–18 (7)	1–30 (14)	0.1–1.5 (0.7)	4–24 (13)	0–4 (1)	2.0–∞ (20)
9–11 yr	50–110 (80)	−15 to +110 (+60)	0.12–0.17 (.14)	0.05–0.09 (.07)	1–16 (6)	1–26 (16)	0.1–1.0 (0.5)	4–24 (14)	0–4 (1)	4.0–∞ (20)
12–16 yr	50–100 (75)	−15 to +110 (+60)	0.12–0.17 (.15)	0.05–0.09 (.07)	1–16 (5)	1–23 (14)	0.0–1.0 (0.3)	4–22 (14)	0–5 (1)	2.0–∞ (9)
> 16 yr	50–90 (70)	−15 to +110 (+60)	0.12–0.20 (.15)	0.05–0.10 (.07)	1–14 (3)	1–23 (10)	0.0–1.0 (0.3)	4–21 (10)	0–6 (1)	2.0–∞ (9)

Adapted from Garson A, Gilette PC, McNamara DG, eds.: A guide to cardiac dysrhythmias in children. New York: Grune and Stratton, 1980.
Mean values are noted in parentheses.

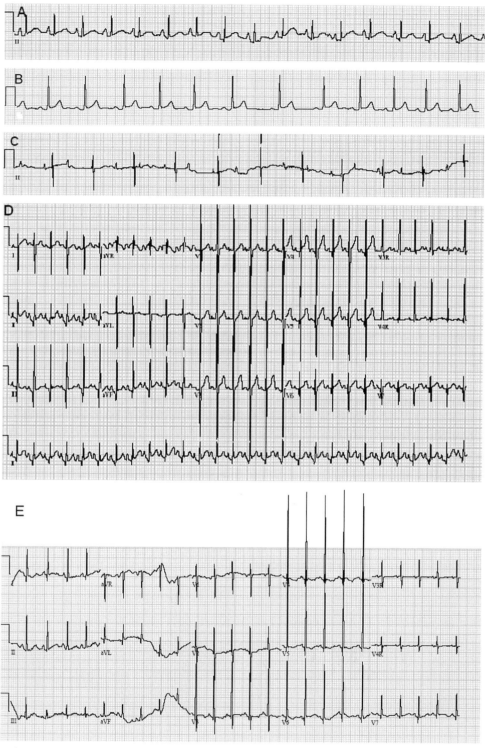

Figure 1-1   **A,** ECG lead II rhythm strip showing normal sinus rhythm. **B,** ECG lead II rhythm strip showing the normal variant of sinus arrhythmia. **C,** ECG lead II rhythm strip showing electrical dissociation between the atria and ventricles consistent with complete heart block. The atrial rate is 130 BPM; ventricular rate is 65 BPM. **D,** 15-lead ECG in a 7-year-old, showing an R/S ratio in $V_1 > 1$ and an R/S ratio in $V_6 < 1$, consistent with right ventricular hypertrophy (RVH). **E,** 15-lead ECG in a 4-year-old showing an R:S ratio in $V_1 < 1$, an R:S ratio in $V_6 > 1$, and an R in V_6 of 30 mm, consistent with left ventricular hypertrophy (LVH).

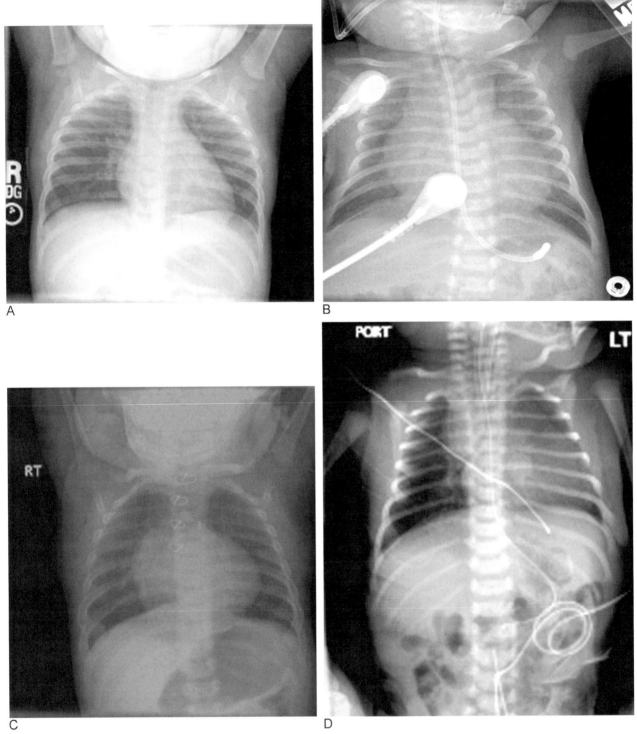

Figure 1-2   A, Posteroanterior (PA) radiograph demonstrating a normal cardiac silhouette, normal cardiothoracic ratio with normal contours, and pulmonary blood flow. Note the slight radio-opaque contour to the left of the trachea causing slight rightward deviation of the airway. This is consistent with a normal left aortic arch. **B,** PA radiograph demonstrating an enlarged cardiothoracic ratio with increased pulmonary blood flow. This type of radiograph is commonly seen in lesions such as a VSD with a large left-to-right shunt. **C,** PA radiograph demonstrating an enlarged heart with decreased pulmonary blood flow. This type of radiograph is commonly seen in lesions, such as TOF, with significant obstruction to pulmonary blood flow. **D,** PA radiograph demonstrating a radio-opaque contour to the right of the trachea (with endotracheal tube in place) causing slight leftward deviation of the airway. This is consistent with a right aortic arch.

Continued

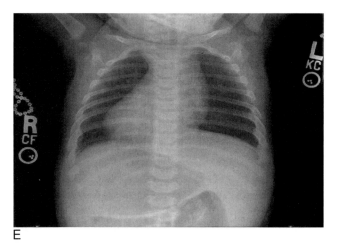

E

Figure 1-2, cont'd **E,** PA radiograph demonstrating the gastric bubble in the left upper quadrant. Note that the apex of the heart is pointing to the right, consistent with dextrocardia.

regurgitation from Ebstein's anomaly; and (5) single ventricle physiology at various stages of Fontan palliation performed for hypoplastic left heart syndrome, tricuspid atresia, or double outlet ventricles.

Exercise tolerance or ability can be limited by an abnormal heart rate response to exercise from chronotropic impairment associated with congenital or acquired heart block or from sinus node dysfunction. In a similar fashion, a variety of arrhythmias can impair exercise ability. These include supraventricular tachycardia (SVT) in patients with structurally normal hearts, as in many patients with WPW syndrome, or SVT in postoperative cardiac patients. Similarly, ventricular tachycardia can impair exercise performance in patients with prolonged QT syndrome, structurally normal hearts, or cardiomyopathies, or patients who have had surgery for congenital heart disease.

Noncardiac causes of exercise intolerance are numerous and may involve the cardiopulmonary system. A primary cause is physical deconditioning, often associated with childhood obesity, decreased levels of regular exercise, or both. Another common obstacle to normal exercise tolerance is the presence of pulmonary disease, which most often relates to obstructive airway disease due to reactive airways, either in the case of true bronchospasm or with exercise-induced asthma. Occasionally, pulmonary function tests will demonstrate restrictive lung disease. This can be seen in patients who have had thoracic surgery, or chest radiation therapy, and in patients with severe skeletal deformities such as scoliosis, pectus excavatum, or both. Primary pulmonary hypertension (PPH) is a rare but critical abnormality of the pulmonary vascular bed of unclear etiology, more common in females, often presenting in adolescence, and often first present as a change in exercise tolerance. Finally, in patients with neuromuscular diseases, including the muscular dystrophies

and mitochondrial conditions, exercise capacity may be limited.

Evaluation

History

The information obtained from a thorough history is a critical part of assessing exercise intolerance. The details of the patient's or family's concerns regarding exercise performance need to be clarified. The onset of the exercise intolerance and its progression require delineation. A differential of exercise intolerance is shown in Table 1-7. In considering exercise intolerance in a pediatric patient, several points have to be considered:

1. Is this a previously well child or a patient with a known cardiac condition?
2. Has the patient ever had surgery or other cardiac intervention?
3. Is the patient medicated for a cardiac condition?
4. Is there a history of cardiopulmonary disease in the family?
5. Does the patient have any other medical problems, particularly of the respiratory system?
6. Are there any known allergies?
7. Is the patient age-appropriate for height, weight, and blood pressure?
8. Does the patient complain primarily of shortness of breath or of easy fatigability with activity?

The details of the history should note the onset of symptoms, the frequency of occurrence, and the specific precipitating factors. Associated features such as palpitations, chest pain, dizziness, or syncope should increase the suspicion of a true cardiac etiology. Other features such as coughing, shortness of breath, color change (e.g., pallor or plethora), perioral tingling, or paresthesia should be evaluated. The history should include questions about recent illness, fever, rash, joint swelling, sore throat, and insect bites, which could implicate an acquired form of cardiac disease (e.g., Lyme disease or rheumatic fever). Families with children who have

Table 1-7	Exercise Intolerance
Symptoms	**Possible Etiologies**
Easy fatuigability	Deconditioning, obesity, anemia, low cardiac output, hypothyroidism, poor nutritional state, anorexia, hypoglycemia, dehydration, diabetes, neuromuscular disease, hypotonia, behavioral.
Shortness of breath ± cough	Reactive airway disease, smoking, pulmonary edema, chronic heart failure, restrictive lung disease, pulmonary hypertension

atopic tendencies may be more prone to exercise-induced reactive airway disease. A thorough review of prescription and nonprescription drug use, cigarette smoking in patients or family members, and illicit substance use should be obtained from the patient.

Physical Examination

The physical examination of the patient presenting with exercise intolerance should be complete, including the vital signs and cardiac examination; the pulmonary, abdominal, and extremity examination; and a neurologic and a musculoskeletal exam. Tachycardia for age, the presence of an irregular heart rate, a new or changing cardiac murmur, a gallop rhythm, or the presence of rales, hepatomegaly, and peripheral edema all strongly point to congestive heart failure. A loud, single S_2 suggests pulmonary hypertension. Careful auscultation for prolonged expiration is important, and if none is appreciated at rest, reassessment should be made after a period of exercise in the office. The reassessment should include resting and post-exercise pulmonary function testing.

In the absence of any specific abnormalities of the general or cardiac examination, the health care provider's attention should be directed to physical deconditioning. The patient's height and weight should be plotted on appropriate growth curves, and the body mass index (BMI) should be calculated and plotted for age. Many families are surprised to find the degree of extra weight being carried by their children. Dietary and activity history should be reviewed in all cases, but especially when the height and weight are inappropriate.

Diagnostic Tests

Testing of the child or adolescent with a history of exercise intolerance should be guided toward the most likely etiologies, but it should include cardiac tests if there is a murmur or if the history suggests a potentially life-threatening cardiac issue, including exercise-related chest pain, palpitations, dizziness, or syncope. A baseline 12-lead ECG can alert the physician to electrical abnormalities that predispose a patient to an exercise-induced arrhythmia, such as WPW, long QT syndrome (LQTS), and hypertrophic cardiomyopathy. Evidence of RVH or LVH could indicate structural heart disease, cardiomyopathy, or pulmonary hypertension. Abnormalities of T waves can be seen in cardiomyopathies. Ambulatory ECG monitoring (Holter monitoring) or event monitoring should be performed in patients with exercise-related palpitations, with use of the device during activities in which exercise intolerance is experienced.

A chest x-ray (CXR) should be performed in any patient with exercise-related shortness of breath (with or without a cardiac murmur), looking for hyperinflation, intrathoracic masses, or cardiomegaly. Attention should be paid to heart size, pulmonary vascular markings, and aortic arch sidedness. Echocardiography in patients with exercise-related symptoms may be diagnostic and can allow the examiner to evaluate cardiac chamber size and contractility, to look for evidence of cardiac hypertrophy or structural heart disease (especially congenital or acquired coronary abnormalities), and to obtain estimates of intracardiac pressure. This is particularly important in the evaluation of pulmonary hypertension. If no cardiac pathology is found by these preliminary tests, formal exercise stress testing may be indicated.

The goal of standard testing is to evaluate the patient at maximal exercise and to make objective assessments of exercise duration, heart rate and blood pressure response to exercise, and aerobic and physical working capacity, along with documentation of arrhythmias or ischemic changes. Additional information can be obtained depending on the type of stress test performed. Metabolic testing includes noninvasive assessment of cardiac output at rest and with exercise, which differentiates primary cardiac dysfunction from pulmonary or neuromuscular conditions or from general deconditioning. Pulmonary stress testing assesses pulmonary function at rest and with exercise, which is useful for exercise-induced asthma or other pulmonary conditions. Reproducing the patient's symptoms with exercise stress testing allows the cardiologist to make a more accurate assessment of cause.

Treatment of Selected Conditions

The primary roles of the evaluating cardiologist are to rule out the unlikely prospect of serious pathology and to provide reassurance and support to the patient and family. Often, the cardiologist makes recommendations for further evaluation or treatment when a noncardiac cause is suspected because of the examination, history, or testing. Deconditioned patients without heart disease may benefit from an exercise prescription to improve physical fitness. Referral to a nutritionist may be helpful in patients with weight issues. Referral to a pulmonary medicine specialist may be indicated for those patients with reactive airway disease. Judicious use of bronchodilator inhalers prior to exercise, or other treatments of reactive airway disease, may relieve symptoms in young athletes.

CHEST PAIN

Background

Chest pain is a common presenting complaint in patients seen by the general pediatrician and in the emergency department and is a common reason for referral to a cardiologist.[11] The sudden occurrence of chest pain in a previously healthy child can be a source of fear and concern for both the child and the family. Extensive public education on the association of chest pain with ischemic heart disease and myocardial infarction in the adult has led to an erroneous assumption that the same holds true for the pediatric patient. The least likely cause of chest pain in children is a cardiac origin. The differential diagnosis of pediatric chest pain is described in Box 1-1.[12]

Box 1-1   Differential Diagnosis of Chest Pain

IDIOPATHIC

MUSCULOSKELETAL

Overuse pain, costochondritis, Tietze's syndrome, cervical ribs, slipping rib, precordial catch syndrome, trauma, child abuse, osteomyelitis, herniated disc, neoplasm

PULMONARY

Reactive airway disease, pneumothorax, pneumomediastinum, pneumonia, chronic cough, pleural effusion, pleurodynia, pulmonary embolism, foreign body aspiration, cystic adenomatoid malformation, primary or secondary adenoma or carcinoma

GASTROINTESTINAL

Esophagitis, esophageal diverticulum, esophageal spasm, esophageal rupture, Mallory-Weiss tear, achalasia, gastroesophageal reflux disease, gastritis, peptic ulcer disease, Zollinger-Ellison syndrome, hiatal hernia, cholecystitis, pancreatitis, subdiaphragmatic abscess

CARDIAC

Anatomic Lesions: Aortic stenosis (subvalvar, valvar, supravalvar), aortic aneurysm with dissection, ruptured sinus of Valsalva, coarctation of aorta, coronary anomalies, mitral valve prolapse, severe pulmonary stenosis, arrhythmogenic right ventricular dysplasia

Acquired Lesions: Cardiomyopathy, endocarditis, myocarditis, rheumatic fever, Lyme, myocardial infarction, coronary vasospasm, Kawasaki disease, pericarditis, postpericardiotomy syndrome, pulmonary hypertension, Eisenmenger's syndrome, Takayasu's arteritis, cardiac tumors, pericardial neoplasm

Arrhythmias: Premature atrial contractions, atrial flutter, atrial fibrillation, supraventricular tachycardia, premature ventricular contractions, ventricular tachycardia

PSYCHIATRIC

Modified from Kocis KC: Chest pain in pediatrics. *Pediatr Clin North Am* 46(2):189-203, 1999.

Characteristics

Understanding the origins and manifestations of chest pain is helpful in guiding the evaluation. The neural fibers that convey pain stem from either cutaneous or visceral sources. Cutaneous pain typically is described as sharp or stabbing in quality and is brief, well-localized, and easily reproduced by palpation. In contrast, visceral pain is diffuse and poorly localized. The qualities ascribed to visceral pain are typically burning, gnawing, pressure, dull, or aching.[13]

The factors associated with the chest pain often predict the etiology. Pain that recurs at night or after ingestion of food or drink is suggestive of esophageal or gastric pathology.[13] Pain that is reproducible with a particular position, movement, or palpation can indicate a musculoskeletal etiology, particularly costochondritis. Environmental factors or physical stress may provoke chest pain in asthmatics. Chest pain related to myocardial ischemia is often associated with exertion.

Epidemiology

Chest pain accounts for 650,000 physician visits per year in patients 10–21 years of age.[14] This constitutes 0.3% of all physician visits. Chest pain can exist as a chronic condition in the pediatric population, with persistent symptoms in 45–69% and 19% of patients having symptoms for more than 3 years.[13]

Etiology

Although it is incumbent on the consulting cardiologist to rule out cardiac causes of chest pain, the very fact that noncardiac causes predominate makes it essential for the practicing cardiologist to be familiar with the other common causes and their clinical presentations. Noncardiac causes primarily arise from three sources: the chest wall (i.e., the musculoskeletal system), the gastrointestinal system, and the pulmonary system. Often, a thorough history delineates the cause without need for further testing or consultation.

Although cardiac causes of chest pain in children are decidedly rare, there are a few general cardiac causes to keep in mind. Lesions resulting in insufficient coronary perfusion either at rest or with exertion include the coronary aneurysm or stenosis associated with Kawasaki's disease; congenital coronary anomalies; and moderate to severe left ventricular outflow tract obstruction, including valvar or subvalvar aortic stenosis and hypertrophic cardiomyopathy (HCM). Inflammatory lesions include pericarditis, postpericardiotomy syndrome, and rheumatic fever. Other cardiac abnormalities associated with chest pain include cardiac neoplasms and arrhythmias.

Evaluation

History

The details of the history should be obtained, paying specific attention to the onset, frequency, and precipitating and relieving factors, as well as the characteristics, duration, and location of the chest pain. Associated features that would heighten suspicion for a true cardiac etiology include exercise intolerance, palpitations or shortness of breath with activity, presyncope or syncope, or a family history of congenital heart disease or sudden cardiac death.

Physical Examination

A complete cardiovascular, respiratory, and abdominal examination should be performed. The physical examination of the patient presenting with chest pain should initially focus on the vital signs. After documenting a stable regular heart rate and rhythm, respirations, and blood pressure, a thorough physical examination should focus on finding noncardiac causes. The initial evaluation should include inspecting for evidence of trauma, bruises, or abrasions on the chest wall. Palpation should focus on bony abnormalities and localized chest swellings and on the site of the pain indicated by the patient. There should be an attempt to reproduce the pain by palpation of the location indicated by the patient. Reproducible pain, particularly at the costochondral junction or over a rib, points to costochondritis as the etiology of the pain.

Diagnostic Tests

Although a broad array of tests exists (Box 1-2) to include or exclude various etiologies, a shotgun approach to the evaluation of chest pain is not advocated. Often, the diagnosis can be made by history alone. In addition, the etiology of many cases of chest pain cannot be determined. Despite this, patients and families take great comfort when a clinician can exclude worrisome pathology, even though a definitive diagnosis cannot be made.

Treatment of Selected Conditions

The primary role of the evaluating cardiologist is to rule out the unlikely prospect of serious cardiac pathology. An equally important role is to provide reassurance and support to the patient and family. In addition, the cardiologist may need to begin definitive therapy for the cause of the pain. Most commonly, treatment takes the form of histamine blockers or proton pump inhibitors (PPIs) for gastroesophageal reflux disease (GERD) or nonsteroidal anti-inflammatory

Box 1-2	Tests Available for the Evaluation of Chest Pain
Cardiac	ECG, CXR, echocardiogram, Holter monitor, exercise stress test, pharmacologic stress test, thallium scan, serum creatinine kinase with myocardial band fraction, serum troponin T, fractionated serum lipid profile, pericardiocentesis, cardiac catheterization, endomyocardial biopsy with PCR
Pulmonary	CXR, CT scan of chest, MRI of chest, pulmonary function tests (PFTs) at rest and with exercise, bronchoscopy, ventilation/perfusion scanning, sweat chloride testing
Gastrointestinal	Gastric lavage, hydrogen ion concentration (pH) probe; upper gastrointestinal (GI) series, upper endoscopy, esophageal manometry, abdominal ultrasound, liver function tests
Musculoskeletal	Skeletal radiographs, CT scan of spine, MRI of spine, nuclear bone scan, muscle enzymes

ECG, Electrocardiogram; *CXR,* chest x-ray.

drugs (NSAIDs) for costochondritis or other musculoskeletal disorders.

PALPITATIONS

Definition

The term *palpitations* has numerous meanings. In medical terms it is defined as "the conscious, unpleasant awareness of one's own heartbeat." This includes the sensation of extra or missed beats, but the same sensation may be related to normal physiologic responses. Evaluation of the patient complaining of palpitations becomes much easier when the clinician realizes that palpitations can be the subjective sensation of normal cardiovascular events.

Etiology

The majority of patients who complain of palpitations have no discernible pathologic process, or else the palpitations represent a physiologic variant with no risk of progression or sudden death. Occasionally, palpitations are the initial manifestation of systemic disease or serious arrhythmia (Box 1-3).

Box 1-3   Causes of Palpitations

Cardiac
  Primary
    Premature atrial contractions
    Premature ventricular contractions
    Supraventricular tachycardia
    Ventricular tachycardia
    Ventricular fibrillation
    Second-degree AV block
    Sinus arrest
  Secondary
    Systemic illness with cardiac effects (hyperthyroidism
      neoplasm, pheochromocytoma)
Fever
Anxiety
Hyperventilation
Exercise
Muscle spasm

Evaluation

History

It is important to determine the onset and duration of the symptoms. The patient should be asked if the episodes begin and end gradually or abruptly, the latter of which is more characteristic of reentrant arrhythmias. Association with factors such as activity or consumption of certain medications, including albuterol or other bronchodilators, decongestants, stimulants for attention deficit disorder, certain psychotropic drugs, or foods that contain caffeine, such as chocolate, coffee, tea, sodas, and herbal stimulants, should be determined. Symptoms of fever or systemic illness (e.g., weight loss, jitteriness, clamminess, increased appetite, and diarrhea associated with hyperthyroidism) should be elicited. One should determine whether there are stressors that might point to a psychogenic etiology for these complaints.

Physical Examination

Palpation of the radial pulse is a part of the physical examination that can indicate abnormalities of cardiac rate or rhythm. The initial evaluation should determine whether there is a normal heart rate, bradycardia, or tachycardia. Next, the clinician should determine whether the pulse is irregular and if there is a discernible pattern of irregularity. Finally, if irregularity is noted, one should determine if the patient's symptoms correlate with the irregularity. A complete cardiovascular examination should be performed. In addition, the clinician should systematically evaluate the patient for evidence of noncardiac medical conditions that can be associated with alterations of heart rate (e.g., anemia, hyperthyroidism, infectious or inflammatory diseases, connective tissue disorders, neoplasia, or pheochromocytoma).

Diagnostic Tests

The extent of the cardiac evaluation depends on the impact that the symptoms have on day-to-day functioning and the likelihood that the symptoms have a cardiac etiology. If the history points to relatively infrequent, well-tolerated episodes that do not cause significant impairment and that appear to be secondary to an external cause, it may be prudent simply to monitor the patient closely and to instruct the patient to limit intake of possible stimulants (e.g., caffeine, chocolate, or sympathomimetic medications such as decongestants) and to increase fluid intake. If episodes are prolonged and frequent without signs of systemic illness, a more extensive evaluation may be necessary.

In either situation, a routine 12-lead ECG and rhythm strip may be helpful to determine the origin of the rhythm, to determine the etiology of any irregularity, to assess the QT interval, and to look for evidence of any conduction abnormality or of preexcitation as seen in WPW syndrome or other arrhythmias. Occasionally, documentation of premature beats (of atrial or ventricular origin) or second-degree AV block occurs, even on asymptomatic recordings. Additional testing that may prove useful includes a variety of ambulatory electrocardiographic monitoring devices.

If the patient's symptoms are frequent, one may choose to monitor him or her as an inpatient through continuous telemetry or as an outpatient with a 24–72 hour ambulatory Holter monitor (three-lead ECG) or an event monitor. The patient is asked to keep a diary to correlate symptoms with objective electrocardiographic data. If the patient's symptoms are relatively infrequent, the test of choice is a portable event monitor. This device can be activated when symptoms occur or can be of a continuous recording modality with activation of the device retaining a period of time before and after activation or with continuous monitoring through satellite technology. The event monitor will document cardiac rate and rhythm during the 30–45 seconds prior to activation and will record the ECG during or after symptoms; these ECG signals are transmitted by telephone for analysis.

For complicated cases in which no etiology has been found with event monitors but the index of suspicion is high, a subcutaneously implanted device may be used. If symptoms occur with exercise, exercise stress testing should be performed. In cases that appear to be potentially threatening, a cardiac catheterization using programmed electrophysiologic testing may be warranted. The etiology of the arrhythmia and the need for intervention with catheter ablation, pacemaker, or implantable cardioverter defibrillator can be determined.

SYNCOPE

Background

Syncope is the sudden and transient loss of consciousness and postural tone that results from inadequate cerebral perfusion. Syncope in children causes great anxiety in parents, teachers, and school officials. These episodes result in a large number of visits to pediatricians, family physicians, and emergency departments and a surprising number of admissions to community and children's hospitals nationwide.[15] Although children may require some cardiac testing, they rarely require the complete cardiovascular assessment that older adults with the same presentation routinely receive, which often culminates in coronary angiography and electrophysiologic testing. The greatest concern regarding syncope is to discern which children might be at risk for sudden cardiac death. The overall incidence of sudden death in children and teenagers is 1–8 in 100,000 patient-years.[16] Some particular features should prompt a more aggressive emergent evaluation, such as syncope with exertion or syncope associated with cardiac symptoms such as chest pain or palpitations; prolonged or frequent syncope; syncope associated with known, preexisting congenital or acquired heart disease; syncope requiring cardiopulmonary resuscitation (CPR) or in patients with known arrhythmia such as LQTS; or a family history of sudden death.

Epidemiology

The reported incidence of syncope is variable, with as many 25–50% of young adults recalling at least one episode in their past. The incidence of those seeking medical attention is about 126 per 100,000.[17] Girls are seen for evaluation more frequently than boys.[18] Data from a group of male college and postgraduate students found an incidence of 15.5%, whereas a study among basic trainees in the U.S. Air Force demonstrated an incidence of 22.3%.[16] The most common forms of syncope are more frequent during adolescence than in early childhood. The single exception is the pallid breath-holding spell of the toddler. Numerous studies have estimated that at least 5% of children between 6 and 18 months of age have demonstrated some form of a breath-holding spell.[15]

Symptoms and Clinical Associations

The child may present with nausea, vomiting, pallor, diaphoresis, dizziness, weakness, or frank syncope. There may be a sensation of an increased heart rate. Premonitory symptoms can occur without a true syncopal event and are referred to as near syncope or presyncope. Presyncope is a sense that one is "about to pass out." Patients often complain of an impending loss of consciousness accompanied by nausea and visual phenomena of blurring, dimming, or partial loss, and also by auditory symptoms of diminished hearing and lightheadedness, but without true syncope. The approach to presyncope is essentially the same as that for syncope.[19]

The description of syncope can be variable with terms such as dizziness, lightheadedness, and presyncope often used for the same symptom complex. Vertigo, disequilibrium, and seizures are often confused with syncope. Dizziness is a symptom that needs better definition to distinguish it from lightheadedness or vertigo. The principal distinction is the description of the sensation of motion. Swaying, whirling, and spinning of the environment or room are characteristics of vertigo. Alteration of balance or perception of the environment or a feeling of spinning often describes dizziness. Hyperventilation can result in lightheadedness. Sensations of dizziness or lightheadedness may be frequently associated with psychological distress, including anxiety, depression, and panic attacks.[19]

Disequilibrium refers to balance problems without vertigo. This sensation is often unrelated to position or movement; the characteristic feature on history is difficulty ambulating. A fairly rare complaint among children, disequilibrium in the young is often caused by vestibular pathology or ataxia.[19]

Making the distinction between a seizure and syncope is important. Absence seizures and temporal lobe epilepsy can be described by younger patients and observers in a manner that appears to be syncope. Both phenomena result in an impairment of consciousness. Seizures tend to occur and to resolve independent of position or posture; however, most pediatric syncope is related to position or volume status and is resolved quickly with supine posture without a postictal state. True vasodepressor syncope (VDS) does not occur in the supine position but may occur while sitting. Standing or rising to standing are the most common positional relationships.

Etiology

Categories of syncope include noncardiac, cardiac, and neurocardiogenic (Box 1-4). Syncope in most young patients will not be life-threatening, but the physician's aim must be to identify the patient at risk for a serious event. If a true syncopal event has occurred, an accurate description of the event is often sufficient to alert the physician to the likely cause.

Box 1-4   Differential Diagnosis of Syncope

AUTONOMIC

Neurocardiogenic
  Reflex or situational
    Breath-holding
      Pallid
      Cyanotic
    Swallowing
    Hair-combing
    Stretch
    Carotid sinus hypersensitivity
    Cough
    Micturition
    Defecation
  Excessive vagal tone or hypervagotonia
Orthostatic
Anemia
Hypovolemia or dehydration
Postural orthostatic tachycardia syndrome
Dysautonomia

CARDIAC

Arrhythmias
  Tachycardias
    Supraventricular tachycardia or Wolff-Parkinson-
      White syndrome
    Atrial flutter
    Atrial fibrillation
    Junctional tachycardia
    Ventricular tachycardia
    Ventricular fibrillation
  Bradycardias
    Sinus
    Asystole
    Atrioventricular block
    Pacemaker malfunction
    Long QT syndrome
    Sinus node dysfunction
    Atrioventricular block

CARDIAC (Cont'd)

  Obstruction
    Outflow
      Aortic stenosis
      Pulmonary stenosis
      Hypertrophic cardiomyopathy
      Pulmonary hypertension
      Hypercyanotic spell
      Eisenmenger's syndrome
    Inflow
      Mitral stenosis
      Tamponade
      Constrictive pericarditis
      Tumor (myxoma)
  Myocardial dysfunction
    Primary
      Idiopathic dilated cardiomyopathy
      Neuromuscular
        Duchenne muscular dystrophy
    Secondary
      Dilated cardiomyopathy (with metabolic causes,
        myocarditis, or anomalous left coronery artery
        from the pulmonary artery)

NEUROLOGIC

Seizure
Migraine
Increased intracranial pressure

METABOLIC

Hypoglycemia
Anorexia nervosa
Drugs, toxins, or electrolyte disorders

PSYCHOGENIC

Hyperventilation or hysteria
Conversion reaction

Noncardiac Syncope

Noncardiac syncope includes neurologic, metabolic, drug or toxin exposure, and psychogenic etiologies.

Neurologic Etiology

Certain neurally mediated or autonomic etiologies of syncope, such as breath-holding spells and VSD, can terminate with tonic-clonic movements, which can cause confusion with a true epileptic seizure. They may be referred to as convulsive syncope or anoxic seizures. Convulsive disorders are easily identified when they have an aura or prodrome, generalized tonic-clonic seizure activity, or a postictal phase with confusion and lethargy.[20]

A syncopal event occurring while the patient is in a recumbent position is likely to be due to a seizure.[16,20] These etiologies can be more difficult to identify when the patient has absence seizures without an aura, loss of motor tone, or postictal confusion. Akinetic seizures or "drop attacks" are most common between 2 and 5 years of age.[20]

Temporal lobe epilepsy (TLE) is usually accompanied by an aura, often a smell or a sense of fear or foreboding, and is longer in duration than absence seizures. TLE is associated with simple or complex semi-purposeful motor activity, also known as "automatism." Loss of consciousness may be more gradual.[20]

Complex partial seizures may involve behavioral changes and may be difficult to diagnose with decreased responsiveness and awareness of self and surroundings.

Basilar artery migraine results in occipital headache, vertigo, visual symptoms, ataxia, confusion, or syncope, or a combination thereof. In the classic scenario, the headache and premonitory aura is severe enough to result in a vagally mediated syncope. In atypical presentations, there is no premonitory headache, but vasoconstriction occurs in the vertebrobasilar arterial supply, leading to syncope without a change in heart rate or blood pressure. Diagnosis may be difficult to make without the input of a neurologist. Basilar artery migraine may account for up to 24% of childhood migraines, especially in adolescent females.[21]

Metabolic Etiology

Hypoglycemia is an uncommon cause of syncope in children.[20] Preceding symptoms of hypoglycemia can be divided between the *neuroglycopenic* and *sympathomimetic* symptoms. The sympathomimetic symptoms consist of tachycardia, mydriasis, and diaphoresis. The neuroglycopenic symptoms consist of irritability, emotional lability, confusion, lethargy, and syncope. Causes of hypoglycemia in children include diabetes, ketotic hypoglycemia, liver enzyme deficiencies, and inborn errors of metabolisms such as medium chain acyl-coenzyme A dehydrogenase (MCAD) deficiency.

Drug and Toxin Exposure

Illicit drugs such as *3,4-methylenedioxy-N-methylamphetamine* (MDMA or Ecstasy), cocaine, or others, as well as a variety of prescribed drugs, can result in syncope from a variety of causes, most commonly from arrhythmias triggered by the drugs or by increasing the likelihood of orthostatic hypotension.

Psychogenic Etiology

Hyperventilation, most commonly associated with unrecognized anxiety or distress, occasionally results in syncope.[20] Although the exact mechanism is not clearly understood, hypocapnia, resulting in alkalosis and reduction in regional cerebral blood flow from cerebral vasoconstriction, plays an integral role. Patients, who are usually adolescents, will rarely provide this aspect of the history and often present with the primary complaint of "chest tightness" or "smothering." A detailed history may uncover frequent panic attacks, which result in hyperventilation episodes and syncope. Hysterical syncope or conversion reaction mimics loss of consciousness and most commonly occurs in adolescents in the presence of an audience. Patients are typically calm when describing the episodes.[20] There are no abnormalities of heart rate, blood pressure, or skin color during the episodes, which may have an unusually long duration. The patient typically falls without injury.[20,22] Position may be supine in these situation. Frequently, an internalized stress can be uncovered by a psychiatrist or

psychologist, and syncope can be resolved with therapy for the underlying issue.

Cardiac Etiology

Syncope without warning is more likely to be cardiac in origin, as is exertional syncope.[16,20] A careful history often reveals that the syncope occurs during or shortly after exercise. Such a history should always be of serious concern to the astute clinician. The catecholamine surge associated with exercise makes a vagally mediated phenomenon unlikely as an explanation for syncope that occurs during the period of exertion.

The exception is the volume-sensitive athlete who has maintained suboptimal hydration throughout exercise and develops hypotension in the face of the peripheral vasodilatation associated with exercise. Such patients should receive the thorough evaluation warranted for exercise-induced syncope before the episodes can be attributed confidently to neurally mediated phenomena.

Causes of exercise-induced or cardiac syncope can be separated into three broad categories. First is low output on a primary cardiac basis from obstruction, including obstructed inflow, as in cardiac tamponade or from cardiac tumors (external or internal), and obstructed outflow, as seen in hypertrophic cardiomyopathy or aortic stenosis. Symptoms from obstructive tumors, such as myxomas, may be paroxysmal and are often associated with changes in position.[20] Obstruction can occur with pulmonary vascular disease and is seen with primary pulmonary hypertension or Eisenmenger's syndrome.

Another cause of cardiac syncope occurs with myocardial dysfunction with poor cardiac contractility associated with primary myopathy. Cardiomyopathy, associated with neuromuscular disorders such as Duchenne's muscular dystrophy, can result in syncope. Cardiomyopathies may be associated with low output, but more commonly, these patients have syncope from associated arrhythmias.[20] Ventricular dysfunction can occur in the presence of inflammatory or ischemic heart disease. Myocarditis from a viral etiology would be the most common in this category. Kawasaki disease is associated early with inflammation of coronaries and myocardium, and later with ischemic coronary disease from coronary aneurysms with stenosis or thrombosis. Other causes of ischemia from coronary anomalies include abnormal-course or intramural coronary artery, anomalous origin from the pulmonary artery, and atherosclerotic coronary disease, particularly with postcardiac transplant arteriopathy or with homozygous familial hypercholesterolemia.

A third major category of cardiac syncope occurs in association with a variety of arrhythmias that interrupt the cardiac output (Fig. 1-3). Rhythm disturbances may decrease cerebral perfusion from a heart rate that is either

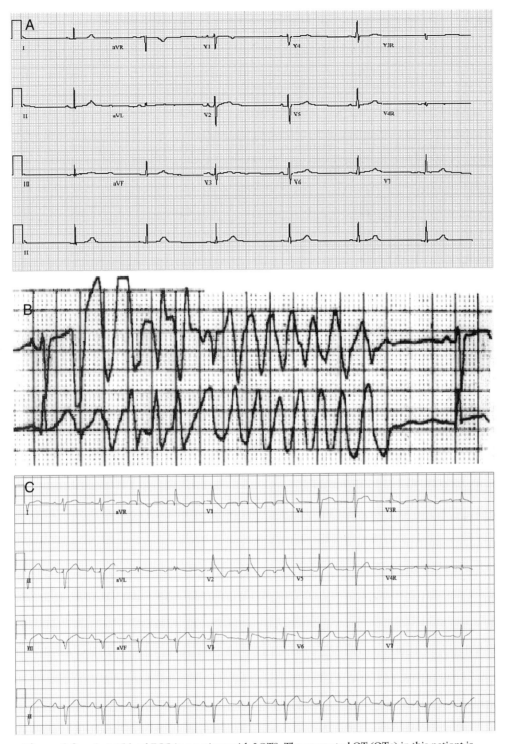

Figure 1-3   **A,** A 15-lead ECG in a patient with LQTS. The corrected QT (QTc) in this patient is 610 ms.(normal < 460 ms). **B,** Rhythm strip demonstrating a coarse wide complex tachycardia with a constantly "twisting axis" consistent with torsades de pointes. **C,** 15-lead ECG demonstrating a right bundle branch block pattern in an 18-year-old and S-T segment elevation in the right precordial leads (V_1-V_3) consistent with the diagnosis of Brugada syndrome.

Continued

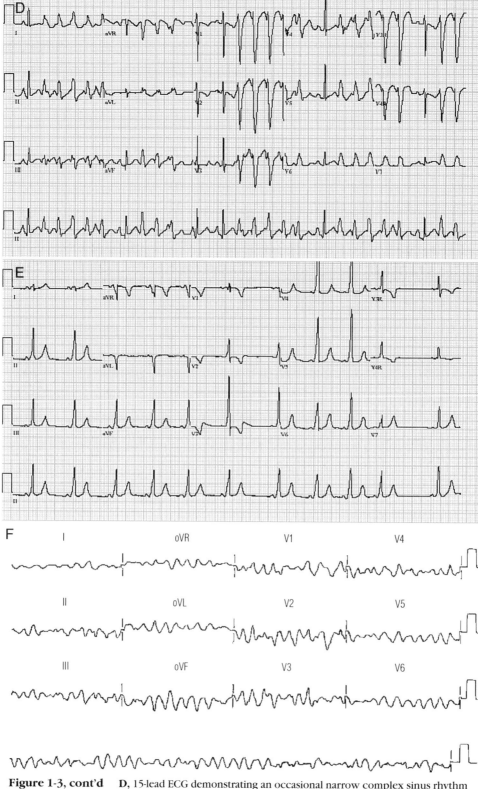

Figure 1-3, cont'd **D,** 15-lead ECG demonstrating an occasional narrow complex sinus rhythm interrupted by a regular wide QRS tachycardia, consistent with ventricular tachycardia. **E,** 15-lead ECG demonstrating a short PR interval, a slurred upstroke of the QRS (delta wave), and absence of septal Q waves (in V_6) diagnostic of the WPW anomaly. **F,** 15-lead ECG demonstrating a coarse, poorly organized wide QRS pattern consistent with ventricular fibrillation.

Continued

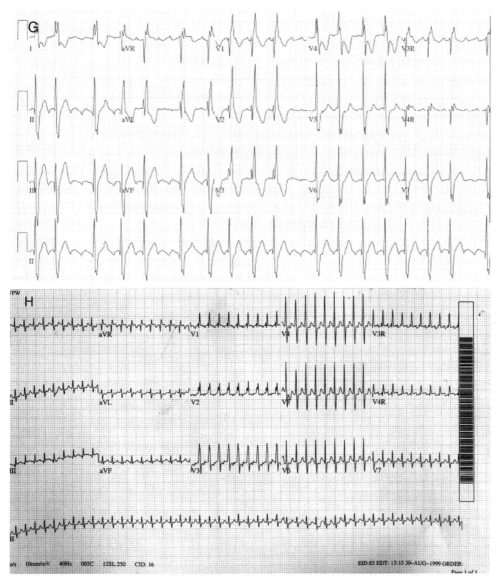

Figure 1-3, cont'd   G, 15-lead ECG demonstrating an irregularly irregular narrow complex tachycardia with an absence of true P waves. There are flutter waves with variable AV conduction. This represents atrial flutter with variable AV block. **H,** ECG of narrow complex tachycardia. There is evidence of retrograde P waves. This is consistent with a diagnosis of supraventricular tachycardia.

too slow or too fast. These include ventricular arrhythmias, seen with arrhythmogenic RV dysplasia, idiopathic or catecholamine-induced ventricular fibrillation/ventricular tachycardia (VF/VT), long QT syndrome with torsades de pointes, Brugada syndrome, VT with structurally normal hearts, and also seen in specific postoperative congenital heart defects, most commonly tetralogy of Fallot or similar lesions. Atrial tachyarrhythmias may result in syncope, as seen in the WPW syndrome, with atrial fibrillation and rapid ventricular response, which can lead to ventricular fibrillation. Atrial flutter with rapid AV conduction, seen after intraatrial repairs of D-TGA or

after the Fontan repair for single ventricle physiology, can result in syncope and sudden cardiac death. Syncope can be seen with supraventricular or ventricular tachycardia (SVT or VT), more commonly in association with a structurally or functionally abnormal heart, although very rapid tachyarrhythmia can cause syncope in the presence of a normal heart. Less frequently, slow rhythms, including high-degree atrioventricular block and sick sinus syndrome with periods of asystole, can also be responsible for syncope. Hypercyanotic "spells" may be seen in conjunction with an existing right-to-left shunt, most commonly described in TOF. A spell frequently begins with an illness or dehydration accompanied by a crying episode. Increased resistance to pulmonary blood flow, combined with decreased resistance to systemic blood flow, can result in a spiraling cycle of cyanosis, hypoxemia, and syncope.

Autonomic Nervous System

Neurally Mediated Syncope

Neurally mediated syncope, also referred to as autonomic, neurocardiogenic, vasovagal or vasodepressor syncope, common or emotional syncope, or reflex syncope, is the most common cause of syncope in the pediatric patient.[20] It includes syncope associated with the following: emotional stress and fear; pain; physical situations such as overheating, physical exhaustion, dehydration, and hypovolemia; anemia; prolonged standing or sitting; and a change in position from supine to standing or kneeling to standing.

Neurally mediated syncope is thought to be mediated by abnormal or heightened autonomic responses to various stimuli. Peripheral vasodilatation occurs with a decrease in blood pressure and a slow heart rate. The prodromal symptoms often consist of lightheadedness, nausea, pallor and diaphoresis, and visual or auditory loss. Usually the patient collapses suddenly and remains unconscious for less than 1 minute unless attempts are made to restore upright posture, which can result in exacerbation of symptoms or can prevent resolution of symptoms. The patient may remain pale, weak or tired, and diaphoretic following the episode.[20] These episodes occur while the patient is standing, sitting, or on changing from a sitting to a standing position but do not occur in the supine position. A number of reflex and compensatory neurocardiovascular mechanisms allow individuals to change position, to adjust to physical exercise, to digest food, and to respond to unexpected or unpleasant mental stresses. These adaptive autonomic nervous system mechanisms preserve arterial blood pressure and cerebral perfusion. Syncope can occur when afferent, central, or efferent portions of the autonomic reflex arc are impaired, myocardial contractility or vascular reactivity is suppressed, hypovolemia is present, hormonal responses are abnormal, or adaptive responses are inadequate.

On standing, pooling of up to 25% of the cardiac output occurs in the lower extremities. A decrease in venous return and, thus, decrease in cardiac output and blood pressure occur. The baroreceptors or stretch receptors detect these changes and relay information to the central nervous system with a resultant decrease in parasympathetic tone, allowing for an increase in heart rate. There is a concomitant increase in sympathetic outflow, which increases norepinephrine secretion and increases peripheral resistance. Blood pressure and cerebral perfusion are preserved.

Abnormalities can occur at one or several parts of this reflex arc. The traditional hypothesis regarding neurocardiogenic syncope is that such episodes arise from vagally mediated hypotension (vasodepressor type), bradycardia (cardioinhibitory type), or both (mixed type), in part associated with vigorous contraction of a relatively empty ventricle.[22] It is generally agreed that there is an increase in parasympathetic tone and inhibition of sympathetic outflow. The initial mechanism relates to a decrease in systemic venous return and excessive vagal stimulation associated with the decrease in ventricular filling. Normal autonomic reflexes do not function normally in these patients. The initial stimulus is venous pooling of blood within the vascular system, the vasodilator effects of adrenaline, decreased production of norepinephrine by the adrenal, an under-representation of α receptors or over-representation or hypersensitivity of β receptors, or else stimulus by a primary neurogenic process.[20,22] In the presence of hypotension, sympathetic activation results in an increase in catecholamine release with more forceful cardiac contractions and subsequent mechanoreceptor stimulation. Although heart rate typically does increase prior to the syncopal episode, cardiac output does not increase sufficiently in response to the decrease in blood pressure.[15,20] Sympathetic withdrawal and increased parasympathetic activity ensue with hypotension, bradycardia, and syncope. A poorly understood central nervous system reflex, in response to pain, fear, the sight of blood, or anxiety, triggers sympathetic inhibition with vasodilatation and parasympathetic activation with bradycardia, resulting in syncope.

Reflex or Situational Syncope

An amplified or inappropriate reflex response to a physiologic stressor can result in syncope. Pallid breath-holding spells are a common pediatric reflex phenomenon, usually beginning in infancy or early childhood. An unexpected, startling stimulus elicits a sudden reflex increase in vagal tone and resultant asystole for up to 15 seconds. As the episode nears conclusion, there may be accompanying tonic-clonic seizure activity. The more common type of breath-holding spell follows a period of crying, terminated with sustained exhalation (often against a closed glottis) and visible cyanosis. This is followed by vagally mediated hypotension and syncope. Reflex syncope may be associated with swallowing, stretching, hair combing, sneezing, and diving. Cough, defecation, and micturition syncope are related to increased intrathoracic pressure, leading to vagally mediated reduction in cardiac output.[20]

Carotid Sinus Syncope

Carotid sinus baroreceptors are located above the common carotid artery, in the internal carotid artery. Shaving or turning the head with a tight collar, anomalies of the cervical vertebrae, or having pressure applied over the carotid sinus can initiate this reflex.

Hypervagotonia

Hypervagotonia, or excessive vagal tone, is primarily seen in 2- to 6-year-olds and is a result of an exaggerated vagal response that is not interrupted by normal reflexes. Generally, there is a vagal stimulus, but not the type that elicits breath holding. Most children with this condition gradually have resolution, but they may require treatment with medication such as atropine for a period of time. They commonly develop vasodepressor syncope as adolescents. Both conditions are most likely manifestations of autonomic nervous system abnormalities or imbalance. Many individuals, especially in late childhood and early adolescence, have increased vagal tone that manifests as a low resting heart rate, junctional rhythm, or varying degrees of AV block, especially during sleep. This is a physiologic variant found in healthy, asymptomatic children and adolescents. Rarely is it of sufficient magnitude to be a cause for syncope.

Postural Orthostatic Hypotension and Syncope

Postural neurally mediated syncope is more common than centrally mediated syncope. Syncope can result from *orthostasis*, defined as a decrease in systolic blood pressure of at least 20 mmHg within 3 minutes of standing, or a lesser change in blood pressure but with associated symptoms. There is an exaggeration of the usual orthostatic pooling during the upright position. An increase in sympathetic activity occurs when the heart contracts vigorously with a relatively empty chamber. This exaggeration in the usual physiologic responses associated with a change in position is often a consequence of hypovolemia, anemia, or medications, or else of an autonomic nervous system (ANS) imbalance. The role of the baroreceptors in maintaining a normal adaptive process has suggested that malfunction of this reflex may be responsible for many instances of postural syncope. Normally, neurohormonal agents aid in blood volume control and maintain peripheral vascular resistance.

Postural orthostatic tachycardia syndrome (POTS) refers to a significant increase in heart rate of greater than 30 beats per minute (bpm) that occurs in some patients with positional change. Although syncope may occur, the major symptom is that of tachycardia, which becomes disabling on its own.

Post-Exercise Syncope

VDS occurs after exercise in patients and is associated with extreme vasodilatation and hypovolemia, usually occurring once exercise stops and sympathetic withdrawal occurs. Other more serious causes of exercise-induced syncope must be excluded before this etiology can be entertained in this subset of patients.

Dysautonomia

Syncope can occur as a manifestation of familial *dysautonomia*, a sympathetic nervous system malfunction (Riley-Day syndrome), in which the normal adrenergic responses do not occur due to a primary autonomic system disorder with abnormal control of heart rate and blood pressure. Inheritance is an autosomal recessive pattern predominantly in children of Ashkenazi Jewish ancestry. Manifestations include sleep apnea, seizures, developmental delay, and temperature instability.

Evaluation

History

The history from the patient and eyewitness observers is invaluable in evaluating the patient with syncope. Of particular importance are the activity and position immediately prior to the episode, as well as sudden changes in position such as rising from supine to standing. Associated symptoms such as dizziness, weakness, nausea, visual blurring or loss of vision, hearing loss, diaphoresis, or epigastric discomfort may be present. Syncope during or immediately following exertion requires careful consideration and evaluation because it may be a harbinger of cardiac disease and a risk for sudden death. Knowing the duration of loss of consciousness as well as the time to full recovery assists in forming the differential diagnosis. Syncope of autonomic origin is usually brief in duration, whereas syncope due to neurologic, metabolic, or psychologic origin (e.g., migraines and convulsive disorders) tends to have more prolonged periods of unconsciousness. Syncope of cardiac cause is less commonly self-limited. A thorough family history should be obtained, particularly for family members with syncope, seizures, deafness, need for pacemaker or arrhythmia medication, or sudden early cardiac or accidental death. If there is a strong family history for sudden, unexplained early death, this may suggest a familial cardiomyopathy or LQTS. Many patients with vasodepressor syncope have a strong family history for similar episodes. In patients suspected of conversion reaction, family, school, or other stresses should be carefully sought in the history. A dietary history is important because those patients, particularly adolescents, with limited fluid intake or salt restriction may be predisposed to orthostatic syncope. Finally, a medication history may suggest drugs—prescribed, over-the-counter, or illicit—as a cause of syncope.[20]

Physical Examination

Particular attention should be paid to changes in the vital signs with postural maneuvers during the physical examination. In a standing adolescent, a systolic blood pressure of less than 80 mmHg, a decrease of 20 mmHg or more from the supine blood pressure measurement, or an increase in heart rate of greater than 20 bpm is diagnostic of *orthostasis*. A complete cardiovascular and neurologic assessment should be performed.

When hyperventilation is suspected as a cause of syncope, asking the patient to hyperventilate for 30–40 seconds will often reproduce the symptoms of concern and clarify the diagnosis. The remainder of the physical examination should be entirely normal.

Diagnostic Tests

The decision regarding which additional diagnostic tests need to be performed should be guided by the results of the history and physical examination. An ECG and rhythm strip, with the primary purpose of evaluating the corrected QT (QTc) interval or finding other ECG abnormalities, may be all that are needed in an otherwise healthy patient who faints after an emotional shock, positional change, or vagal stimuli. Further studies are required if any of the following apply (Box 1-5)[15]:

- The syncope is exercise-induced, occurring during or immediately after exercise.
- The syncope is preceded by chest pain, palpitations, or a sensation of an increased or decreased heart rate.
- There is evidence of seizure activity or loss of bowel or bladder control.
- The faint is atypical for vasodepressor syncope.
- The syncope is recurrent, significantly impairs day-to-day function, or both, or results in injury.
- Physical findings suggest a specific organic etiology.
- There is a family history of unexplained sudden or accidental death (e.g., drowning or a car accident with a young person).

Tilt Table Testing

Tilt table testing provides a passive method of assuming upright posture to 60–80 degrees in a controlled environment and increases the yield of diagnostic evaluation of syncope by identifying many patients prone to develop postural neurally mediated syncope.[15,20,22] Tremendous

---

Box 1-5 Tests Available for Evaluation of Syncope

Initial laboratory studies may include serum electrolyte levels, fasting blood glucose levels, and hemoglobin levels.

Cardiac: Echocardiography and color Doppler studies, 24-hour Holter monitor, event monitor, exercise stress testing, myocardial perfusion testing, tilt table testing, cardiac MRI, cardiac catheterization with coronary angiography, electrophysiology (EP) studies

Neurologic: CT/MRI brain scan, ophthalmologic assessment, vestibular testing, electroencephalogram (EEG) or video EEG monitoring

---

physiologic change is associated with assuming an upright posture; these changes may be more prominent in individuals prone to syncope.

In tilt table testing, the patient assumes a supine position initially and, after a rest of 5–15 minutes, is brought to an upright position of approximately 80 degrees. Blood pressure and heart rate are recorded each minute and continuous ECG monitoring occurs. An upright position is maintained for 15–20 minutes and, if no symptoms or changes in the vital signs occur, the patient is brought to the supine position and isoproterenol, ~1 µg/minute (0.025 µg/kg/minute for children weighing less than 40 kg), is infused. The patient is again brought to the upright position for 15–20 minutes and the heart rate and blood pressure are monitored carefully.[16,20] The isoproterenol dose is serially increased every 10 minutes to achieve a heart rate of 120–160 bpm or until symptoms occur or the maximum dose is reached (up to a maximum of 2–4 µg/minute or 0.1 µg/kg/minute).[16,23] The table is returned to the supine position when there is reproduction of symptoms (even without change in vital signs), asystole or severe bradycardia (< 40 bpm), or severe systolic hypotension (< 60 mmHg), or if 20 minutes has elapsed.[16,20]

Positive responses to tilt testing may be divided into three subsets. A cardioinhibitory response is a sudden onset of bradycardia or asystole without preceding hypotension.[20] A vasodepressor response is hypotension with less significant changes in heart rate.[20] Lastly, the mixed type includes both a cardioinhibitory and vasodepressor response.[20,23] But this may well be an artificial subdivision without a true pathophysiologic or clinical implication. Although most patients have spontaneous resolution of symptoms over time or can be treated with dietary change or medication, there is a subset of patients with a "malignant" response and prolonged asystole, in whom pacemaker insertion is recommended to be beneficial.[20,23] Among teenagers, the specificity of tilt testing without isoproterenol is 83–100% (low rate of false positives).[23] The sensitivity at baseline is a dismal 43–57% (high rate of false negatives). Sensitivity improves with addition of the isoproterenol infusion to 70–100%,[23] but this may reduce the specificity of the test. The reproducibility of syncope or presyncope is variable in the pediatric patient, limiting the value of tilt table testing. The reproducibility of an initial negative test is fairly high, at 85–100%.[23] The unpleasant experience of a positive tilt test may influence the response to subsequent testing.

Treatment of Neurally Mediated Syncope

There are a variety of therapeutic options for children and teenagers with neurally mediated syncope. A trial of an initial therapy is often more practical than performing a tilt table test on every youngster with syncope that sounds neurocardiogenic in origin, because up to 75% will respond to dietary therapies. This includes augmentation of fluid (1–2 oz/kg/day) and dietary salt intake, as well as the avoidance of caffeine or other diuretics, especially alcohol. Patients who relate symptoms to periods of inadequate hydration may require dietary counseling only, but patients who suffer from repetitive episodes or episodes accompanied by seizures or bodily injury clearly require more definitive testing and therapy.[16] It is prudent to reserve such testing for cases where the history is unclear, where empiric conservative therapy is unsuccessful, or where the family circumstances result in heightened concern regarding sudden cardiac death. Additional medications should be reserved for those with repetitive or refractory syncope, those with asystole that is sudden and without warning, and those who sustain injury with their episodes.

When medication is needed, the first choice is generally fludrocortisone and a high-sodium, high-fluid diet. In patients with marked tachycardia prior to syncope, β-adrenergic blocking agents may be helpful. Midodrine, an α-adrenergic stimulator, is effective in many patients and is often combined with fludrocortisone. Selective serotonin reuptake inhibitor (SSRI) therapy has been shown to be effective in some patients, but it should be carefully monitored in light of recent information regarding the association of some SSRIs with an increased risk of suicide in children. Controlled trials comparing the efficacy of these interventions in children are lacking.

Therapy should be individualized.[16] The use of the tilt table test to evaluate the efficacy of various treatment strategies has been controversial at best. General guidelines of treatment should include avoidance or careful monitoring of fludrocortisone and high-sodium diets in patients with resting systemic hypertension. It may be advisable to obtain routine electrolytes and blood pressure measurements for patients, both prior to starting fludrocortisone and 1–2 weeks later. Potassium loss can be seen with the use of this medication, and a high-potassium diet should be suggested. In addition, β-blocking agents should be avoided in children with asthma and diabetes mellitus and may not be well-tolerated in those with a depressive disorder. Failure of one agent necessitates adding or switching to another. Fortunately, neurally mediated syncope is not considered to be a life-threatening condition unless the patient is in a circumstance in which loss of consciousness is dangerous, such as driving, swimming, crossing the road, or climbing a ladder. Patients can be counseled on how to avoid situations that predispose them to fainting, thus making them less prone to injury. The benign nature of this condition, with no serious underlying cardiac pathology, led to a good long-term prognosis, with many patients improving over time, especially by the end of adolescence.

MAJOR POINTS

- A focused history with concentration on symptoms related to growth and development and exercise intolerance or respiratory issues, combined with a thorough family history, forms the basis of the pediatric cardiac evaluation.
- Physical examination includes a general assessment of "wellness" and presence of dysmorphology as well as accurate vital signs. The components of the cardiac examination include inspection of the precordium and extremities, palpation of the precordium and pulses, and auscultation. The splitting of S2 is a vital component of cardiac auscultation and provides valuable clues to the presence or absence of disease.
- Innocent murmurs are common in childhood and are easily distinguished by the experienced pediatrician from pathologic murmurs by using history and physical exam.
- Diastolic murmurs and the presence of a thrill indicate pathology.
- Ancillary cardiac testing in the community may include a 12-lead ECG, a chest radiograph, or both. The ECG is a relatively sensitive tool with variable specificity.
- The ECG is an important part of the evaluation of the child or adolescent with syncope, palpitations, and chest pain.
- For maximum benefit, ECGs on children should be read by pediatric cardiologists and echocardiograms should be performed and read by pediatric cardiologists.
- Exercise intolerance is a common symptom with etiologies that include deconditioning, obesity, pulmonary disease, musculoskeletal disease, and cardiovascular disorders. When the history suggests a cardiovascular cause, the patient may require echocardiography and exercise stress testing.
- Chest pain is a common pediatric symptom. Noncardiac causes predominate. A thorough history and physical examination often delineates the cause. Cardiac consultation and testing should be geared toward those with exercise-related symptoms or family history of cardiac disease.
- The majority of pediatric patients with palpitations have no significant pathology. Most palpitations represent benign ectopy or a physiologic variant with no risk of progression or sudden death. For the patient with exercise-related symptoms, syncope, or a family history of sudden death, further testing is indicated.
- Syncope is an important and common pediatric and adolescent complaint. Categories of syncope include noncardiac, cardiac, and neurocardiogenic. Noncardiac causes such as neurologic, drug, metabolic, and psychogenic causes need to be excluded. Cardiac etiologies such as outflow tract obstruction (HCM or aortic stenosis), coronary anomalies, and arrhythmia are evaluated by clinical history, physical examination, ECG, and echocardiography.
- VDS is a common cause of syncope, distinguished by history and physical exam. Its etiology is multifactorial and often responds to simple measures such as maintenance of adequate hydration and sodium intake.

REFERENCES

1. Duff DF, McNamara DG: History and Physical Examination of the Cardiovascular System. In Garson A, Bricker JT, McNamara DG (eds): *The Science and Practice of Pediatric Cardiology, 1st ed.* Philadelphia: Lea & Febiger, 1990, pp 671–691.

2. Moller JH: Clinical History and Physical Examination. In Moller JH, Hoffman JIE (eds): *Pediatric Cardiovascular Medicine.* Philadelphia: Churchill Livingstone, 2000, pp 97–110.

3. Nadas AS: History, Physical Examination and Routine Tests. *Pediatric Cardiology, 3rd ed.* Philadelphia: W.B. Saunders, 1972, pp 1–20.

4. Goldman HI, Maralit A, Sun S, Lanzkowsy P: Neonatal cyanosis and arterial oxygen saturation. *J Pediatr* 82(2):319–24, 1973.

5. Danford DA, McNamara DG: Innocent Murmurs and Heart Sounds. In Garson A, Bricker JT, McNamara DG (eds): *The Science and Practice of Pediatric Cardiology, 1st ed.* Philadelphia: Lea & Febiger, 1990, pp 1919–1929.

6. Miao CY, Zuberbuhler JS, Zuberbuhler JR: Genesis of vibratory functional murmurs. *Am J Cardiol* 60(14):1198–1199, 1987.

7. Leatham A: Auscultation of the heart. *Pediatr Clin North Am* 5(4):839–870, 1958.

8. Levine SA: The systolic murmur: its clinical significance. *JAMA* 101:436–438, 1933.

9. Leatham A: A classification of systolic murmurs. *Br Heart J* 17:574, 1955.

10. Newburger JW, Rosenthal A, Williams RG, et al: Noninvasive tests in the initial evaluation of heart murmurs in children. *N Engl J Med* 308(2):61–64, 1983.

11. Selbst SM, Ruddy RM, Clark BJ, et al: Pediatric chest pain: a prospective study. *Pediatrics* 82(3):319–323, 1988.

12. Kocis KC: Chest pain in *pediatrics. Pediatr Clin North Am* 46(2):189–203, 1999.

13. Duster MC: Chest Pain. In Garson A, Bricker JT, McNamara DG (eds): *The Science and Practice of Pediatric Cardiology,* 2nd ed. Baltimore: Lippincott Williams & Wilkins, 1998, pp 2213–2217.

14. Driscoll DJ: Chest Pain in Children and Adolescents. In Allen HD, Gutgesell HP, Clark EB, Driscoll DJ (eds): *Moss and Adams' Heart Disease in Infants, Children, and Adolescents,* 6th ed. Philadelphia: Lippincott Williams & Wilkins, 2001, pp 1379–1382.

15. Park MK: Syncope. *Pediatric Cardiology for Practitioners,* 3rd ed. Philadelphia: Mosby, 1996, pp 452–461.

16. Kanter RJ: Syncope and Sudden Death. In Garson A, Bricker JT, McNamara DG (eds): *The Science and Practice of Pediatric Cardiology,* 2nd ed. Baltimore: Lippincott Williams & Wilkins, 1998, pp 2169–2199.

17. Driscoll DJ, Jacobsen SJ, Porter CJ, Wollan PC: Syncope in children and adolescents. *J Am Coll Cardiol* 29(5):1039–1045, 1997.

18. Tanel RE, Walsh EP: Syncope in the pediatric patient. *Cardiol Clin* 15(2):277–294, 1997.

19. Lewis DA, Dhala A: Syncope in the pediatric patient: the cardiologist's perspective. *Pediatr Clin North Am* 46(2):205–219, 1999.

20. Scott WA. Syncope and the Assessment of the Autonomic Nervous System. In Allen HD, Gutgesell HP, Clark EB, Driscoll DJ (eds): *Moss and Adams' Heart Disease in Infants, Children and Adolescents,* 6th ed. Philadelphia: Lippincott Williams & Wilkins, 1998, pp 443–451.

21. Hockaday JM: Headache in children. In Olesen J, Tfelt-Hansen P, Welch KMA (eds): *The Headaches.* New York: Raven Press, 1993, p 795.

22. Mark AL: The Bezold-Jarisch reflex revisited: clinical implications of inhibitory reflexes originating in the heart. *J Am Coll Cardiol* 1(1):90–102, 1983.

23. Thilenius OG, Quinones JA, Husayni TS, Novak J. Tilt test for diagnosis of unexplained syncope in pediatric patients. *Pediatrics* 87(3):334–338, 1991.

Critical Heart Disease in the Newborn

ILANA ZELTSER

SARAH TABBUTT

INTRODUCTION

In the United States, congenital heart disease (CHD) occurs in 8/1000 live births, and the subpopulation with critical CHD is roughly 3.5/1000 live births. In other terms, approximately 32,000 children each year are born with CHD, and 14,000 of them are born with critical heart lesions. Prompt recognition, diagnosis, management, and treatment of neonates with CHD significantly decrease overall mortality and prevent untoward secondary damage to other organ systems.

Fetal Circulation

With an understanding of fetal circulation and the physiologic changes that occur at birth, one can appreciate why critical heart disease is readily tolerated in utero but is uniformly fatal postnatally without intervention. Furthermore, appreciation of perinatal physiology allows for the early recognition of critical heart disease and offers insight into management and treatment strategies.

In the fetus, the ventricles work in concert to deliver blood to systemic tissues, and the placenta serves as the organ of oxygen delivery. Through a series of central shunts and preferential streaming patterns, oxygenated blood is directed to vital, metabolically demanding organs. In contrast, deoxygenated blood is diverted to organs with lower oxygen consumption and to the placenta for exchange of metabolites between mother and fetus. To better appreciate how this is achieved, it is easiest to divide the fetal circulation into two components: (1) oxygen-rich blood delivery to metabolic active tissues and (2) deoxygenated blood returned to the placenta.

The umbilical vein carries oxygenated blood from the placenta to the inferior vena cava through the ductus

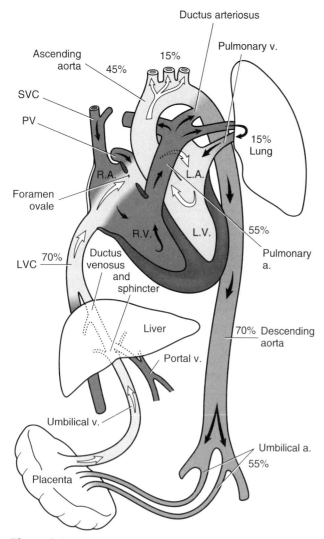

Figure 2-1 Diagram of the fetal circulation showing the four sites of shunt: placenta, ductus venosus, foramen ovale, and ductus arteriosus. Intravascular shading is in proportion to oxygen saturation, with the lightest shading representing the highest PO_2. The numerical value inside the chamber or vessel is the PO_2 for that site in mmHg. The percentages outside the vascular structures represent the relative flows in major tributaries and outlets for the two ventricles. The combined output of the two ventricles represents 100%. *a*, Artery; *v*, vein; *IVC*, inferior vena cava; *PV*, pulmonary vein; *SVC*, superior vena cava. (Modified with permission from Guntheroth WG, et al: Physiology of the Circulation: Fetus, neonate, and child. In Kelley VC, ed: Practice of Pediatrics, vol 8. Philadelphia: Harper & Row, pp 1982–1983.)

venous, with a fraction of this flow to the hepatic circulation (Fig. 2-1). Upon entering the right atrium, oxygenated blood preferentially streams across the foramen ovale and enters the left atrium, where it mixes with pulmonary venous return before entering the left ventricle. From the left ventricle (LV), the ascending aorta delivers this oxygen-rich blood to the coronary arteries, the head and neck vessels, and the upper extremities. Only a small

portion of left ventricular cardiac output traverses the aortic arch and supplies flow to the thoracic aorta.

The most deoxygenated blood returns to the heart from the upper body through the superior vena cava and from the myocardium through the coronary sinus, where it is directed across the tricuspid valve into the right ventricle (RV). Because fetal lungs do not function in the oxygenation of blood and pulmonary vascular resistance (PVR) is elevated, only a small portion of blood ejected from the right ventricle enters the pulmonary circulation. The majority of right ventricular output is directed from the main pulmonary artery across the ductus arteriosus and into the descending aorta. Although a small portion of descending aortic flow supplies organs that have a low metabolic demand, such as the gut, kidneys, and lower extremities, the majority of flow returns to the low-resistance placenta through two umbilical arteries.

Fetal circulation allows survival to term in the presence of severe structural heart disease. For example, in the case of hypoplastic left heart syndrome, the right ventricle assumes the responsibility of supplying both the descending aorta in the normal fashion, as well as the head, neck, and coronary arteries by retrograde perfusion through the ductus arteriosus. Pulmonary venous return is diverted from the left atrium across the foramen ovale into the right atrium and, from there, into the right ventricle. Thus, the hypoplastic left ventricle is not essential to fetal circulation and vitality.

Another distinctive feature of fetal circulation is the pivotal role of the placenta, a well-vascularized, low-resistance vascular bed where oxygenation and metabolite exchange occurs. The placenta is not an efficient organ for gas exchange, and so the fetus adapts by producing fetal hemoglobin, which has a higher affinity for oxygen molecules, compared with adult hemoglobin.

Transitional Circulation

Regulation of flow across a vascular bed is dictated by the hydraulic equivalent of Ohm's law, and thus pulmonary blood flow (Qp) is equal to the change in pressure across the pulmonary vascular bed ($P_{pa} - P_{pv}$) divided by the PVR:

$$Qp = (P_{pa} - P_{pv}) / PVR$$

At birth, with separation of the umbilical cord, the responsibility of oxygenation shifts from the placenta to the lungs. In order for this to occur, PVR must fall rapidly. Physical expansion of the lungs and the replacement of fluid-filled alveoli with gaseous molecules change the surface tension within the alveoli, generating a negative pressure. This negative force promotes the dilation and distention of the pulmonary arteries, thereby decreasing PVR. Mechanical distention of the lungs also promotes local production of prostacyclin, a pulmonary artery vasodilator, further increasing antegrade Qp and decreasing PVR. In addition, the increased oxygen tension in the pulmonary artery acts as a vasodilator both directly and through its ability to stimulate nitric oxide production. The cumulative effect of all these forces is a substantial reduction in PVR in the immediate postnatal period.

When the placenta is removed from the circulation, blood return to the heart through the inferior vena cava is significantly diminished, causing right atrial pressures to fall. Coincidentally, the increase in Qp brings about an increase in pulmonary venous return and subsequent elevation in left atrial pressures. With the left atrium being at a higher pressure than the right atrium, the flap over the foramen ovale closes and there is no longer intraatrial communication. In addition, there is a dramatic reduction in the production of prostaglandin E_2 (by the placenta) and an increase in its metabolism (by the lungs). This, in combination with increased oxygen content in the blood, provides the stimulus for the ductus arteriosus to constrict.

With the disruption of the uteroplacental circulation, the neonatal circulation transitions to a series configuration, thereby establishing separate systemic and pulmonary circulations postnatally. Through the closure of central shunts that were essential to fetal life, the RV exclusively supplies Qp, and the LV assumes sole responsibility for providing systemic circulation. During fetal life, the ductus arteriosus is patent and unrestrictive, and so pulmonary and aortic pressures are equal. Once the duct closes, pulmonary artery pressures significantly decrease as the resistance in the pulmonary vascular bed falls. Within the first 24 hours of life, pulmonary artery pressures are approximately one-half of aortic pressures.

Normal Neonatal Circulation

Cardiac output (CO) is directly proportional to the heart rate (HR) and stroke volume (SV): $CO = SV \times HR$. Stroke volume is dependent on three determinants: (1) preload, or the distention of the ventricle prior to systole, (2) afterload, or the resistance to ejection from the ventricle, and (3) myocardial contractility. Compared with the mature adult heart, neonatal myocardium is relatively stiff and has fewer contractile myofibrils. A newborn is relatively incapable of increasing its cardiac output by augmenting stroke volume, and instead relies primarily on increases in heart rate to supply the required cardiac output.

Because neonatal myocytes are deficient in sarcoplasmic reticulum calcium stores, newborn cardiac output is exquisitely sensitive to calcium.

PREOPERATIVE CARE: GENERAL PRINCIPLES

The outcome of a newborn with critical congenital heart disease ultimately depends on the timely assessment and accurate diagnosis of the underlying defect, as well as the prompt evaluation of potential secondary end-organ damage. Communication among obstetrical, medical, surgical, and nursing disciplines is absolutely imperative to provide the most appropriate care in the newborn period.

Fetal Diagnosis

Fetal echocardiography (echo) has become a vital tool in the diagnosis of congenital heart disease. Prenatal diagnosis of critical congenital heart disease avoids the hemodynamic compromise often accompanying postnatal diagnosis.[1,2] The current recommended timing for fetal echo is 16–20 weeks gestation, and indications for the procedure include a host of fetal, maternal, and familial risk factors associated with congenital heart disease. Though fetal echo can detect a large percentage of defects, certain anomalies, including coarctation of the aorta, small ventricular septal defects, atrial septal defects, and anomalous pulmonary venous return, may evade even the most detailed prenatal evaluations.

Delivery Room Stabilization

Communication among caretakers is necessary to determine the optimal location for delivery, taking into account both neonatal and maternal concerns. In general, lesions that mandate delivery near a pediatric tertiary cardiac care center include (1) those that require immediate surgery or cardiac catheterization, (2) those that require ductal patency for Qs, and (3) those that require ductal patency for Qp. Spontaneous delivery at term is generally recommended because a full-term infant is easier to manage medically from cardiovascular, respiratory, and nutritional standpoints.

Delivery room resuscitation should abide foremost by the general guidelines for neonatal resuscitation. The airway should be stabilized. Medications should be readily available to correct acidosis, profound metabolic abnormalities, and significant hypovolemia. Inotropic agents, specifically epinephrine and atropine, as well as prostaglandin, should be available and administered when indicated.

With the exception of a handful of lesions, newborns with critical CHD do not present critically ill immediately at birth. This is due to the persistence of fetal physiology within the first hours of life. That said, neonates with congenital heart disease are less likely to tolerate acute hypoxemia, acidosis, and bradycardia. Therefore, the most skilled practitioners available should perform all procedures on the baby in the delivery room.

Oxygen must be used with caution in the neonate with congenital heart disease, particularly those with single-ventricle physiology. Oxygen is a potent pulmonary vasodilator and will increase Qp at the expense of the systemic circulation. Oxygen administration should be minimized in ductal-dependent congenital heart disease. Conversely, oxygen should be administered when there is concurrent underlying lung disease and may be required in newborns with cyanotic right-sided obstructive lesions and cyanotic transposition of the great arteries, where the arterial partial pressure of oxygen (PaO_2) is less than 30 mmHg. In general, arterial oxygen saturations should be maintained between 80% and 85%, which in a neonate with single-ventricle physiology and good cardiac output translates to a balanced circulation with a Qp:Qs ratio of 1:1.

After the airway has been appropriately assessed and secured if necessary, vascular access should be obtained by the placement of umbilical arterial and venous catheters. Those infants with ductal-dependent circulation should be started on prostaglandin E_1 (PGE_1) before there is chance for the ductus to close spontaneously. If the ductus remains patent, lower-dose PGE_1 is sufficient (0.01 µg/kg/min). If the ductus has spontaneously closed or has constricted, a higher initial of dose PGE_1 is often necessary (0.05–0.1 µg/kg/min). Potential side effects of PGE_1 include hypotension, hypoventilation, apnea, and temperature elevation. Volume expanders and dopamine (3–5 µg/kg/min) may be needed to maintain adequate systemic perfusion. When intubation is warranted, the infant should be given atropine, sedation, and muscle relaxants immediately prior to the procedure in order to minimize the risk of procedure-related bradycardia, hypoxia, and acidosis.

Initial Evaluation of the Neonate with Suspected CHD

Although an increasing number of neonates are diagnosed with congenital heart disease in utero, the majority of infants born with severe cardiac lesions do not come to medical attention until after birth. *Critical congenital heart disease, by definition, includes all cardiovascular lesions that would result in neonatal demise unless immediate intervention to palliate or correct the anatomic defect is undertaken.* The timing of and symptomatology upon presentation of neonates with critical CHD depends on (1) the nature and severity of the anatomic defect and (2) the impact of the normal physiologic alterations that occur during the first week of life with the closure of the ductus arteriosus and the fall in PVR. Even though there are numerous different cardiac lesions, there are many similarities in their clinical presentation. Signs and symptoms of severe heart disease in the newborn period include cyanosis, discrepant pulses and blood pressures, congestive heart failure, and cardiogenic shock.

The initial evaluation of any newborn suspected of having critical congenital heart disease includes a thorough physical exam, four-extremity blood pressures, preductal and postductal saturations, a hyperoxia test, a chest radiograph, electrocardiogram (ECG) and an echo, even in the event of a prenatal diagnosis (Box 2-1). Features particular to individual lesions will be discussed in detail later in this chapter. General principles regarding blood pressure, pulse oximetry, and cyanosis will be discussed below.

Blood pressure measurements should be obtained in all four extremities. A difference of greater than 10 mmHg in upper compared to lower-extremity blood pressure suggests the presence of aortic coarctation, aortic arch hypoplasia, or interrupted aortic arch. It should be noted that blood pressure measurements are highly specific but not often sensitive for diagnosing arch obstruction. First, in the event of low cardiac output and systemic hypotension blood pressure, discrepancies are diminished. That is, coarctation may be present in the absence of significant blood pressure gradient. Hypotension should be corrected, and cardiac output should be maximized prior to interpretation of blood pressure differences. Second, if the ductus arteriosus is widely patent, a blood pressure difference between upper and lower extremities may not be noted, despite underlying coarctation. A complete assessment of the newborn with cyanosis includes preductal and postductal measurements of oxygen saturation.

Differential cyanosis exists when preductal (i.e., upper-extremity) saturations are higher than those found postductal (i.e., in lower extremities). This phenomenon occurs when the great vessels are normally aligned and deoxygenated blood from the pulmonary artery crosses into the descending aorta through the ductus arteriosus.

Differential cyanosis is seen with aortic arch obstruction (interrupted aortic arch, critical coarctation) or pulmonary hypertension. *Reverse differential cyanosis* is when the preductal saturation is lower than the postductal saturation (Fig. 2-2). This occurs exclusively in children with the physiology of transposition of the great arteries when oxygenated blood from the pulmonary artery enters the descending aorta through the ductus arteriosus. Reverse differential cyanosis can be seen in transposition of the great arteries with aortic arch obstruction (interrupted aortic arch, critical coarctation) or pulmonary hypertension.

Cyanosis

Central cyanosis can be detected when the absolute concentration of deoxygenated hemoglobin is at least 5 g/dL

Box 2-1 Basic Evaluation of the Newborn for Congenital Heart Disease

EXAM:

Systolic murmur: Consider valvar stenosis (pulmonic or aortic) or tricuspid or mitral regurgitation
Diminished pulses:
  Diminished lower extremity pulse: Coarctation
  Diminished four-extremity pulse: Left-sided obstructive lesions
Tachypnea:
  High Qp:Qs
  Diminished left ventricular function

ECG:

Check for sinus rhythm
Superior axis: consider atrioventricular canal or tricuspid atresia (single ventricle)

CHEST X-RAY:

Severe cardiomegaly: consider neonatal Ebstein's or cardiomyopathy
Look for right aortic arch
Look for normal abdominal situs (stomach on left)
Hypoxemia with normal lung fields: Consider congenital heart disease
Progressive interstitial pattern: Consider obstruction to pulmonary venous return

CUTANEOUS OXYGEN SATURATIONS:

Differential cyanosis: Consider pulmonary hypertension, coarctation, or interrupted arch
Reverse differential cyanosis: Consider the above with transposition of the great arteries

ARTERIAL BLOOD GAS:

Hyperoxia test: PaO_2 in right radial artery on 100% FiO_2 with less than 150 mmHg: Consider intracardiac mixing
Hypoxemia that improves markedly with oxygen: Consider lung disease

Qp, Pulmonary blood flow; *PaO₂,* arterial partial pressure of oxygen; *Qs,* systemic blood flow; *FiO₂,* fractional concentration of oxygen in inspired gas.

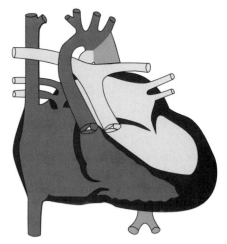

Figure 2-2   Reverse differential cyanosis occurs when the preductal oxygen saturation is lower than the postductal oxygen saturation. This occurs solely in the presence of the physiology of transposition of the great arteries and right-to-left ductal blood flow, as seen in pulmonary hypertension, coarctation, or interrupted aortic arch.

in a child with a normal hemoglobin level. The best indicator of cyanosis is the mucous membranes, which are free of pigmentation and have a rich vascular supply. Central cyanosis should not be confused with acrocyanosis, a common physical finding in newborns in which there is blueness of the extremities due to peripheral vasoconstriction. Whether or not cyanosis is manifested depends on (1) the hemoglobin and (2) factors that alter the affinity of hemoglobin (temperature, serum pH, level of 2,3-diphosphoglycerate, and the percentage of fetal vs. adult hemoglobin). For example, a newborn with polycythemia (hemoglobin of 20 g/dL) with an arterial saturation of 80% will have 4 g/dL of deoxygenated hemoglobin and will therefore appear cyanotic. In contrast, an anemic newborn (hemoglobin of 10 g/dL) with an arterial saturation of 80% will have only 2 g/dL of deoxygenated hemoglobin and will likely not appear cyanotic.

The differential diagnosis for causes of hypoxemia includes abnormalities in the cardiovascular, pulmonary, neurologic, and hematologic systems. In all neonates with hypoxemia and a suspicion of CHD, the hyperoxia test is a useful diagnostic tool to identify those neonates with a cardiovascular etiology of their hypoxemia. If a right radial arterial PaO_2 on 100% fractional inspired oxygen is less than 150 mmHg, critical congenital heart disease is likely present. In such a scenario, the infant is presumed to have ductal-dependent CHD and should be immediately started on a PGE_1 infusion to maintain ductal patency until the underlying anatomy can be accurately determined. Patients passing a hyperoxia test with critical CHD include those with critical aortic stenosis, critical coarctation, and interrupted aortic arch.

Stabilization and Transport

Once the diagnosis of critical CHD is made, attention should continue to focus on the basic principles of neonatal life support and maintenance of a patent ductus arteriosus. An airway must be stabilized, vascular access must be secured, volume status, and inotropic support must be maintained, and systemic and pulmonary circulations must be balanced.

In general, if respiratory distress, profound cyanosis, acidosis, or apnea are present, the neonate should undergo endotracheal intubation and mechanical ventilation. Administration of sedation and neuromuscular blockade prior to intubation is the preferred strategy for several reasons. First, the increased catecholamine secretion associated with intubation might potentially lead to significant arrhythmias and pose a hemodynamic threat to the underlying "at-risk" myocardium. Second, vagally mediated bradycardia from manipulation of the laryngoscope, acute hypoxia, and hypercarbia are often not well-tolerated in the face of a myocardium with little reserve. Finally, sedation and neuromuscular blockade will reduce overall systemic oxygen consumption and improve mixed oxygen saturation and oxygen delivery to vital tissues.

PGE_1 is administered in nearly all cases of critical CHD. As the ductus becomes patent, profound hypoxia generally improves and metabolic acidosis improves. Less commonly, administration of PGE_1 may not improve the clinical condition. When this occurs, one must suspect one of the following underlying conditions: (1) total anomalous pulmonary venous return with obstruction, (2) hypoplastic left heart syndrome with an intact atrial septum, or (3) transposition of the great arteries with an intact ventricular septum and restrictive atrial communication. If one of the above is suspected, echocardiography should be performed immediately to confirm the diagnosis, in which case either urgent catheterization or surgical intervention is indicated.

Once the infant has been stabilized, it is often necessary to transport the neonate to a tertiary center that specializes in management and treatment of congenital heart disease. In order to facilitate a successful transport, direct and detailed communication among the referring hospital, the transport team, and the receiving hospital is of crucial importance.

Confirming the Diagnosis

Once the infant has been stabilized, confirmation of the underlying diagnosis is sought prior to formulating a definitive management plan. Echo is a useful tool in defining anatomic detail and in providing information regarding physiology and myocardial function. Although necessary, echo should be considered an invasive procedure. The newborn is prone to temperature instability and may become hypothermic if left exposed for prolonged periods of time. In addition, certain views require that the probe be manipulated in ways that might compromise respiratory effort or impede venous return to the heart. For example, suprasternal notch imaging that best visualizes the aortic arch requires hyperextension of the neck and may compromise the airway. Therefore, echo performed on a critically ill infant should be accompanied by a cardiorespiratory monitor with a dedicated bedside nurse present to assess the patient's status at all times.

With the advances in the technology of echo and the advent of color Doppler, most anatomic and hemodynamic information can be reliably obtained from a thorough echocardiogram. The role of cardiac catheterization is reserved for those instances where (1) anatomic detail could not be delineated fully by echo (e.g., distal pulmonary architecture, aorticopulmonary collaterals, and aberrant coronary arteries) or (2) transcatheter therapeutic intervention is required.

Evaluation of Additional Organ Systems

Cardiovascular

For most patients with critical CHD whose ductal patency is maintained with PGE_1, attention to balancing Qs and Qp is essential. This is particularly important for patients with single-ventricle physiology and complete intracardiac mixing. In these patients, systemic venous return (desaturated blood) and pulmonary venous return (saturated blood) usually completely mix within the heart. In this situation, and particular of single-ventricle physiology, there is competitive Qp and Qs blood flow and the relative resistances to flow govern the ratio of distribution of flow between the two circuits (Fig. 2-3). Resistance to Qp is encountered on several levels, including (1) subvalvar or valvar pulmonary stenosis, (2) pulmonary arteriolar resistance, and (3) elevated pulmonary venous and left atrial pressures. Resistance to Qs likewise occurs at multiple levels, including (1) subvalvar or valvar aortic stenosis, (2) aortic arch hypoplasia or coarctation, and (3) systemic vascular resistance.

The management goal of patients with single ventricle physiology is to provide adequate pulmonary blood flow without compromising systemic oxygen delivery and tissue perfusion. Knowing that aortic and pulmonary arterial saturations are equal in a complete mixing lesion, the ratio of Qp to Qs can be calculated using a modification of the Fick principle:

$$Qp:Qs = \frac{\text{aortic saturation} - \text{mixed venous saturation}}{\text{pulmonary venous saturation} - \text{pulmonary arterial saturation}}$$

Ideally, in the patient with good cardiac output (mixed venous oxygen saturation of 60%) and fully saturated pulmonary veins, an arterial oxygen saturation of 80% represents balanced Qp and Qs, Qp:Qs = 1. For these patients, therapies that lower PVR (e.g., oxygen, hyperventilation, and metabolic alkalosis) must be avoided. It is important to realize that ventricular workload in single ventricle physiology is Qp + Qs. All considered, a Qp:Qs ratio of 1:1 is generally considered optimal, balanced physiology: systemic oxygen delivery is appropriately maintained at the minimal ventricular workload expense.

Patients with unbalanced physiology can be broadly categorized into two categories (1) inadequate Qp,

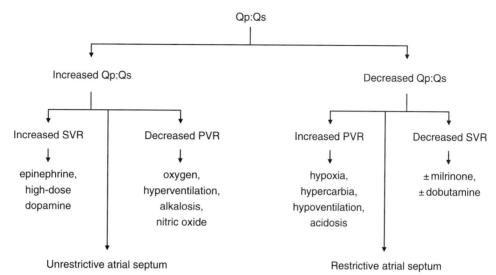

Figure 2-3   The balance between Qp and Qs blood flow is dependent on the relative resistances of the systemic (SVR) and pulmonary vasculature (PVR). Maneuvers that lower PVR (oxygen, hyperventilation, and alkalosis) will increase Qp:Qs at the expense of systemic perfusion. Maneuvers that increase PVR (hypoxia, hypercarbia, acidosis) will decrease Qp:Qs and improve systemic perfusion. Other factors being equal, an unrestrictive atrial septum will encourage pulmonary blood flow, whereas restriction at the atrial septum will help to limit pulmonary blood flow.

resulting in hypoxemia, and (2) excessive Qp, resulting in systemic hypoperfusion. As mentioned previously, inadequate Qp (low Qp:Qs) results from increased resistance to flow into the pulmonary vascular bed. Management options to increase Qp should focus on the underlying reason causing diminished flow. For example, patients with hypoxemia on the basis of restrictive atrial communication with hypoplastic left heart syndrome should undergo a transcatheter or surgical septostomy.

Excessive Qp (high Qp:Qs) often results in systemic hypoperfusion. Clinical manifestations include hypotension, acidosis, and decreased end-organ perfusion, possibly leading to necrotizing enterocolitis, renal insufficiency, and compromised cerebral blood flow. High Qp:Qs can result from either increased systemic vascular resistance (SVR) or diminished PVR. Elevated SVR can be the result of increased endogenous catecholamines (e.g., agitation) or secondary to exogenous vasoactive agents (e.g., epinephrine or high-dose dopamine). Excessive inotropic support, especially those with α-agonist properties, should be minimized. Strategies that decrease PVR should be avoided (oxygen or hyperventilation). Persistent pulmonary overcirculation may require endotracheal intubation to control ventilation, to reduce systemic oxygenation consumption, and to allow delivery of inspired gas mixtures to manipulate the balance between SVR and PVR. Adequate sedation and even paralysis lower systemic metabolic demands and decrease SVR. Permissive hypoventilation to elevate the arterial partial pressure of carbon dioxide ($PaCO_2$) to 40–50 mmHg has been effective in inducing a respiratory acidosis and

increasing PVR but can result in unwanted atelectasis. Supplemental inspired gas mixtures (nitrogen or carbon dioxide) administered during controlled mechanical ventilation have been shown to decrease Qp:Qs. In a prospective crossover analysis, hypoxia (17% FiO_2) resulted in no change in mixed cerebral oxygenation and no improvement in systemic oxygen delivery, whereas hypercarbia (i.e., P_ICO_2 of 20 mmHg) increased both systemic oxygen delivery and mixed cerebral oxygenation (Fig. 2-4).[3]

Genetic

It has been estimated that approximately 25% of all infants with CHD have at least one associated extracardiac malformation. A broad spectrum of genetic etiologies has been identified, but many remain unknown.

One of the more recent areas of focus in cardiac developmental genetics is the role of chromosome 22q11. Defects in this genetic locus were originally described as part of DiGeorge syndrome or velo-cardiofacial syndrome. Deletions in 22q11 can result in conotruncal abnormalities, including tetralogy of Fallot (TOF), truncus arteriosus, type B interrupted aortic arch, and malalignment-type ventricular septal defects (VSDs).[4] Therefore, all infants with conotruncal defects should have fluorescent *in situ* hybridization analysis for deletions in 22q11. Clinically, this is particularly relevant because the associated deficiencies of the parathyroid can result in abnormalities in calcium homeostasis; associated deficiencies of the thymus can result in immunodeficiency, generally characterized by

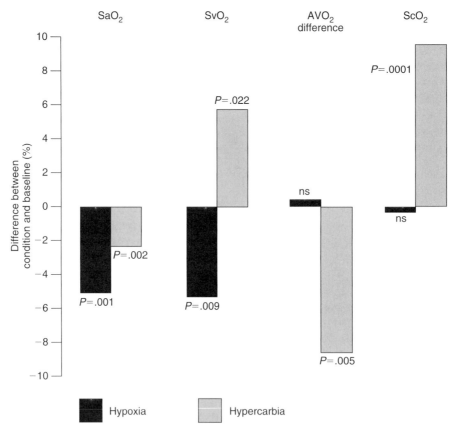

Figure 2-4   Inspired gases can be employed to decrease Qp:Qs. In a prospective crossover analysis, hypoxia (17% FiO_2) decreased arterial (SaO_2) and superior vena cava venous (SvO_2) co-oximetry; no change was observed in mixed cerebral oxygenation (ScO_2) or systemic oxygen delivery (AVO_2 difference). Hypercarbia (P_ICO_2 at 20 torr) increased both systemic oxygen delivery and mixed cerebral oxygenation. (Modified with permission from Tabbutt S, Ramamoorthy C, Montenegro LM, et al: Impact of inspired gas mixtures on preoperative infants with hypoplastic left heart syndrome during controlled ventilation. *Circulation* 104[Suppl I]:I159–I164, 2001.)

defects in T-cell production.[5] Serum calcium levels should be followed in patients with DiGeorge syndrome.

Other chromosomal abnormalities or syndromes[6] seen in infants with congenital heart disease include the following. Turner's syndrome can be seen in females with coarctation or hypoplastic left heart syndrome (HLHS) variants and is associated with an increased incidence of chylous pleural effusion; infants with trisomy 21 often have ventricular septal defects, particularly the atrioventricular canal type, and also have a 2-5% incidence of duodenal atresia; VACTERL association (vertebral abnormalities, anal atresia, cardiac malformations, tracheoesophageal fistula and/or esophageal atresia, renal agenesis and dysplasia, and limb defects) is often seen with tetralogy of Fallot.

Finally, abnormalities in systemic venous pathways and abnormalities in thoracic and abdominal organ sidedness may represent heterotaxy syndrome, which is frequently associated with complex single ventricle anatomy often

with limited Qp, which also can be associated with functional asplenia and intestinal malrotation.

Central Nervous System

Imaging studies of the central nervous system (CNS) may be required to complete the preoperative evaluation. If the infant is thought to have a genetic syndrome that has CNS involvement, a cranial magnetic resonance imaging (MRI) study often is indicated. The presence of significant underlying CNS abnormalities may (1) impact on the decision of whether or not to proceed with surgical intervention, (2) guide perioperative treatment strategies, and (3) anticipate potential postoperative complications (e.g., seizures). Preoperative cranial MRI studies in infants with critical CHD otherwise thought to be at low risk demonstrate an increased incidence of periventricular leukomalacia (16%) (Fig. 2-5).[7] The long-term clinical implications of these findings remain undefined.

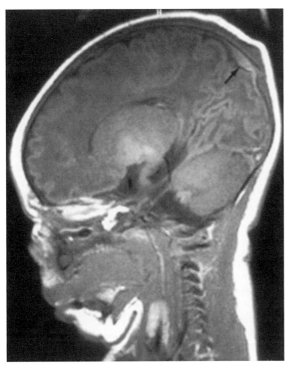

Figure 2-5   Preoperative T1-weighted sagittal image from a subject with hypoplastic left heart syndrome demonstrates the presence of subdural blood *(arrow)* but is otherwise normal. (From Mahle WT, Tavani F, Zimmerman RA, et al: An MRI study of neurological injury before and after congenital heart surgery. *Circulation* 106[12 Suppl 1]:I109-I114, 2002.)

Imaging studies of the CNS are indicated in the premature neonate if there is concern that the infant suffered hypoxic-ischemic injury secondary to presentation in shock. An ultrasound of the brain can detect the presence of intracranial hemorrhage. A cranial MRI can detect hypoxic-ischemic injury.

Renal

Neonates who present in cardiogenic shock will invariably have concurrent signs of end-organ damage. Similarly, neonates with ductal-dependent CHD are at risk for pulmonary overcirculation and inadequate systemic oxygen delivery resulting in end-organ damage or ischemia. Infants with acute renal failure will typically present oliguric or anuric and will have associated elevations in their blood urea nitrogen and creatinine. Intravascular volume status, ductal patency, myocardial function, and a balanced Qp:Qs must be readdressed whenever there is suspicion of inadequate systemic perfusion. Because of the increased risk of compromised systemic perfusion in these patients, umbilical arterial catheter placement should be noted, avoiding placement of the tip at the level of the renal arteries.

Finally, structural abnormalities of the kidneys may be part of a broader genetic syndrome. When a structural abnormality is suspected, or if there is underlying renal dysfunction, a renal ultrasound is indicated.

Gastrointestinal

Infants with critical CHD and decreased systemic perfusion, systemic hypotension, or low diastolic blood pressure are at risk of developing necrotizing enterocolitis (NEC).[8] NEC is especially a concern in the premature infant. Because enteral feeds maintain the vitality of the intestinal mucosa and allow for higher caloric intake, any infant susceptible to developing NEC should be fed enterally with great caution and usually only after the umbilical arterial catheter is removed. At many centers, enteral feeding is avoided in the preoperative newborn with ductal-dependent CHD.

Hepatic dysfunction is common in the infant presenting in shock with critical CHD. This dysfunction most commonly improves within several days but often is associated with a coagulopathy. Recovery of synthetic liver function and correction of the coagulopathy are preferred before proceeding to surgery.

Prematurity

Primary reparative or palliative cardiac surgery in the neonate can be performed in infants weighing as little as 1200-1500 g and offers the advantage of decreasing the morbidity associated with the primary cardiac lesion.[9,10]

Generally, infants with evidence of surfactant deficiency should receive surfactant replacement. Special consideration should be given to readministration of surfactant replacement in these infants after cardiopulmonary bypass.

Timing of Surgery

Neonatal surgery prevents untoward cumulative damage to secondary organs that would otherwise be sustained if surgery were delayed. The medical and surgical team caring for the neonate must collectively decide on the optimal timing of the surgery. In the event that the neonate presents with evidence of myocardial depression and end-organ ischemia, when possible, surgical correction or palliation should be delayed until medical management can optimize cardiac function and allow for end-organ recovery. If the possibility of sepsis or infection exists, cultures should be obtained and appropriate antibiotic treatment administered. Ideally, clinical evidence of clearing the infection should be present prior to surgery. In general, the more stable the neonate preoperatively, the lower the intraoperative risk and postoperative morbidity.

PREOPERATIVE CARE: LESION-SPECIFIC MANAGEMENT

A very practical approach to critical CHD is to consider lesions in terms of the timing of presentation and categorizing them as follows: (1) "shock" in the delivery room, (2) "symptoms" on the first day of life, and (3) "symptoms" in the first week of life. Understanding the physiology that dictates the timing of presentation of severe CHD is the key to prompt diagnosis and appropriate management. In each section, specific lesions will be discussed in detail in terms of pathophysiology, clinical presentation, diagnostic assessment, and treatment.

Shock in the Delivery Room

With the disruption of the uteroplacental circulation, the newborn circulation resembles a series configuration, with the right side of the heart functioning to deliver blood to the pulmonary bed for oxygenation and the left side responsible for distributing oxygenated blood for peripheral consumption. If oxygenated blood cannot be adequately presented to the systemic circulation, cardiogenic shock rapidly ensues, resulting in infant demise. As a general principle, *cardiac lesions that are unstable in the delivery room represent abnormalities of oxygen delivery that are often not stabilized by PGE$_1$ alone and require immediate intervention in order to sustain life*.

Hypoplastic Left Heart Syndrome with Intact Atrial Septum

When left ventricular hypoplasia (HLHS) (Fig. 2-6) and an intact atrial septum (IAS) are present, effective egress from the left atrium is not possible. Unless a decompressing vein is present, there is no means by which the pulmonary venous return can leave the left atrium. Pulmonary venous obstruction develops and pulmonary hypertension ensues. HLHS with an open atrial septum is discussed later in this chapter.

At the time of delivery, infants with HLHS/IAS present with profound cyanosis, metabolic acidosis, respiratory distress, and cardiovascular collapse. Patients are critically ill, markedly tachypneic, and often have a PaO$_2$ of less than 20 mmHg. Their cardiovascular exam is significant for a single, loud second heart sound and the absence of a murmur. The chest x-ray (CXR) demonstrates pulmonary venous congestion and a normal cardiac silhouette. Echo confirms the diagnosis with careful examination of left-sided heart structures and interrogation of the atrial septum.

As is true for all infants with HLHS, prostaglandin should be administered immediately to ensure ductal patency and systemic perfusion. Immediate resuscita-

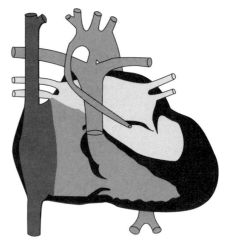

Figure 2-6   Physiology of hypoplastic left heart syndrome. In the situation of aortic atresia, cerebral and coronary arterial blood flow arises retrograde from the patent ductus arteriosus. Increased restriction at the atrial septum decreases Qp:Qs. A patient with an intact or near-intact atrial septum presents with shock in the delivery room because of obstructive pulmonary venous return and inadequate systemic output.

tion includes endotracheal intubation, vascular access, correction of metabolic acidosis, and oxygen, as needed. Once the diagnosis of HLHS/IAS is made, prompt left atrial decompression is necessary. Emergent transcatheter (balloon and blade atrial septostomy) or surgical (atrial septectomy or stage 1 reconstruction) intervention must be performed to decompress the left atrium and allow for oxygenated blood to reach the circulation. Despite early and aggressive intervention, survival of infants with HLHS/IAS is poor and may be related to increased pulmonary venous tone developing in utero.[11]

Transposition of the Great Arteries with Restrictive or Intact Atrial Septum

In a newborn with D-transposition of the great arteries (D-TGA), the aorta is connected to the RV, and the pulmonary artery is connected to the LV. The systemic and pulmonary circulations function in parallel rather than in series, resulting in recirculated Qp and a deficiency of oxygen supply to the tissues. When the atrial septum is intact or very restrictive, mixing between the two circulations only can occur at the level of the ductus arteriosus and results in significantly impaired oxygen delivery to the tissues.

D-TGA/IAS presents at delivery with profound cyanosis and associated metabolic acidosis. The pre- and postductal saturations may demonstrate reverse differential cyanosis (see Fig. 2-2). Despite the intracardiac pathology, the cardiac exam is essentially unremarkable. Arterial blood gas analysis suggests a combined picture of metabolic and respiratory acidosis, with a PaO_2 generally less than 25 mmHg. The CXR shows a narrow mediastinal shadow, the ECG is usually normal, and the echo confirms diagnosis.

Treatment of the severely hypoxic patient with D-TGA involves optimizing the mixed venous oxygen content and ensuring adequate mixing of the two parallel circulations. PGE_1 should be initiated immediately to maintain ductal patency. Maximizing oxygen delivery to the tissues can be accomplished through various maneuvers such as (1) decreasing oxygen consumption through sedation and paralysis, (2) optimizing oxygenation with mechanical ventilation and supplemental oxygen, (3) increasing oxygen delivery by increasing cardiac output with inotropic agents (dopamine at 3–5 µg/kg/min), and (4) optimizing blood oxygen-carrying capacity by keeping the hemoglobin above 13 g/dL. An emergent balloon atrial septostomy (echocar- diography- or fluoroscopy-guided) must be performed to allow for adequate mixing at the atrial level (Fig. 2-7). Once the baby has recovered, definitive surgical correction is performed by "switching" the great arteries: the aorta is reconnected to the LV and the pulmonary artery to the right, with reimplantation of the coronary arteries into the neoaorta.

Following transcatheter or surgical stabilization of newborns presenting in the delivery room with HLHS/IAS or D-TGA/IAS, end-organ function must be assessed to determine the optimal timing of palliative or definitive surgical intervention.

Symptoms on the First Day of Life

To review, normal physiology at birth is characterized by a dramatic decrease in PVR leading to a concomitant increase in pulmonary blood flow, with the lungs assuming the responsibility of oxygenation and ventilation. Critical CHD that presents prior to ductal closure includes derangements in physiology at two levels: (1) cardiovascular structures resulting in mechanical airway compromise (e.g., severe Ebstein's and TOF with absent pulmonary valve), and (2) inability to deliver oxygenated blood to target systemic tissues (e.g., total anomalous pulmonary venous return with obstruction and D-TGA with restrictive atrial septum).

Airway Compromise
Severe Ebstein's Anomaly of the Tricuspid Valve
Ebstein's anomaly is characterized by abnormality of the tricuspid valve wherein the septal and posterior leaflets are deformed and displaced inferiorly into the RV. These leaflets are usually rudimentary and thick-

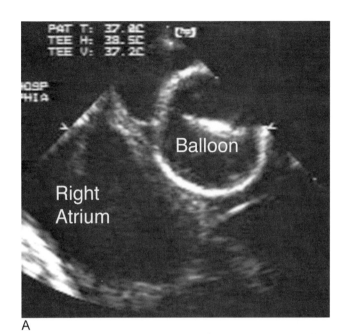

A

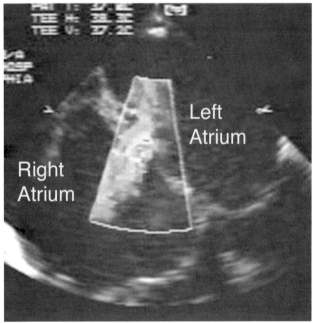

B

Figure 2-7   Echocardiographic images of a balloon atrial septostomy for transposition of the great arteries. **A,** A deflated balloon catheter is advanced across the atrial septum to the left atrium, where it is inflated with 2–3 mL of saline. **B,** The inflated balloon is pulled abruptly across the atrial septum to the right atrium and immediately deflated. After removal of the balloon, the atrial septal defect created can be seen easily on color flow Doppler.

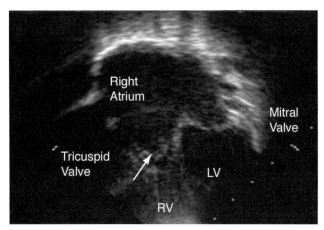

Figure 2-8   Echocardiographic pictures from a subxyphoid projection of Ebstein's anomaly of the tricuspid valve. The leaflets of the tricuspid valve are displaced inferiorly, resulting in a functionally hypoplastic right ventricle *(RV)*. *LV,* Left ventricle.

ened and often have abnormal tethered attachments to the ventricular septum. The portion between the true valve annulus and the downwardly displaced leaflets is referred to as the atrialized portion of the RV. In the most severe form of this disease, the tricuspid valve is severely incompetent, resulting in profound right atrial enlargement (Fig. 2-8).

In this most severe form, newborns often present with airway compression from the profound cardiomegaly, functional pulmonary atresia, and resultant right-to-left atrial-level shunt resulting in cyanosis and ductal-dependent pulmonary blood flow. Neonatal Ebstein's can be associated with anatomic pulmonary atresia. Even in those newborns with a functional pulmonary valve, the combination of a small RV cavity, severe tricuspid regurgitation, and elevated PVR often result in functional pulmonary atresia. Deoxygenated blood is diverted from the right atrium across the foramen ovale and into the systemic circulation.

A neonate with severe Ebstein's anomaly typically presents in the immediate newborn period with respiratory failure and marked cyanosis. The lungs fields are usually clear to auscultation. The cardiac exam is significant for a systolic regurgitant murmur, heard best at the left lower sternal border consistent with tricuspid regurgitation. CXR demonstrates impressive cardiomegaly. ECG demonstrates right atrial enlargement as evidenced by characteristic peaked P waves in lead II. Widening of the QRS complex consistent with a right bundle branch pattern may be evident. Wolff-Parkinson-White (WPW) syndrome is seen in 20–30% of patients with Ebstein's disease. Even in the absence of WPW, patients with

Ebstein's are predisposed to a variety of atrial arrhythmias. Echo confirms the diagnosis.

Infants should be intubated immediately to relieve the compromised ventilation caused by airway compression. PGE_1 must be administered to maintain ductal patency to ensure adequate pulmonary blood flow. Vascular access should be secured; volume expansion, inotropic support, and bicarbonate should be administered judiciously. Anemia should be corrected in an attempt to maximize oxygen-carrying capacity. In the event that tachyarrhythmias are present, adenosine can be used acutely to convert reentrant supraventricular tachycardia to normal sinus rhythm. Functional pulmonary atresia may be overcome by lowering PVR. If cyanosis worsens as the ductus arteriosus becomes restrictive after discontinuing PGE_1, it may be necessary to decrease PVR by using oxygen or nitric oxide.[12] Surgical options for severe neonatal Ebstein's anomaly include modified Blalock-Taussig shunt placement with atrial reduction procedure or heart transplantation. Despite aggressive medical management, the mortality rate remains quite high for the severe form of this disease.[13]

TOF with Absent Pulmonary Valve

Congenital absence of the pulmonary valve (i.e., rudimentary ridges of pulmonic valve tissue) is a rare defect. It often is associated with an anterior malalignment VSD and mixed pulmonary valve disease (obstruction and regurgitation) resulting in massive dilation of the proximal pulmonary arteries. This entity has been termed TOF with absent pulmonary valve. The pulmonary trunk and its main branches are often of aneurysmal proportion, resulting in the most severe form with airway obstruction and associated tracheobronchomalacia. In addition, often there are distal pulmonary artery stenoses.

Severely affected infants present immediately after birth with evidence of respiratory failure. The physical exam reveals tachypnea, subcostal retractions, and cyanosis. The CXR may appear hyperinflated with evidence of decreased pulmonary blood flow. The cardiac exam demonstrates a characteristic "to-and-fro" murmur at the left upper sternal border, consistent with pulmonary outflow obstruction and regurgitation. The second heart sound is single and heard most loudly at the base of the heart. Right ventricular hypertrophy is present on the ECG, but may be difficult to distinguish from normal right-sided voltages in the immediate newborn period. Echo confirms the diagnosis.

These infants require immediate intubation to ensure adequate ventilation and oxygenation. The prognosis for infants with this disease depends in part on the extent of tracheobronchial abnormalities secondary to the massively dilated branch pulmonary arteries. Infants who present immediately with respiratory distress have a worse prognosis than their counterparts without respiratory symptoms at birth. Some babies have compression of their airways that can be surgically relieved with plication of the pulmonary arteries. Others have more diffuse abnormalities of the airway architecture and, despite surgical intervention, continue to require long-term ventilatory management strategies.[14]

Obstruction to Pulmonary Venous Return

Completion of gas exchange occurs at the alveolar level; fully oxygenated blood returns to the left atrium through four pulmonary veins, two veins from each side draining the upper and lower segments of each lung field. From the left atrium, blood flows into the left ventricle and is ejected into the systemic circulation. If a structural heart lesion obstructs oxygenated blood from entering the systemic circulation, within several hours of life, progressive hypoxemia and resultant metabolic acidosis ensue.

In total anomalous pulmonary venous return (TAPVR) with obstruction, there is no connection between the pulmonary veins and the left atrium. The pulmonary veins form a confluence behind the left atrium, which decompresses through a vertical vein, usually inferiorly below the diaphragm, and empties either into the portal system or into the ductus venosus before ultimately returning to the right atrium. There exists complete mixing of systemic and pulmonary venous return within the right atrium. When the vertical vein enters the portal system, obstruction to pulmonary venous return is primarily caused by increased resistance to flow as blood is forced through the hepatic sinusoids before entering the inferior vena cava (Fig. 2-9). In the case where pulmonary venous return drains into the ductus venosus, constriction of the ductus venous after birth dramatically increases the resistance. In either scenario, elevated pressure in the pulmonary venous channel is transmitted to the pulmonary capillary bed.

Neonates with TAPVR with obstruction usually present within the first hours to days of life, and the greater the degree of obstruction, the earlier the appearance of clinical manifestations. Infants typically demonstrate cyanosis and evidence of respiratory distress secondary to pulmonary venous congestion. On physical examination, the infant is ill-appearing with evidence of cyanosis and marked tachypnea. TAPVR is a complete mixing lesion; therefore, saturations in the aorta and pulmonary arteries are equal and there is no discrepancy between pre- and postductal saturations. Cardiovascular findings are minimal and the only abnormality appreciated on exam is accentuation of the pulmonary component of the second heart sound. Other features of pulmonary venous congestion are present, including bilateral rales at the lungs' bases. CXR reveals very characteristic features of a normal cardiac silhouette and progressive pulmonary venous congestion. The ECG is typically unremarkable

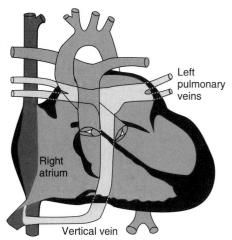

Figure 2-9 Physiology of infradiaphragmatic total anomalous pulmonary venous return. The pulmonary veins return to a complex behind the left atrium, decompressed by a vertical vein through the diaphragm and ductus venosus to the right atrium. There is complete mixing of pulmonary and systemic venous return in the right atrium. Obstruction to pulmonary venous return occurs as the vertical vein passes past the diaphragm through hepatic sinusoids or at the ductus venosus.

when the intracardiac anatomy is normal. Echo confirms diagnosis. The location of each pulmonary vein should be carefully documented, the pulmonary venous confluence pathway of the decompressing vein delineated, and sizing of the left sided heart structures determined. Although left-sided structures may appear small, they most commonly tolerate the full cardiac output postoperatively.

Treatment for TAPVR is surgical repair, which should be performed as soon as possible. If the infant is critically ill and immediate surgery is not an option, the infant can be stabilized with venoatrial extracorporeal membrane oxygenation while awaiting surgery. Endotracheal intubation should be performed to maximize oxygenation and ventilation. Sedation and neuromuscular blockade will minimize oxygen consumption and peak inspiratory airway pressures. Vascular access should be secured, volume status maintained, and electrolyte corrections and inotropic support administered if necessary. Although these patients are cyanotic, prostaglandin administration has been reported to worsen the hemodynamic state by further increasing pulmonary blood flow.

Symptoms in the First Week of Life

Postnatal closure of the ductus arteriosus occurs in two stages. Within 12 hours after birth, contraction and thickening of the walls of the ductus arteriosus result in its functional closure. The second stage of closure usually takes place over the next week or so as ductal tissue involutes and is ultimately replaced by fibrous connective tissue, sealing the lumen permanently and producing the ligamentum arteriosum. "Ductal-dependent" blood flow describes abnormalities of cardiac physiology with obligatory flow across the ductus to maintain systemic or pulmonary perfusion. Patients with ductal-dependent blood flow typically present within the first few days to weeks of life with evidence of cyanosis or systemic hypoperfusion. These lesions can be broadly considered in two categories: (1) left-sided obstructive lesions with ductal-dependent Qs, and (2) right-sided obstructive lesions with ductal-dependent Qp.

In addition, patients with significant left-to-right shunting may present with symptoms of congestive heart failure as the PVR falls during the first week of life. An example of this physiology is truncus arteriosus.

Lesions with Ductal-Dependent Systemic Blood Flow

Although there are multiple levels at which obstruction can occur along the left ventricular outflow tract, neonates with left-sided obstructive disease present with similar clinical manifestations suggestive of cardiogenic shock. Signs and symptoms include pallor, "dusky" appearance, cool extremities, "thready" pulses, diaphoresis, tachycardia, and tachypnea. These findings reflect an underlying state with inadequate systemic perfusion, progressive metabolic acidosis, and cardiovascular collapse. Infants presenting in this manner are often considered to be septic, and a complete septic work-up is often initiated. The practitioner must consider the possibility of ductal-dependent heart disease, especially when infants present during the first month of life. In addition to antibiotic therapies, one should consider the administration of prostaglandins promptly until a complete cardiac evaluation can be obtained.

Hypoplastic Left Heart Syndrome

HLHS is a spectrum of left-heart obstructive lesions resulting in the underdevelopment of the mitral valve, LV, left ventricular outflow tract, aortic valve, and aorta. Physiologically, the right ventricle is responsible for maintaining both pulmonary and systemic circulation. Adequate systemic perfusion is dependent on the patency of the ductus arteriosus (see Fig. 2-4). Without treatment, HLHS is uniformly fatal.

The majority of neonates with HLHS present within the first week, manifesting signs and symptoms of shock: tachycardia, tachypnea, hypotension, cool extremities, poor perfusion, and diminished peripheral pulses. The cardiac exam demonstrates a dominant right ventricular impulse, a normal first heart sound, and a single second heart sound. Occasionally, neonates will have a ductal flow murmur best appreciated at the left upper sternal border. A gallop rhythm can be present, as can evidence of an enlarged liver, both signs of heart failure. Distal extremities are cool and pulses often are difficult to palpate. Metabolic acidosis and hypoglycemia usually are

present and indicate inadequate systemic perfusion. Arterial blood gas analysis reveals metabolic acidosis and a failed hyperoxia test. The ECG can be normal. The CXR typically demonstrates cardiomegaly with increased pulmonary vascular markings. Echo not only establishes the diagnosis but provides important clinical information regarding right ventricular function, tricuspid regurgitation, and restriction to atrial-level shunting. HLHS is a combination of mitral stenosis or atresia and aortic stenosis or atresia (Fig. 2-10).

Therapy for preoperative infants with HLHS is outlined above (see Evaluation of Additional Organ Systems: Cardiovascular). Specifically, ductal patency must be maintained (by urgent administration of PGE_1) and pulmonary overcirculation and systemic hypoperfusion must be avoided. Management strategies should be focused on manipulating PVR and SVR in a manner that maintains the precarious balance between pulmonary and systemic circulations. The goal should be to maintain an arterial pH of 7.4, a PO_2 of 40 mmHg, and a pCO_2 of 40 mmHg. To avoid pulmonary overcirculation, administration of oxygen, a potent pulmonary vasodilator, should be avoided in the absence of lung disease. Hyperventilation and metabolic alkalosis decrease PVR and should be avoided. Finally, controlled ventilation may be necessary to reduce systemic oxygenation consumption and to allow delivery of inspired gas mixtures. Specifically, administration of inspired carbon dioxide has been shown to increase systemic oxygen delivery, while at the same time decreasing the relative Qp (see Fig. 2-4).[3]

Since the initial introduction of the Norwood procedure in the early 1980s,[15] survival for patients with HLHS has significantly improved, with reported stage 1 survival at over 90%.[16] The overall goal of the initial surgery is to provide (1) unobstructed flow from the single RV to the systemic circulation, (2) decompression of the left atrium and pulmonary venous return, and (3) adequate and controlled pulmonary blood flow through a systemic-to-pulmonary arterial shunt. The stage 1 palliation is the first of a series of staged surgical reconstruction and entails (1) creation of a neoaorta from the native pulmonary artery and the aorta arising from the RV, (2) excision of the intra-atrial septum, and (3) creation of a systemic-to-pulmonary artery shunt to assure adequate pulmonary blood flow. More recently, many centers have transitioned to using an RV–to-pulmonary-artery conduit to provide pulmonary blood flow.[17] It has not been determined whether this physiology improves pulmonary artery growth, augments coronary blood flow, or improves overall survival.[18]

Critical Aortic Stenosis

Critical valvar AS is present when the LV is unable to provide adequate antegrade cardiac output and the systemic circulation is reliant on flow from the RV through a patent ductus arteriosus. Critical AS most often is caused by fusion of the valve leaflets, resulting in a slit-like aortic

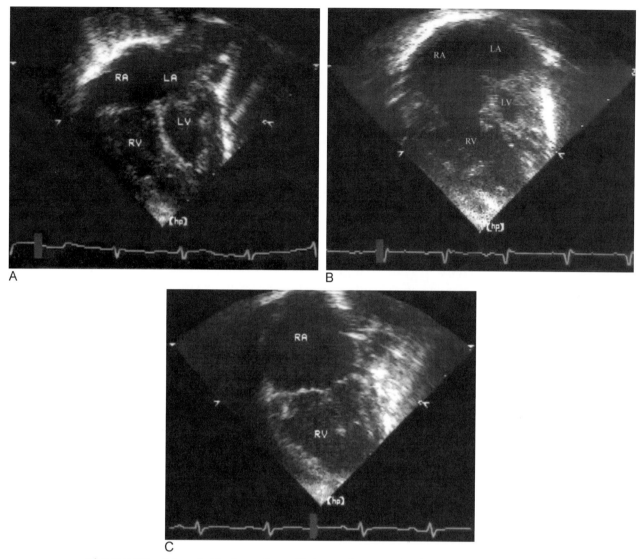

Figure 2-10   Subxyphoid echocardiographic images demonstrating three variations of hypoplastic left heart syndrome: **A,** mitral stenosis and aortic stenosis, with a hypoplastic left ventricle (LV); **B,** mitral stenosis and aortic atresia, with a very hypoplastic LV; and **C,** mitral atresia and aortic atresia, with near absence of the LV. *RV,* Right ventricle, *RA,* right atrium, *LA,* left atrium.

orifice. The valve leaflets can be myxomatous and immature, and often are unicommissural (Fig. 2-11). Severe obstruction to egress from the left ventricle results in an undue pressure strain on the left ventricle, leading to ventricular hypertrophy and, ultimately, heart failure. As the LV becomes increasingly stiff and non-compliant, the end-diastolic pressure rises, resulting in pulmonary edema.

As the ductus arteriosus closes, the infant will become symptomatic with signs of inadequate systemic blood flow and metabolic acidosis, including pallor, tachypnea, tachycardia, and lower extremity hypotension. The cardiovascular exam may reveal a systolic ejection click and a gallop rhythm. A systolic ejection murmur is typically appreciated at the right upper sternal border, with the quality of the murmur reflecting the cardiac output. In infants with significant heart failure, a murmur is often not appreciated, reflecting minimal antegrade flow from the left ventricle; as myocardial performance improves and more blood is ejected across the stenotic valve, the murmur becomes appreciably louder. A systolic regurgitant murmur of mitral insufficiency may be heard at the left axilla. The ECG typically demonstrates evidence of left ventricular hypertrophy. The CXR shows cardiomegaly and increased pulmonary venous markings consistent with pulmonary edema. Diagnosis is confirmed by echocardiography. One must be mindful to assess for evidence of associated left-sided hypoplasia (mitral valve, LV, aortic arch). Depending on the constellation of findings associated with critical AS, the neonate can be assessed accurately for candidacy for a biventricular vs. single ventricle palliation.[19,20]

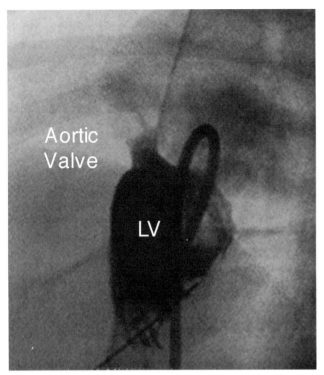

Figure 2-11   An angiographic picture of a contrast injection in the left ventricle *(LV)* in an infant with critical aortic stenosis. There is a tiny jet of antegrade flow across the aortic valve.

PGE₁ should be initiated immediately to ensure ductal patency. In the most severe form of this disease, with significant cardiac dysfunction, the myocardium is vulnerable to arrhythmia and caution should be used with volume administration, inotropic agents, and endotracheal intubation. If it has been determined that the infant is an acceptable candidate for a biventricular repair, transcatheter balloon valvuloplasty should be performed. After successful balloon dilation, PGE₁ can be discontinued and inotropic support should slowly be weaned as ventricular function gradually improves. Development of significant aortic regurgitation, particularly in the face of persistent aortic stenosis, may lead to a Ross procedure.

Critical Coarctation of the Aorta

Coarctation of the aorta most commonly occurs at the insertion site of the ductus arteriosus into the descending aorta. Coarctation of the aorta can be difficult to appreciate in the face of a widely patent ductus arteriosus. With closure of the ductus arteriosus, the entire cardiac output must cross the area of coarctation to enter the descending aorta. In the case of critical coarctation, severe obstruction is present and the left ventricle cannot supply adequate antegrade flow to the descending aorta. Ultimately, congestive heart failure results and cardiogenic shock ensues.

Newborns with critical coarctation usually present in the first 6 weeks (typically in the first 7–10 days) of life with evidence of tachypnea, tachycardia, and severe hypotension. If the ductus is partially open, preductal saturations will be higher than postductal saturations and there will be evidence of upper extremity hypertension and diminished palpable femoral pulses. If the ductus has completely closed, no discrepancy between saturations will be noted and femoral pulses often will be absent. Frequently, a gallop rhythm is appreciated on auscultation. If the ductus is still patent but severely restrictive, occasionally a systolic murmur is appreciated at the left upper sternal border with radiation to the back and left axilla. Bibasilar rales and hepatomegaly are generally present and consistent with signs of CHF. An ECG often demonstrates left or right ventricular hypertrophy, or both. CXR confirms the presence of cardiomegaly and pulmonary edema. Echo establishes diagnosis with demonstration of a critical narrowing of the isthmus, sometimes extending into the transverse arch. Attention should be made to investigate other potential left-sided structural abnormalities such as bicuspid aortic valve, subaortic stenosis, and mitral valve abnormalities.

Initial management strategies focus on maintaining ductal patency and supporting systemic perfusion. PGE₁ should be initiated, metabolic acidosis corrected, and volume expansion and inotropic support administered. Patients presenting late may require a higher of dose PGE₁ (up to 0.2 μg/kg/min) necessitating support for associated side effects (e.g., ventilation for apnea and dopamine for hypotension). Preductal and postductal blood pressures and oximetry should be monitored frequently, and evidence of end-organ damage must be investigated. If the ductus arteriosus opens, attention must be placed to avoid pulmonary overcirculation. Many institutions prefer surgical correction by a thoracotomy. Current surgical strategy entails resection of the discrete region of narrowing and primary repair with an end-to-end anastomosis, if possible. Results of surgical repair of neonatal coarctation of the aorta are excellent. Only 15% require subsequent transcatheter balloon dilation for recoarctation, with increased risk for those with younger age and smaller transverse aortic arch.[21]

Lesions with Ductal-Dependent Pulmonary Blood Flow

Lesions with severe right ventricular outflow tract obstruction are considered critical when there is obligate left-to-right shunting across the ductus arteriosus to insure adequate pulmonary blood flow. Although heterogeneous in etiology, most neonates with ductal-dependent pulmonary blood flow present with evidence of hypoxemia within a few weeks of life. This section will focus on those right-sided lesions with ductal-dependent pulmonary blood flow that have underlying biventricular physiology, including critical pulmonary stenosis, many forms of pulmonary atresia with intact ventricular septum, and severe TOF. In addition, severe Ebstein's anomaly of the tricuspid valve and tetralogy of Fallot with absent pulmonary valve, previously described because of their frequent association with mechanical airway obstruction, are examples of ductal-dependent Qp. Other right-sided obstructive lesions include single ventricle with pulmonary atresia and tricuspid atresia.

Critical Pulmonary Valve Stenosis

In classic critical pulmonary valve stenosis (PS), the valve leaflets are diffusely thickened and fused together, forming a slit-like opening. In most infants with critical PS, secondary right ventricular hypertrophy occurs with right ventricular pressures often suprasystemic. In addition, an intra-atrial communication provides necessary right-to-left flow.

Patients with critical PS typically present within the first week of life with evidence of cyanosis and hypoxia. The cardiac exam reveals a single second heart sound. The systolic murmur of pulmonary stenosis may be quite soft or even absent, reflecting diminished flow across the right ventricular outflow tract. More often, a systolic regurgitant murmur of tricuspid insufficiency is appreciated at the left midsternal border. The ECG typically features right ventricular hypertrophy and a right axis deviation. The CXR usually demonstrates decreased pulmonary blood flow. Echo confirms the diagnosis with attention to the size of the tricuspid valve and right ventricular cavity. In the most severe form of the disease, antegrade flow across the pulmonary valve may not be appreciated and valve patency noted by a small regurgitant jet.

Treatment involves administration of PGE_1 to ensure ductal patency. With the ductus widely patent, care must be taken to avoid maneuvers that increase pulmonary blood flow to the point at which systemic perfusion is jeopardized. Balloon valvuloplasty (occasionally in association with radio-frequency ablation of the plate-like pulmonary valve) is the preferred treatment for critical valvar pulmonary stenosis. Immediately following successful intervention, there is often significant dynamic subvalvar obstruction and volume expansion; β-blocking agents or intermittent PGE_1 may be necessary to avoid profound cyanosis and to maintain cardiac output. If cyanosis persists, a small aortopulmonary shunt or stenting of the ductus arteriosus may be required. Balloon dilation of the pulmonary valve should be performed with caution in the presence of significant tricuspid regurgitation.

Pulmonary Atresia, Including RV-Dependent Coronary Circulation

Pulmonary atresia with an intact ventricular septum (PA/IVS) describes plate-like atresia of the pulmonary valve with no ventricular septal defect and no right ventricular outflow. Pulmonary blood flow is dependent on left-to-right flow across the ductus arteriosus. Associated findings include a small right ventricular (RV) cavity, tricuspid valve (TV) hypoplasia, and RV-to-coronary artery fistulous connections. Patients with stenosis or occlusion of the native antegrade coronary blood flow are considered to have RV-dependent coronary circulation, in which a portion of the myocardium is supplied by the deoxygenated

blood from the RV (Fig. 2-12). For these infants, maintaining RV preload and RV intracavitary pressure and avoiding low mixed venous oxygenation are vital to preserving myocardial performance. In the event of myocardial ischemia, management strategies should include minimizing myocardial oxygen consumption (with judicious use of inotropic agents), maximizing myocardial oxygen delivery by decreasing systemic oxygen extraction (with sedation, muscle relaxants, and mechanical ventilation), avoiding pulmonary overcirculation (with controlled ventilation and inspired carbon dioxide), and optimizing hemoglobin.

Preoperative physiology is similar to that of other lesions with ductal-dependent pulmonary blood flow. Complete mixing of systemic and pulmonary venous return occurs at the left atrial level, and the ratio of pulmonary to systemic blood flow is governed by the ratio of pulmonary to systemic vascular resistances. The cardiovascular exam is remarkable for a single S_2. A continuous murmur from RV to coronary fistula may be appreciated in infancy. Echocardiography is important to confirm the anatomy and to delineate the size of the tricuspid valve. Heart catheterization is important to define the presence of RV-dependent coronary circulation.

In the absence of RV-dependent coronary circulation, the surgical strategy is to maximize RV growth; the RV is decompressed with a transannular RV outflow tract patch and a Blalock-Taussig shunt is placed to ensure adequate pulmonary blood flow. In the presence of RV-dependent coronary circulation, RV pressure must be maintained to avoid coronary hypoperfusion and myocardial ischemia; shunt placement is undertaken in isolation.[22,23]

Severe Tetralogy of Fallot ("Blue Tet")

Anatomically, tetralogy of Fallot (TOF or tet) results from anterior and cephalic displacement of the infundibular portion of the ventricular septum. This deviation causes (1) anterior deviation of the aorta over the ventricular septum, (2) disruption in the continuity between the infundibular and muscular portion of the ventricular septum, resulting in a large unrestrictive VSD, (3) obstruction to flow across the right ventricular outflow tract and pulmonary valve, and (4) systemic pressure in the right ventricle with associated hypertrophy.

The clinical diversity of physiology seen in patients with TOF reflects the degree and directionality of shunting at the level of the VSD. This, in turn, reflects the relative impedance to flow from the right ventricle to either the pulmonary or the systemic vascular bed. The degree of cyanosis reflects the ratio of pulmonary versus systemic blood flow. A "blue tet" describes the infant with severe subpulmonic obstruction and hence a significant amount of right-to-left flow across the VSD at baseline.

Blue tet often presents with marked cyanosis. Pulse oximetry is equal in all extremities and demonstrates oxygen saturations of 70–80% in room air. Arterial blood gas analysis demonstrates hypoxemia. The cardiac exam is remarkable for a normal first heart sound and a single

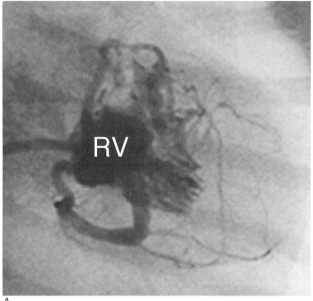

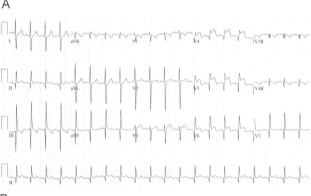

Figure 2-12 The coronary blood flow of patients with the most severe form of pulmonary atresia with intact ventricular septum (PA/IVS) is dependent on the high-pressure right ventricle (*RV*). Flow across the atrial septum is right to left. **A,** An angiogram of a contrast injection in the tiny RV demonstrates near-complete filling of the coronaries through fistulous connections. **B,** The ECG of the same baby, presenting with profound anemia with cyanosis. The associated low systemic mixed venous oxygen saturation resulted in inadequate oxygen delivery to the myocardium and is reflected in marked S-T segment elevation in the left lateral leads.

second heart sound. A harsh, systolic ejection murmur along the left mid-to-upper sternal border is typically present, with the degree of intensity correlating to the severity of the right ventricular outflow tract obstruction. If a murmur is not audible, one must be concerned that there is essentially no flow across the pulmonary outflow tract.

An ECG typically shows right ventricular hypertrophy and right axis deviation of the frontal QRS complex; these findings are not always evident on a newborn's ECG. The CXR classically demonstrates a small or absent main pulmonary artery with decreased pulmonary blood flow, and over time the development of a "boot-shaped" heart. Diagnosis is confirmed by echocardiography with

specific anatomical features noted, including additional VSDs, a degree of right ventricular outflow tract and pulmonary valve narrowing, and proximal coronary artery anatomy. The degree of obstruction across the right ventricular outflow tract should be documented; careful documentation of additional stenosis at the level of the pulmonary valve and branch pulmonary arteries allows for complete understanding of the degree of right ventricular outflow tract obstruction. When there is minimal antegrade flow across the right ventricular outflow tract, left-to-right flow across the ductus arteriosus from the descending aorta into the pulmonary arteries can be appreciated as a continuous murmur.

Ideally, and most commonly, surgical repair can be performed electively at several months of age to avoid associated morbidities of newborn heart surgery.[24] A smaller subset present with significant right ventricular outflow tract obstruction and may require newborn surgical repair. Treatment of the cyanotic newborn with TOF involves initiation of PGE$_1$ to provide adequate pulmonary blood flow. In the absence of a patent ductus arteriosus, infants should be calmed, and oxygen and sedation should be provided as needed. Acidosis should be corrected and volume expansion administered. Intubation, oxygenation, and ventilation may be necessary. If marked hypoxia persists, α-agonists that increase systemic vascular resistance are indicated (e.g., phenylephrine), and agents that decrease systemic vascular resistance should be avoided (e.g., warming blankets and benzodiazepines). Finally, if hypoxia progresses to metabolic acidosis, surgical repair should be undertaken. If necessary, venoarterial extracorporeal membrane oxygenation (ECMO) can be used to bridge the patient to surgery. Palliation with a systemic-to-pulmonary artery shunt may be indicated for premature infants, in the presence of significant lung disease, or in the presence of an anomalous left coronary artery crossing the right ventricular outflow tract.

Lesions with Large Left-to-Right Shunts
Patients with large left-to-right shunts may develop symptoms of congestive heart failure and compromised systemic circulation in the first week of life. Examples include patients with (1) truncus arteriosus or (2) a VSD with arch obstruction.

Truncus Arteriosus
During embryonic life, the truncus arteriosus normally divides into the aorta and the pulmonary artery. This occurs during the third and fourth gestational week by the development of conotruncal ridges that grow in a caudal, spiral fashion, septating the common trunk into the more anterior and leftward aorta and the posterior and rightward pulmonary artery. Failure of septation results in truncus arteriosus, characterized by the persistence of a single great vessel originating from the heart and giving rise to

the aorta, at least one pulmonary artery, and at least one coronary artery. The truncal valve is often dysmorphic, and though most commonly tricommissural, quadricuspid and bicuspid variations are not usual. The associated truncal valve insufficiency, stenosis, or both can complicate surgical repair and postoperative recovery.

A number of classification schemes have been used to describe the various origins of the pulmonary arteries from the truncus in combination with aortic arch anomalies. In the Van Praagh classification scheme, type A is associated with a VSD and type B is not. Type 1 describes the main pulmonary artery is absent arising from the truncus (incidence of 1A is 50%). In type 2, the main pulmonary artery is absent and the two branch pulmonary arteries arise directly from the truncus (incidence of 2A is 21%). In type 3, a single branch pulmonary artery arises from the truncus, and the ductus arteriosus gives rise to the contralateral branch pulmonary artery (incidence of 3A is 8%). Type 4 has an associated interrupted aortic arch (incidence of 4A is 12%).[25]

Infants with truncus arteriosus typically present in the neonatal period with clinical signs of pulmonary overcirculation and CHF, including tachypnea, tachycardia, and a widened pulse pressure. The cardiovascular exam is significant for a single S_2 and often for an ejection click. The degree of systolic ejection and diastolic murmurs reflects the functionality of the truncal valve. A continuous murmur may be heard secondary to diastolic run-off into the pulmonary arteries. An electrocardiogram may be normal or may demonstrate biventricular hypertrophy. Diffuse S-T changes may reflect coronary insufficiency secondary to low diastolic perfusion pressure. Diagnosis is confirmed by echocardiography. Attention should be paid to the proximity of the coronary arteries to the pulmonary artery, the architecture of the truncal valve, and identifying additional VSDs. Twenty-five percent have a right aortic arch, increasing the likelihood of a deletion of 22q11.

Infants with truncus arteriosus are best served by early surgical repair and have a low expected mortality (4% at 3 years).[26] Preoperative management focuses on balancing Qp:Qs and avoidance of maneuvers that decrease pulmonary vascular resistance. The pulmonary artery run-off and low diastolic pressures in infants with truncus arteriosus can result in coronary ischemia and ventricular fibrillation. Systemic vasodilators, such as benzodiazepines or α-blockers, which further decrease diastolic blood pressure, should be avoided or used with extreme caution. Postoperatively, these infants can demonstrate labile PVR, particularly those whose surgical repair has been delayed. Inhaled nitric oxide may be useful in the older infant with hemodynamically significant pulmonary hypertension.[27,28] Persistence of the patent foramen ovale in the early postoperative course can aid in cardiac output at the expense of cyanosis. Those infants with associated 22q11 deletion may have significant calcium requirements.

VSD with Arch Obstruction

Infants with a posterior malalignment VSD and arch obstruction often present in shock with a large left-to-right shunt and systemic hypoperfusion. Maintenance of ductal patency may be necessary for hemodynamic stabilization. Particularly in the face of a patent ductus arteriosus, these patients should be managed similarly to those with HLHS. Surgical approach includes VSD closure and arch repair.

CONCLUSION

Survival for infants with critical congenital heart disease has improved dramatically over the past few decades, with surgical mortality approaching less than 5% for most lesions.[16] The focus of care has transitioned to optimizing long-term neurological and cardiovascular outcomes. Emphasis on the timing of diagnosis and attention to the details of perioperative care are of utmost importance in maximizing overall quality of life.

MAJOR POINTS

- As the newborn separates from the placenta, oxygenation and ventilation are dependent on the infant; PVR falls, and the ductus arteriosus begins to close.
- Cardiac output is proportional to heart rate and stroke volume. The infant's stroke volume is fairly fixed, and cardiac output is predominantly heart rate-dependent.
- Newborns are deficient in calcium stores in their sarcoplasmic reticulum. They are very responsive to calcium administration.
- Potential side effects of PGE_1 are hypotension, central hypoventilation, and fever.
- Reverse differential cyanosis is only seen with the physiology of transposition of the great arteries.
- A failed hyperoxia test (PaO_2 <150 mmHg in the right radial artery) is consistent with an intracardiac mixing lesion. Congenital heart lesions with normal hyperoxia tests include coarctation, aortic stenosis, and isolated interrupted aortic arch.
- Many factors impact Qp:Qs. Oxygen, hyperventilation, alkalosis, and inspired nitric oxide increase Qp:Qs. Hypoventilation and inspired carbon dioxide decrease Qp:Qs.
- Cardiac lesions that are unstable in the delivery room represent abnormalities of oxygen delivery that are often not stabilized by PGE_1 alone and require immediate intervention (HLHS with intact atrial septum, TGA with intact atrial septum, or TAPVR with severe obstruction).
- Neonatal Ebstein's anomaly and TOF with absent pulmonary valve syndrome can result in immediate respiratory compromise caused by compression of the airways by the large right atrium or large central pulmonary arteries, respectively.

Continued

<table>
<tr><td colspan="2">

MAJOR POINTS—CONT'D

- Patients with left-sided obstructive lesions (e.g., critical AS, HLHS, or critical coarctation of the aorta) can present in shock in the first few weeks of life with diminished pulses and a profound metabolic acidosis. Coarctation can present in the first several months.
- Patients with ductal-dependent Qp on PGE$_1$ are also at risk for pulmonary overcirculation and systemic hypoperfusion.
- Patients with truncus arteriosus often have low systemic diastolic pressures and are at risk for pulmonary overcirculation. They have an increased preoperative incidence of ventricular fibrillation.

</td></tr>
</table>

REFERENCES

1. Cohen MS: Fetal diagnosis and management of congenital heart disease. *Clin Perinatol* 28(1):11–29, 2001.
2. Verheijen PM, Lisowski LA, Stoutenbeek P, et al: Prenatal diagnosis of congenital heart disease affects preoperative acidosis in the newborn patient. *J Thorac Cardiovasc Surg* 121:798–803, 2001.
3. Tabbutt S, Ramamoorthy C, Montenegro LM, et al: Impact of inspired gas mixtures on preoperative infants with hypoplastic left heart syndrome during controlled ventilation. *Circulation* 104[suppl I]:I159–I164, 2001.
4. Perez E, Sullivan KE: Chromosome 22q11.2 deletion syndrome (DiGeorge and velocardiofacial syndromes). *Curr Opin Pediatr* 14(6):678–683, 2002.
5. Jawad AF, McDonald-McGinn DM, Zackai E, Sullivan KE: Immunologic features of chromosome 22q11.2 deletion syndrome (DiGeorge syndrome/velocardiofacial syndrome). *J Pediatr* 139:715–723, 2001.
6. Goldmuntz E: The epidemiology and genetics of congenital heart disease. *Clin Perinatol* 28(1):1–10, 2001.
7. Mahle WT, Tavani F, Zimmerman RA, et al: An MRI study of neurological injury before and after congenital heart surgery. *Circulation* 106(12 Suppl 1):I109–I114, 2002.
8. McElhinney DB, Hedrick HL, Bush DM, et al: Necrotizing enterocolitis in neonates with congenital heart disease: risk factors and outcomes. *Pediatrics* 106:1080–1087, 2000.
9. Reddy VM, McElhinney DB, Sagrado T, et al: Results of 102 cases of complete repair of congenital heart defects in patients weighing 700–2500 grams. *J Thorac Cardiovasc Surg* 117:324–331, 1999.
10. Wernovsky G, Rubenstein SD, Spray TL: Cardiac surgery in the low-birth-weight neonate. New approaches. *Clin Perinatol* 28(1):249–264, 2001.
11. Mahle WT, Rychik J, Gaynor JW, et al: Restrictive interatrial communication after reconstructive surgery for hypoplastic left heart syndrome. *Am J Cardiol* 88(12):1454–1457, 2001.
12. Atz AM, Munoz RA, Adatia I, Wessel DL: Diagnostic and therapeutic uses of inhaled nitric oxide in neonatal Ebstein's anomaly. *Am J Cardiol* 91(7):906–908, 2003.
13. Celermajer DS, Cullen S, Sullivan ID, Spiegelhalter DJ, et al: Outcome in neonates with Ebstein's anomaly. *J Am Coll Cardiol* 19(5):1041–1046, 1992.
14. McDonnell BE, Raff GW, Gaynor JW, et al: Outcome after repair of tetralogy of Fallot with absent pulmonary valve. *Ann Thorac Surg* 67:1391–1396, 1999.
15. Norwood WI, Lang P, Hansen DD: Physiologic repair of aortic atresia-hypoplastic left heart syndrome. *N Engl J Med* 308:23–26, 1983.
16. Tweddell JS, Hoffman GM, Fedderly RT, et al: Patients at risk for low systemic oxygen delivery after the Norwood procedure. *Ann Thorac Surg* 69:1893–1899, 2000.
17. Sano S, Ishino K, Kawada M, et al: Right ventricle-pulmonary artery shunt in first-stage palliation of hypoplastic left heart syndrome. *J Thorac Cardiovasc Surg* 126:504–510, 2003.
18. Tabbutt S, Dominguez TE, Ravishankar C, et al: Outcomes after the stage 1 reconstruction comparing the right ventricular to pulmonary artery conduit with the modified Blalock-Taussig shunt. *Ann Thorac Surg* 80:1582–1591, 2005.
19. Cohen MS and Rychik J: The small LV: how small is too small. *Pediatric Cardiac Surgery Annual of the Seminars in Thoracic and Cardiovascular Surgery, vol II*:189–202, 1999.
20. Rhodes LA, Colan SD, Perry SB, et al: Predictors of survival in neonates with critical aortic stenosis. *Circulation* 84(6):2325–2335, 1991.
21. Giglia TM, Jenkins KJ, Matitiau A, et al: Influence of right heart size on outcome in pulmonary atresia with intact ventricular septum. *Circulation* 88(5 part 1): 2248–2256, 1993.
22. McElhinney DB, Yang SG, Hogarty AN, et al: Recurrent arch obstruction after repair of isolated coarctation of the aorta in neonates and young infants: is low weight a risk factor? *J Thorac Cardiovasc Surg* 122(5):883–890, 2001.
23. Rychik J, Levy H, Gaynor JW, et al: Outcome after operations for pulmonary atresia with intact ventricular septum. *J Thorac Cardiovasc Surg* 116:924–931, 1998.
24. Brizard CP, Mas C, Sohn YS, et al: Transatrial-transpulmonary tetralogy of Fallot repair is effective in the presence of anomalous coronary arteries. *J Thorac Cardiovasc Surg* 116(5):770–779, 1998.
25. Van Praagh R, Van Praagh S: The anatomy of common aorticopulmonary truck (truncus arteriosus communis) and its embryologic implications: a study of 57 necropsy cases. *Am J Cardiol* 16:406–425, 1965.
26. Jahangiri M, Zurakowski D, Mayer JE, et al: Repair of the truncal valve and associated interrupted arch in neonates with truncus arteriosus. *J Thorac Cardiovasc Surg* 199:508–514, 2000.
27. Journois D, Pouard P, Mauriat P, et al: Inhaled nitric oxide as a therapy for pulmonary hypertension after operations for congenital heart defects. *J Thorac Cardiovasc Surg* 107:1129–1135, 1994.
28. Wessel DL, Adatia I, Giglia TM, et al: Use of inhaled nitric oxide and acetylcholine in the evaluation of pulmonary hypertension and endothelial function after cardiopulmonary bypass. *Circulation* 88:2128–2138, 1993.

Cyanotic Heart Disease

AMY H. SCHULTZ

JACQUELINE KREUTZER

Cyanotic congenital heart disease can be defined most broadly as malformations of the heart causing venous blood to be returned to the arterial side of the circulation without being oxygenated in the lungs. Return of venous blood to the arterial circulation without oxygenation in the lungs is referred to as *right-to-left shunting*. Within the great diversity of malformations composing cyanotic heart disease, the amount of right-to-left shunting of blood varies considerably, resulting in a continuum of degrees of arterial desaturation.

CYANOSIS

Cyanosis, as the term is currently used, refers to a visible bluish discoloration of the skin and mucous membranes due to arterial oxygen desaturation of any cause. Jean-Baptiste De Senac first proposed in 1749 that cyanosis resulted from mixture of arterial and venous blood, caused by an abnormal communication between the two sides of the heart, which he noted in an autopsy specimen. Lundsgaard took a particular interest in this phenomenon and published a series of papers in the early 20th century, in which he investigated cyanosis caused by a variety of cardiac and pulmonary conditions.[1,2] He noted that arterial puncture was considered inadvisable and measured the oxygen content of venous blood in his subjects. He inferred that the visible phenomenon of cyanosis was due to the concentration of deoxygenated hemoglobin in capillary blood and hypothesized the deoxyhemoglobin concentration of capillary blood to be the average of the concentrations in the arterial and venous circulations. Using these assumptions, among others, he proposed that cyanosis could be perceived if the concentration of capillary deoxyhemoglobin exceeded 5 gm/dL, a threshold which continues to be quoted in textbooks today. A corollary of his observations was that the ability to perceive cyanosis depends on the hemoglobin concentration. Patients with lower hemoglobin concentrations must have a lower percentage saturation to achieve the same threshold amount of deoxyhemoglobin.

In the current era, the easiest way to measure oxygen saturation is by pulse oximetry and, consequently, the relationship of cyanosis to arterial deoxyhemoglobin concentration is of greater interest. Goss et al.,[3] in a study of adults with pulmonary diseases, reported that central cyanosis was apparent when the concentration of arterial deoxyhemoglobin was at least 1.5 gm/dL. This amount corresponds to an arterial saturation of 88% at a hemoglobin concentration of 12 gm/dL or 90% at a hemoglobin concentration of 15 gm/dL. Other studies have documented the perception of cyanosis to be unreliable until arterial desaturation is profound. Goldman et al.[4] found that neonates with arterial saturations of 85–89% were rated as cyanotic in the lips only approximately 55% of the time. This percentage increased to approximately 70% at arterial saturations of 75–79% and exceeded 90% only at saturations of less than 75%. There was also a significant rate of false positives, with 28% of neonates with saturation of over 90% rated as cyanotic.

Cyanosis attributable to congenital heart disease (CHD) has generally been thought of as *not* associated with respiratory distress, unlike cyanosis due to lung disease. Exceptions to this rule are as follows:

1. Truly profound cyanosis, with partial pressure of oxygen (PaO_2) in the 20s or less, in which case hyperpnea is stimulated.
2. Cyanosis associated with poor systemic perfusion, resulting in inadequate tissue oxygen delivery, metabolic acidosis, and compensatory tachypnea. This scenario is commonly seen with left heart obstructive lesions if the ductus arteriosus becomes restrictive. The pulses will be poor and the extremities cool.
3. Cyanosis associated with obstruction of pulmonary venous drainage resulting in pulmonary edema, such as is seen in obstructed total anomalous pulmonary venous return. Significant pulmonary edema is usually readily apparent by chest x-ray.
4. Cyanosis associated with CHF resulting from a large amount of pulmonary blood flow.

True or "central" cyanosis should be distinguished from *acrocyanosis*, a bluish discoloration limited to the extremities, related to sluggish peripheral blood flow. Acrocyanosis is not associated with arterial desaturation and the mucous membranes should be pink. Pulse oximetry easily distinguishes between true arterial desaturation and acrocyanosis and should be employed whenever the distinction is in question. Normal values for

infants and children are 97% and above in room air. Newborns achieve saturations in this range fairly consistently by 2 hours of life, with mean pulse oximetry readings on admission to the newborn nursery of 97%.[5] When the question of right-to-left shunting of blood is raised, the hyperoxia test is required (see Chapter 2).

Differential Cyanosis

Differential cyanosis refers to differences in arterial oxygenation in different parts of the body, caused by shunting through a patent ductus arteriosus (PDA) from the pulmonary artery to the aorta. This phenomenon occurs when all of the following are present:

1. One ventricle supplies the circulation proximal to the PDA.
2. The other ventricle supplies at least some blood to the circulation distal to the PDA.
3. The ventricles contain blood with differing oxygen saturations.

In *usual differential cyanosis*, the right arm saturation is higher than the leg saturation. Deoxygenated right ventricular blood shunts from the pulmonary artery to the distal aorta because of either elevated pulmonary vascular resistance or obstruction of the arch proximal to the PDA. Examples of this scenario include persistent pulmonary hypertension of the newborn, interrupted aortic arch, critical coarctation of the aorta, and PDA with Eisenmenger's syndrome.

In *reverse differential cyanosis*, the leg saturation is higher than the right arm saturation. This scenario occurs when there is transposition physiology with a PDA and pulmonary artery hypertension. Aortic arch obstruction proximal to the PDA (coarctation of the aorta or interrupted aortic arch) accentuates the differential in saturations. The proximal arch vessels are supplied by deoxygenated right ventricular blood, whereas oxygenated left ventricular blood is pumped to the pulmonary artery and some passes through the PDA to the descending aorta. Either of these patterns may be altered by abnormal aortic arch branching patterns, particularly when a subclavian artery arises aberrantly from the descending aorta.

Consequences and Complications of Chronic Right-to-Left Shunting

Chronic cyanosis results in clubbing of the extremities and polycythemia. Polycythemia helps to normalize oxygen delivery to the tissues by increasing the hemoglobin concentration of blood and, thus, its oxygen-carrying capacity. For example, 100 mL of blood with a hemoglobin concentration of 12 gm/dL and an oxyhemoglobin saturation of 100% carries the same amount of oxygen as 100 mL of blood with a hemoglobin concentration of 15 gm/dL and an oxyhemoglobin saturation of 80%.

Although polycythemia does increase oxygen-carrying capacity, there is a dramatic increase in blood viscosity as the hematocrit exceeds approximately 70%.[6] Iron deficiency also increases viscosity because of the rigidity of iron-deficient erythrocytes.[7] Symptoms of this *hyperviscosity syndrome* can include general malaise, anorexia, headache, visual disturbances, dyspnea, chest pain, and joint pain. Evidence of iron deficiency should be sought and treated if present. The hematocrit should be monitored carefully once iron therapy is instituted as an abrupt increase in hematocrit can result. Acute dehydration can increase hematocrit and can trigger symptoms, which can be relieved by rehydration. If neither iron deficiency nor dehydration is present and the hematocrit exceeds 65%, *symptomatic* hyperviscosity syndrome can be treated by phlebotomy with isovolumic replacement under careful monitoring.[8] Rapid volume shifts can precipitate a hypoxemic crisis and this therapy is *not* indicated solely on the basis of hematocrit. In the setting of iron deficiency, phlebotomy will only exacerbate the underlying disorder.

Chronic right-to-left shunting is associated with stroke, brain abscess, and scoliosis. Stroke occurred in 1.6% of children followed with cyanotic heart disease at Boston Children's Hospital between 1950 and 1970.[9] In patients less than 4 years of age, stroke was associated with decreased mean corpuscular hemoglobin concentration, which was felt to be indicative of iron deficiency, whereas in older patients, stroke was associated with more severe hypoxemia and polycythemia. Both venous and arterial occlusions were noted at autopsy. Routine phlebotomy, as described above for symptomatic hyperviscosity syndrome, does not reduce the incidence of stroke.

Brain abscess usually presents in a subacute fashion, often without fever. Typical presenting complaints are headache, lethargy, changes in mental status, vomiting, and seizures. Site-specific focal deficits may be noted. Brain abscess occurred in 2% of the patients with cyanotic CHD followed at Boston Children's Hospital between 1960 and 1973.[10] More profound cyanosis was identified as a risk factor, whereas brain abscess is felt to be extremely rare under 2 years of age. Organisms isolated included a variety of oral, gastrointestinal, and respiratory flora.

Scoliosis is very common in patients with cyanotic CHD and frequently develops during adolescence, such that the prevalence is approximately 70% in cyanotic patients over 13 years of age.[11] The prevalence in this age group also increases with decreasing oxygen saturations. The confounding effect of surgical incisions was not completely addressed in this study, but no association was seen between the side of the thoracotomy incision and the direction of the thoracic curvature.

Patients with cyanotic CHD are at risk for subacute bacterial endocarditis. Antibiotic prophylaxis should be prescribed for indicated procedures and good dental hygiene should be maintained. Among congenital heart defects, higher risk appears to be associated with sites with high-pressure gradients and those in the systemic circulation.[12]

It is difficult to study whether arterial hypoxemia, in and of itself, has adverse neurodevelopmental consequences since chronic cyanosis is often accompanied by other potential confounders, such as multiple cardiac surgeries and interventions, chronic CHF, and other congenital anomalies and genetic syndromes. Newburger et al.[13] demonstrated an inverse relation between age at Mustard procedure for repair of transposition of the great arteries and intelligence quotient (IQ), and this finding was attributed to a longer duration of cyanosis. The age at operation was between 6 months and 6 years and the hypoxemia was profound, with an average preoperative arterial saturation of 68%. A study by Aram et al.[14] supported this conclusion, whereas a study by Oates et al.[15] in predominantly younger children, did not. Certainly, there is concern that chronic cyanosis may be one of many risk factors for neurodevelopmental impairment. The current approach of repair or palliation in early infancy would be expected to lessen any impact of chronic cyanosis.

PATHOPHYSIOLOGY OF RIGHT-TO-LEFT SHUNTING

Causes of Right-to-Left Shunting

Right-to-left shunting can occur either because hemodynamic forces favor right-to-left flow across a communication between the two sides of the circulation [such as an atrial septal defect (ASD), a ventricular septal defect (VSD), or a PDA] or because the anatomy of the heart dictates return of venous blood to the arterial circulation. Anatomic and physiologic factors that provide the substrate for right-to-left shunting are listed below. There is some overlap among these categories.

1. **Factors favoring right-to-left shunting across communications between the right and left sides of the circulation:**
   a. **Atretic or stenotic pathways:** the usual flow of blood is impaired by obstruction within the heart or great vessels and blood shunts right-to-left through a communication to bypass the obstruction. For example, in pulmonary atresia with intact ventricular septum, blood shunts right-to-left across and interatrial communication to bypass the right ventricle. In interrupted aortic arch, blood shunts from the pulmonary artery to the descending aorta through the PDA, circumventing the interruption. Stenotic lesions

exist on a continuum of severity and those at the mild end may not result in right-to-left shunting. At the severe end of the spectrum, the physiology may be dependent on ductus arteriosus flow to provide pulmonary or systemic blood flow, and single-ventricle physiology results.

b. **Abnormal right ventricular compliance:** in the absence of anatomic obstruction of the atrioventricular valves, the direction and magnitude of shunt through an ASD is determined by the relative ventricular compliances (see Chapter 4). If the right ventricle is poorly compliant, right-to-left shunting at the atrial level will result.

c. **Elevated pulmonary vascular resistance:** in the absence of anatomic obstruction of the semilunar valves or great vessels, the direction and magnitude of shunt through a VSD or PDA is determined by the relative pulmonary and systemic vascular resistances (see Chapter 4). If the pulmonary vascular resistance is elevated, such as in persistent pulmonary hypertension of the newborn or Eisenmenger's syndrome, right-to-left shunting at the ventricular or great artery level will result.

2. **Single ventricle physiology:** the cardiac anatomy dictates that there is complete mixing of systemic and pulmonary venous return. As detailed further below, many complex lesions result in this physiology.

3. **Abnormal anatomic alignments or connections:** the segments of the heart (i.e., veins, atria, ventricles, and great arteries) are aligned such that blood flows from the systemic veins to the arterial system without traversing the lungs. For example, this occurs in D-transposition of the great arteries because the aorta arises from the right ventricle and the pulmonary artery from the left ventricle (Fig. 3-1). Another rare example is connection of the superior vena cava to the left atrium rather than to the right atrium.

Determinants of the Degree of Cyanosis

The degree of cyanosis is primarily determined by the ratio of oxygenated and deoxygenated blood that mixes together and then passes to the arterial circulation. Conceptually, one can imagine taking a gallon of red paint and adding one drop of blue paint, resulting in a color essentially the same as the original red paint. If one took a gallon of blue paint and added one drop of red paint, the resulting color would be nearly identical to the blue paint. Mixing a half a gallon each of red and blue paints would result in a purple color, halfway between

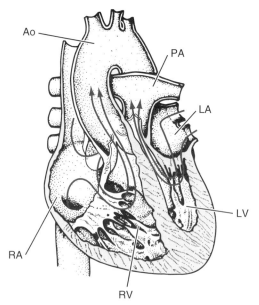

Figure 3-1   Schematic drawing of D-transposition of the great arteries with intact ventricular septum. Arrows indicate pathway of blood flow, demonstrating that systemic venous return is directed to the aorta without traversing the lungs. Intercirculatory mixing occurs only at the atrial level unless the ductus arteriosus is patent. *RA*, right atrium; *LA*, left atrium; *RV*, right ventricle; *LV*, left ventricle; *Ao*, aorta; *PA*, pulmonary artery. (From Friedman WF, Silverman N: Congenital heart disease in infancy and childhood. In Braunwald E, Zipes DP, Libby P [eds]: *Heart Disease: A textbook of cardiovascular medicine,* 6th ed. Philadelphia: WB Saunders, 2001.)

the red and blue. Every shade along the continuum between red and blue could be generated by mixing various proportions of red and blue paint. A similar situation exists with the mixture of fully oxygenated (colloquially termed "pink") blood returning from the pulmonary veins and partially deoxygenated ("blue") systemic venous blood. If a large amount of fully oxygenated blood is mixed with a small amount of systemic venous blood, the resulting arterial blood will be only mildly desaturated. If the ratio is reversed, the arterial blood will be significantly desaturated.

Two factors can affect the ratio of oxygenated and deoxygenated blood that mixes together: the amounts of oxygenated and deoxygenated blood and the efficacy of mixing. In most cyanotic lesions, once venous blood shunts into the arterial side of the circulation, it mixes freely with the oxygenated blood. The amount of blood going to the systemic circulation is regulated by homeostatic mechanisms within a relatively narrow range, so the ratio of oxygenated to deoxygenated blood is determined primarily by the *amount of pulmonary blood flow*. Less pulmonary blood flow results in more profound cyanosis. Some authors have termed this scenario "pulmonary blood flow-dependent cyanosis." In contrast, in lesions with *transposition physiology*, mixing of oxygenated and deoxygenated blood is not complete. The degree of cyanosis is more affected by the *extent of mixing* than the absolute amount of pulmonary blood flow. A large amount of blood may be pumped to the lungs, but if none of the oxygenated pulmonary venous return reaches the arterial circulation, cyanosis will be profound. Some authors have therefore termed cyanosis in lesions with transposition physiology "pulmonary blood flow-independent cyanosis." In addition, complex lesions can also exhibit "streaming." Despite a large communication at the ventricular level, there is incomplete mixing of systemic and pulmonary venous return and the saturation of blood reaching the aorta and pulmonary artery differ. The systemic venous return flows predominantly into one great vessel, whereas the pulmonary venous return is delivered predominantly to the other.

The final saturation of arterial blood is also affected by how "pink" the pulmonary venous blood is and how "blue" the systemic venous blood is. Pulmonary edema or pulmonary parenchymal disease can result in the pulmonary venous return being less than fully saturated. When blood passes through the tissue capillary beds, oxygen is extracted according to the needs of the tissues. The saturation of systemic venous blood is determined by the starting arterial saturation, the oxygen demands of the tissues, the amount of blood supplied to the tissues (i.e., the cardiac output), and the blood's oxygen carrying capacity (i.e., hemoglobin concentration). Low arterial oxygen saturation, high tissue oxygen demand (such as occurs with fever), low cardiac output, and anemia all result in lower systemic venous saturations. When a patient with cyanotic heart disease presents with greater than usual cyanosis, it is useful to go through the mechanistic differential diagnosis outlined in Table 3-1.

It should also be apparent that "pinker" is not always better from a hemodynamic standpoint. In patients with single ventricle physiology, a high systemic saturation occurs because of a very high ratio of pulmonary to systemic blood flow (Table 3-2; see also Chapter 11 for a discussion of shunt calculations). Pulmonary blood flow is much greater than usual, and in some anatomic circumstances there may be significant diastolic runoff of blood flow from the aorta into the pulmonary artery, resulting in poor systemic tissue perfusion. Symptoms and signs of heart failure usually are present when the ratio of pulmonary to systemic blood flow exceeds 2:1.

Classifications of Cyanotic Congenital Heart Disease

Cyanotic CHD includes what can be a baffling array of different lesions, so a mental organization of some sort is important to the clinician. Traditionally, cyanotic CHD has been subclassified by the amount of pulmonary blood flow (increased, normal, or decreased), as assessed by chest x-ray (Table 3-3).[16] There is a fair amount of overlap among categories. In the era when the definitive diagnostic test was an invasive cardiac catheterization and patients tended to present later with more developed physical examination and chest x-ray findings, this classification served clinicians well. In the current era, many patients are diagnosed in the first few days of life, when typical chest x-ray findings may not be present; pulmonary vascular resistance may not have fallen sufficiently to promote increased pulmonary blood flow in lesions such as truncus arteriosus and transposition of the great arteries, and the ductus arteriosus may still be patent, normalizing pulmonary blood flow in those lesions otherwise associated with decreased pulmonary blood flow. The availability of specific anatomic diagnosis by echocardiography has made clinicians less reliant on the chest x-ray for diagnostic categorization of the cardiac lesion. An alternative listing of cyanotic lesions, grouped by anatomic level of right-to-left shunting, is given in Table 3-4.

Table 3-1	Determinants of the Degree of Cyanosis: Why Is My Patient with Cyanotic Congenital Heart Disease Bluer than Usual?	
Mechanism	**Specific Reason**	**Diagnostic Test(s)**
Decreased pulmonary blood flow	Increasing obstruction to pulmonary blood flow	Change in physical exam findings, echocardiography (ECHO)
Poor mixing of systemic and pulmonary venous return in transposition of the great arteries	Restrictive ASD or PDA	ECHO
Low pulmonary venous saturation	Pulmonary edema or pneumonia	Respiratory rate, lung exam, chest x-ray
Low systemic venous saturation	Low hemoglobin	Hemoglobin
	Increased tissue oxygen demand (e.g., fever)	Temperature
	Low cardiac output (e.g., dehydration or myocardial dysfunction)	Clinical assessment

ASD, Atrial septal defect; *PDA*, patent ductus arteriosus.

Table 3-2   The Cost of a High Systemic Saturation in Single Ventricle Physiology*

Systemic Arterial Saturation	Systemic Venous Saturation	Pulmonary Venous Saturation	Qp:Qs	Work Imposed on the Single Ventricle (Qp + Qs)
65%	40%	98%	0.75:1	1.75 cardiac outputs
73%	48%	98%	1:1	2 cardiac outputs
86%	61%	98%	2:1	3 cardiac outputs
90%	65%	98%	3:1	4 cardiac outputs
92%	67%	98%	4:1	5 cardiac outputs

Qp, Pulmonary blood flow; *Qs*, systemic blood flow; *Qp:Qs*, the ratio of pulmonary to systemic blood flow.
*The systemic venous saturation is usually approximately 25 percentage points lower than the systemic arterial saturation if the cardiac output and hemoglobin are normal.

Table 3-3   Classification of Cyanotic Congenital Heart Disease by the Amount of Pulmonary Blood Flow Seen on Chest X-Ray

Increased Pulmonary Blood Flow	Normal or Decreased Pulmonary Blood Flow
Tricuspid atresia with large VSD	Tricuspid atresia with restrictive VSD
Total anomalous pulmonary venous return	Pulmonary atresia with intact ventricular septum
Truncus arteriosus	Ebstein's anomaly
D-transposition of the great arteries	D-transposition of the great arteries with pulmonary stenosis
Taussig-Bing anomaly	Double outlet right ventricle with pulmonary stenosis
Tetralogy of Fallot with minimal right ventricular outflow tract obstruction	Tetralogy of Fallot
Tetralogy of Fallot with pulmonary atresia and increased collateral flow	Tetralogy of Fallot with pulmonary atresia
Single ventricle without pulmonary stenosis	Single ventricle with pulmonary stenosis
Interrupted aortic arch with PDA	Vena cava to left atrium communication
Hypoplastic left heart syndrome	ASD with Eisenmenger's syndrome
	VSD with Eisenmenger's syndrome
	PDA with Eisenmenger's syndrome

VSD, Ventricular septal defect; *PDA*, patent ductus arteriosus; *ASD*, atrial septal defect.

SPECIFIC FORMS OF CYANOTIC CONGENITAL HEART DISEASE

Table 3-5 lists the prevalence of selected subtypes of cyanotic CHD identified during the first year of life in two different studies. The practitioner is most likely to encounter dextrotransposition of the great arteries (D-TGA), tetralogy of Fallot (TOF), and hypoplastic left heart syndrome. Specific anatomic lesions are addressed below in order of decreasing prevalence, with special attention to their neonatal presentations.

Transposition of the Great Arteries

Transposition of the great arteries (TGA) is defined anatomically as a malformation in which the aorta arises from the right ventricle and the pulmonary artery arises from the left ventricle. In the most common form of TGA, D-TGA, the atria and ventricles are otherwise normal. The aortic valve is positioned anterior and to the right of the pulmonary valve. When blood returns from the systemic veins, it passes into the right atrium, the right ventricle, and then into the aorta without being oxygenated in the lungs. When blood returns from the pulmonary veins, it passes into the left atrium, the left ventricle, and then into the pulmonary artery, to be returned again to the lungs (see Fig. 3-1). This parallel, rather than series, circulation of blood through the heart is termed *transposition physiology*, and is obviously incompatible with life without mixing of blood from the two circuits. The medical and surgical management of D-TGA is described in Chapters 2 and 14, respectively.

Other forms of anatomic TGA exist, although they are much less common than D-TGA. In levotransposition of the great arteries (L-TGA), also called congenitally corrected

Table 3-4 Forms of cyanotic congenital heart disease organized by level of shunting

Site of Shunting	Lesion	Reason for Shunting
Atrial level	Connection of SVC or IVC to left atrium	Obligatory connection
ASD	Tricuspid atresia	Atretic tricuspid valve with no other outflow from RA
ASD	Critical pulmonic stenosis	Severe RV hypertrophy results in poor RV compliance and elevated RV filling pressures
ASD	Pulmonary atresia with intact ventricular septum	No RV outlet
ASD	Ebstein's anomaly	Poor RV compliance
ASD	ASD with Eisenmenger's syndrome	RV hypertrophy secondary to pulmonary hypertension results in poor RV compliance
ASD	Total anomalous pulmonary venous return	Elevated RA pressure with low LA pressure
Ventricular level	Single ventricle (with common inlet or double inlet)	All blood mixes in ventricle, and both systemic and pulmonary vascular beds are supplied from one ventricle
VSD	Tetralogy of Fallot	VSD with obstruction to flow to the pulmonary artery
VSD	VSD with Eisenmenger's syndrome	VSD with elevated PVR
Conotruncus*	Truncus arteriosus	One great vessel comes off both ventricles and therefore receives both ventricular outputs
Conotruncus*	D-transposition of the great arteries	The aorta arises from the RV, so venous blood passes from RA to RV to aorta
Conotruncus*	Double outlet right ventricle with transposition of the great arteries (i.e., Taussig-Bing anomaly)	Both great vessels come off the RV, but the pulmonary artery is closer to the LV while the aorta is very rightward and therefore gets blue blood
Conotruncus*	Double outlet right ventricle with subaortic VSD and pulmonic stenosis	Aorta comes off RV and there is obstruction to pulmonary blood flow
PDA	Hypoplastic left heart syndrome and variants	Obstruction to aortic flow proximal to PDA favors right-to-left PDA flow
PDA	Interrupted aortic arch	Interruption of the aorta favors right-to-left PDA flow to the aorta distal to the interruption, while LV supplies the aorta proximal to the interruption.
PDA	Coarctation of the aorta	Obstruction within aorta proximal to PDA favors right-to-left PDA flow to descending aorta
PDA	Critical aortic stenosis	Obstruction to flow across aortic valve favors right-to-left PDA flow, supplying both ascending and descending aorta
PDA	Persistent pulmonary hypertension of the newborn†	Elevated pulmonary vascular resistance favors right-to-left PDA flow, with or without RV dysfunction, resulting in abnormal RV compliance and right-to-left atrial-level shunting

*The conotruncus refers to the junction between the ventricles and the great arteries.
†Not a form of congenital heart disease, but frequently in the differential diagnosis of the cyanotic newborn

SVC, Superior vena cava; *IVC,* inferior vena cava; *ASD,* atrial septal defect; *VSD,* ventricular septal defect; *PDA,* patent ductus arteriosus; *RA,* right atrium; *LA,* left atrium; *RV,* right ventricle; *LV,* left ventricle.

TGA, the right atrium drains to a right-sided morphologic *left* ventricle, which ejects to the pulmonary artery, whereas the left atrium drains to a left-sided morphologic *right* ventricle, which ejects to the aorta. Thus, the patient has anatomic TGA, but *not* transposition physiology and, in the absence of additional complicating intracardiac defects, may not be cyanotic. More complex anomalies may also exhibit TGA, for example, tricuspid atresia with TGA. These forms of TGA will not be further discussed here.

Surgical correction for D-TGA by arterial switch operation (see Chapter 14) is undertaken in the first few days of life unless complicating anatomic factors dictate another approach. Several older series reported approximately 15% mortality for this procedure; most major centers now expect a surgical mortality under 5%.[19,20] Center volume

has been shown to be inversely related to surgical mortality.[20] General physical and psychosocial health status is not different from the general population at 8 years of age in patients with D-TGA after an arterial switch operation.[21] Reintervention is required in 10–15% of patients within 2 years of the initial operation for development of supravalvar pulmonary stenosis (PS). Coronary occlusion occurs in a few percent of patients and usually is asymptomatic, but several large series report sudden death (presumably secondary to coronary complications) in less than 1% of patients.[19] Consequently, many cardiologists will perform an exercise stress test with myocardial perfusion imaging in patients with repaired D-TGA prior to competitive interscholastic sports participation. Prior to the 1980s, the surgical approach to D-TGA was an

Table 3-5   Prevalence of Subtypes of Cyanotic CHD Identified in the First Year of Life in the New England Regional Infant Cardiac Program Study, 1968–1974[17] and The Baltimore-Washington Infant Study, 1981–1989.[18]

Lesion	NERICP # per 100,000 Live Births	BWIS # per 100,000 Live Births
D-transposition of the great arteries	21.8	20.1
Tetralogy of Fallot	19.6	26.0
Hypoplastic left heart syndrome	16.3	17.8
Heterotaxy syndrome	8.8	9.2*
Severe[†] valvar pulmonic stenosis	7.3	7.1
Pulmonary atresia with intact ventricular septum	6.9	5.8
Total anomalous pulmonary venous return	5.8	6.6
Tricuspid atresia	5.6	3.6
Single ventricle	5.4	‡
Severe[†] valvar aortic stenosis	4.1	4.3
Double outlet right ventricle	3.2	6.7
Truncus arteriosus	3.0	4.9
Severe[†] Ebstein's anomaly	§	2.8

*Patients classified in BWIS as having defects of laterality and looping, excluding those with ʟ-transposition of the great arteries or dextrocardia with situs inversus.
†Patients who died or required catheterization or surgery in the first year of life; not all patients in this group will be cyanotic.
‡Category not specified separately in BWIS.
§Category not specified separately in NERICP.
NERICP, New England Regional Infant Cardiac Program; *BWIS*, Baltimore-Washington Infant Study.

intra-atrial baffle or an *atrial* level switch, the Mustard or Senning procedures, respectively. These procedures achieved physiologic correction with low mortality but have been associated with sudden death, high rates of late postoperative atrial arrhythmias, and right ventricular failure in a minority of patients.

Tetralogy of Fallot

The four components tetralogy of Fallot (TOF) are a VSD, an over-riding aorta, pulmonary stenosis, and right ventricular hypertrophy (Fig. 3-2). However, TOF can be reduced to a single unifying anatomic malformation: underdevelopment of the right ventricular infundibulum (i.e., the outflow portion of the right ventricle).[22] Underdevelopment of the infundibulum results in hypoplasia of the pulmonary outflow tract and, consequently, PS. Pulmonary stenosis can be at the subvalvar, valvar, and supravalvar levels (Fig. 3-3A). The infundibulum also contributes to the development of the ventricular septum; the infundibular portion of the septum lies between the right and left ventricular outflow tracts. When the infundibulum is hypoplastic, the infundibular septum is displaced anteriorly (toward the right ventricular outflow tract) and a large VSD results, which is accompanied by a large aorta over-riding the VSD (Fig. 3-3B). The right and left ventricular pressures are equalized by the large VSD, and secondary right ventricular hypertrophy results. Right aortic arch is present in about 25% of cases of TOF.[23]

There are additional notable variants of TOF. The variant of TOF with pulmonary atresia often has tiny central (i.e., true) pulmonary arteries, with arterial supply to segments of lung arising from a variable number of major collateral vessels off the aorta. These collateral vessels do not have the histologic characteristics of normal pulmonary arteries, and pulmonary vascular disease or severe stenosis frequently develops. Thus, TOF with pulmonary atresia and major aortopulmonary collaterals is a difficult disease to treat and has a considerably worse prognosis than uncomplicated TOF. Another variant, TOF with absent pulmonary valve, is associated with markedly dilated central pulmonary arteries in utero; however, the intraparenchymal pulmonary arteries may be small. Severe bronchomalacia can result from compression of the bronchi by the large central pulmonary arteries, and the prognosis of these patients may be limited by their ventilatory difficulties. Finally, particularly in trisomy 21, complete atrioventricular canal (CAVC) and TOF can coexist.

The etiology of TOF is heterogeneous and in many cases idiopathic, although specific genetic causes are increasingly recognized. Approximately 16% of patients with TOF in a hospital-based series had a microdeletion of chromosome 22q11.[24] In the population-based Baltimore–Washington Infant Study, 7% of cases of TOF had trisomy 21.[18] TOF occurs in patients with Alagille syndrome, VACTERL association (vertebral abnormalities, tracheoesophageal fistula and/or esophageal atresia, renal agenesis and dysplasia, and limb defects) syndrome, and many other rarer genetic syndromes associated with

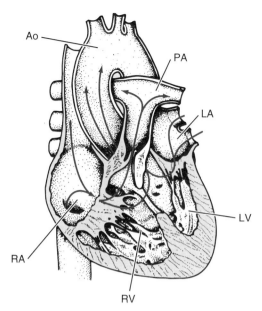

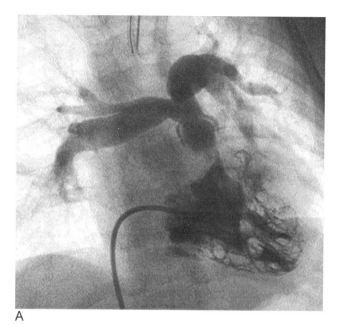

A

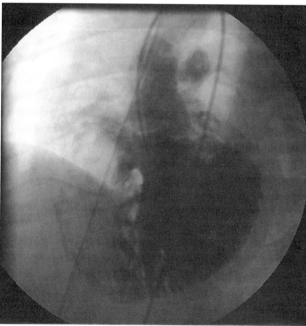

B

Figure 3-2   Schematic drawing of tetralogy of Fallot with subpulmonic stenosis and valvar PS. The arrows indicate the direction of blood flow. A substantial right-to-left shunt exists across the VSD. *RA,* right atrium; *LA,* left atrium; *RV,* right ventricle; *LV,* left ventricle; *Ao,* aorta; *PA,* pulmonary artery. (From Friedman WF, Silverman N: Congenital heart disease in infancy and childhood. In Braunwald E, Zipes DP, Libby P [eds]: *Heart Disease: A textbook of cardiovascular medicine,* 6th ed. Philadelphia: WB Saunders, 2001.)

CHD. Still, most patients with TOF have no other identified anomalies.

TOF exists along a continuum of severity of PS, which in turn determines the patient's physiology. Patients with little PS display the physiology of a large VSD and are prone to heart failure. Patients with severe PS may be ductal-dependent for pulmonary blood flow; that is, they may have insufficient pulmonary blood flow once the ductus arteriosus closes, resulting in profound cyanosis. The latter patients are described in Chapter 2, and require surgical intervention in the neonatal period. Patients with an intermediate degree of PS will have acceptable oxygen saturations in the absence of heart failure and may be repaired electively. The degree of PS can progress with time, causing the patient to become more cyanotic and to experience hypercyanotic spells.

TOF can be diagnosed prenatally by fetal echocardiography; outflow tract views increase the sensitivity of ultrasound over a simple four-chamber view. Most patients with TOF present clinically with a systolic murmur attributable to pulmonic or subpulmonic stenosis. The VSD is large, has no pressure gradient across it, and does not generate a murmur. On physical examination, if there is little PS and a large *left-to-right* shunt through the VSD (the so-called pink tetralogy), the patient will become tachypneic as the pulmonary vascular resistance falls. There may be no visible cyanosis, and desaturation by pulse oximetry is minimal. These patients will

Figure 3-3   Angiograms from a patient with tetralogy of Fallot. **A,** Right ventricular injection shows multiple levels of right ventricular outflow tract obstruction. There is narrowing below the valve because of infundibular muscle (i.e., subpulmonic stenosis). The pulmonary valve annulus is small and the valve leaflets are thickened and doming, consistent with valvar PS. There are stenoses of the proximal right (RPA) and left pulmonary arteries (LPA). **B,** Left ventricular injection seen from a long axial oblique projection demonstrates contrast passing through a large malalignment-type VSD under the aortic valve and an overriding aorta. This patient also had additional defects in the muscular ventricular septum.

develop hepatomegaly if they have symptomatic heart failure. Most commonly, TOF is accompanied by a significant degree of PS, a normal respiratory rate, and cyanosis. As pulmonary blood flow decreases, oxygen saturation, measured by pulse oximetry, decreases.

Across the spectrum of patients with TOF, the right ventricular impulse is increased and the second heart sound is usually single. A harsh systolic murmur is present along the left upper sternal border radiating across the precordium and to the back. An ejection click may be generated by a dilated aortic root or by an abnormal pulmonary valve. In TOF with an absent pulmonary valve, a "to-and-fro" murmur is heard from systolic ejection of blood across the right ventricular outflow tract and from diastolic regurgitation of the same. In contrast, patients with TOF with pulmonary atresia and multiple collaterals have no flow across the right ventricular outflow tract and thus no systolic ejection murmur. There may be continuous murmurs over the back, corresponding to flow through collaterals, but these are often subtle in the newborn period. If the degree of cyanosis is mild, TOF with pulmonary atresia and major collaterals may go undiagnosed for a prolonged period of time.

The electrocardiogram (ECG) in TOF characteristically demonstrates right ventricular hypertrophy, including right axis deviation. If left axis deviation with counterclockwise looping is present preoperatively, one should consider the diagnosis of TOF with CAVC. On chest x-ray, the classic finding of the "boot-shaped heart" is attributed to a combination of right ventricular prominence and hypoplasia of the main pulmonary artery segment. This finding usually is evident in older children but may not be apparent in newborns, especially if a thymus is present. The degree of pulmonary blood flow is reflected in the prominence of the pulmonary vascular markings, which usually are decreased in TOF but may be increased in "pink" TOF. A right aortic arch may be apparent. Echocardiography provides a definitive anatomic diagnosis.

Special attention is paid to the coronary artery anatomy because the anterior descending coronary artery arises from the right coronary and crosses the right ventricular outflow tract in about 4% of patients.[23] This anatomic feature complicates the surgical repair. Typically, an incision is made across the right ventricular outflow tract to relieve obstruction, but if the anterior descending coronary crosses the outflow tract, a conduit must be placed from the right ventricle to the pulmonary artery instead.

Cardiac catheterization is not indicated preoperatively in most patients with uncomplicated TOF and can confer a significant risk of precipitating a hypercyanotic spell.

Hypercyanotic spells ("Tet spells") result in an acute increase in right-to-left shunting. Although the precise precipitating cause has been debated over the years, likely any stimulus which either increases right ventricular outflow tract obstruction or decreases systemic vascular resistance will tip the balance of blood flow towards more right-to-left shunting, less pulmonary blood flow, and increased cyanosis. Such stimuli can include increased catecholamines, dehydration, exercise, and sedatives with systemic vasodilatory properties. Clinically, increased cyanosis, hyperpnea, and agitation are observed. Although most spells are self-limited, there is the potential for a vicious cycle to be set up as hypoxemia leads to increased agitation, metabolic acidosis, and worsening hypoxemia. Spells should be managed initially with the knee-chest position (to increase systemic vascular resistance), removal of noxious stimuli, and allowing a familiar caregiver to comfort the child. For spells that do not resolve promptly, oxygen, morphine (given subcutaneously, intramuscularly, or intravenously), intravenous volume, intravenous phenylephrine, and intravenous β-blockers can be used. In the extreme, management is escalated to intubation, heavy sedation, and paralysis. Occurrence of a hypercyanotic spell is an indication for prompt surgical repair.

Surgical repair of TOF is reviewed in Chapter 14. In the current era, primary repair is undertaken on infants at most major centers, rather than initial palliation with a shunt. In brief, repair involves closure of the VSD and relief of right ventricular outflow tract obstruction. Frequently, the annulus of the pulmonary valve is significantly hypoplastic and is enlarged with a patch (i.e., the "transannular patch" technique), which results in free pulmonic insufficiency. Even if all obstruction to right ventricular outflow is relieved, the physical examination of a patient after repair of TOF usually reveals a "to-and-fro" murmur due to increased systolic ejection volume through the right ventricular outflow tract and diastolic pulmonary insufficiency. The postoperative ECG usually displays a right bundle branch block pattern.

In uncomplicated TOF, repair is a low-mortality procedure with excellent short- and long-term term results. Surgical mortality is approximately 2%. In a cohort of patients with TOF operated on at the Mayo Clinic between 1955 and 1960, the 32-year actuarial survival was 86%, whereas that in a control population without CHD was 96%.[25] In contrast, less than 5% of patients with unrepaired TOF survive to adulthood. In the Mayo Clinic study, 77% of survivors were in New York Heart Association functional class I (i.e., asymptomatic), 17% in class II (i.e., symptoms with ordinary levels of physical activity), and 6% in class III (i.e., symptoms with minimal exertion). Pulmonary insufficiency is usually well-tolerated for many years, although decades of pulmonary insufficiency may result in right ventricular dilation and dysfunction. Indications for pulmonary valve replacement in this patient population are controversial; ideal prostheses are currently not available. Late ventricular arrhythmias can develop, typically more than 20 years after repair, and are associated with a risk of sudden death.[26] The duration of the QRS complex on ECG is a predictor of risk and periodic Holter monitoring and exercise stress testing to screen for asymptomatic ventricular arrhythmias is indicated.

Left Heart Obstructive Lesions

The spectrum of left heart obstructive lesions includes hypoplastic left heart syndrome, critical valvar aortic stenosis, interrupted aortic arch, and critical coarctation. These lesions share an inability to adequately perfuse some or all of the systemic arterial circulation once the ductus arteriosus closes. Right-to-left shunting occurs at the ductal level, whereas the ductus arteriosus remains patent, although cyanosis may not be perceptible in these lesions because the amount of pulmonary blood flow tends to be large. In critical coarctation, the degree of right-to-left shunting may be minimal or absent. The diagnosis and preoperative management of these lesions are discussed in Chapter 2, and surgical management is addressed in Chapter 14.

Heterotaxy Syndrome

Heterotaxy syndrome is not a specific anatomic form of CHD. Rather, it is a syndrome of inconsistency of sidedness of multiple abdominal and thoracic organs that is associated with CHD in nearly all cases. *Situs inversus totalis*, in which all organs are present in the mirror image of the normal configuration, is not a subset of heterotaxy syndrome. The spleen is the abdominal organ most consistently abnormal in heterotaxy syndrome. It can be absent, rudimentary, present as multiple small splenuli, present but located in the right upper quadrant, or rarely present and normally located.[27] The predominant splenic morphologies, asplenia and polysplenia, have been associated with constellations of cardiac and pulmonary abnormalities. Although there is significant overlap between the asplenia and polysplenia syndromes, this division does provide a helpful starting point for a mental organization of the complex abnormalities in heterotaxy syndrome.

Asplenia syndrome is often thought of as "bilateral right-sidedness," which has intuitive appeal for practitioners who can remember that the spleen is normally a left-sided structure. About 95% of patients with asplenia syndrome have bilateral right bronchial morphology, 81% have bilateral trilobed lungs, and 79% have a symmetrical liver.[27] The CHD is typically complex; characteristic elements, which may all coexist, include an unroofed coronary sinus, a total anomalous pulmonary venous connection to a systemic vein, a common atrioventricular canal, a double outlet right ventricle or transposition of the great arteries, and pulmonary stenosis or atresia (Fig. 3-4). The inferior vena cava (IVC) is intact.

Polysplenia syndrome, by analogy, is often thought of as "bilateral left-sidedness." About 72% of patients with polysplenia syndrome have bilateral bilobed lungs, 68%

have bilateral left bronchial morphology, and 67% have a symmetrical liver.[27] The CHD can be complex, but simpler heart disease is also seen. Some patients have isolated absence of the intrahepatic portion of the IVC [also known as interrupted IVC; the inferior venous return drains to the superior vena cava (SVC) through

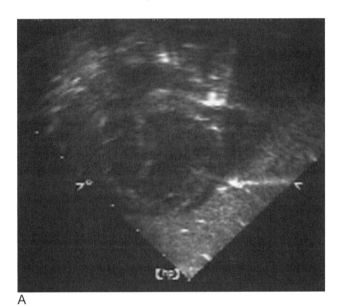

A

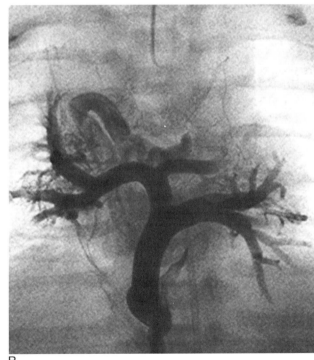

B

Figure 3-4 Common inlet single right ventricle in a patient with heterotaxy syndrome (asplenia). **A,** Subcostal echocardiographic view of a single ventricle with common inlet and right ventricular morphology. The aorta can be seen arising from the single right ventricle. **B,** Angiogram of the pulmonary venous confluence that drained anomalously below the diaphragm (i.e., infradiaphragmatic TAPVR).

Continued

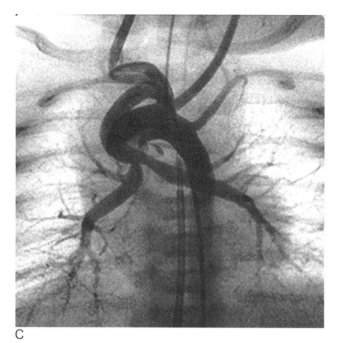

C

Figure 3-4, cont'd   C, Injection into the ascending aorta demonstrates that the RPA and LPA are filled from a right-sided ductus arteriosus arising from the base of the innominate artery. There is atresia of the main pulmonary artery.

the azygous vein instead] but normal intracardiac anatomy. Typical features of CHD in polysplenia syndrome include interrupted IVC, total or partial anomalous pulmonary venous return to the right atrium, complete or partial atrioventricular (AV) canal, and normally related great arteries or double outlet right ventricle.

The etiology of heterotaxy syndrome is likely heterogeneous.[28] Although most cases are sporadic, some families have been reported with multiple members with abnormalities of sidedness. Autosomal dominant, autosomal recessive, and X-linked inheritance patterns have been reported. Penetrance and expressivity are variable: in some affected families, members with both heterotaxy syndrome and *situs inversus totalis* are observed, as are obligate carriers with normal situs.

Even if splenic tissue is present in the heterotaxy syndromes, splenic function can be abnormal. Therefore, patients should be treated with antibiotic prophylaxis unless adequate splenic function can be demonstrated. In addition, patients with heterotaxy should be screened for malrotation of the gut by an upper gastrointestinal (GI) series because malrotation is a common association. Extrahepatic biliary atresia is seen rarely, predominantly in those with polysplenia syndrome. Patients with heterotaxy syndrome who require palliation to a Fontan circulation have a poorer prognosis than those with other forms of CHD palliated in this fashion, likely due to the high frequency of common AV valves and anomalous pulmonary venous return in heterotaxy syndrome.

Common AV valves are more likely to develop insufficiency, whereas any obstruction to pulmonary venous return is detrimental in a Fontan circuit.

Critical Pulmonic Stenosis

In critical PS, the pulmonary valve is so severely stenotic that ductal patency is required to provide sufficient pulmonary blood flow, and right-to-left atrial level shunting occurs. This entity and its management are described in detail in Chapter 2. Critical PS can usually be treated with transcatheter balloon pulmonary valvuloplasty with excellent long-term results, although occasionally a Blalock-Taussig shunt is required until right ventricular hypertrophy regresses and compliance improves.

Pulmonary Atresia with Intact Ventricular Septum

In pulmonary atresia with intact ventricular septum (PA/IVS), the pulmonary valve is atretic, there is no VSD, and there are varying degrees of hypoplasia of the right ventricle and the tricuspid valve (Fig. 3-5). The notation emphasizing intact ventricular septum is to distinguish PA/IVS from pulmonary atresia with VSD, a term that is sometimes used to refer to TOF with pulmonary atresia. In a minority (5–10%) of cases of PA/IVS, Ebstein's anomaly of the tricuspid valve is also present.[29] Fistulous connections from right ventricular sinusoids to the coronary arteries are present in some patients and are particularly likely to be found when the right ventricle is very small and hypertensive. In approximately 20% of cases with coronary artery fistulae, there are stenoses or even interruptions in the coronary arteries impeding antegrade flow from the aorta, and an important amount of myocardial perfusion is supplied from the right ventricle by fistulae.[29] This physiologic situation is termed *right ventricular-dependent coronary circulation* (Fig. 3-6).

Systemic venous blood returns to the right atrium, and from there most crosses a patent foramen ovale (PFO) to the left atrium. Depending upon the sizes of the tricuspid valve and the right ventricle, some amount of blood enters the right ventricle. Since the pulmonary valve is atretic, the only egress from the right ventricle is either by tricuspid regurgitation or by right ventricular sinusoids connecting to the coronaries. The systemic and pulmonary venous returns mix in the left atrium and then continue to the left ventricle and the aorta. The pulmonary arteries are supplied from the ductus arteriosus and the degree of cyanosis is determined primarily by the ratio of pulmonary to systemic blood flow. Clearly, if the ductus arteriosus begins to close, profound hypoxemia will result. In RV-dependent coronary circulation, the portions of the coronaries supplied from the right ventricle

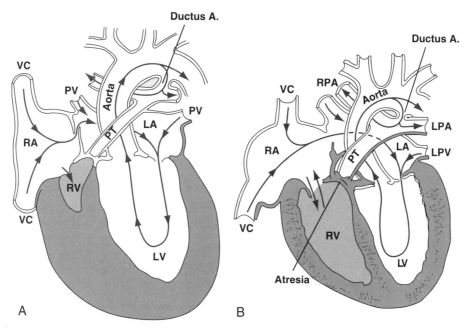

Figure 3-5   Schematic drawings of two examples along the continuum of pulmonary atresia with intact ventricular septum. In both cases, the pulmonary valve is atretic. **A,** There is a tiny RV cavity, a very small tricuspid valve annulus, and little tricuspid regurgitation. This morphology is likely to be associated with RV-dependent coronary circulation. **B,** A more well-developed RV cavity and tricuspid valve annulus are present, as well as tricuspid regurgitation. Arrows indicate the pathway of blood flow. *VC,* vena cava; *RA,* right atrium; *RV,* right ventricle; *LA,* left atrium; *LV,* left ventricle; *Ductus A.,* ductus arteriosus; *PV,* pulmonary vein; *RPA,* right pulmonary artery; *LPA,* left pulmonary artery; *PT,* pulmonary trunk; *LPV,* left pulmonary vein. (Redrawn from Edwards JE: Congenital malformations of the heart and great vessels. In Gould SE [ed]: *Pathology of the Heart,* 2nd ed. Springfield, IL: Charles C. Thomas Publisher, 1960.)

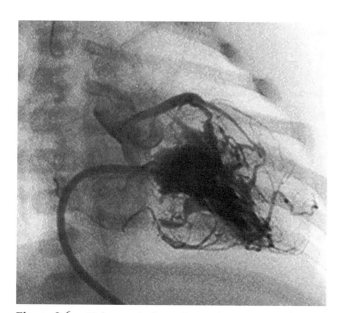

Figure 3-6   Right ventricular angiogram in a patient with PA/IVS and RV-dependent coronary circulation. Contrast injected into the diminutive right ventricle (RV) fills the coronary arteries retrograde through multiple fistulae. The proximal left coronary is continuous, as evidenced by contrast reaching the left main coronary and the aortic root, but there are interruptions in the right coronary and the distal left coronary system.

are perfused with deoxygenated blood, the diastolic perfusion pressure is low, and myocardial ischemia can occur.

PA/IVS can be diagnosed prenatally by fetal echocardiography; a screening ultrasound four-chamber view will be abnormal due to the hypoplastic right ventricle. Interestingly, in some cases, PS has been observed to progress to pulmonary atresia in utero on serial echocardiograms,[30] leading some to term this progression "acquired congenital heart disease." In particular, this phenomenon has been reported in the recipient twin in twin-twin transfusion syndrome. Postnatally, most patients present with cyanosis, and over 90% are identified in the first three days of life. Pulse oximetry is low, but other vital signs are normal unless profound hypoxemia (i.e., partial pressure of oxygen [pO$_2$] in the 20s or below) leads to metabolic acidosis and compensatory hyperpnea. Central cyanosis is observed. Cardiac examination will demonstrate a single second heart sound (S$_2$) and in some cases a holosystolic murmur of tricuspid regurgitation. Nonspecific systolic murmurs attributed to ductal flow or increased left ventricular stroke volume have been described. Flow through the ductus arteriosus may or may not result in a continuous murmur in the immediate neonatal period. In older children, continuous murmurs may be heard related to coronary fistulae. The pulses should be normal unless the left ventricular output is compromised by metabolic acidosis.

The ECG may demonstrate right atrial enlargement, particularly if there is significant tricuspid regurgitation. The QRS axis commonly falls between 60 and 135 degrees. Voltage criteria for left ventricular hypertrophy or a lack of the usual neonatal right ventricular voltage dominance is typical of patients with diminutive right ventricles. However, patients with PA/IVS can also meet ECG criteria for right ventricular hypertrophy. The chest x-ray does not conform to particular pathognomic findings. The pulmonary vascularity is usually normal to reduced, related to the amount of pulmonary blood flow. If there is severe tricuspid regurgitation with dilation of the right atrium, cardiomegaly is seen, but otherwise the heart size usually appears normal.

The diagnosis of PA/IVS is made by transthoracic echocardiography, although cardiac catheterization and angiography are still required in most patients to define the coronary anatomy. The size of the tricuspid annulus, a qualitative assessment of right ventricular hypoplasia, the degree of tricuspid regurgitation, and an estimate of the right ventricular pressure are important pieces of information from the echocardiogram.

The mainstay of initial management is prostaglandin E_1 infusion to maintain patency of the ductus arteriosus, which is the only source of pulmonary blood flow. (Additional details on medical stabilization of neonates with ductal-dependent pulmonary blood flow can be found in Chapter 2.) An initial surgical or transcatheter procedure in the neonatal period establishes an alternate source of pulmonary blood flow. Surgical procedures may include a Blalock-Taussig shunt, a patch across the right ventricular outflow tract to relieve obstruction, or both. Most patients are treated surgically, but when there is membranous pulmonary atresia, transcatheter radiofrequency perforation of the atretic pulmonary valve and balloon valvotomy may be used. The management of patients with PA/IVS may lead to a complete two ventricle circulation, a so-called one-and-a-half ventricle repair, or a Fontan palliation. Further description of these procedures and factors dictating which pathway is pursued is presented in Chapter 14. Current decisionmaking strategies depend chiefly on the size of the right ventricle, as measured by the tricuspid valve annulus size,[29] and the presence or absence of RV-dependent coronary circulation. PA/IVS remains a challenging lesion to treat, with an overall survival of 64% at 4 years; a small tricuspid valve and RV-dependent coronary circulation are identified risk factors for death.[29] Some patients with severe occlusive coronary disease may be considered for neonatal heart transplantation.

Total Anomalous Pulmonary Venous Return

In total anomalous pulmonary venous return (TAPVR), the confluence of the pulmonary veins fails to incorporate into the posterior wall of the left atrium and instead drains by other routes to the systemic venous system. The alternative drainage can be to veins inferior to the diaphragm (i.e., infradiaphragmatic), to abnormal sites in the heart such as the coronary sinus (i.e., cardiac), to veins above the diaphragm (i.e., supradiaphragmatic), or to multiple sites (i.e., mixed). In addition, the drainage can be obstructed or unobstructed, leading to different clinical presentations. Obstruction of pulmonary venous drainage results in pulmonary edema, and unobstructed TAPVR results primarily in CHF. Medical and surgical management of TAPVR are described in Chapters 2 and 14, respectively. Surgical mortality for repair of TAPVR has declined, and in a recent series from Children's Hospital of Philadelphia, was 5% in patients operated on since 1995.[31] The chief late complication is recurrent pulmonary venous obstruction, which occurs in approximately 10% of patients within the first few years after the repair and frequently becomes evident within months. It is more common in the infracardiac and mixed types and portends a poorer prognosis. Recurrent obstruction can result either from stenosis at the anastomosis of the confluence to the left atrium or from progressive stenosis of the intrapulmonary portions of the veins.

Tricuspid Atresia

In tricuspid atresia, a membrane or, more commonly, a muscular plate is present in the expected location of the tricuspid valve (Figs. 3-7 and 3-8), such that there is no flow from the right atrium to the right ventricle. The inflow portion of the right ventricle is typically missing, resulting in a variable degree of right ventricular hypoplasia. Blood reaches the right ventricle only from the left ventricle, through a VSD. Tricuspid atresia is further characterized by (1) whether the great vessels are normally related to the ventricles (i.e., the aorta arises from the left ventricle and the pulmonary artery arises from the right ventricle) or transposed (i.e., the aorta arises from the right ventricle and the pulmonary artery arises from the left ventricle), and (2) what degree of restriction of pulmonary blood flow is present (Fig. 3-7).[32] If the great vessels are normally related, the amount of pulmonary blood flow is determined both by the size of the VSD and by the degree of PS that is present. A smaller VSD generally is associated with a more hypoplastic right ventricle and more PS. Very rarely, tricuspid atresia is accompanied by pulmonary atresia and a nearly nonexistent right ventricular cavity. More

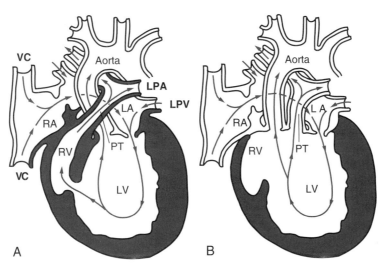

A   B

Figure 3-7   Schematic drawings of **A,** tricuspid atresia with normally related great arteries, a small VSD, a diminutive RV, and PS; **B,** tricuspid atresia with transposition of the great arteries and no outflow tract obstruction. Arrows indicate the pathway of blood flow. *VC,* vena cava; *RA,* right atrium; *LA,* left atrium; *RV,* right ventricle; *LV,* left ventricle; *LPV,* left pulmonary vein; *LPA,* left pulmonary artery; *PT,* pulmonary trunk. (From Friedman WF, Silverman N: Congenital heart disease in infancy and childhood. In Braunwald E, Zipes DP, Libby P [eds]: *Heart Disease: A textbook of cardiovascular medicine,* 6th ed. Philadelphia: WB Saunders, 2001.)

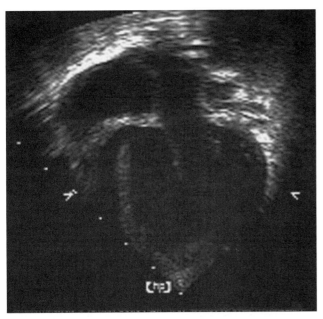

Figure 3-8   Apical echocardiographic view of tricuspid atresia. In this case, a plate of cardiac muscle is seen in the expected location of the tricuspid valve. There is a large VSD in the inlet portion of the ventricular septum, and the right ventricle is hypoplastic. The outflow tracts are not seen in this view. *RA,* right atrium; *LA,* left atrium; *RV,* right ventricle; *LV,* left ventricle.

complex and rarer forms of CHD, including atresia of the tricuspid orifice, exist but will not be discussed further.

All blood returning to the right atrium must pass through a PFO or ASD to the left atrium, where it mixes with the pulmonary venous return and subsequently empties into the left ventricle. In tricuspid atresia with normally related great vessels, some left ventricular blood is ejected to the aorta, and some passes through a VSD to the right ventricle and from there to the pulmonary artery. Because there is complete mixing of systemic and pulmonary venous return, the degree of cyanosis is primarily determined by the ratio of blue blood mixing with pink blood. This ratio is equal to the ratio of pulmonary blood flow to systemic blood flow. If the VSD is large and there is no PS, there will be a large amount of pulmonary blood flow, minimal cyanosis, and these patients will be prone to heart failure. Along a continuum, as the VSD gets smaller and the PS more significant, pulmonary blood flow decreases and increasing cyanosis is present. These patients may be prone to hypercyanotic spells. When the pulmonary valve is atretic, pulmonary blood flow is supplied only by a PDA.

Tricuspid atresia may be suspected from a hypoplastic right ventricle on a screening ultrasound four-chamber view and can be diagnosed prenatally by fetal echocardiography. Postnatally, the degree of restriction to pulmonary blood flow will determine the clinical presentation and physical findings. Most patients present with a murmur or cyanosis. On physical examination, the patient will be tachypneic if there is a large amount of pulmonary blood flow. Desaturation by pulse oximetry increases as the amount of pulmonary blood flow decreases; cyanosis will be apparent if the patient is sufficiently desaturated. The left ventricular impulse is prominent, but the right ventricular impulse is diminished or absent. A thrill may be palpable if the VSD is restrictive. The first heart sound

(S_1) is single, but one or two components of S_2 may be audible. Most commonly, the murmur heard is harsh, holosystolic, arises from the VSD, and is heard best along the left sternal border. However, the murmur can also be one of systolic ejection, arising primarily from the turbulence in the right ventricular outflow tract. A highly restrictive muscular VSD can result in a less than holosystolic murmur. Hepatomegaly can be present in the setting of CHF, caused by excessive pulmonary blood flow.

The ECG characteristically demonstrates left superior deviation of the QRS axis (i.e., 0 to −90 degrees), right atrial enlargement, and left ventricular hypertrophy. Patients with normally related great arteries and increased pulmonary blood flow or patients with coexistent transposition of the great arteries may have a normal QRS axis. According to the amount of pulmonary blood flow, the chest x-ray can either show a normal heart size and decreased pulmonary vascular markings or a variable degree of cardiomegaly and increased pulmonary vascular markings. The main pulmonary artery segment may be diminished; conversely, the right atrial border may be prominent if the main pulmonary artery is dilated.

Definitive diagnosis of the defect is achieved by transthoracic echocardiography. Cardiac catheterization is rarely needed in the newborn period and usually is reserved for defining hemodynamics and anatomy later in infancy, prior to surgical intervention.

Patients with tricuspid atresia require palliation to a Fontan-type circulation (Chapter 14), which can involve one or more intermediate operations. In fact, the principle currently known as the Fontan circulation was first conceived and successfully executed as a palliation for tricuspid atresia. Management after diagnosis focuses on preserving an appropriate amount of pulmonary blood flow to ensure that the patient will be a good candidate for this palliation. Neonates with excessive cyanosis upon ductal closure are treated with a modified Blalock-Taussig shunt to augment pulmonary blood flow. Patients with evidence of excessive pulmonary blood flow are treated with a pulmonary artery band. Depending on the type of VSD, the VSD may become more restrictive with time. Patients may become markedly cyanotic as the VSD becomes restrictive and pulmonary blood flow decreases, even if pulmonary blood flow was initially increased. Patients with tricuspid atresia require careful monitoring of oxygen saturations until they undergo superior cavopulmonary anastomosis at approximately 4–6 months of age. Subsequently, a total cavopulmonary anastomosis, also known as a Fontan completion, follows after 2 years of age.

Single Ventricle

Single ventricle as an *anatomic entity* should be distinguished from *single ventricle physiology*, a condition met by many forms of complex CHD. A formal anatomic definition describes single ventricle as a malformation in which both atrioventricular valves (i.e., "double inlet") or a common atrioventricular valve enter into one ventricle, and there is only one identifiable ventricular sinus (*see* Fig. 3-9). In contrast, single ventricle physiology describes the situation in which the systemic and pulmonary venous returns mix completely within the heart, such that the aorta and the pulmonary artery receive blood with equal saturations. For example, both tricuspid atresia and pulmonary atresia exhibit single ventricle physiology, but neither meets the anatomic definition of single ventricle.

An anatomic single ventricle is accompanied by further complexities of the outflow tracts and semilunar valves. The great vessels usually arise from the heart in an abnormal fashion and an associated obstruction of variable severity at the pulmonary or aortic levels is commonly present.

The single ventricle can be classified as having left or right ventricular morphology. The *single left ventricle* accounts for about three-quarters of cases,[33] typically with a small outlet chamber from which the aorta arises (Fig. 3-10). Restriction at the level of the septal defect between the single ventricle and the outlet chamber (also known as the bulboventricular foramen) can cause subaortic stenosis or subpulmonary stenosis, depending on which vessel arises from the outlet chamber. In the presence of subaortic stenosis, coarctation of the aorta and hypoplasia of the aortic arch can occur. Other patients can have pulmonary stenosis or atresia. It is more common to see two atrioventricular valves (i.e., double inlet) than one atrioventricular valve (i.e., common inlet).

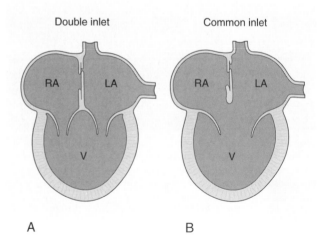

Figure 3-9   Schematic drawing of two forms of anatomic single ventricle. Ventricular morphology is not specified for the purposes of this figure. **A,** double inlet; **B,** common inlet. *RA,* right atrium; *LA,* left atrium; *V,* ventricle. (From Mertens LL, Hagler DJ: Tricuspid atresia and single ventricle. In Crawford MH, DiMarco JP [eds]: *Cardiology,* London: Mosby, 2001.)

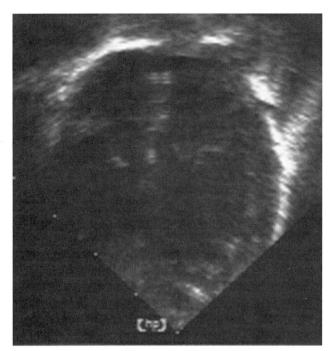

Figure 3-10   Apical echocardiographic view of a double inlet single left ventricle. This patient also had transposition of the great arteries, aortic valve stenosis, and hypoplasia of the aortic arch (not shown).

Most *single right ventricles* have associated pulmonary stenosis or atresia, a common atrioventricular valve, and findings consistent with heterotaxy syndrome (i.e., anomalies of the systemic venous return, anomalous pulmonary venous connections, ambiguous atrial situs, a common atrium, a double outlet right ventricle, and pulmonary stenosis or atresia; see Fig. 3-4).[33]

There are single ventricle variants that do not meet the strict definition of anatomic single ventricle, typically severely unbalanced atrioventricular canal defects. Either the left or right ventricle is dominant, with hypoplasia of the other chamber. An unbalanced common atrioventricular canal with a dominant right ventricle is the most frequent type, commonly associated with heterotaxy (i.e., asplenia syndrome).

The hemodynamic characteristics and clinical presentation in patients with single ventricle depend on whether there is pulmonary or subpulmonary stenosis, aortic or subaortic stenosis, atrioventricular valve regurgitation or stenosis, or ventricular dysfunction. Patients without PS have increased pulmonary blood flow and develop signs of CHF without significant cyanosis. Patients with PS exhibit cyanosis according to the degree of obstruction. Patients with either pulmonary atresia, aortic atresia, or severe hypoplasia of the aortic arch have a ductal-dependent circulation and require treatment with prostaglandin E_1 until surgical intervention. Subaortic obstruction is most commonly due to the small

size of the bulboventricular foramen. It can sometimes present acutely following a sudden decrease of the preload and ventricular volume following a volume unloading operation (i.e., Stage II operation or bidirectional Glenn) or after pulmonary arterial banding. Associated arch obstruction in patients with subaortic stenosis can be severe, requiring a management approach similar to those patients with hypoplastic left heart syndrome.

Single ventricle can be diagnosed prenatally by screening ultrasonography, in which the four-chamber view will be distinctly abnormal, and can be characterized in great detail by fetal echocardiography. Most patients with single ventricle present in the newborn period with either signs of CHF or cyanosis. Those with PS develop similar clinical manifestations to patients with TOF. If the PS is mild, the patient may be acyanotic and may develop CHF as pulmonary vascular resistance falls. Patients with systemic outflow tract obstruction may present with cardiovascular collapse if the lesion is not recognized before the ductus arteriosus constricts. A stenotic semilunar valve generates a systolic ejection murmur, and a systolic regurgitant murmur originates from a regurgitant common AV valve.

In single left ventricle, the frontal QRS axis of the ECG depends on the ventricular loop. Patients with ventricular D-loop (i.e., a rightward bulboventricular outlet chamber) have left ventricular hypertrophy with a QRS axis frequently in the left inferior quadrant. Patients with ventricular L-loop (i.e., a leftward bulboventricular outlet chamber) have Q waves in the right precordial leads with an inferior and rightward QRS axis. Patients with single right ventricle have right ventricular hypertrophy and commonly a superior QRS axis with a counterclockwise loop. In heterotaxy, those with asplenia syndrome or dextroisomerism can have two sinus nodes, whereas those with polysplenia or levoisomerism may lack a sinus node and therefore have a low atrial rhythm.

On chest x-ray, findings depend on the presence or absence of PS. When PS is present, patients will have no cardiomegaly and diminished pulmonary vascular markings. Otherwise, there will be cardiomegaly and increased pulmonary vascular markings. The cardiac silhouette commonly has abnormal mediastinal densities, suggesting abnormal great vessel orientation.

A detailed anatomic diagnosis is made by transthoracic echocardiography, including determination of visceral situs, systemic venous connections, atrioventricular and ventriculo-arterial alignments and connections, and morphology and function of the single ventricle. Doppler interrogation of all valves, septal defects, and the aortic arch should be performed to identify any obstruction and to provide hemodynamic information. The area of the bulboventricular foramen should be carefully evaluated to rule out potential restriction after volume-unloading surgical procedures or pulmonary artery banding. In patients with poor echocardiographic windows, particularly adults with single ventricle, transesophageal echocardiography may be necessary. Magnetic resonance imaging now allows quantification of ventricular function in single ventricle and can also provide detailed anatomic definition.

Although cardiac catheterization is rarely needed for the initial anatomic diagnosis, it is still performed to provide anatomic and hemodynamic information necessary to make management decisions prior to a bidirectional Glenn or Fontan procedure. Interventional cardiac catheterization procedures, such as balloon dilation of branch pulmonary artery stenoses or embolization of decompressing vessels, are commonly performed in patients with single ventricle at various stages with the aims of optimizing hemodynamics and improving long-term outcome.

The management of patients with pure and variant forms of single ventricle is similar. Various surgical staging procedures are performed, ending with a Fontan procedure (see Chapter 14). Most patients require neonatal surgery to address inadequate pulmonary blood flow, excessive pulmonary blood flow, or obstructed systemic arterial outflow. If left untreated, more than half of the patients with single ventricle will not survive the first month of life. Patients with increased pulmonary blood flow can develop pulmonary vascular disease. Most adult survivors with single ventricle without interven-tion have a moderate degree of PS. Complete heart block can develop, particularly in those with L-loop ventricles, requiring a pacemaker. Significant insufficiency of the atrioventricular valves is poorly tolerated in the patients with univentricular hearts and can lead to progressive ventricular dysfunction. Patients with heterotaxy have a worse prognosis due to the higher incidence of PS, hypoplastic pulmonary arteries, pulmonary venous anomalies, predominance of a single right ventricle versus a left ventricle, or insufficiency of the atrioventricular valves, all of which can predispose to the development of ventricular dysfunction.

Double Outlet Right Ventricle

Double outlet right ventricle (DORV) is a heterogeneous collection of lesions that share one morphologic feature, namely that both the aorta and the pulmonary artery arise from the right ventricle (Fig. 3-11). Within this category, anatomy and physiology can be quite variable. Two of the more common forms that result in cyanosis are described below. The most widely used classification system focuses on the proximity of the VSD to one or both great vessels. This anatomic relationship determines both the physiology observed and the surgical approach possible.

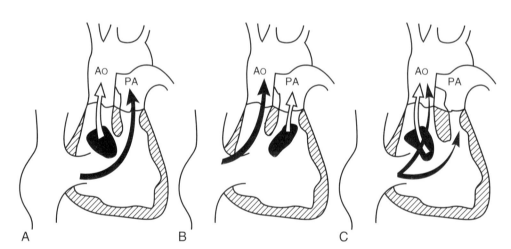

Figure 3-11   Three major forms of double outlet right ventricle (DORV), illustrated with the anterior free wall of the right ventricle removed. **A,** DORV with a subaortic VSD and no PS: oxygenated blood *(open arrow)* from the left ventricle (LV) is directed preferentially to the aorta *(Ao),* whereas the deoxygenated systemic venous return *(solid arrow)* is directed to the pulmonary artery *(PA).* This lesion does *not* result in cyanosis; the physiology is that of a large VSD. **B,** DORV with subpulmonic VSD (i.e., Taussig-Bing anomaly): oxygenated blood flows preferentially from the LV to the PA, whereas deoxygenated systemic venous return is directed to the aorta, resulting in cyanosis. **C,** DORV with subaortic VSD and PS: subpulmonic stenosis results in restricted pulmonary blood flow with mixing of oxygenated and deoxygenated blood in the aorta. The subaortic VSD also directs the limited pulmonary venous return to the aorta, resulting in variable degrees of cyanosis. (Redrawn from Silka MJ: Double outlet right ventricle. In McMillan JA, DeAngelis CD, Feigin RD, Warshaw JB [eds]: *Oski's Pediatrics: Principles and Practice,* 3rd ed. Philadelphia: Lippincott Williams & Wilkins, 1999.)

There are no pathognomonic ECG abnormalities in DORV. Right ventricular hypertrophy is commonly seen beyond the newborn period. The pulmonary vascular markings and heart size on the chest x-ray will reflect the amount of pulmonary blood flow. The superior mediastinum may appear narrow, similar to the appearance of D-TGA.

Transthoracic echocardiography establishes the diagnosis definitively. In all forms of DORV, it is important to establish the relationship of the great vessels to each other and to the VSD. The type and size of the VSD are important as some may become restrictive. The aortic arch and the coronary arteries should be carefully defined. Cardiac catheterization is reserved for clarification of unresolved anatomic questions and balloon septostomy, if indicated.

Double Outlet Right Ventricle with Subpulmonary VSD

In double outlet right ventricle with subpulmonary VSD, or Taussig-Bing anomaly, the great vessels are side-by-side, but the aorta is the more *rightward* great vessel. The pulmonary artery lies closer to the VSD, with resultant transposition physiology (Fig. 3-11B). Although mixing of systemic and pulmonary venous return takes place to some degree in the right ventricle, there is streaming of systemic venous return to the aorta, whereas the left ventricular (i.e., pulmonary venous) blood tends to be ejected across the VSD to the pulmonary artery. Associated arch obstruction is not uncommon. Coronary artery anatomy should be defined for surgical planning since an arterial switch operation is likely to be required.

Although most patients present with cyanosis, those with arch obstruction can present with decreased femoral pulses or shock, similar to left heart obstructive lesions. Symptoms of CHF develop within a few weeks of birth. On physical examination, pulse oximetry will be low, and cyanosis is present. There may be reverse differential cyanosis. If shock or CHF has intervened, tachypnea and tachycardia are also noted. The precordium is hyperdynamic if the amount of pulmonary blood flow is large. After the first few days of life, S_2 can be heard to split. As pulmonary vascular resistance falls and pulmonary blood flow increases, a holosystolic VSD murmur may be heard at the left lower sternal border, related to the large volume of blood ejected from the left ventricle, although usually the VSD itself is large. CHF may be accompanied by such signs as a gallop or hepatomegaly. If arch obstruction is present, as the ductus arteriosus closes, the femoral pulses will diminish.

The preoperative management strategy is the same as that used for D-transposition of the great arteries (see Chapter 2). Patients may require balloon atrial septostomy for preoperative stabilization if mixing is inadequate at the ventricular level. In addition, if arch obstruction is present, patency of the ductus arteriosus must be maintained to provide adequate systemic outflow. Surgical repair is undertaken in the first few days of life. The preferred approach is to baffle the left ventricular output to the pulmonary valve and to perform an arterial switch procedure. Any arch obstruction is addressed at the same operation. If anatomic factors preclude the use of the native aortic valve as an outflow tract, a Damus-Kaye-Stansel anastomosis with a modified Rastelli procedure can be performed, which involves anastomosing both native outflow tracts to each other, baffling the left ventricle to both outflow tracts, and placing a conduit from the right ventricle to the pulmonary arteries. These procedures are described in further detail in Chapter 14. Outcomes are generally good, although reoperation may be required for late development of left ventricular outflow tract obstruction, caused by restriction at the VSD, right ventricular outflow tract obstruction, or conduit revision.

Double Outlet Right Ventricle with Subaortic VSD and Pulmonary Stenosis

In DORV with subaortic VSD and PS (also known as the "tetralogy type" of DORV) both great vessels arise from the right ventricle, but the VSD sits directly below the aorta and there is obstruction to pulmonary outflow (Fig. 3-11C). The presentation is similar to TOF, with cyanosis resulting from decreased pulmonary blood flow and streaming of venous blood to the aorta, aligned to the right ventricle. However, since the aorta is typically closer to the VSD, the cyanosis may not be as marked as in forms of DORV with transposition physiology. If the subpulmonary obstruction is severe, cyanotic spells can occur. Physical examination findings will be similar to TOF. These patients are unlikely to develop CHF.

In DORV with PS, like TOF, the degree of cyanosis is determined by the severity of PS, which determines the amount of pulmonary blood flow. In patients with severe PS, cyanosis could be severe following ductal closure. Most patients can be monitored for a few months before requiring intervention. Palliative surgery with a Blalock-Taussig shunt can be considered as an initial option if cyanosis is severe, followed later by complete repair with the Rastelli procedure. The Rastelli procedure involves baffling of left ventricular blood through the VSD to the aorta with placement of a right ventricular to pulmonary artery conduit (see Chapter 14). Patients require monitoring for conduit obstruction and late development of left ventricular outflow tract obstruction caused by restriction at the VSD.

Truncus Arteriosus

Truncus arteriosus occurs when a single great vessel, the truncus, emerges from the heart and gives direct rise to both the aorta and the pulmonary arteries. The truncus overrides a large VSD. The truncal valve is most often tricuspid (69% of cases), but can be quadricuspid (22%), bicuspid (9%), and very rarely can have one or five cusps.[34] Truncal valve insufficiency (50%) or stenosis (5–10%), a right aortic arch (21–36%), or an interrupted aortic arch (11–19%) can occur.[34] Two classification systems exist for truncus arteriosus (Fig. 3-12): the Collett and Edwards classification (i.e., types I, II, and III; originally proposed type IV is TOF with pulmonary atresia and major aortopulmonary collaterals) and the Van Praagh classification (i.e., types A1–A4). In both systems, the chief distinguishing feature is from where the pulmonary arteries arise. Van Praagh type A4 represents truncus arteriosus with interrupted aortic arch.

With recent advances in cytogenetic techniques, approximately 35% of patients with truncus arteriosus have been demonstrated to have a microdeletion of chromosome 22q11, and those with concomitant arch anomalies (i.e., right aortic arch or aberrant subclavian artery) have an even higher frequency of 22q11 microdeletion.[24] In addition, other studies have demonstrated associations between maternal diabetes[18] or fetal retinoic acid exposure[34] and truncus arteriosus.

Cyanosis in truncus arteriosus results from mixing of systemic and pulmonary venous return as blood is ejected into a single great vessel. The degree of cyanosis is determined primarily by the amount of pulmonary blood flow, which dictates the ratio of systemic and pulmonary venous blood mixing together. Because the pulmonary arteries arise directly from the aorta and pulmonary artery stenosis is rare, pulmonary blood flow can be torrential, particularly as the pulmonary vascular resistance progressively falls. Consequently, cyanosis is usually mild and signs of CHF appear early. In addition, aortic diastolic pressure is usually low due to diastolic runoff into the pulmonary arteries, potentially compromising coronary and mesenteric blood flow. Truncal valve insufficiency will exacerbate this situation. Truncus arteriosus has been shown to be a risk factor for necrotizing enterocolitis among full-term infants with CHD.[35] In the era before neonatal repair, pulmonary vascular disease developed as early as 3–4 months of age in patients with truncus arteriosus due to high flow and high pressure in the pulmonary arteries, in combination with cyanosis.

Truncus arteriosus can be diagnosed prenatally by fetal echocardiography, although a four-chamber ultrasound view may appear normal unless outflow tract views are included. Postnatally, patients may present with a murmur of truncal stenosis or insufficiency, symptoms of heart failure, or cyanosis, although the last is usually mild and may not be easily perceived. On physical examination, tachypnea is present in patients with heart failure and pulse oximetry may demonstrate desaturation. The

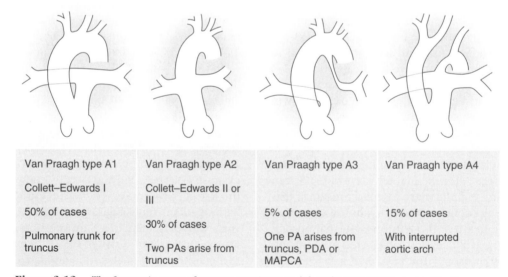

Van Praagh type A1	Van Praagh type A2	Van Praagh type A3	Van Praagh type A4
Collett–Edwards I	Collett–Edwards II or III		
50% of cases	30% of cases	5% of cases	15% of cases
Pulmonary trunk for truncus	Two PAs arise from truncus	One PA arises from truncus, PDA or MAPCA	With interrupted aortic arch

Figure 3-12　The four main types of truncus arteriosus and their frequencies. Two classification schemes are shown. In Van Praagh type A1 and Collett-Edwards type I, a main pulmonary trunk arises from the truncus. In Van Praagh type A2 and Collett-Edwards type II or III, the right and left pulmonary arteries (PAs) arise separately from the truncus. Van Praagh type A3 is not included in the Collett–Edwards classification scheme; one branch PA arises from the truncus, the other from a ductus arteriosus or aortopulmonary collateral. In Van Praagh type A4, also not included in the Collett-Edwards scheme, associated interrupted aortic arch is present. *PDA,* patent ductus arteriosus; *MAPCA,* major aortopulmonary collateral artery. (From Momma K: Tetralogy of Fallot and truncus arteriosus. In Crawford MH, DiMarco JP [eds]: *Cardiology.* London: Mosby, 2001.)

precordium is hyperdynamic due to the volume load on the heart, and the pulses are bounding secondary to the diastolic runoff into the pulmonary arteries. S_2 is single and an ejection click is common. A grade II to III systolic murmur is usually heard along the left sternal border, arising from the outflow tract, and is accompanied by a diastolic regurgitant murmur if truncal valve insufficiency is present. Continuous murmurs are uncommon unless there are stenoses of the branch pulmonary arteries. In patients with heart failure, hepatomegaly is noted and a third heart sound (S_3) gallop may be present.

Biventricular hypertrophy is usually present on the ECG, although isolated right or left ventricular hypertrophy can be seen. In the first few days of life, it is possible for an infant to have normal ECG. The chest x-ray shows cardiomegaly and increased pulmonary vascular markings within a few days of birth. Definitive diagnosis can be established by transthoracic echocardiography and is usually sufficient for preoperative evaluation. In certain cases, cardiac catheterization may be performed to clarify the anatomy of the branch pulmonary arteries, coronary arteries, ventricular septum, or aortic arch. In older patients, cardiac catheterization is necessary to evaluate for pulmonary vascular disease.

Truncus arteriosus repair is discussed in detail in Chapter 14. Surgical mortality as low as 5% has been reported by some major centers.[36] Because the repair requires use of a conduit between the right ventricle and the pulmonary arteries, reoperation is necessary as the patient grows to upsize the conduit. Long-term prognosis is significantly affected by other anomalies and developmental delay if the patient has a 22q11 microdeletion.

Ebstein's Anomaly

Ebstein's anomaly is a defect of the development of the right ventricle, characterized primarily by varying degrees of inferior displacement of the septal and posterior leaflets of the tricuspid valve (Fig. 3-13). The anterior leaflet is large and "sail-like," often with abnormal chordal attachments. The portion of the right ventricle between the true tricuspid annulus and the hinge point of the displaced leaflets becomes "atrialized," in that it is functionally part of the right atrium although histologically it is ventricular tissue. All of the right ventricular myocardium is thin; however, the abnormality is more pronounced in the atrialized portion. Nearly all patients have a coexisting ASD or PFO. Ebstein's anomaly can be associated with accessory atrioventricular conduction pathways and the Wolff-Parkinson-White syndrome (see Chapter 10).

Normally, the tricuspid valve leaflets form by delamination from the right ventricular myocardium; the anterior leaflet delaminates earlier in gestation than the posterior and septal leaflets. Ebstein's anomaly is thought to occur because of incomplete delamination, but the underlying mechanism of failure is unclear. Although initial case reports and registries indicated the

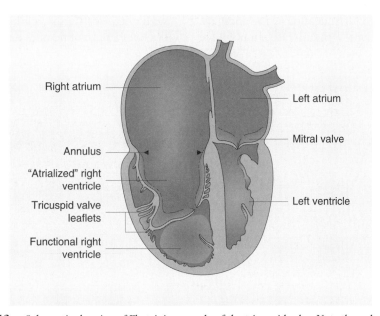

Figure 3-13   Schematic drawing of Ebstein's anomaly of the tricuspid valve. Note the enlarged right atrium, the "atrialized" portion of the right ventricle between the tricuspid valve annulus and the hinge point of the septal leaflet of the tricuspid valve, and the diminutive functional right ventricle. (From Shaughnessy R: Ebstein's anomaly. In Crawford MH, DiMarco JP [eds]: *Cardiology*. London: Mosby, 2001.)

risk of Ebstein's anomaly was very high after maternal exposure to lithium (an estimated relative risk of 400), subsequent cohort studies demonstrated a much lower risk (a relative risk of 1.5–3.0).[37] Some familial cases have been reported. Overall, recognized Ebstein's anomaly is rare, accounting for less than 1% of CHD.[38]

The pathophysiology of Ebstein's anomaly is highly variable because of the wide spectrum of morphologic abnormalities. At one end of the spectrum, the anomaly may be incidentally discovered; at the other extreme, Ebstein's anomaly can cause hydrops fetalis and intrauterine demise. Elements of the pathophysiology of this lesion can include tricuspid regurgitation and, less commonly, tricuspid stenosis; atrial-level shunting; right ventricular dysfunction; secondary left ventricular dysfunction; and, in the most severe cases, functional or anatomic right ventricular outflow tract obstruction. Atrial-level shunting can be in either direction, depending on the rest of the cardiac physiology. In more severely affected patients, when right-to-left shunting occurs at the atrial level, Ebstein's anomaly fits into the category of cyanotic CHD. The most severely affected patients, those with Ebstein's anomaly who are symptomatic in the neonatal period, are described in Chapter 2.

Ebstein's anomaly can be detected prenatally by fetal echocardiography, especially in the most severe cases wherein referral for fetal echo is prompted by other evidence of hydrops fetalis. Neonates with severe Ebstein's anomaly present in the delivery room with respiratory distress and severe cyanosis caused by the combination of associated pulmonary hypoplasia and right-to-left shunting. Beyond that time period, an abnormal physical examination often leads to identification of the anomaly. Patients with cyanotic forms of the disease should have

decreased pulse oximetry values, and if the right-to-left shunt is of sufficient magnitude, visible cyanosis and, after months to years, digital clubbing. In patients with chronically low systemic cardiac output, a ruddy appearance may be noted, caused by compensatory polycythemia. Auscultation characteristically reveals widely split first and second heart sounds, multiple systolic clicks generated by the redundant tricuspid valve leaflet, and a holosystolic murmur of tricuspid regurgitation at the left lower sternal border. If the right-sided filling pressures are elevated, hepatomegaly or an elevated jugular venous pressure may be noted. Uncommonly, patients will present with supraventricular tachycardia and will be found on subsequent workup to have Ebstein's anomaly.

There are several characteristic ECG abnormalities, including right axis deviation, right bundle branch block, low-voltage QRS complexes in the right precordial leads, right atrial enlargement, and first degree AV block (Fig. 3-14). Preexcitation (i.e., Wolff-Parkinson-White syndrome) can also be noted, caused by accessory AV conduction pathways. The chest x-ray demonstrates a spectrum of degrees of cardiomegaly, although those sufficiently severely affected to have cyanosis will likely have significant cardiomegaly.

Transthoracic echocardiography demonstrates inferior displacement of the insertion of the septal leaflet of the tricuspid valve. In addition, tricuspid regurgitation, tricuspid stenosis, right ventricular outflow tract obstruction, atrial septal anatomy, direction of atrial level shunting, chamber sizes, and ventricular function can be assessed. In older patients, exercise testing can define exercise capacity and can document arterial desaturation with exercise. Cardiac catheterization can be useful for documentation of hemodynamics and cardiac output.

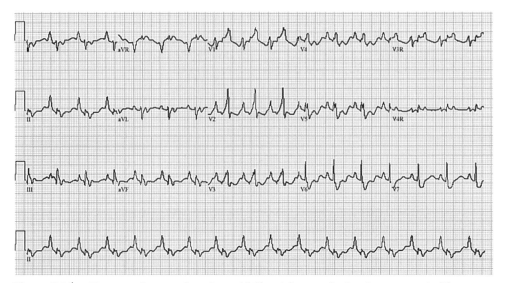

Figure 3-14   Electrocardiogram of a patient with Ebstein's anomaly, showing many typical features including right atrial enlargement, right axis deviation, and right bundle branch block.

The natural history of Ebstein's anomaly is related to the severity of the malformation in a given patient. Those with cyanosis are at the more severe end of the spectrum. Initially, acyanotic patients can develop cyanosis over time. There is a high mortality among symptomatic neonates and surgical intervention in this group generally has not been beneficial.

In older patients, surgical management is tailored to the individual and is more successful.[39] Those patients with severe symptoms despite medical therapy are candidates for tricuspid valvuloplasty and ASD closure. The tricuspid valvuloplasty is frequently accompanied by a right atrial reduction, right ventricular plication, and, if the valvuloplasty creates tricuspid stenosis, a bidirectional Glenn anastomosis (see Chapter 14). Some patients with severe Ebstein's anomaly are converted to a Fontan circulation. Patients with Ebstein's anomaly are susceptible to a variety of tachyarrhythmias, including ventricular tachycardia, atrioventricular reciprocating tachycardia due to accessory pathways, and atrial fibrillation. Radiofrequency catheter ablation therapy (see Chapter 10) can be performed when clinically indicated. Sudden death was reported in 2.5% of patients with Ebstein's anomaly, studied in one large series.[40]

Anomalous Connection of Large Systemic Veins to the Left Atrium

Very rarely, the right superior vena cava (RSVC), a persistent left superior vena cava (LSVC), or the inferior vena cava (IVC) can drain directly to the left atrium in the absence of any other structural heart disease. (Note: persistence of the LSVC is relatively common, but the LSVC usually drains to the coronary sinus. Unless the coronary sinus is unroofed, blood from an LSVC to coronary sinus returns to the *right* atrium.) The fixed right-to-left shunt results in mild cyanosis, with saturations in a newborn typically in the upper 80s to low 90s. No other abnormal cardiovascular physical findings are present. Diagnosis can be established by transthoracic echocardiography; bubble studies using injections in various extremities can be particularly helpful. Alternatively, the abnormal connection can be demonstrated by angiography or magnetic resonance imaging. These anomalies are repaired electively by intra-atrial baffle procedures or reimplantation. Repair is deferred if the defect is diagnosed in the neonatal period because cyanosis is usually minimal and larger patient size facilitates the repair.

EISENMENGER'S SYNDROME IN ACYANOTIC DEFECTS

Eisenmenger's syndrome refers to the development of pulmonary vascular disease and resultant right-to-left shunting in patients with CHD. Obliterative changes in the pulmonary capillaries and arterioles occur in these vessels after chronic exposure to elevated pressure and flow. Pulmonary vascular resistance climbs as vessels are destroyed, ultimately resulting in reversal of the shunt in originally acyanotic septal defects such as ASD, VSD, and PDA. Pulmonary vascular disease can develop in patients with complex cyanotic heart disease. In fact, cyanosis is thought to accelerate its development, such that patients with D-TGA or truncus arteriosus can develop pulmonary vascular disease within the first year of life if not surgically corrected.

Patients with Eisenmenger's syndrome are unable to augment cardiac output in response to exercise without an increase in the right-to-left shunt and may have inadequate systemic cardiac output at rest. Consequently, they present with fatigue and dyspnea, dizziness, or syncope on exertion. In addition, as right ventricular dysfunction develops, signs and symptoms of right-sided CHF become evident. Persistent cyanosis leads to polycythemia, which, if profound, can cause symptoms of hyperviscosity such as headache, dizziness, and visual disturbances. Right-to-left shunting puts these patients at risk for brain abscess and systemic embolization. In addition, hemoptysis may occur in patients with longstanding pulmonary hypertension.

Physical findings consistent with pulmonary hypertension include a right ventricular heave along the left lower sternal border and a palpable pulmonic valve closure (P_2) in the second left intercostal space. P_2 is loud, and if pulmonary hypertension is advanced, S_2 is single. A systolic ejection click arising from the dilated pulmonary artery may be present. Two types of murmurs may be heard as secondary consequences of pulmonary hypertension: pulmonary regurgitation, which causes a diastolic regurgitant murmur at the left sternal border, and tricuspid regurgitation, which causes a harsh holosystolic murmur at the lower left and right sternal borders. Both murmurs will be relatively high-pitched due to the elevated right-sided pressures. When right ventricular failure is present, dyspnea, tachycardia, elevated jugular venous pressure, gallops, hepatomegaly, and peripheral edema may be noted.

ECG demonstrates right axis deviation and right ventricular hypertrophy, often with a strain pattern. Chest x-ray shows dilated central pulmonary arteries and, at late stages, decreased peripheral vessels. In patients with VSD and PDA, the heart is usually of normal size, whereas in those with ASD there is cardiomegaly from prior right ventricular dilation.

Eisenmenger's syndrome has a much better natural history than primary pulmonary hypertension, with 54% of patients with VSD and Eisenmenger's syndrome in the Second Natural History study still alive 20 years after diagnosis of Eisenmenger's syndrome.[41] The septal defect should not be closed once irreversible pulmonary vascular disease is established as it provides a mechanism to maintain systemic cardiac output if pulmonary vascular resistance increases acutely. Pregnancy should be avoided because of a maternal mortality of approximately 45%.[42] Likewise, noncardiac surgery is associated with a mortality of approximately 19% and, if necessary, should be undertaken with specialized anesthesia and an intensive care unit support.[42]

Medical treatment of Eisenmenger's syndrome includes supportive therapy and avoidance of stimuli that may worsen pulmonary hypertension. A pulmonary hypertensive crisis is a spiral of increased right-to-left shunting, worsening hypoxia, and increased pulmonary vascular resistance that can be precipitated by factors including acute volume depletion, drugs that lower systemic vascular resistance, and alveolar hypoxia. Supportive drug therapy includes digitalis and careful use of diuretics in those patients with signs of heart failure. Pulmonary vasodilators are used if a beneficial response is demonstrated in the catheterization laboratory. In this category, the longest experience is with calcium-channel blockers, but newer drugs including various forms of prostaglandin analogs and endothelin receptor antagonists are being studied. Supplemental oxygen may be useful in certain settings, including during exercise in those patients with significant exercise-associated desaturation, in patients with right heart failure, during plane flights, and certainly in the setting of intercurrent lower respiratory tract infections. Nighttime oxygen has been advocated by some authors. Low-dose warfarin (i.e., international normalized ratio [INR] 1.5–2.0) is used by some practitioners to prevent intracardiac or venous thrombosis in these patients who are polycythemic and often relatively sedentary. Either systemic or pulmonary embolism can have grave consequences. The risk of bleeding, including hemoptysis, must be weighed against the potential benefits of anticoagulation. Oral contraceptives, hormone replacement therapy, dehydration, and iron deficiency should be avoided due to their association with hypercoagulability and hyperviscosity. If iron deficiency and acute dehydration are ruled out and the hematocrit exceeds 65%, phlebotomy with replacement of volume can be performed for symptoms of hyperviscosity in a carefully monitored environment. Patients should avoid living or vacationing at high altitude; they should also avoid drugs (such as appetite suppressants) associated with the development of pulmonary hypertension.

Eisenmenger's Syndrome Associated with Atrial Septal Defect

Eisenmenger's syndrome is uncommon in patients with isolated ASD. Most series of adults diagnosed with ASD in adulthood find that 6–15% have elevated pulmonary vascular resistance at cardiac catheterization.[43,44] Pulmonary vascular disease attributable to ASD is thought to be very rare in childhood. Eisenmenger's syndrome in ASD usually occurs after 20 years of age and is seen predominantly in women, an epidemiology interestingly similar to that of primary pulmonary hypertension. On physical examination, arterial desaturation is present if the right ventricle is less compliant than the left ventricle, resulting in right-to-left shunting at the ASD. Longstanding desaturation leads to clubbing. No murmur is attributable to flow across the ASD, but the other findings of pulmonary hypertension described above will be present.

Eisenmenger's Syndrome Associated with Ventricular Septal Defect

The risk of developing Eisenmenger's syndrome in a patient with a VSD depends on the magnitude of the shunt and the pulmonary artery pressure early in the patient's course, factors that are related to the size of the defect. Patients usually have a history of CHF early in life, related to a significant left-to-right shunt. Eisenmenger's syndrome can develop in children with large VSDs by early childhood.[45] On physical examination, arterial desaturation is present if the pulmonary vascular resistance is higher than the systemic vascular resistance, resulting in right-to-left shunting at the VSD. Chronic desaturation results in clubbing. The holosystolic murmur of a VSD becomes much diminished or abolished as right and left ventricular pressures equalize. The other signs of pulmonary hypertension described above are present.

Eisenmenger's Syndrome Associated with Patent Ductus Arteriosus

The precise risk of Eisenmenger's syndrome associated with PDA is difficult to define for many reasons. Routine surgical closure of these defects, when associated with symptoms or typical physical findings, has been the practice for over 50 years. PDA exists along a continuum of degrees of restriction to pressure and flow, and the shunt can be difficult to quantify even by cardiac catheterization. Finally, since the decline of maternal rubella syndrome because of routine vaccination, *large* PDAs are uncommon beyond the first few days of life. What is clear is that Eisenmenger's syndrome caused by a large PDA can develop by age 4–7 years.[46]

On physical examination, differential cyanosis is present, with the right upper extremity receiving fully oxygenated blood while deoxygenated blood shunts across the PDA and reaches the lower extremities. Clubbing is likewise differential, with the right hand spared. The murmur attributable to the PDA first loses the diastolic component as the pulmonary vascular resistance rises, and later the systolic component is abolished as well. Consequently, in severe pulmonary vascular disease, no murmur will be attributable to the PDA, but the findings of pulmonary hypertension described above will be present.

Eisenmenger's Syndrome's in Complete Common Atrioventricular Canal

Eisenmenger's syndrome can also occur in patients with complete common atrioventricular canal. Patients with Down syndrome are at higher risk of pulmonary vascular disease and tend to develop this complication earlier. The physiology is similar to that of Eisenmenger's syndrome in VSD.

POSTOPERATIVE PHYSIOLOGY

Most patients with complex cyanotic lesions undergo repair or palliation in infancy, many within the first few days of life. Therefore, the practitioner is more likely to encounter patients with postoperative findings than those with the classic unoperated findings that have populated textbooks for many years. A wide variety of lesions that are unsuitable for complete correction are now palliated to the Fontan circulation, often in three stages (see Chapter 14). The following discussion reviews the physiology and typical physical findings of patients at each stage of this palliation.

Lesions with Functionally Single Ventricle After a Systemic-to-Pulmonary Artery Shunt

In this physiologic state (also referred to as "Stage I" physiology in pediatric cardiology circles), blood is pumped from a functionally single ventricle to the aorta, which supplies both the systemic circulation and the pulmonary circulation. The pulmonary circulation is fed through a tube graft, typically from the base of the innominate artery to the central pulmonary arteries (i.e., a modified Blalock-Taussig shunt) and is the physiologic equivalent of a somewhat restrictive PDA. An alternative means of supplying pulmonary blood flow, which has been gaining popularity recently, is the placement of a 4- to 5-mm ventricular-to-pulmonary artery conduit (the Sano modification). In either approach, the ventricle is by definition volume-loaded because it supplies both the systemic and pulmonary circulation; the degree of volume overload depends on the amount of pulmonary blood flow (see Table 3-2). The more cyanotic patients have less pulmonary blood flow and less volume load, so they have fewer symptoms and signs of CHF and better growth. The opposite is true of less-cyanotic patients with this physiology.

On physical examination, pulse oximetry is typically between 70% and 85% in room air and the baseline value should be noted for future reference. Those with higher saturations are more likely to have tachypnea. In those whose initial palliation involved an arch repair, it is important to determine that the lower extremity blood pressures are not lower than those in the upper extremity. Recurrent arch obstruction occurs in about 10% of neonates who required an arch repair initially. If a classic Blalock-Taussig shunt, utilizing the subclavian artery instead of a tube graft, was performed, the blood pressure in the affected arm will be unreliable. The classic procedure is rarely performed today. Increased respiratory effort will be observed in those with larger volume loads, but the chest is usually clear. The precordial impulse is hyperdynamic. The most typical feature of the exam, if a Blalock-Taussig shunt is used, is a prominent continuous murmur arising from the shunt (commonly loudest under the right clavicle), which may obscure S_2. If heard, S_2 is single, because there is not ejection by two ventricles into separate systemic and pulmonary circulations. If a ventricular to pulmonary artery conduit is used, a systolic ejection murmur, with or without a diastolic regurgitant murmur, can be heard arising from the conduit. A gallop may be audible in the setting of a large volume load. If atrioventricular valve regurgitation is present, it may add to the systolic component of the murmur. The liver is enlarged in proportion to the degree of CHF. The femoral pulses should be carefully sought in patients with a history of arch repair. Frequently, the femoral pulses are bounding in patients with shunt physiology because of diastolic runoff from the aorta into the pulmonary arteries.

Specific ECG findings depend on the underlying lesion, but it is common to see atrial enlargement and ventricular hypertrophy. Chest x-ray typically shows mild to moderate cardiomegaly, with pulmonary vascular markings in proportion to the amount of blood flow.

Lesions with Functionally Single Ventricle after a Superior Cavopulmonary Anastomosis

A superior cavopulmonary anastomosis connects the superior vena cava directly to the pulmonary artery (also referred to as "Stage II" physiology in pediatric cardiology circles). Specific operative techniques include the Glenn, the bidirectional Glenn, and the Hemi-Fontan (see Chapter 14). The systemic to pulmonary artery shunt is ligated at the same operation. Blood is no longer pumped to the pulmonary vascular bed, but rather it flows passively and silently from the SVC into the pulmonary arteries. Inferior vena cava blood returns to the right atrium, the ventricle, and the aorta without being oxygenated in the lungs. The important physiologic consequence is that the ventricle now pumps only the systemic cardiac output, and therefore symptoms and signs of heart failure usually improve or resolve. All the techniques involve surgery in the vicinity of the sinus node. Sinus node dysfunction is a known long-term complication but is not usually symptomatic in early childhood.

On physical examination, pulse oximetry is typically in the 80s in room air and respiratory rate is normal. The baseline pulse oximetry value should be noted for future reference. Heart rate may be lower than expected for age if there is sinus node dysfunction. In the early postoperative period, frequently there is mild facial edema caused by the acute change in venous pressure, but this resolves within days to weeks. Inspection of jugular veins will demonstrate absence of the usual pulsations and may indicate elevated pressure. The precordium is quiet, and the second heart sound is single. In the absence of atrioventricular or semilunar valve pathology, there should be no murmurs or gallops. The liver is not enlarged, and peripheral pulses are no longer bounding.

ECG findings will vary with the underlying lesion, but signs of atrial enlargement may resolve. In a single right ventricle, criteria for right ventricular hypertrophy or biventricular hypertrophy will persist since the right ventricle is operating at high pressure. Cardiomegaly should resolve or improve after a superior cavopulmonary anastomosis.

Lesions with Functionally Single Ventricle After a Fontan Completion (Total Cavopulmonary Anastomosis)

A Fontan completion involves incorporating the IVC blood into the pulmonary circulation. Flow is passive and frequently a fenestration is created at the operation between the Fontan pathway and the atrium to allow a small amount of deoxygenated blood to shunt from the venous circulation to the heart (see Chapter 14). The purpose of the fenestration is to decrease venous pressure and to augment preload to the ventricle in the immediate postoperative period. The fenestration is designed to be closed later by a transcatheter device if it does not close spontaneously to eliminate the risk of paradoxical embolism. In Fontan physiology, the ventricle pumps a normal systemic cardiac output and the amount of pulmonary blood flow, which is entirely passive, equals the systemic blood flow minus any small amount that shunts across the fenestration.

On physical examination, pulse oximetry is typically in the high 80s to low 90s if the fenestration is patent. If the fenestration has closed, pulse oximetry will usually be 93% or above. Even with no right-to-left shunt, some patients with a Fontan circulation have sufficient V:Q mismatch to have saturations in the lower 90s. For future reference, it is important to know what saturation is normal for a patient with a Fontan when he or she is

well. Also, significant desaturation implies a baffle leak, decompressing vessels, or development of pulmonary arteriovenous malformations. The heart rate may be low if sinus node dysfunction is present. The respiratory rate is normal. Jugular veins lack the normal pulsations, and the height of the blood column may be elevated. The precordium is quiet and S_2 is single. In the absence of atrioventricular or semilunar valve pathology, there should be no murmurs or gallops. Pulses are normal. In a well-functioning Fontan circulation, the liver is not enlarged significantly. (Progressive hepatomegaly is worrisome for rising Fontan circuit pressures and failure of the Fontan.) Ascites or lower-extremity edema are particularly ominous signs and are often associated with protein-losing enteropathy, a known, although infrequent, complication of the Fontan circulation.

ECG and chest x-ray findings parallel those described for the superior cavopulmonary anastomosis above. Cross-sectional studies have shown that although serum albumin is usually normal, ALT and AST are mildly elevated (at less than two times above the upper limit of normal) in the majority of patients.[47]

Predicting longterm outcome in patients with a Fontan circulation is difficult. A multitude of factors, including surgical techniques, myocardial preservation techniques, intensive care unit management strategies, and age at operation have changed constantly over the past several decades.

Some consistent patterns have emerged and should give the primary practitioner a good idea of what to expect for their patient with a Fontan circulation.[47] When formal exercise testing is performed, patients with a Fontan circulation have diminished exercise capacity. Cardiac catheterization usually reveals a mildly depressed cardiac index. Subjectively, the majority of patients and their physicians identify either no functional limitations or only slight functional limitations. Sinus node dysfunction and atrial arrhythmias are common. In a cross-sectional study of Fontan survivors[47] at a median of 5.4 years of follow-up, 9.4% of patients had a pacemaker and the prevalence of atrial flutter increased with duration of follow-up, reaching 33% at 10 years. Protein-losing enteropathy is reported in 2.6–13.4% of long-term Fontan survivors,[48-50] and late stroke in 4%.[48] Institutional management style varies, but many cardiologists maintain patients with Fontan circulations on antiplatelet or anticoagulant therapy because of the chronic venous stasis and the risk of stroke associated with this physiology. Afterload reduction therapy is also advocated by some, but no randomized controlled trials have been completed that examine this question. Overall, the majority of patients with a Fontan circulation have good functional status, a remarkable achievement given the severity of the underlying heart disease in this group. Through research efforts and innovation, practitioners are optimistic that outcomes will continue to improve for current and future generations of patients with single ventricle physiology.

MAJOR POINTS

- Cyanotic congenital heart disease, broadly defined, includes any malformations of the heart causing venous blood to be returned to the arterial side of the circulation without being oxygenated in the lungs.
- Cyanosis is a visible bluish discoloration of the skin and mucous membranes caused by arterial oxygen desaturation of any cause.
- The intensity of cyanosis is related to the concentration of arterial deoxyhemoglobin and depends on both the percent saturation of hemoglobin and the hemoglobin concentration.
- Cyanosis is not perceived consistently until desaturation is profound.
- Complications of chronic right-to-left shunting include stroke, brain abscess, scoliosis, and hyperviscosity syndrome.
- Right-to-left shunting occurs either because hemodynamic forces favor right-to-left flow across a communication between the two sides of the circulation or because the anatomy of the heart dictates return of venous blood to the arterial circulation.
- In most cyanotic lesions, the degree of cyanosis is primarily determined by the ratio of pulmonary to systemic blood flow.
- In cyanotic lesions with transposition physiology, the degree of cyanosis is determined primarily by the extent of mixing of systemic venous and pulmonary venous blood.
- A wide variety of cardiac malformations result in right-to-left shunting.
- Many forms of cyanotic congenital heart disease with only one functional ventricle are managed using the Fontan palliation, wherein all systemic venous blood flows passively to the lungs.
- Eisenmenger's syndrome results in a reversal of the direction of shunting in acyanotic cardiac malformations and, consequently, cyanosis.

REFERENCES

1. Lundsgaard C: Studies on cyanosis. *J Exp Med* 30:259–293, 1919.
2. Lundsgaard C, Van Slyke DD: Cyanosis. *Medicine* 2:1–76, 1923.
3. Goss GA, Hayes JA, Burdon JG: Deoxyhaemoglobin concentrations in the detection of central cyanosis. *Thorax* 43:212–213, 1988.
4. Goldman HI, Maralit A, Sun S, Lanzkowsy P: Neonatal cyanosis and arterial oxygen saturation. *J Pediatr* 82:319–324, 1973.
5. Levesque BM, Pollack P, Griffin B, Nielsen HC: Pulse oximetry: what's normal in the newborn nursery? *Pediatric Pulmonol* 30:406–412, 2000.
6. Wells R: Syndromes of hyperviscosity. *N Engl J Med* 283:183–186, 1970.
7. Linderkamp O, Klose HJ, Betke K, et al: Increased blood viscosity in patients with cyanotic congenital heart disease and iron deficiency. *J Pediatr* 95:567–569, 1979.
8. Perloff JK, Rosove MH, Sietsema KE, et al: Cyanotic Congenital Heart Disease: A Multisystem Disorder. In Perloff JK, Child JS (eds): *Congenital Heart Disease in Adults,* 2nd ed. Philadelphia: W.B. Saunders, pp 199-226, 1998.
9. Phornphutkul C, Rosenthal A, Nadas AS, Berenberg, W: Cerebrovascular accidents in infants and children with cyanotic congenital heart disease. *Am J Cardiol* 32:329–334, 1973.
10. Fischbein CA, Rosenthal A, Fischer EG, et al: Risk factors of brain abscess in patients with congenital heart disease. *Am J Cardiol* 34:97–102, 1974.
11. Roth A, Rosenthal A, Hall JE, Mizel M: Scoliosis and congenital heart disease. *Clin Orthop Relat Res* 93:95–102, 1973.
12. Morris CD, Reller MD, Menashe VD: Thirty-year incidence of infective endocarditis after surgery for congenital heart defects. *JAMA* 279:599–603, 1998.
13. Newburger JW, Silbert AR, Buckley LP, Fyler DC: Cognitive function and age at repair of transposition of the great arteries in children. *N Engl J Med* 310:1495–1499, 1984.
14. Aram DM, Ekelman BL, Ben-Shachar G, Levinsohn MW: Intelligence and hypoxemia in children with congenital heart disease: fact or artifact? *J Am Coll Cardiol* 6:889–893, 1985.
15. Oates RK, Simpson JM, Cartmill TB, Turnbull JA: Intellectual function and age of repair in cyanotic congenital heart disease. *Arch Dis Child* 72:298–301, 1995.
16. Perloff JK. *The Clinical Recognition of Congenital Heart Disease,* 4th ed. Philadelphia: W.B. Saunders, 1994.
17. Report of the New England Regional Infant Cardiac Program. *Pediatrics* 65:375–461, 1980.
18. Ferencz C, Loffredo CA, Rubin JD, et al: Epidemiology of congenital heart disease: The Baltimore-Washington Infant Study 1981-1989. *Perspectives Pediatric in Cardiology,* 4, 1993.
19. Hutter PA, Kreb DL, Mantel SF, et al: Twenty-five years' experience with the arterial switch operation. *J Thorac Cardiovasc Surg* 124:790–797, 2002.
20. Scott WA, Fixler DE. Effect of center volume on outcome of ventricular septal defect closure and arterial switch operation. *Am J Cardiol* 88:1259–1263, 2001.
21. Dunbar-Masterson C, Wypij D, Bellinger DC, et al: General health status of children with D-transposition of the great

arteries after the arterial switch operation. *Circulation* 104:I138–1142, 2001.

22. Van Praagh R, Van Praagh S, Nebesar RA, et al: Tetralogy of Fallot: Underdevelopment of the pulmonary infundibulum and its sequelae. *Am J Cardiol* 26:25–33, 1970.

23. Neches WH, Park SC, Ettedgui JA: Tetralogy of Fallot and tetralogy of Fallot with pulmonary atresia. In Garson Jr. A, Bricker JT, Fisher DJ, Neish SR (eds): *The Science and Practice of Pediatric Cardiology,* 2nd ed. Baltimore: Williams & Wilkins, pp 1383–1411, 1998.

24. Goldmuntz E, Clark BJ, Mitchell LE, et al: Frequency of 22q11 deletions in patients with conotruncal defects. *J Am Coll Cardiol* 32:492–498, 1998.

25. Murphy JG, Gersh BJ, Mair DD, et al: Long-term outcome in patients undergoing surgical repair of tetralogy of Fallot. *N Engl J Med* 329:593–599, 1993.

26. Gatzoulis MA, Balaji S, Webber SA, et al: Risk factors for arrhythmia and sudden cardiac death late after repair of tetralogy of Fallot: a multicentre study. *Lancet* 356:975–981, 2000.

27. Van Praagh S, Santini F, Sanders SP: Cardiac malpositions with special emphasis on visceral heterotaxy (asplenia and polysplenia syndromes). In Nadas AS, Fyler DC (ed): *Nadas' Pediatric Cardiology.* Philadelphia: Hanley & Belfus, pp 589–608, 1992.

28. Kosaki K, Casey B: Genetics of human left-right axis malformations. *Sem Cell Devel Biol* 9:89–99, 1998.

29. Hanley FL, Sade RM, Blackstone EH, et al: Outcomes in neonatal pulmonary atresia with intact ventricular septum. A multiinstitutional study. *J Thoracic Cardiovasc Surg* 105:406–423, 1993.

30. Cohen MS: Fetal diagnosis and management of congenital heart disease. *Clin Perinatol* 28:11–29, 2001.

31. Kirshbom PM, Myung RJ, Gaynor JW, et al: Preoperative pulmonary venous obstruction affects long-term outcome for survivors of total anomalous pulmonary venous connection repair. *Ann Thoracic Surg* 74:1616–1620, 2002.

32. Epstein ML: Tricuspid atresia. In Allen HD, Clark EB, Gutgesell HP, Driscoll DA (eds): *Heart disease in infants, children and adolescents,* 6th ed. Philadelphia: Lippincott Williams & Wilkins, pp 799–809, 2001.

33. Van Praagh R, Plett JA, Van Praagh S: Single ventricle. Pathology, embryology, terminology and classification. *Herz* 4:113–150, 1979.

34. Mair DD, Edwards WD, Julsrud PR, et al: Truncus arteriosus. In Allen HD, Gutgesell HP, Clark EB, Driscoll DA (eds): *Moss and Adams' Heart Disease in Infants, Children, and Adolescents,* 6th ed. Philadelphia: Lippincott Williams & Wilkins, pp 910–923, 2001.

35. McElhinney DB, Hedrick HL, Bush DM, et al: Necrotizing enterocolitis in neonates with congenital heart disease: risk factors and outcomes. *pediatrics* 106:1080–1087, 2000.

36. Thompson LD, McElhinney DB, Reddy M, et al: Neonatal repair of truncus arteriosus: continuing improvement in outcomes. *Ann Thorac Surg* 72:391–395, 2001.

37. Cohen LS, Friedman JM, Jefferson JW, et al: A reevaluation of risk of in utero exposure to lithium. *JAMA* 271:146–150, 1994.

38. MacLellan-Torbert SG, Porter CJ: Ebstein's anomaly of the tricuspid valve. In Garson Jr. A, Bricker JT, Fisher DJ, Neish SR (eds): *The Science and Practice of Pediatric Cardiology,* 2nd ed. Baltimore: Williams & Wilkins, pp 1303–1315, 1998.

39. Danielson GK, Driscoll DJ, Mair DD, et al: Operative treatment of Ebstein's anomaly. *J Thoracic Cardiovasc Surg* 104:1195–1202, 1992.

40. Watson H: Natural history of Ebstein's anomaly of tricuspid valve in childhood and adolescence: an international cooperative study of 505 cases. *Br Heart J* 36:417–427, 1974.

41. Kidd L, Driscoll DJ, Gersony WM, et al: Second Natural History Study of congenital heart defects. Results of treatment of patients with ventricular septal defects. *Circulation,* 87:I38–51, 1993.

42. Vongpatanasin W, Brickner ME, Hillis LD, Lang RA: The Eisenmenger syndrome in adults. *Ann Int Med* 128:745–755, 1998.

43. Craig RJ, Selzer A: Natural history and prognosis of atrial septal defect. *Circulation,* 37:805–815, 1968.

44. Steele PM, Fuster V, Cohen M, et al: Isolated atrial septal defect with pulmonary vascular obstructive disease: long-term follow-up and prediction of outcome after surgical correction. *Circulation* 76:1037–1042, 1987.

45. Weidman WH, Blount SG, Jr., DuShane JW, et al: Clinical course in ventricular septal defect. *Circulation,* 56:156–69, 1977.

46. Coggin CJ, Parker KR, Keith JD: Natural history of isolated patent ductus arteriosus and the effect of surgical correction: twenty years' experience at The Hospital for Sick Children, Toronto. *Can Med Assoc J* 102:718–720, 1970.

47. Gentles TL, Mayer JE, Jr., Gauvreau K, et al: Fontan operation in five hundred consecutive patients: factors influencing early and late outcome. *J Thorac Cardiovasc Surg* 114:376–391, 1997.

48. Burkhart HM, Dearani JA, Mair DD, et al: The modified Fontan procedure: Early and late results in 132 adult patients. *J Thoracic Cardiovasc Surg* 125:1252–1259, 2003.

49. Feldt RH, Driscoll DJ, Offord KP, et al: Protein-losing enteropathy after the Fontan operation. *J Thoracic Cardiovasc Surg* 112:672–680, 1996.

50. Gentles TL, Gauvreau K, Mayer JE, et al: Functional outcome after the Fontan operation: factors influencing late morbidity. *J Thorac Cardiovasc Surg* 114:392–403, 1997.

CHAPTER 4

Acyanotic Congenital Heart Defects

VIJAYA M. JOSHI

SEPEHR SEKHAVAT

The term *acyanotic heart defects* refers to a heterogeneous group of lesions, broadly categorized into "shunt" or "non-shunt" lesions. *Shunt* lesions are those in which fully oxygenated blood bypasses the systemic circulation and reenters the pulmonary circulation. The *non-shunt* lesions include *obstructive* or *regurgitant* valvar lesions.

LEFT-TO-RIGHT SHUNT LESIONS

General Physiologic Principles

Shunt lesions allow blood that leaves the pulmonary veins (and thus is fully oxygenated) to reenter the pulmonary arteries and to bypass the peripheral vessels and organs. This results in a variable amount of excess pulmonary blood flow. The physiologic effects of left-to-right shunts depend on three main factors: (1) the location of the shunt, (2) the size of the defect, and (3) the relative pulmonary and systemic vascular resistances or (for atrial-level shunts) the relative ventricular compliances. The net excessive pulmonary blood flow and pressure in the pulmonary vascular bed together result in the patient's signs and symptoms.

After the newborn infant's first breath, the pulmonary vascular resistance (PVR) drops precipitously, then gradually approaches that of adult levels at around 1 month of age. In large ventricular or arterial level defects, the drop in PVR usually occurs more gradually and may take 2–3 months to reach the nadir.

Normally, after closure of the ductus arteriosus and the foramen ovale, blood flows through the pulmonary and systemic vascular beds in a series circuit. The right ventricle (RV) pumps the same amount of blood as the left, with beat-to-beat adjustment. The cardiac output—at rest, approximately 4 L/min/m^2—is determined by the body's metabolic needs. Akin to Ohm's law of electric circuits, blood pressure is a product of flow and vascular resistance.

The prototypical example of a left-to-right shunt is a ventricular septal defect (VSD). The actual amount of blood that crosses the VSD depends on the size of the defect and the relative difference between the PVR and the systemic vascular resistance (SVR). With each systolic contraction, blood in the left ventricle (LV) can travel across the aortic valve to the systemic circulation, or it can go through the VSD and across the pulmonary valve into the pulmonary circulation. In a septal defect as large as the aortic valve, the defect itself offers no flow obstruction. Therefore, the shunted pulmonary flow will be inversely related to the PVR.

The systemic output to the body is usually maintained, and the LV continues to pump 4 L/min/m^2 to the body. If, for example, the LV is pumping an additional 4 L/min/m^2 through the VSD, it does a total work of 8 L/min/m^2. Note that the RV has 4 L/min/m^2 returning from the systemic circulation that flows into the lungs. A total of 8 L/min/m^2 passes through the pulmonary circulation and returns to the left atrium (LA) and to the LV. This substantially high pulmonary venous return to the LV is referred to as *volume loading.* Cardiovascular structures dilate with increased volume loading (and hypertrophy with pressure, volume loading, or both). All parts of the circuit receiving excessive flow from the left-to-right shunt will dilate. The patient in this example has 8 L/min/m^2 of pulmonary blood flow (Qp), whereas systemic blood flow (Qs) remains 4 L/min/m^2. The relative amount of pulmonary versus systemic blood flow is expressed as Qp:Qs. In this case, the ratio is 8:4, or 2:1. Note that this extra pulmonary blood is already fully saturated with oxygen and provides no physiologic benefit.

As mentioned earlier, PVR drops more gradually than normal in patients with a large VSD or PDA and can take 2–3 months to reach the nadir. Patients who live at a high altitude with lower ambient oxygen tension can have an even longer period before PVR drops to adult levels. The development of symptoms depends on the degree of excessive pulmonary blood flow, the pressure in the pulmonary arteries, and the response of the body to this pressure-flow alteration. These responses will be discussed with the specific lesions.

Patent Foramen Ovale

The foramen ovale is patent at birth in normal babies. After birth, the rise in pulmonary venous return and the increase in left atrial pressure usually results in closure of the foramen ovale. When the flap of septum primum tissue seals to the rim of the fossa ovale (i.e., septum secundum), the atrial septum becomes intact. But incomplete closure results in patent foramen ovale (PFO), which is relatively common beyond infancy. Pooled analysis of autopsy studies shows a prevalence of PFO in 17–35% of adults.[1] The degree of left-to-right shunting is typically small and patients are asymptomatic. The cardiac exam, electrocardiogram (ECG), and chest x-ray are normal. PFO is often recognized as an incidental finding on echocardiography (echo) and has been discovered with increasing frequency as ultrasound technology improves over time.

In the evaluation of embolic stroke, the presence of a PFO raises the concern of a causal role. Any embolus originating in the deep systemic veins is usually filtered by the pulmonary circulation. With a PFO, such emboli could potentially travel from the right atrium, across the atrial defect, and into the systemic and cerebral circulations. Transient increases in the right atrial pressure, such as during a Valsalva effort, could result in a brief right-to-left shunt and, hence, the paradoxical travel of an embolus.

Atrial Septal Defect

(See Table 4-1.)

Figure 4-1A shows the anatomic landmarks of the atrial septum. Understanding of these landmarks helps one appreciate the three major types of atrial septal defects (ASDs) shown in Figure 4-1B. The *ostium secundum* defect is by far the most common. This defect is caused by an absence or a deficiency of the tissue of the thin septum primum that forms a curtain over the fossa ovale (with a continuum between small secundum defects and PFO). *Ostium primum ASD* is a defect in the atrioventricular (AV) canal septum, which normally separates the AV valves. Defects of the *sinus venosus* type reside in the posterior septum and occur near the superior vena cava junction with the right atrium. Very rarely,

Table 4-1 Atrial Septal Defects	
Types and associations	Ostium secundum: most common
	Ostium primum (i.e., partial AV canal): associated with cleft mitral valve
	Sinus venosus: associated with partial anomalous pulmonary venous return
Symptoms	Minimal to none: CHF is very rare
Signs	Widely split, fixed S_2
	Pulmonary ejection murmur at LUSB, well-transmitted to the back
	With significant shunting, a diastolic murmur (i.e., "relative tricuspid stenosis") at LLSB
ECG	If small, normal
	Right axis deviation
	Right atrial enlargement
	rSR' in V_1 (RV volume overload)
	"Superior" axis with counterclockwise loop, characteristic of ostium primum defects
Chest x-ray	Increased pulmonary blood flow
	Dilated right atrium, right ventricle, and main PA
Management	Closure if high Qp:Qs (i.e., > 1.5) by surgery or with transcatheter device

LUSB, Left upper sternal border; *LLSB,* Left lower sternal border.

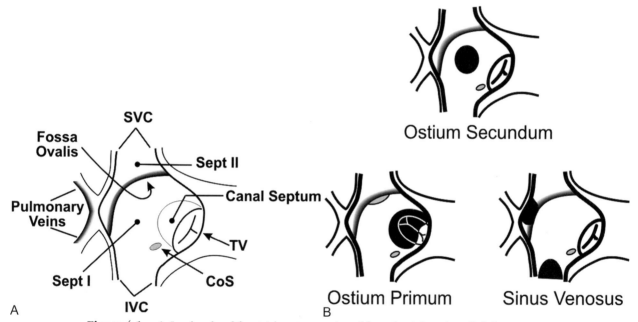

Figure 4-1   A, Landmarks of the atrial septum as viewed from the right atrium. *CoS,* Coronary sinus; *IVC,* inferior vena cava; *Sept I,* septum primum; *Sept II,* septum secundum; *SVC,* superior vena cava; *TV,* tricuspid valve. **B,** Types of ASDs, as viewed from the right atrium. (Courtesy of Paul M. Weinberg, MD, adapted from Braunwald E [series ed], Freedom RM [vol. ed]: *Atlas of Heart Diseases,* Vol. XII: *Congenital Heart Disease.* Current Medicine: Philadelphia, 1997.)

they reside near the inferior vena cava (IVC) junction. Partial anomalous pulmonary venous connection often accompanies these lesions.

The direction of shunting at the atrial level is determined by the *ventricular compliances.* The relatively higher compliance of the RV leads to left-to-right shunting. The right ventricle, the pulmonary vasculature, and the right atrium dilate to accommodate the increase in blood flow. Note that pulmonary arterial pressures usu-

ally remain low, and the additional flow and cardiac work are well-tolerated.

Symptoms

Young children rarely develop symptoms. On finding an ASD in infants with failure to thrive, the clinician should continue the search for a cause of poor weight gain. In these infants, ASD closure rarely results in improved weight gain or growth.[2] Children and infants who develop bronchial or pulmonary disorders as a consequence of prematurity, infection, or asthma may have exacerbated symptoms due to the ASD. In extremely unusual cases, a child may develop frank congestive heart failure (CHF). Older children may present with dyspnea and fatigue with exertion, especially when compared to peers or siblings. These symptoms become more prominent with age. Pulmonary vascular obstructive disease has been reported in infancy but is distinctly unusual. After the teen years, the probability of developing pulmonary vascular obstructive disease steadily increases, but it remains a little less than 10%. The risk appears greater in women.[3] Some patients may develop an atrial arrhythmia in adolescence, with the incidence increasing markedly in middle age.

Physical Exam

In early infancy, the exam may be entirely normal. In older, lean patients, palpation may reveal a prominent RV heave. In older infants and beyond, auscultation usually reveals the widely and usually fixed split second sound (S_2) superior and to the left of the base of the heart. This is caused by the large stroke volume ejected by the right ventricle into a now large-capacity pulmonary circuit, causing the pulmonic second sound (P_2) to occur late. A pulmonary ejection murmur is common. In patients with relatively large shunts, generally with a Qp:Qs of > 2:1, the increased blood flow through the tricuspid annulus results in a diastolic flow murmur of relative tricuspid stenosis, which can be appreciated at the left edge of the lower sternum.

Diagnostic Studies

Beyond early infancy, the ECG usually shows right axis deviation and an rSR' pattern in V1 (i.e., incomplete right bundle branch block) that is typical of RV volume overload. P waves that are peaked and measure > 3 mm in lead II correlate with right atrial enlargement. Criteria for right ventricular hypertrophy (RVH) can be found. Teenagers and older patients may present with atrial arrhythmias, and patients with sinus venosus defects may develop sinus node dysfunction. The "superior" or far left QRS axis is a signature for the ostium primum ASD.

Chest x-ray classically demonstrates increased pulmonary flow and dilated right atrium, RV, and main pulmonary artery. The degree of enlargement of these structures correlates with the degree of the shunt.

Echo confirms the diagnosis and demonstrates the anatomic details allowing for further classification and management. In newborn infants, the distinction between a widely PFO and a small secundum atrial septal defect may be difficult to ascertain by echo.

Management

Patients who have no symptoms need not be restricted, and SBE prophylaxis is not necessary in isolated ASD.

The smaller the defect and the younger the age at diagnosis, the more likely there will be spontaneous closure. However, sinus venosus and primum defects do not close spontaneously. Surgical closure has been the standard treatment; defects can be closed by approximating the margins or by using a patch of pericardium. In recent years, there has been widespread use of transcatheter closure of secundum ASD. Defects that are moderate to small and have well-defined rims are most amenable to device closure, but long-term follow-up data, particularly in pediatric patients, are lacking. An estimated high pulmonary-to-systemic flow ratio (i.e., Qp:Qs >1.5), especially when the RV is dilated, is an indication for ASD closure. As small secundum defects may close spontaneously, treatment can often be deferred until the child is at least 4 years old if transcatheter technique is anticipated. At experienced centers, operative mortality is less than 1%.

Because of the posterior location of sinus venosus defects and the associated partial anomalous pulmonary venous return, surgical closure remains the treatment of choice. Pericardium is used to close the defect, as well as to baffle the anomalous pulmonary vein or veins into the left atrium.

Ventricular Septal Defect

(See Table 4-2.)

The anatomy of the ventricular septum as seen from the RV (Fig. 4-2A) allows for understanding the classification of ventricular septal defects (Fig. 4-2B). The small membranous septum is located near the annulus of the tricuspid valve septal leaflet. It forms the nexus of the inlet septum inferiorly, the muscular (or trabecular septum) represented by the septal band, and the outlet septum (i.e. infundibular septum or crista supraventricularis).

For any VSD, the area of the hole compared to the area of the aortic valve best predicts physiology. As a simplistic but useful guide, defects less than one third the size of the aortic annulus are considered small, one third to two thirds of the size are moderate, and greater than two thirds are large. For larger defects, the amount of shunting depends on the relative ratio of PVR and SVR.

Perimembranous (i.e., conoventricular) defects are the most common form of VSD. The defect extends from the membranous septum into its adjoining regions. Many of these defects, even large ones, can become smaller or can close completely. Tissue associated with the septal leaflet of the tricuspid valve fills the defect and occasionally creates a windsock-like tube that extends in to the RV chamber; this process happens most commonly in the first 6 months of life. On the LV aspect of the ventricular septum, perimembranous defects are located just inferior to the aortic valve and the supporting structure of the

Table 4-2 Ventricular Septal Defects

Types	Muscular: may close spontaneously
	Perimembranous: may close spontaneously (by associated tricuspid valve tissue or aneurysm formation)
	Malalignment: often associated with left or right outflow tract obstruction (as in tetralogy of Fallot); do not close spontaneously
	Inlet: associated with ostium primum ASD and AV canal. Do not close spontaneously
Symptoms	If small with minimal shunt (i.e., Qp:Qs < 1.5): none
	If moderate to large (i.e., Qp:Qs > 1.5): CHF with increased work of breathing, difficulty feeding, diaphoresis, and poor growth
Signs	Holosystolic murmur at LLSB ± thrill
	If significant shunting: CHF with tachycardia, tachypnea, pallor, and hepatomegaly
	If pulmonary hypertension is present: single loud second sound
ECG	If small: normal
	If significant shunt: LVH, possible LAD
	If pulmonary hypertension: RVH ± LVH
	In AV canal: superior, far left or right, or QRS axis with counterclockwise loop
Chest x-ray	Cardiomegaly, possible pulmonary edema, flat diaphragms, hyperexpanded lungs
	Increased pulmonary vascular markings
Management	Maximize nutrition (especially fortify caloric intake)
	Consider medications (i.e., diuretics, digoxin, or ACE inhibitors)
	SBE prophylaxis
	If growth can be maintained, wait ~6 months for VSD to become restrictive
	Surgical closure indicated sooner for significant symptoms and failure to thrive despite medical management

ASD, Atrial septal defect; *AV,* atrioventricular; *Qp,* pulmonary blood flow; *Qs,* systemic blood flow; *CHF,* congestive heart failure; *LLSB,* lower left sternal border; *LVH,* left ventricular hypertrophy; *RVH,* right ventricular hypertrophy; *ACE,* angiotensin-converting enzyme; *SBE,* subacute bacterial endocarditis; *VSD,* ventricular septal defect.

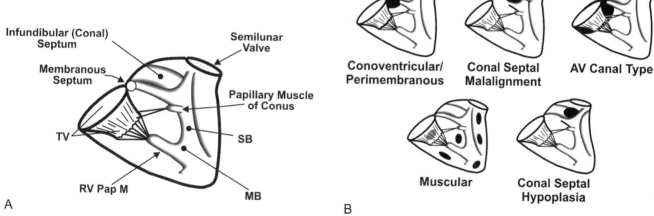

Figure 4-2   A, Landmarks of the ventricular septum as viewed from the right ventricle. *MB,* Moderator band; *RV Pap M,* papillary muscle of the right ventricle; *SB,* septal band; *TV,* tricuspid valve. **B,** Types of ventricular septal defects as seen from the right ventricle. See text for details. (**A-B,** Courtesy of Paul M. Weinberg, MD, adapted with permission from Braunwald E [series ed], Freedom RM [vol. ed]: *Atlas of Heart Diseases,* Vol. XII: *Congenital Heart Disease.* St Louis: Mosby–Year Book, 1997.)

aortic valve is absent along the VSD. With rare frequency, the right leaflet of the aortic valve can prolapse into the defect, resulting in aortic regurgitation.

Muscular defects are located within the muscular or trabecular septum. They are subclassified based on the anatomic location (e.g., apical or midmuscular). It is not unusual to incidentally discover small defects with echocardiography of premature infants. Small and moderate defects have high rates of spontaneous closure. The anatomic characteristics of some defects make them difficult to close surgically, for example, apical defects and the rare "Swiss cheese septum" with multiple muscular defects, which require individualized approaches to management. The apical defect is one type of VSD for which transcatheter device closure may become the intervention of choice.

Inlet defects are found in the posterior septum, inferior to the membranous septum at the junction of the atrioventricular valves, and extend the full superoinferior length of the tricuspid valve. Most are seen in endocardial cushion defects (e.g., common AV canal). Although rarely, they can be described as isolated inlet or "canal-type" defects.

Malalignment defects result when the superiorly located infundibular (i.e., conal) septum fails to align with and to join the trabecular septum at the septal band. This type of VSD may be associated with coarctation of the aorta or interruption of the aortic arch. It can also occur in cyanotic lesions such as tetralogy of Fallot and transposition of the great arteries.

Conal septal hypoplasia defects are defects in, as opposed to malalignment of, the infundibular septum. They are referred to as "subpulmonary," based on their proximity to the pulmonary valve when viewed from the RV, but this can be misleading because they are actually in proximity to both semilunar valves. In fact, when viewed from the LV, the aortic valve can appear to sit at the edge of the defect with the right aortic valve leaflet partly filling it. This may cause prolapse of the valve leaflet and aortic regurgitation (although, because of the relative infrequency of conal septal defects in Western populations, this occurs less commonly than with conoventricular defects).

Symptoms

Newborns with VSDs are usually well, and, if the VSDs are small, they will remain well. With moderate to large defects, infants may develop signs of congestive failure as the PVR falls and left-to-right shunting increases. The baby's breathing can range from mild tachypnea to labored. The newborn who initially feeds vigorously can evolve to one who fatigues, with a drop in the volume consumed and an increase in the time needed to feed. Diaphoresis with feeding is a manifestation of increased sympathetic output caused by the increased cardiac work. Cyanosis or a gray color suggests a more complex problem. By 2 months of age, the infant can show poor weight gain. Congestive heart failure in these patients is manifested as tachycardia, increased work of breathing, diaphoresis, failure to thrive with poor feeding, and liver enlargement. The infant with a large defect, who may be fragile but compensated, can deteriorate rapidly with an infection such as bronchiolitis or pneumonia.

Physical Exam

Small defects usually present with a murmur in the early newborn period. With moderate to large VSDs, it is not unusual for a newborn to have no murmur, because high PVR prevents significant shunting across the defect. As the PVR drops, the murmur can be discovered at a subsequent exam in infancy. The murmurs typically have a harsh quality and pansystolic duration that may obscure distinct first and second heart sounds. The loudest location of the murmur depends on the trajectory of the turbulent shunt, but it is usually heard to the left of the mid or lower sternum. Small muscular defects can sound squeaky rather than harsh and may have dynamic systolic closure causing a short murmur (i.e., early systolic) that ends before S_2.

If the pulmonary artery (PA) pressure is high, especially in the presence of a large VSD, the S_2 will sound single and loud. Truly large defects can be a diagnostic challenge as the patient may not have a significant murmur, and the recognition of a loud single second heart sound requires quiet conditions and an experienced examiner. Since these infants are repaired relatively early, a precordial bulge in the left thorax, caused by longstanding LV volume overload, is rarely seen.

The murmur intensity does not correlate with defect size. High flow or high velocity can be associated with increased intensity. A diastolic apical rumble confirms the presence of a large shunt causing excessive flow through a mitral valve that has not substantially dilated. A third heart sound (S_3) gallop sometimes accompanies clinical heart failure.

Diagnostic Studies

With small defects, the ECG remains normal. Moderate defects usually demonstrate left ventricular hypertrophy (LVH). Criteria for RVH may be notable, especially after the first few months of life. Large defects have biventricular hypertrophy and often have left atrial enlargement. RVH alone suggests that PVR may be high or that there is also RV outflow obstruction (e.g., acyanotic tetralogy of Fallot). When the ECG shows a superior (i.e., far left) QRS axis, suspect a canal-type VSD, although mild left axis deviation (i.e., −30 to +30 degrees) can be seen with small conoventricular VSDs.

On chest x-ray, cardiomegaly, left atrial enlargement, and increased pulmonary blood flow correlate directly with the amount of left-to-right shunting. Pulmonary edema correlates with symptoms of congestive heart failure, especially tachypnea. If pulmonary vascular obstructive disease has developed (i.e., Eisenmenger's syndrome), the heart size may be only minimally enlarged, the main pulmonary artery is dilated and the pulmonary blood flow may appear normal or decreased. Advanced cases show "pruning" of the pulmonary vessels, characterized by large hilar PA branches with smaller peripheral vessels and dark peripheral lung fields, secondary to decreased pulmonary blood flow.

Echo is diagnostic and, along with the clinical data, can provide sufficient information to proceed with management, including surgery. The ECHO study can define the location and number of defects and also can demonstrate the physiologic consequences, such as atrial and ventricular dilation. Using a combination of color flow mapping and continuous wave Doppler, pressures can be estimated. For example, a 70 mmHg peak pressure difference between the LV and RV in a child with normal blood pressure is consistent with normal RV pressure and a restrictive defect. The child's cooperation, obtained by natural or pharmacological means, is essential to obtaining a complete and accurate diagnostic study.

Since the 1990s, the frequency of cardiac catheterization for VSD has decreased. For the young child with an isolated VSD, diagnostic catheterization is rarely needed. Catheterization has an important role in complex lesions or when the clinician needs to quantify the shunt and the PVR, especially after 9–12 months of age or in those cases in which catheter closure devices can be used.

Management

Patients with moderate to large defects may develop CHF and growth failure and are medically managed with diuretics, angiotensin-converting enzyme (ACE) inhibitors, and digoxin. This treatment helps to relieve symptoms, allows the child to grow, and gives time to allow the defect to become smaller or to close. Supplemental nutrition, such as high-calorie formula, should be instituted early if a large shunt is present, because metabolic demands are increased. Up to 150–200 kcal/kg/day may be needed for adequate growth. On occasion, one can initiate tube feedings to relieve the work of feeding; this is usually employed as a bridge to surgery. As anemia aggravates heart failure, the clinician should have a low threshold to supplement with iron. During the late autumn, palivizumab (i.e., antirespiratory syncytial virus monoclonal antibody) immunization series should be considered, especially in premature infants or those with significant shunting. A multicenter trial found a 45% reduction in hospitalization in infants with significant congenital heart defects.[4]

In infants with a large perimembranous or muscular VSD, medical management can allow for adequate growth before surgery is required. The defect may spontaneously close or may get smaller. In symptomatic infants with the other types of VSD, little advantage is gained by waiting.

Most infants with a significant left-to-right shunt (i.e., Qp:Qs of 2:1 or greater) should undergo surgical closure before 1 year of age and much earlier if they have symptoms. Recent advances in transcatheter devices may make nonsurgical closure of VSDs more common in the near future. When PVR exceeds 50% of SVR, surgical risk rises, as does the risk of residual pulmonary hypertension.

After surgical closure, there is a 10% risk of having a residual defect. Usually, such defects are considerably smaller than the original and are not of hemodynamic consequence. Also, because of the proximity of the conduction system to the VSD, there is a risk, approaching 1%, of postoperative complete heart block. The vast majority of patients who have had a successful repair and recovery will have normal long-term cardiac function and will need no exercise restrictions. Older children with small VSDs also need no physical restrictions. Those who have pulmonary vascular obstructive disease should limit themselves to low-intensity work and play. All individuals with VSDs (and those with postrepair residual defects) should observe subacute bacterial endocarditis (SBE) prophylaxis and should pay special attention to dental hygiene.

Common Atrioventricular Canal (i.e., Endocardial Cushion defect or AV Septal Defect)

Fusion of the superior and inferior endocardial cushions allows for the normal development of separate mitral and tricuspid valves. Common atrioventricular canal (CAVC) defects result from incomplete fusion and loss of the crux of the four cardiac chambers. The degree of fusion failure determines where in a spectrum the resulting defect will fall. *Complete* CAVC is at the extreme end of the clinical spectrum and is the most common form. In complete CAVC, a common AV valve sits over both ventricles. There is a primum ASD and an inlet VSD, with shunting occurring at the atrial and ventricular levels. The common AV valve usually has four or five leaflets, with a superior and inferior bridging leaflet crossing through the VSD. The LV outflow tract is relatively elongated by the bridging superior leaflet of the common AV valve, resulting in the classic "goose neck" appearance on angiography and echo.

In some cases of AV canal, AV valve leaflet tissue and attachments "fill" the inlet VSD. If there is still a residual but restrictive VSD, a *transitional* atrioventricular canal (AVC) results. If the VSD is effectively closed, the end result is an ostium primum ASD and a cleft in the anterior "mitral" leaflet (i.e., what would have become the mitral valve, had the common AV valve leaflet divided into mitral and tricuspid tissue). This is called *incomplete* AVC and represents the opposite end of the spectrum from complete CAVC.

In describing the CAVC, particular attention should also be paid to *ventricular balance*. Usually, the common AV valve is equally committed to both ventricles, with equal numbers of leaflet attachments into each chamber. Both ventricles are well-developed and of good size, resulting in a "balanced" AVC. In some cases, the AV valve can be "unbalanced" toward one ventricle, resulting in hypoplasia of the other ventricle and more complex lesions.

CAVC is often associated with other congenital abnormalities, most notably trisomy 21, as well as the asplenic type of heterotaxy syndrome.

Symptoms

Newborns are usually asymptomatic. Infants with incomplete AV canal have ASD physiology unless there is significant left AV valve regurgitation. Infants with large VSD components develop symptoms similar to those with isolated VSD unless the PVR remains high. AV valve regurgitation may hasten the development of heart failure symptoms.

Physical Exam

A newborn or young infant may have no murmur because the PVR is still elevated and there is little left-to-right shunting in the first days to weeks of life. Patients with complete CAVC or significant AV valve regurgitation may appear thin and undernourished. Work of breathing is increased and the heart rate is faster than expected. The precordium often feels hyperactive. S_2 is narrowly split and P_2 is loud. Since the VSD is large, its murmur tends to be soft, transmitted to the pulmonary outflow region, or it may be completely absent. A blowing pansystolic murmur at the apex and in the back is found in AV valve regurgitation. A transitional AV canal may cause loud harsh "restrictive"-sounding VSD murmurs because of the small size of the VSD component. The patient with an incomplete AV canal and a competent mitral valve will have a physical exam similar to that for ASD. Growth of children with trisomy 21 should be plotted on the appropriate growth charts.

Diagnostic Studies

The defect in the canal portion of the septum displaces the conduction system, which causes leftward deviation of the QRS axis on ECG from −30 degrees to −120 degrees, with counterclockwise looping. The "superior axis" is a hallmark of this defect. P-wave abnormalities can be common, depending on age. The QRS complex may show rSR' from RV dilation. Biventricular hypertrophy is common with CAVC.

Chest x-ray findings are similar to ASD or VSD, with enlargement of the cardiac silhouette and increased pulmonary vascular markings.

Echo is essential to defining the anatomy, valve function, and associated lesions. Special attention should be paid to features such as ventricular balance and AV valve regurgitation. Cardiac catheterization is needed when PVR is in question or in the presence of a more complex lesion.

Management

In symptomatic patients, initial medical management should begin with anticongestive therapy (e.g., digoxin and furosemide). Children with incomplete CAVC and no AV valve regurgitation usually do not require medical management. A diuretic such as furosemide should be the first choice in symptomatic AV valve regurgitation. Afterload reduction with ACE inhibitors may further benefit the patient.

Children without significant "mitral" (i.e., left AV valve) regurgitation can have elective surgery with a wide degree of latitude. Infants with complete CAVC who develop symptoms will benefit from medicines and nutrition as discussed in the section on VSD. In the ideal case, infants should have surgical repair by 6 months of age. Because of the large VSD, pulmonary artery pressures will be high and pulmonary vascular obstructive disease can develop before 1 year of age, especially in the patients with Down syndrome. Surgeons usually close the mitral cleft at the initial operation; however, patients may require another operation later in life for mitral regurgitation or, rarely, mitral stenosis. A few incomplete AVC patients develop subaortic stenosis related to abnormal endocardial cushion tissue in the subaortic region.

Patent Ductus Arteriosus

(See Table 4-3.)

Patent ductus arteriosus (PDA) accounts for up to 10% of congenital heart defects found in term infants. In preterm infants, the incidence is inversely proportional to gestational age. The ductus arteriosus is a normal fetal structure connecting the main pulmonary artery near the origin of the left pulmonary artery to the descending aorta. In utero, it shunts more than 80% of the flow that goes through the main pulmonary artery to the descending aorta. During fetal life, prostaglandins promote ductal

Table 4-3 Patent Ductus Arteriosus		
Types	Premature infant, usually with respiratory distress syndrome	Term infant or older child
Symptoms	Multiple nonspecific symptoms including poor feeding	Increased work of breathing, poor growth, poor feeding
Signs	Specific signs may be obscured by other clinical issues (e.g., respiratory distress syndrome)	Continuous murmur and bounding pulses
ECG	Similar to VSD (see Table 4-2)	
Chest x-ray	Similar to VSD (see Table 4-2)	
Management	Early treatment with indomethacin. If treatment is contraindicated or fails, then surgery	Catheter device or surgical closure

patency. As the fetus comes closer to term, oxygen becomes more potent in its ability to constrict the duct. The ductal wall muscle constricts after birth as prostaglandin levels decrease, and partial pressure of oxygen (PaO_2) increases with functional closure of the ductus within 12–48 hours. The closing ductus appears cone-shaped, with the smaller end on the pulmonary side. Persistent patency of the ductus causes shunting from the aorta to the pulmonary arteries. As the PVR drops, the PDA shunts blood left to right in both systole and diastole. The pulmonary vascular bed, left heart, and ascending aorta dilate proportionately to the net shunt.

Symptoms

Symptoms generally mimic those of VSD. Patients with small PDAs are asymptomatic, whereas infants and young children with a large shunt tend to have increased heart rates and work of breathing.

Physical Exam

On examination, there is a hyperactive precordium and occasionally a systolic thrill at the left upper sternal border. Bounding peripheral pulses and a widened pulse pressure are characteristic. P_2 is usually normal unless there is pulmonary hypertension. Auscultation reveals a continuous murmur of varying intensity between the left clavicle and the upper sternum. The murmur is often characterized as having a "machinery" quality. It must be confirmed in the supine position to differentiate it from venous hum, which is best heard in the upright position. In the newborn and the young infant, when pulmonary resistance has begun to drop but is still higher than in the older child, the murmur may be systolic only, and located at the lower left sternal border, similar to that of a VSD. One clue to the presence of a PDA is the "bag of rocks," or multiple systolic clicks from fluttering of the pulmonary valve from the opposing streams of blood (i.e., antegrade across the valve and retrograde through the duct). There may be an apical diastolic rumble when the shunt is large (usually > 2:1). The physical exam may not rule out a PDA in the very-low-birth-weight baby on mechanical ventilation, and echo is necessary to confirm the presence of a PDA.

Should the natural history progress to the development of pulmonary vascular obstructive disease, the increased PVR can shift the shunt to right to left, from pulmonary artery to aorta. The result is differential cyanosis: the lower half of the body is blue, whereas the upper half remains fully saturated. This occurs in infants with persistent pulmonary hypertension.

Diagnostic Studies

Findings on ECG are similar to VSD. Small to moderate PDA may have normal ECG. With a large PDA, there can be LVH or biventricular hypertrophy (BVH). RVH alone may be found if the PVR is elevated.

The chest x-ray is similar to VSD, appearing normal in small to moderate PDA. In more significant shunts with increased pulmonary blood flow, there can be varying degrees of cardiomegaly, with enlargement of the left atrium, LV, and ascending aorta. If PVR is elevated, the heart size is normal, but there is prominence of the MPA segment and hilar vessels.

With echo, the size and shape of the PDA can be assessed. Dilation of the left atrium and the LV occurs in the presence of a significant shunt. Color and two-dimensional (2D) Doppler provide additional data on the direction and magnitude of shunting.

Natural History

In the term infant, a PDA found beyond the first few days of life has a low probability of spontaneous closure. CHF and recurrent respiratory infections can occur if the shunt is large. In large, untreated defects, pulmonary vascular obstructive disease may develop. PDA incurs a relatively high lifetime risk of SBE.

Management

Premature infants should be treated soon after diagnosis. The initial treatment of choice is intravenous indomethacin, which blocks prostaglandin synthesis and induces ductal closure. The initial dose is 0.2 mg/kg; if the PDA does not close, two additional doses (0.1–0.25 mg/kg) every 12–24 hours should be given, based on size and age. The medication is contraindicated in patients with active bleeding, low platelet count, intracranial hemorrhage, renal insufficiency, or necrotizing enterocolitis. Surgery is recommended in these cases and generally is performed by a lateral thoracotomy, often at the bedside. In term infants with PDA, indomethacin is ineffective.

Older patients with PDA do not require exercise restriction unless there is pulmonary hypertension. SBE precautions should be observed. In the era of liberal use of echo, the "silent" PDA is increasingly discovered. These are usually tiny and the risk of SBE appears less than the audible PDA. There is still debate regarding the risk-to-benefit ratio of closing the incidentally found PDA.

In older patients, closure of PDA with catheter-delivered devices has become increasingly common. Stainless steel coils are the standard device for closure, although specially shaped PDA closure devices have been recently approved in the United States. Surgical closure by a lateral thoracotomy remains the standard option, especially for the large PDA. Video-assisted thorascopic techniques are available at some centers.

NON-SHUNT LESIONS

General Physiologic Principles

Physiologically, non-shunt acyanotic heart defects can be subdivided into *obstructive* and (valvar) *regurgitant* lesions. As the name implies, in obstructive lesions there is resistance to blood flow. Akin to Ohm's Law in electronics (i.e., $V = I \times R$, where V is voltage, I is current, and R is resistance), any resistance in flow produces a pressure gradient across that resistance (i.e., $\Delta P = Q \times R$, where ΔP is the pressure gradient, Q is blood flow, and R is resistance). A ventricle proximal to a stenosis generates a greater pressure load to overcome the obstruction. This is referred to as a *pressure load* on the ventricle. Blood flow across the obstruction becomes turbulent; this produces the murmur. In severe cases, the obstruction either can impede blood flow, or, over time, the ventricle can fail because of the excessive work load demanded of it, or both. In addition, with stenosis in a blood vessel (such as coarctation of the aorta or stenosis of the semilunar valves), there is poststenotic dilation of the vessel. If there is stenosis of an AV valve, as pressure increases, the atrium will dilate. This, in turn, causes an increase in pressure in "upstream" veins as well.

In valvar regurgitant lesions, the involved ventricle has to pump an extra volume of blood to compensate for the regurgitation. This constitutes a *volume load* on the ventricle. The ventricle dilates to accommodate the volume, and structures across the lesion also become dilated. For example, in mitral regurgitation, the LV has to pump a full cardiac output through the aorta as well as any regurgitant volume across the incompetent mitral valve. The LV thus becomes dilated, as does the left atrium as it is forced to accept the regurgitant volume. If the regurgitation is severe enough, the ventricle will not be able to provide adequate cardiac output.

Although non-shunt acyanotic heart defects are divided physiologically into obstructive and regurgitant lesions, clinically the two types are sometimes seen together, for example, in an abnormal aortic valve that is both stenotic and insufficient. For the purposes of organization, the lesions described here are grouped by anatomic location.

Bicuspid Aortic Valve

When closed, the normal aortic valve forms a pattern with three leaflets that, from above, looks somewhat like the Mercedes-Benz symbol. The valve annulus is in fibrous continuity with the annulus of the mitral valve below. In bicuspid aortic valve (BAV), two of the valve leaflets are partially fused, resulting in an eccentric and smaller-than-normal orifice.

BAV is the most common congenital heart defect.[5] It has been found in 0.5% of Italian school children who were not suspected of having heart defects. BAV patients are prone to develop stenosis alone or combined with insufficiency or, less commonly, insufficiency alone. Physical findings often are subtle; the only finding may be a systolic ejection click caused by the opening of the relatively rigid aortic valve leaflets. BAV is not detected in childhood in many individuals. The more severe the disease, the more likely it is to be appreciated on auscultation. In mild cases, significant valve dysfunction may never develop, or not until the adult years. The risk of endocarditis mandates antibiotic prophylaxis for relevant procedures.

Aortic Stenosis

(See Table 4-4.)

Aortic valve stenosis (AS) presents in two clinical settings. Infants with severe or "critical" aortic stenosis present

Table 4-4 Aortic Stenosis (Valvar)		
Typical time of presentation (i.e., type)	Infant/critical AS (usually unicuspid)	Older patients (usually bicuspid)
Symptoms	Mild CHF to shock	Initially none; may progress to CHF, syncope, chest pain, or arrhythmias
Signs	Crescendo-decrescendo systolic ejection murmur at RUSB or LUSB or RUSB, may radiate to carotids	
	Diastolic murmur if associated aortic insufficiency	
	Severe: thrill, narrowed pulse pressure	
ECG	Moderate to severe: LVH, possibly with strain	
	ST depression on exercise stress testing	
Chest x-ray	Mild: no significant findings	
	Moderate to severe: prominent ascending aorta; cardiomegaly, pulmonary congestion if there is LV failure	
Management	SBE prophylaxis	
	No restriction of activity if mild to moderate gradient with normal EST and ECG	
	Balloon valvuloplasty for catheter gradient > 50–60 mmHg	
	Surgery: Ross, homograft, or prosthetic valve replacement	

CHF, Congestive heart failure; *RUSB,* right upper sternal border; *LUSB,* left upper sternal border; *LVH,* left ventricular hypertrophy; *EST,* exercise stress test; *AS,* aortic stenosis; *LV,* left ventricular.

acutely ill shortly after birth. Patients in the second group tend to be diagnosed because of physical findings (e.g., a murmur or intermittent symptoms) and are often diagnosed in the outpatient setting during a routine exam.

In severe neonatal AS, the valve is often unicuspid. In infants and children without critical AS, the valve is usually bicuspid. Boys tend to have a several-fold higher incidence of AS than girls. Due to the small orifice size, a higher velocity of flow is required through it to achieve adequate cardiac output; the smaller the orifice size, the greater the velocity of flow needed. When the orifice area becomes less than half of normal, the LV systolic pressure begins to exceed that in the aorta, and the high velocity of blood being forced through the aortic valve orifice causes turbulence of blood flow.

As the severity of AS increases, the LV walls hypertrophy. This preserves LV systolic function and minimizes wall stress as the systolic pressure load rises. Those in whom the AS becomes severe cannot substantially increase stroke volume with increasing metabolic demands, and CHF results. The coronary flow may not sufficiently supply the hypertrophied myocardium, particularly the subendocardium.

Supravalvar aortic stenosis can occur due to stenosis at the level of the junction of the sinuses of Valsalva with the ascending aorta or due to a long segment hypoplasia of the ascending aorta. This finding is seen in Williams syndrome. *Subaortic stenosis* can be caused by fibrous membranous tissue in the left ventricular outflow tract (LVOT), which is often associated with an active or spontaneously closed VSD or caused by muscular tunnel-like narrowing of the LVOT. Hypertrophic cardiomyopathy variants can develop dynamic subaortic stenosis.

Symptoms

The subset of infants with critical AS present in a spectrum from mild CHF to shock due to LV dysfunction. The ventricular dysfunction leads to elevated left atrial pressure and pulmonary edema. Those who have poor ventricular function tend to have a less intense murmur, although they may have a gallop.

After early infancy, patients are less likely to present with heart failure. AS tends to progress with age, although at varying rates. Rapid progression is more likely to occur during the first 2 years of life or during puberty. Mild AS that seems stable over most of a decade can progress dramatically over the course of puberty.

Symptoms have a low correlation with the degree of AS. Similarly, indirect diagnostic tests such as ECG and exercise testing have a frustrating degree of variability for a given degree of AS. Clinically, those who remain untreated for severe AS can present with heart failure, syncope, ventricular arrhythmias, or sudden death.

Physical Exam

After the newborn period, the murmur grade correlates with the degree of AS, assuming that ventricular contractility remains normal. There is frequently a suprasternal notch thrill. There may be a thrill at the right upper sternal border (RUSB) in cases of severe AS. The murmur is a crescendo-decrescendo systolic ejection murmur heard at the base of the heart, usually at the RUSB. Depending on the projection of the jet, one may hear it best at the left upper sternal border LUSB. The murmur often radiates into the carotids and may be preceded by an ejection click.

Diagnostic Studies

ECG findings vary significantly in newborns and infants with AS. Characteristically, in the child with moderate to severe AS, LVH is manifested by inappropriately tall voltages in the limb and left precordial leads or by deep S waves in V_1. LVH with strain occurs when the LVH findings are found along with T-wave inversion, with or without ST-segment depression in V_5 or V_6; this can suggest severe AS.

With exercise testing, these patients can develop a blunted systolic blood pressure response. The ECG findings of ST segment depression in the inferior or lateral precordial leads suggest ischemia.

On chest x-ray, the subtle finding of a dilated ascending aorta may be the only finding but is not definitive. In the presence of CHF, cardiomegaly, pulmonary venous congestion, and pulmonary edema may be seen.

Two-dimensional echo can reveal the aortic valve morphology (i.e., bicuspid or unicuspid). Frequently, leaflet thickening and "doming" are seen. LV function and hypertrophy are quantified. Associated aortic regurgitation can be displayed using color Doppler, and 2D Doppler is used to determine the gradient across the stenosis. Both the peak and mean gradients are usually obtained. The mean pressure gradients obtained by echo tend to correlate better with the peak-to-peak gradients recorded in the catheterization laboratory. The grading of the severity of AS has traditionally been based on the pressure gradient across the valve.[6] Table 4-5 is a composite of the grades given to various pressure gradients. Classifications by valve area, often favored for adults, are used less commonly in pediatrics.

Management

In patients with good ventricular systolic function, medications provide little benefit for AS. The timing of intervention to relieve the AS has to be individualized for the patient. The 1994 Bethesda Conference has provided conservative guidelines for allowing participation in competitive sports.[7] Children with AS with 25–49 mmHg gradients must have a normal exercise test and mild LVH on their ECG to have no restrictions. Otherwise, they should be restricted to lower-intensity sports. Our center

Table 4-5 Classification of Aortic Valve Stenosis by Peak Catheterization-Determined Pressure Gradients				
Degree of AS (Older)	Trivial	Mild	Moderate	Severe or critical
Degree of AS (Newer)	Mild	Moderate	Moderate to severe	Severe or critical
Pressure gradient	< 25 mmHg	25–49 mmHg	50–79 mmHg	> 80 mmHg

usually intervenes when a patient will have a predicted catheter gradient of > 50–60 mmHg. The patient with symptoms such as syncope or an abnormal exercise test may be treated at a lower threshold.

Performing cardiac catheterization purely for diagnostic purposes is now uncommon in AS. Generally, the diagnostic testing is now done as a prelude to anticipated balloon valvuloplasty. In patients with more than mild aortic regurgitation, surgery is the preferred first procedure. If balloon valvuloplasty does not sufficiently relieve the stenosis or results in significant aortic regurgitation, surgery is indicated. If the pulmonary valve is normal, a Ross procedure, consisting of translocating the pulmonary root and valve into the aortic position and replacement of the removed pulmonary portion with a cadaveric pulmonary homograft, is frequently used. These autograft valves can grow with the patient.[8] Unfortunately, there is a long-term risk of neoaortic valve regurgitation and pulmonary homograft stenosis. An aortic valve homograft or prosthetic aortic valve is another surgical solution. However, the young child can outgrow these implanted valves, requiring repeat surgery. Prosthetic valves require anticoagulation, with a desired international normalized ratio (INR) level between 2.5 and 3.5.

Coarctation of the Aorta

Discrete narrowing of the distal aortic arch results in obstruction to flow and coarctation. The severity of coarctation and associated lesions determines whether the patient presents as a neonate with "critical" coarctation. Older classifications conceptualized a preductal (i.e., neonatal or severe) form and a postductal form presenting beyond neonatal life. Functionally this is useful, but it is not anatomically accurate. The region of arch obstruction is usually caused by narrowing from a shelf of tissue from the greater curvature of the arch opposite the site of ductal insertion. This shelf involves the intima and media of the vessel wall.

In fetal life, the aortic isthmus (i.e., the portion between the left subclavian artery and the ductal insertion) carries less than 10% of the total cardiac output. Left sided lesions proximal to this region can significantly reduce this flow and can impair arch development. BAV is found in the majority of coarctation

patients. Additional left-sided lesions associated with coarctation include aortic valve stenoses, VSDs, and mitral valve anomalies such as parachute valve or mitral arcade (often with mitral stenosis). The male-to-female ratio is approximately 5:1. Turner's syndrome should be considered in all female patients.

Symptoms

Pediatric patients with coarctation usually present in one of three different settings. Critical or "ductal-dependent" coarctation presents in the first few days to weeks of life. These infants present with cyanosis (especially of the lower body, from right-to-left ductal shunting) and, as the ductus closes, ventricular failure or shock.

The second group of infants, with slightly less severe coarctation, present with heart failure symptoms of poor feeding, failure to thrive, and increased work of breathing. If a PDA is still present, left-to-right shunting occurs. Reduced ventricular function results from an inability to tolerate the pressure load.

The third group has a less severe form of coarctation and may have minimal or no significant symptoms in childhood. Good ventricular function is maintained, and adequate flow is present below the region of obstruction. With growth and time, collateral arteries from the major branches of the aorta above the obstruction develop and divert flow to the lower descending aorta. This third group may present with heart murmurs, hypertension, symptoms of fatigue, or endocarditis.

Physical Exam

High blood pressure in the arms, along with lower blood pressure in the legs, is the cardinal finding in coarctation. Sometimes cuff pressures are unobtainable in the legs. One observes either absent or attenuated femoral pulses. A delay between the radial and femoral pulse may be noted because of the slow rise of the lower pulse. This femoral pulse finding is the single most diagnostically useful part of the physical exam.

Variations in arterial anatomy warrant observing pulses and blood pressures in all four limbs. Stenosis or hypoplasia of the left subclavian artery origin can result in a low pressure in the left arm. Aberrant origin of the right subclavian below the coarctation may explain a low pressure in the right arm. Patients with multiple collaterals may have only a small gradient between the arms and legs.

On auscultation, the patient might have a systolic ejection click or murmur from an associated bicuspid aortic valve. Tachycardia and a gallop can be found in the infants with heart failure. A systolic or continuous murmur (with a soft diastolic component) can be heard in the left axilla or left posterior chest. This continuous murmur suggests the presence of intercostal collaterals. In girls with coarctation, one should consider Turner's syndrome.

Diagnostic Studies

In the young infant, the ECG may show RVH. By a few weeks to months of age, LVH is common. BVH may be present if pulmonary artery hypertension occurs.

In the infant with heart failure, the chest x-ray tends to show cardiomegaly and pulmonary edema. In older children, the heart size is usually normal, but rib notching from enlarged collateral vessels may be noted.

ECHO in the young child usually provides sufficient information to proceed with treatment. LV size and function should be carefully assessed. Infants with clinical heart failure have diminished LV function; otherwise, one usually finds good to hyperdynamic LV systolic function. Outside of the newborn period, most have LVH. Special attention should be paid to the morphology and function of other left-sided structures, particularly the mitral and aortic valves. The transverse aortic arch tends to be small but is unlikely to be obstructed. Most cases have a shelf-like projection of the aortic wall from the greater curvature of the arch, found at the level of the ductal ampulla (residing on the lesser curvature side). This results in the classic "number 3" image. Less commonly, long segment or tubular hypoplasia of the isthmus may be found. Doppler data demonstrate turbulent flow with high velocity in systole and a run-off pattern in diastole. Pressure gradients can be estimated from these data.

Older children and adults often have suboptimal images of the distal arch, warranting additional imaging. MRI, or CT scan can be utilized with excellent demonstration of the morphology of the arch and collaterals. With MRI, velocity mapping can provide pressure gradient estimates. Intracardiac morphology and function can be clarified.

Management

Management of the infant with severe critical coarctation is discussed in Chapter 2. Infants who present with signs of heart failure can be managed with digoxin, diuretics, and possibly dopamine. Primary surgical repair is recommended in infants because of the high incidence of recoarctation with catheter balloon angioplasty. Additionally, there is up to a 5% incidence of aneurysm

development in the intermediate follow-up period with balloon angioplasty.[9] In general, the residual blood pressure gradient across the arch is higher with angioplasty than with surgery. Balloon angioplasty could be considered in selected patients for whom surgery is a relatively high risk. This would include patients with severe LV dysfunction, pulmonary hypertension, pulmonary disease, or recent intracranial hemorrhage. Balloon angioplasty with simultaneous stent placement should be considered in teenagers and adults with discrete coarctation. Surgery for discrete coarctation usually involves resection of the narrowed segment and variations of an end-to-end anastomosis that allow for subsequent arch growth. For recurrent coarctation, there is consensus for a catheter angioplasty (with stent placement in older patients) because of its efficacy and better safety record.

The older the patient is at the time of coarctation repair, the greater the likelihood of chronic systemic hypertension. Postoperative hypertension can be treated with β-blockers and ACE inhibitors. High blood pressure in postoperative infants who do not have a significant residual pressure gradient often improves over a few months, and the medications can be gradually weaned. These patients should be followed at regular intervals to manage residual hypertension and to screen for recurrent coarctation. Those who have had balloon angioplasty or surgery need follow-up for aneurysm development. All patients with a history of repaired coarctation who are likely to play competitive high-intensity sports should have an exercise stress test at least once before starting and periodically with growth. These children and adolescents, whose blood pressure may be in the normal or borderline-high range at rest, may have an exaggerated blood pressure response to exercise.

Aortic Insufficiency

(See Table 4-6.)

Aortic insufficiency (AI) results form incomplete closure of the aortic valve. BAV with stenosis may develop AI. Patients with perimembranous or conal septal hypoplasia VSD may present with AI, which may be an indication for VSD closure even in small defects. Subaortic stenosis directs a turbulent jet of blood toward the aortic valve and over time can lead to AI. Endocarditis, usually of a congenitally abnormal valve, or rheumatic fever should be considered when a child presents with a new finding of AI. In patients with a dilated aortic root or mitral valve prolapse, Marfan and Ehlers-Danlos syndromes should be considered.

In order to maintain adequate cardiac output with AI, the left ventricle has to increase stroke volume proportionate to the additional volume burden. The LV becomes dilated and hypertrophied.

Table 4-6 Aortic Insufficiency

Associations	Bicuspid aortic valve; rheumatic fever; VSDs (i.e., conoventricular or conal septal hypoplasia); Marfan syndrome and other connective tissue disorders
Symptoms	Mild: no symptoms
	Moderate to severe: CHF with exercise intolerance; atypical angina; syncope; sudden death
Signs	Soft diastolic murmur at left mid-sternal border, heard better when patient upright or leaning forward
	Systolic murmur if associated aortic stenosis
	Moderate to severe: hyperdynamic precordium, precordial impulse displaced laterally; widened pulse pressure and bounding pulses
ECG	LVH, possibly with strain
Chest x-ray	Moderate to severe: cardiomegaly; left atrial enlargement if LV dysfunction or associated mitral insufficiency
Management	SBE prophylaxis
	Restriction from isometric exercise (e.g., football, weight lifting, wrestling)
	Consider afterload reduction
	Surgery if LV dysfunction (i.e., Ross, homograft, or prosthetic valve replacement)

Symptoms

Patients who initially have mild AI will be asymptomatic. They may only slowly progress, remaining compensated and without symptoms for decades. Endocarditis or recurrent rheumatic fever can result in rapid deterioration if severe AI develops. With increasing severity, the patient usually develops symptoms, including fatigue early in exercise, increased perspiration, and shortness of breath, suggesting the development of CHF. Patients with severe AI may develop atypical angina.

Physical Exam

The patient with mild AI usually has a diastolic murmur audible from the base to the left midsternal border and occasionally toward the apex. The murmur is usually soft and is more prominent if the patient is sitting upright or leaning forward. With significant insufficiency, the precordial impulse becomes hyperdynamic and positioned laterally. A click and an early systolic ejection murmur suggest a BAV. With increasing severity, bounding pulses develop in association with a wide pulse pressure, caused by a decrease in the diastolic pressure.

Diagnostic Testing

Cardiomegaly occurs on chest x-ray. With moderate AI, cardiomegaly can be seen on chest x-ray. Ventricular dysfunction or associated mitral regurgitation (caused by LV dilatation) results in left atrial enlargement or pulmonary edema. On ECG, LVH is typical. Inverted T waves or left atrial enlargement correlate with ventricular dysfunction.

Echo is useful to define the valve morphology, the LV dimensions, and ventricular function. Although the chamber is expected to dilate to some extent, a significantly dilated LV end-systolic diameter correlates with ventricular failure, as does a low shortening fraction. MRI has a role in the patient who has poor image windows for echo. It can quantify ventricular function and the degree of AI.

For the patients whose AI is not well-demonstrated by noninvasive means, there are well-defined angiographic quantification criteria for grading AI by cardiac catheterization.

Management

Patients with more than mild AI should avoid strenuous isometric exercises such as football, weight lifting, or wrestling. Such activities cause acute increases in systemic vascular resistance and thus increase systolic blood pressure; this can worsen the AI and hasten its progression. Afterload-reducing agents such as ACE inhibitors are frequently used for medical management, although there is no solid clinical evidence that medications benefit patients with AI. The exception has been adults who also have hypertension.[10] The timing of surgery in a patient without symptoms needs to be based on the details of the individual patient and can provide a management dilemma. Patients with moderate AI should undergo surgery if ventricular function is even mildly impaired. Occasionally, the aortic valve can be repaired, depending on the details of its morphology. If it is not repairable, the options include a Ross procedure or valve replacement with an allograft or a prosthetic valve.

Pulmonary Stenosis

Pulmonary stenosis (PS) may occur at the valvar, subvalvar, or supravalvar levels. In addition, there may be RV outflow tract (RVOT) obstruction caused by an abnormal RV muscle bundle (i.e., double-chambered RV). In *valvar* defects, the pulmonary valve leaflets are thickened, with fused or absent commissures (Table 4-7). The RV can be normal in size, although in cases of neonatal critical PS, the RV is variably hypoplastic. Patients with Noonan's syndrome have a characteristic pulmonary valve dysplasia. *Subvalvar* (i.e., infundibular) PS is rare in isolation but is usually seen with in patients with tetralogy of Fallot.

Table 4-7	**Pulmonary Stenosis (Valvar)**
Symptoms	Mild: none
	Moderate to severe: exertional dyspnea, right heart failure, sudden death
Signs	Moderate to severe: RV tap and thrill. Systolic ejection murmur at LUSB with radiation to back and/or axillae.
ECG	Moderate to severe: RAD, RVH (with strain if severe), possible RAE
Chest x-ray	Moderate to severe: enlarged MPA segment
Management	SBE prophylaxis
	Balloon valvuloplasty for moderate, severe or critical (neonatal) PS
	Surgical relief

Supravalvar PS can involve main or proximal branch pulmonary arteries either discretely or caused by segmental hypoplasia, and is associated with congenital rubella; Williams syndrome; LEOPARD syndrome (lentigines, ECG abnormalities, ocular hypertelorism, pulmonary stenosis, abnormalities of genitalia, retardation of growth, and deafness); or Alagille syndrome.

Symptoms and Natural History

Patients with mild PS are asymptomatic. In severe cases, patients may present with exertional dyspnea, easy fatigability, right heart failure, or, rarely, sudden death. Newborns with critical PS have tachypnea, poor feeding, and cyanosis from an atrial-level right-to-left shunt.

Children ≤2 years of age with mild to moderate PS may develop increased stenosis, requiring intervention. Patients with gradients <25 mmHg (i.e., mild PS) are unlikely to have progression of the stenosis. In the newborn with mild to moderate PS, the prognosis can be initially difficult to predict since the pulmonary vascular resistance may not have declined sufficiently to accurately determine the gradient across the valve. Some newborns with "immature valves" and very mild PS can resolve spontaneously. Older infants and children with mild PS rarely have worsening of the PS. The risk for infective endocarditis is relatively low. Right heart failure may develop in patients with severe PS. Sudden death during vigorous physical activity has been reported in patients with severe PS.

Physical Exam

Most patients are acyanotic and well-developed. There may be a RV tap and a systolic thrill at the LUSB. In cases of valvar PS, there is a systolic ejection click at the LUSB. S_2 may be widely split with a diminished P_2. The murmur is heard in systole and has a characteristic "crescendo-decrescendo" quality. It is best heard at the LUSB and radiates into to the back and axillae. The loudness and length of the murmur generally correspond to the severity of the stenosis.

Diagnostic Studies

The ECG is normal in mild PS, whereas in moderate PS there is right axis deviation (RAD) and RVH. In severe PS, there may be right atrial enlargement (RAE) and RVH with strain. Neonates with critical PS may show LVH since the RV is hypoplastic and LV forces are dominant.

The chest x-ray shows a normal heart size (in the absence of CHF). The MPA segment is enlarged. Pulmonary vascular markings are usually normal.

Echo can show thickened pulmonary valve leaflets with restricted systolic excursion (i.e., "doming"). Poststenotic MPA dilatation is seen. Dysplastic valves have a characteristic thickening and immobile leaflets. Doppler evaluation can estimate the peak instantaneous pressure gradient across the narrowed orifice by using the simplified Bernoulli equation. There is not a strict consensus in grading the stenoses. Generally, a gradient < 40 mmHg is considered mild, 40–70 is moderate, and > 70 mmHg is considered severe PS. The Doppler peak instantaneous gradient overestimates the "peak-to-peak" gradients obtained at cardiac catheterization.

Management

SBE prophylaxis should be observed. Patients who have an RV systolic pressure greater than half systemic (usually, a catheter-measured gradient > 50 mmHg) should undergo treatment. Balloon valvuloplasty by catheterization is the procedure of choice for valvar PS and usually provides good results except for dysplastic pulmonary valves in which the commissures are already open. If the catheter technique does not provide adequate reduction in PS or if sub-PS is present, surgery will be required. Immediately after relief of the PS, some patients will have transient muscular dynamic RVOT obstruction caused by the sudden decompression of a hypertrophied ventricle (i.e., "suicide RV"). Newborns with critical PS require urgent intervention regardless of the valve gradient.

Pulmonary Insufficiency

Significant congenital pulmonary insufficiency (PI) is relatively uncommon in pediatrics and usually occurs in association with other lesions. In the modern era of surgery, PI is increasingly encountered in the postoperative state, for example, in patients with tetralogy of Fallot who have undergone repair with a transannular patch. The RV and PA dilate over time due to the volume load. Although this is better tolerated than aortic insufficiency, patients with long-standing severe PI can develop symptoms of exercise intolerance and easy fatigability and, potentially, can suffer sudden cardiac death from ventricular arrhythmias. On exam, patients have a decrescendo diastolic murmur that is heard best along the left sternal border. The murmur is usually low-pitched unless there is pulmonary hypertension. Chest x-ray shows a dilated RV and a prominent PA segment, and the ECG shows RVH or right bundle branch block. The incidental finding of very mild PI by color-flow echo Doppler is a normal variant.

Mitral Stenosis

Isolated congenital mitral stenosis (MS) is uncommon in pediatrics. The presence of any left-sided obstructive lesions (e.g., AS or coarctation of the aorta) warrants careful evaluation of the mitral valve to insure its adequacy. In some cases, mitral stenosis is caused not only by a small annular orifice, but also by a small effective orifice due to structural abnormalities of the chordae, by the papillary muscles, or both. Examples include mitral valve *arcade* (in which the chordae are short or nonexistent) and *parachute* mitral valve (in which there is only one papillary muscle). In these cases, there is restriction of blood flow at the subannular level. Mitral stenosis secondary to rheumatic fever is rare in the United States but may be seen in children and adolescents from other countries.

Rarely, MS may occur in association with a supravalvar mitral ring, AS, and coarctation, described as Shone's complex.

Significant MS causes an increase in left atrial pressure, and the LA dilates. The increased pressure is transmitted to the pulmonary veins and can lead to pulmonary venous congestion and pulmonary edema, causing the typical symptoms of the disease. Pulmonary venous hypertension can, in turn, lead to reflex pulmonary artery constriction and pulmonary artery hypertension.

Symptoms and Physical Exam

If the MS is moderate to severe, patients will present with symptoms of pulmonary venous congestion, such as orthopnea and dyspnea on exertion. On examination, patients may have tachypnea or respiratory distress. Auscultation reveals a mid-diastolic rumble, loudest at the apex, and in some cases, an opening snap.

Diagnostic Studies

Chest x-rays show pulmonary venous congestion and pulmonary edema. Deviation of a nasogastric tube to the right (caused by a dilated left atrium pushing the esophagus to the right) is a classic finding on chest films. The ECG may show LA enlargement. Atrial fibrillation may develop in older patients with long-standing

mitral stenosis. In patients who have developed pulmonary artery hypertension, there can be prominence of the PA segment on chest films and evidence of RVH on the ECG.

Echo can provide critical data regarding the degree and type of stenosis. Two-dimensional imaging can show the morphology and function of the mitral valve apparatus. Thickened, poorly mobile leaflets suggest a history of rheumatic disease, whereas the presence of only a single papillary muscle would indicate parachute mitral valve. Color Doppler can help define the level of obstruction, whereas pulse or continuous-wave Doppler imaging can estimate the mean gradient across the valve.

Management

Patients with mild MS rarely need treatment. Initial medical management of MS generally involves diuretics to relieve pulmonary edema and to reduce symptoms. Surgical valvuloplasty can succeed in selected patients; patients with severe MS generally require mitral valve replacement with a prosthetic valve and need anticoagulation for life. In infants and small children in whom the mitral annulus is too small to accommodate the prosthesis, the device may be placed in the supra-annular position.

Mitral Regurgitation

Because of congenital or acquired abnormalities, the mitral valve can be regurgitant, and, as a result, during systole, the LV pumps a fraction of the blood back into the left atrium. The LA and LV become dilated with moderate to severe degrees of regurgitation because the regurgitant blood represents a volume load. The mitral valve annulus may become dilated, which worsens the degree of mitral regurgitation (MR). Over time, progressive dilatation of the LA may result in atrial arrhythmias, particularly atrial flutter or fibrillation. In addition, with severe degrees of regurgitation, the LA pressure increases, which increases pulmonary venous pressure, resulting in pulmonary venous congestion.

Congenital cleft mitral valves, all of which are endocardial cushion defects but only a very few not forms of CAVC, can initially be competent but develop gradually, increasing regurgitation. Isolated mitral valve prolapse (MVP) is unusual in infants and usually presents in the older child or adolescent. The redundant pliable valve leaflets flex posterior to the valve annulus into the left atrium in systole, leading to incompetence and MR. MVP is associated with Marfan syndrome, Ehlers-Danlos syndrome, or other connective tissue disorders. In addition, diseases such as lupus, rheumatic heart disease, or bacterial endocarditis can result in rapid development of MR.

Symptoms

Patients with mild to moderate MR may not have symptoms. At higher grades of MR, infants have poor weight gain and increased work of breathing; older children can develop fatigue, shortness of breath, or palpitations. Some individuals with excellent ventricular function may tolerate quite significant MR for years without symptoms. If MR is left untreated, pulmonary hypertension, atrial arrhythmias, and CHF can develop. These patients are prone to have more frequent and severe pulmonary infections.

Physical Exam

The typical MR murmur is pansystolic and loudest at the apex, with radiation to the left axilla. It is higher pitched and has a blowing quality, compared with a VSD murmur. MVP can result in a midsystolic click noted between the apex and sternum; this can be best appreciated by having the patient rise from a squatting to a standing position. A low-pitched mid-diastolic rumble may be heard at the apex, representing increased flow across the mitral valve in diastole. Patients with severe MR may have a palpable LV heave and an audible gallop.

Diagnostic Studies

With increasing severity of MR, ECG shows LVH and left atrial enlargement (LAE). Older patients with long-standing MR may exhibit atrial fibrillation. Chest x-ray shows an enlarged left heart border and LA. With LA enlargement, the left bronchus may deviate superiorly.

ECHO shows a dilated LV and LA. Abnormal structure of the mitral valve can often be appreciated (e.g., a cleft or the thickened leaflets of rheumatic heart disease). Color Doppler shows the regurgitant jet, and the severity of regurgitation can be assessed. In the older patient, transesophageal echocardiography (TEE) may be needed to demonstrate vegetations if endocarditis is suspected.

Management

SBE prophylaxis should be observed. In moderate to severe cases, afterload-reducing agents such as ACE inhibitors can improve cardiac output. If the LA is markedly dilated or if pulmonary congestion develops, diuretics are indicated. Patients with moderate-to-severe or severe MR should have surgical repair or replacement of the valve. Ideally, the patient should have valve repair while the ventricular function is preserved. Placing a prosthetic valve in a young child commits the child to anticoagulation as well as a subsequent reoperation to replace the valve, necessitated by growth of the child. In infants with CAVC, most surgeons will address the cleft in the mitral valve at the time of the canal repair, even if there is minimal regurgitation. With rheumatic mitral regurgitation, there is a significant incidence of spontaneous resolution over several years.

MAJOR POINTS

- Acyanotic congenital heart defects can be subdivided into *left-to-right shunt* lesions and *non-shunt* lesions. The non-shunt lesions can in turn be divided into *obstructive* and *regurgitant* lesions.
- Left-to-right lesions cause volume loading of the heart and pulmonary overcirculation. Involved cardiac structures become dilated in response to the volume load. Symptoms of CHF are generally related to the amount of blood that is shunted to the lungs and to increased pulmonary pressure.
- In obstructive lesions there is a resistance to blood flow, which causes a pressure gradient across the obstruction. The pressures proximal to the obstruction are elevated in order to produce normal pressures distal to it; corresponding proximal structures hypertrophy to achieve this increased pressure (i.e., *pressure load*). There is turbulent blood flow and poststenotic dilation of vessels.
- In regurgitant lesions, the structures on either side of the lesion have to accommodate an increased volume of blood (i.e., *volume load*). They become dilated in response to the increased volume; this causes the majority of symptoms in affected patients.
- With severe obstruction or regurgitation, cardiac output can become compromised, and over time, involved ventricles may fail.

REFERENCES

1. Meier B, Lock JE: Contemporary management of patent foramen ovale. *Circulation* 107(1):5–9, 2003.

2. Mainwaring RD, Mirali-Akbar H, Lamberti JJ, Moore JW: Secundum-type atrial septal defects with failure to thrive in the first year of life. *J Card Surg* 11(2):116–120, 1996.

3. Steele PM, Fuster V, Cohen M, et al: Isolated atrial septal defect with pulmonary vascular obstructive disease: long-term follow-up and prediction of outcome after surgical correction. *Circulation* 76(5):1037–1042, 1987.

4. Feltes TF, et al (for the Cardiac Synagis Group): Palivizumab prophylaxis reduces hospitalization due to respiratory syncytial virus in young children with hemodynamically significant congenital heart disease. *Pediatr* 14:532–540, 2003.

5. Basso C, Boschello M, Perrone C, et al: An echocardiographic survey of primary school children for bicuspid aortic valve. *Am J Cardiol* 93(5):661–663, 2004.

6. Wagner HR, Ellison RC, Keane JF, et al: Clinical course of aortic stenosis. *Circulation* 56(2):147–156, 1977.

7. Graham JP, Bricker TT, James FW, Strong WB: 26th Bethesda Conference: Recommendations for determining eligibility for competition in athletes with cardiovascular abnormalities. *J Am Coll Cardiol* 24(4):845–899, 1994.

8. Rao PS, Galal O, Smith PA, Wilson AD: Five- to nine-year follow-up results of balloon angioplasty of native aortic coarctation in infants and children. *J Am Coll Cardiol* 27(2):462–470, 1996.

9. Simon P, Aschauer C, Moidl R, et al: Growth of the pulmonary autograft after the Ross operation in childhood. *Eur J Cardiothorac Surg* 19(2):118–121, 2001.

10. Borer JS, Bonow RO: Contemporary approach to aortic and mitral regurgitation. *Circulation* 108(20):2432–2438, 2003.

CHAPTER 5

Cardiomyopathy

P. NELSON LE

MARYANNE R.K. CHRISANT

Dilated Cardiomyopathy
Hypertrophic Cardiomyopathy
Restrictive Cardiomyopathy
Noncompaction Cardiomyopathy
Myocarditis
Summary

Cardiomyopathy is defined as disease of the myocardium. It is uncommon and accounts for only 1% of all pediatric cardiac disease. Originally used to describe myocardial disease not attributable to coronary artery disease, the definition has been revised to now refer to structural and functional abnormalities of the myocardium that are not secondary to hypertension, congenital heart disease, valvular abnormalities, or pulmonary vascular disease.

There are three main classifications of cardiomyopathy, representing primary disease of the heart muscle: dilated, hypertrophic, and restrictive. These diagnoses differ in their clinical presentation, management, and prognosis. A fourth type, spongiform or noncompaction cardiomyopathy, may have features of each type (e.g., a spongy-appearing, hypertrophied but poorly contractile ventricle). This chapter reviews the signs and symptoms, etiologies, diagnostic modalities and findings, therapeutic options, and long-term outcomes of these classifications of cardiomyopathy.

Myocarditis, or inflammation of the myocardium, causes systolic dysfunction, low cardiac output, and, often, arrhythmia. Patients present with heart failure, and the underlying process may be misidentified as dilated cardiomyopathy. Myocarditis is discussed at the end of this chapter.

DILATED CARDIOMYOPATHY

Dilated cardiomyopathy (DCM) is the most common myocardial disease in childhood. Different studies have reported the incidence to range from 0.4 to 8.0 cases per 100,000 people, with a prevalence of 36 cases per 100,000 people. The hallmark of DCM is systolic dysfunction. From this clinical finding stem the characteristic presenting signs and symptoms and the classic diagnostic features. With a better understanding of the pathophysiology and etiology of DCM, management of these patients has been tailored to better treat these symptoms and prevent life-threatening sequelae.

In children, the etiology of the majority of cases remains unidentified or idiopathic. Severe infections and overwhelming systemic inflammation may cause severe systolic dysfunction and may masquerade as DCM. Myocarditis may also be mistaken for DCM. The estimated percentage ranges from 2% to 15% (diagnosed by endomyocardial biopsy) as a percentage of DCM cases; the percentage is slightly higher in children less than 2 years of age. In children, coronary artery disease occurs rarely and then as a feature of a systemic process such as Kawasaki disease, hypercholesterolemia, and vascular abnormalities (such as infantile coronary calcinosis). With the advent of molecular investigation, familial forms of DCM have been described.

There are multiple patterns of inheritance in familial DCM, with autosomal dominant being the most common. Because of derangements in immune regulatory mechanisms seen in a large percentage of patients with DCM, there is a strong suggestion that loci for human leukocyte antigens on chromosome 6 may serve as markers for susceptibility. Thus far, no specific gene has been marked responsible for autosomal dominant familial DCM. However, six genes are under investigation; one of these genes is on chromosome 15q14 and is known to code for actin. Neuromuscular diseases due to genetic mutations, such as that found in Xp21, located in the dystrophin gene locus, cause Duchenne's syndrome and Becker's muscular dystrophy; both of these disorders have cardiomyopathy as a prominent feature. Another X-linked disorder, Barth syndrome, is caused by a mutation in Xq28 responsible for the tafazzin gene. Barth syndrome has cardiac muscle and skeletal muscle involvement and can present with dilated or noncompaction cardiomyopathy.

DCM has also been seen to develop after exposure to chemotherapeutic agents, mainly anthracyclines, some environmental toxins, and recreational drugs such as cocaine. Inborn errors of metabolism have been associated with DCM; some of these disorders follow a mitochondrial inheritance pattern.

Regardless of the etiology, depressed cardiac function is the common feature in all forms of DCM. Initially, cardiac output is maintained despite decreasing contractile function by increased end-systolic and end-diastolic volumes creating increased wall tension. The increased wall tension stimulates myocyte hypertrophy and normalizes cardiac output. In order to accommodate this increased volume, the ventricle dilates. As the contractile function continues to diminish, the dilation and wall tension continue to increase because of pooling of intracavitary blood. At this point, the increased wall tension decreases myocardial efficiency and increases myocardial oxygen consumption. Eventually, this compensatory mechanism is not sufficient to maintain adequate cardiac output. Additional stress, such as febrile illnesses or exercise, may bring out symptoms. Diminished cardiac output results in hypoperfusion of organs and may cause end-organ damage. Decreased renal blood flow activates the renin-angiotensin system to help maintain perfusion pressure by promoting fluid retention, vasoconstriction of peripheral vasculature, and potentiating catecholamines. At the expense of an increased afterload, vasoconstriction maintains perfusion to vital organs. The sympathetic nervous system is stimulated and results in an increase in heart rate and contractility. The failing ventricle continues to dilate because of poor antegrade blood flow. The stretch on the cardiac myocytes distorts the conduction system, and the patient is susceptible to both atrial and ventricular arrhythmias. The progression of symptoms is dependent on the acuity of the decompensation.

The diagnosis of DCM, also referred to as congestive cardiomyopathy, is made from history, physical exam, and testing. Commonly, the initial presenting symptom is respiratory distress secondary to pulmonary edema from congestive heart failure. In infants, a history of decreased oral intake, poor weight gain, diaphoresis, irritability, easy fatigability, or increasing tachypnea during feeding is classic. Failure to thrive is often a chief complaint. In older patients, orthopnea, paroxysmal nocturnal dyspnea, dyspnea on exertion, and exercise intolerance may be elicited in the history. A recent misdiagnosis of bronchitis or asthma is not uncommon. This is either due to pulmonary congestion or to an enlarged heart compressing bronchioles and causing atelectasis. In some cases, palpitations or syncope can be the presenting symptom.

The physical exam findings depend on the severity of the disease, the rate of progression of systolic dysfunction, and the development of congestive heart failure. Tachypnea and tachycardia are two cardinal findings. Pallor may be present; mottled, cold extremities clearly indicate marginal cardiac output. Jugular venous distension, hepatomegaly, and peripheral edema are signs of poor systolic function and venous congestion. These physical findings are more easily identifiable in older children. External jugular vein distention is indicative of elevated right atrial pressure, and internal jugular vein distention (i.e., prominent v wave) reflects the severity of tricuspid regurgitation. On auscultation, the heart sounds may be diminished or muffled. There may be a systolic murmur, depending on the degree of mitral regurgitation. Mitral regurgitation is usually a result of a dilated mitral valve annulus or papillary muscle dysfunction. Third heart sounds (i.e., gallop rhythms) are often present. Palpation of the precordium usually reveals a diffuse and displaced left ventricular impulse. With advancing pulmonary edema, wheezing and rales may be heard. In infants, intercostal retractions and diaphoresis are commonly seen, whereas rales are less commonly heard. The physical findings in patients with chronic heart failure are not as reflective of severity of systolic dysfunction. With long-standing subclinical elevation of left ventricular filling pressures, the pulmonary vasculature and lymphatic drainage are able to acclimate to this change in hemodynamics. Patients may look relatively well, with reasonable growth and development and few symptoms. With the additional burden of a viral illness or other physiologic stress, these patients are at risk for acute cardiac decompensation, hypotension, and shock. Full resuscitation, including intravenous inotropic support and mechanical ventilation, is often necessary at this state. A thorough physical exam must be performed to asses for the presence of associated syndromes. Metabolic, neurologic, and genetic evaluations are appropriate in patients with idiopathic DCM (Box 5-1).

DCM often is first suspected after discovering cardiomegaly on a chest x-ray. The cardiomegaly is caused by left atrial and left ventricular enlargement or by biatrial enlargement when biventricular myopathy is present. Depending on the degree of diminished function, pulmonary venous congestion, pulmonary edema, or Kerley B lines, or a combination thereof, may be present. In cases in which there is severe cardiomegaly, segmental atelectasis may be seen, caused by compression of a mainstem bronchus. It is important to review the chest x-ray thoroughly since certain syndromes associated with DCM have skeletal abnormalities (Fig. 5-1).

The most characteristic finding on electrocardiogram is sinus tachycardia. Left ventricular hypertrophy, left atrial enlargement, and nonspecific ST segment and T-wave abnormalities are common. Because there has

Box 5-1   Clinical Findings in Dilated Cardiomyopathy

SIGNS AND SYMPTOMS

- Respiratory distress secondary to congestive heart failure
- Decreased oral intake
- Poor weight gain
- Irritability
- Diaphoresis
- Easy fatigability
- Resting tachypnea and/or increasing tachypnea during feeding
- Failure to thrive
- Orthopnea
- Paroxysmal nocturnal dyspnea
- Dyspnea on exertion
- Exercise intolerance
- Palpitations
- Syncope

PHYSICAL EXAM FINDINGS

- Tachycardia
- Tachypnea
- Hypotension
- Pallor
- Displaced and/or diffuse left ventricular point of maximal impulse
- Diminished or muffled heart sounds
- Third heart sounds or gallop rhythm
- Systolic murmur depending on degree of mitral regurgitation
- Jugular venous distention
- Wheezing and/or rales
- Hepatomegaly
- Peripheral edema
- Shock in severe congestive heart failure

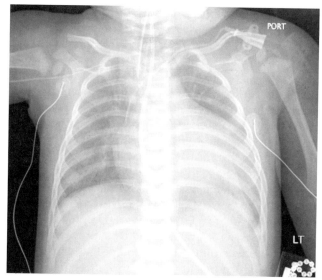

Figure 5-1   Chest x-ray with cardiomegaly in a patient with DCM.

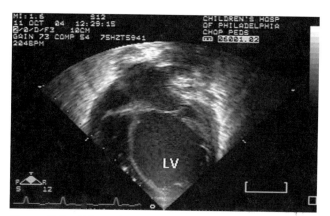

Figure 5-2   Echocardiogram demonstrating an enlarged left ventricle *(LV)* in a patient with DCM.

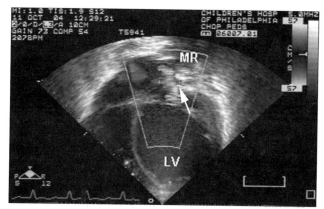

Figure 5-3   With this Doppler, there is a jet *(arrow)* representing mitral regurgitation *(MR)* from a dilated left ventricle *(LV)*.

been some association with the Wolff–Parkinson–White syndrome, delta waves may be seen in some patients. It is unclear if atrial or ventricular arrhythmias predominate, but patients with DCM can have supraventricular tachycardia, ventricular tachycardia, and ventricular fibrillation.

Echocardiography is useful for evaluation of function in patients with DCM. Besides demonstrating a dilated left ventricle and left atrium, the echocardiogram will show a decreased shortening fraction, decreased mean circumferential fiber shortening, and increased ratio of left ventricular pre-ejection period to ejection time (Fig. 5-2). Because of the distortion of the left-sided structures, there often is regurgitation across a stretched mitral valve (Fig. 5-3).

Although rarely used as a primary diagnostic tool for DCM, cardiac catheterization still has a role in delineating coronary anatomy and left-sided obstructive lesions. An aortic root injection is vital in evaluating these patients because an anomalous left coronary artery from the pulmonary artery (ALCAPA) can cause myocardial ischemia and subsequent dilation. Because of the increased afterload, severe left-sided obstructive lesions such as coarctation can cause weakening of the myocardium and abnormal systolic function. Hemodynamic evaluation can provide an accurate assessment of the gradient across the lesion and can indicate whether surgical intervention is necessary. Another use of cardiac catheterization in DCM patients is to obtain an endomyocardial biopsy. Biopsy specimens can differentiate DCM from acute myocarditis. In some forms of DCM, a biopsy can determine the etiology and therapy can then be tailored appropriately.

Blood tests in the evaluation of DCM provide valuable information regarding etiology and prognosis. Genetic testing for mutations in the genes localized for familial DCM should be pursued. Mutations in the dystrophin gene should be analyzed. Urine organic acids and amino acids should be ordered to screen for Barth syndrome. Mitochondrial gene mutations may reveal an underlying mitochondrial cytopathy.

The main goals of treatment in patients with DCM are supportive therapy and prevention of complications such as thromboembolic events and significant arrhythmias; patients who do not have end-stage disease may graduate to an optimized oral regimen that has the potential to slow disease progression. Supportive therapy focuses on improving cardiac function and treating signs and symptoms of congestive heart failure. Dopamine, dobutamine, and milrinone are the three inotropes of choice for an acute decompensation. Dopamine at renal doses can improve renal perfusion and can enhance diuresis. Milrinone is an afterload-reducing agent and decreases the amount of work on the left ventricle. Dobutamine is a pure β agonist, increases myocardial contractility, and is a mild peripheral vasodilator. These medications are discussed in detail elsewhere in this text. Diuresis is essential to controlling signs and symptoms of congestive heart failure. Intravenous diuretic therapy is used during an acute decompensation and can be transitioned over to oral therapy once the systemic or venous congestions, or both, are better managed. It is critical to monitor electrolytes during initiation or escalation of diuretic therapy since electrolyte imbalances can lead to life-threatening arrhythmias.

Optimized oral therapy for symptomatic pediatric patients with dilated cardiomyopathy includes digoxin, an angiotensin-converting enzyme (ACE) inhibitor, an oral diuretic, an aldosterone-antagonist (usually spironolactone), and a beta-receptor antagonist (usually carvedilol or metoprolol). The humoral regulation afforded by ACE inhibition, aldosterone inhibition, and beta-receptor blockade is the cornerstone of heart failure therapy. Data from the adult heart failure literature attest to the therapeutic and survival benefits of these medications.

Optimized therapy for symptomatic pediatric patients may forestall progression of cardiomyopathy.

Patients with DCM often have life-threatening arrhythmias and the use of antiarrhythmics is common. For tachyarrhythmias, amiodarone has been shown to be effective and safe in children. Many antiarrhythmics are proarrhythmic and must be used with caution. Cardioversion or defibrillation is necessary if the arrhythmia does not resolve on its own and is life-threatening. For bradyarrhythmias, temporary pacing may be required. The use of sequential atrioventricular pacing remains a controversial topic. In many cases of arrhythmias in DCM patients, correction of electrolyte or metabolic derangements and augmenting cardiac function is sufficient treatment.

Due to the severe dilation of the ventricle and potential for hemostasis, patients with DCM are placed on anticoagulation therapy to prevent thromboembolic events. Aspirin is usually the first line for prevention of thrombus formation; however, patients with severe dysfunction may better benefit from more aggressive therapy. If a thrombus is identified, heparin therapy should be initiated. Once anticoagulation has been achieved, the patient can be transitioned to warfarin for outpatient management.

Unfortunately, many patients with DCM have progressive ventricular dysfunction and require further support. Ventricular-assist devices are often implanted. Although some patients recover sufficient function and may be weaned off the device, most patients remain on the ventricular-assist device until transplantation. In some cases, extracorporeal membrane oxygenation (ECMO) therapy is used while waiting for transplant.

HYPERTROPHIC CARDIOMYOPATHY

After dilated cardiomyopathy, hypertrophic cardiomyopathy (HCM) is the second most common form in children. Although the true prevalence of HCM is unknown, there are estimated to be 10 to 100 cases per 100,000 people. HCM is a class of heterogeneous diseases of myocyte contractile proteins. Historically, the classical definition of HCM has been excessive septal hypertrophy that may or may not lead to outflow tract obstruction. With a better understanding of the etiologies and pathophysiology of HCM, many types of this cardiomyopathy have been identified. Some of these include idiopathic hypertrophic subaortic stenosis (IHSS), apical HCM, and symmetrical HCM. In the past decade, the discovery of genetic defects potentially causing or contributing to the development of HCM has improved the diagnosis and management of this disease.

The onset of symptoms usually occurs in early adulthood for most patients with HCM. Many patients will report chest pain, palpitations, dyspnea, or syncope. Chest pain may be attributed to subendocardial or myocardial ischemia. Palpitations may be due to atrial or ventricular arrhythmia or ectopy. Dyspnea is indicative of increased left atrial pressure and may be a sign of increasing outflow tract obstruction or mitral regurgitation. Syncope is concerning for severe outflow tract obstruction and atrial or ventricular arrhythmia. These clinical manifestations are signs of worsening disease and require intervention. The most severe complication from HCM is sudden unexpected death. The overall incidence has been reported at between 4% and 6% in children and adolescents and between 1% and 4% in adults. Between the ages of 12 and 35 years and in young athletes, HCM is the most common cause of sudden death. In a recent study of causes of sudden death in 387 young athletes, hypertrophic cardiomyopathy was the etiology in 26.4% of the cases.

Ventricular arrhythmia is thought to be the underlying mechanism. Even with a better understanding of the mechanisms leading to sudden death, it remains difficult to predict which patients with HCM will present with sudden death. Many factors have been offered as prognostic indicators for being at higher risk for sudden death. Of these, the most compelling is previous history of aborted sudden death or family history of sudden death. Other factors include (1) exercise-induced hypotension, (2) myocardial scarring and perfusion defects, (3) inducible ventricular tachycardia by electrophysiologic study, and (4) decreased left ventricular ejection fraction and increased left ventricular end-diastolic pressure. Nonsustained ventricular tachycardia has been associated with an increased risk. The factors that have not been associated with increased risk for sudden death are presence or absence of symptoms, severity of left ventricular outflow tract obstruction, or abnormal signal-averaged electrocardiogram. Left ventricular hypertrophy by itself has not been proven to be a good predictor of sudden death.

The clinical manifestations of HCM can be explained by three distinct mechanisms. These three findings are diastolic dysfunction, outflow tract obstruction, and mitral regurgitation. For many patients, the first clinical manifestation is a systolic murmur heard on routine examination. This murmur is due to the progressive ventricular wall hypertrophy, causing partial ventricular cavity obliteration and outflow tract obstruction. This obstruction is dynamic and is dependent on the filling pressures, afterload, and force of contractility. Unlike patients with aortic stenosis, which is a fixed obstruction to blood flow, the obstruction seen in patients with HCM changes in severity depending on the force of the contraction and the dimensions of the left ventricle. Normally, blood pressure is maintained during vasodilation by an increase in cardiac output. In patients with HCM, outflow tract obstruction may prevent an increase in cardiac output, resulting in hypotension and syncope. The obstruction is dynamic, because in resting states, it is less or is not present. The obstruction becomes clini-

cally evident with increased contractility or smaller left ventricle (LV) dimensions. In patients with HCM, a classic finding on physical examination is augmentation of the systolic murmur while standing, caused by decreased filling pressures leading to smaller left ventricle volume and an increased gradient across the outflow tract.

Mitral regurgitation can be seen in patients with HCM. This finding is confirmed by echocardiogram because it is usually mild in severity. The mechanism behind the mitral regurgitation is thought to be malpositioning of the mitral valve anteriorly during mid-systole, which interferes with mitral valve closure. The systolic anterior motion (SAM) of the mitral valve contributes to the outflow tract obstruction.

As the ventricle continues to hypertrophy, diastolic dysfunction becomes clinically significant. With decreased compliance, higher pressures are required to fill the ventricle. These high pressures are transmitted, resulting in higher left atrial, pulmonary venous and arterial, right ventricular, and right atrial pressures. Patients with severe diastolic dysfunction usually present with signs of congestive heart failure (i.e., dyspnea on exertion, resting tachypnea, orthopnea, hepatomegaly, and increased jugular venous pressure) (Box 5-2).

HCM traditionally has been inherited in a Mendelian autosomal dominant pattern with incomplete penetrance. Over 90% of reported cases are considered to be inherited. Relatives of affected patients often carry the genetic mutation but do not have echocardiographic evidence of HCM. Recent genetic studies over the past decade have implicated specific genetic mutations encoding sarcomeric proteins as major contributors to the development and progression of this disease.

Box 5-2 Clinical Findings in Hypertrophic Cardiomyopathy

SIGNS AND SYMPTOMS
- Chest pain
- Palpitations
- Dyspnea
- Syncope
- Sudden death
- In severe cases, signs of pulmonary congestion (i.e., dyspnea on exertion, resting tachypnea, orthopnea, and paroxysmal nocturnal dyspnea)

PHYSICAL EXAM FINDINGS
- Systolic murmur, loudest when standing or after exercise
- Jugular venous distention
- Hepatomegaly
- Peripheral edema

These proteins include β-myosin heavy-chain, cardiac troponin T and troponin I, α-tropomyosin, myosin binding protein C, and regulatory and essential myosin light chain. There have been over 30 point mutations identified in the β-myosin heavy-chain gene. Some other loci that have been implicated are 14q1, 1q31 (i.e., troponin T), 11p13–q13, and 15q2 (i.e., α-tropomyosin). Depending on the mutation, severity of myocyte hypertrophy, disarray, and fibrosis can vary phenotypically.

One important revelation in the pathophysiology of HCM is the handling of calcium by cardiac myocytes. Intracellular calcium is known to regulate contractile function and relaxation by its coordinated release and sequestration from the sarcolemma and sarcoplasmic reticulum. As the cardiac myocyte begins to hypertrophy, there is an increase in release of intracellular calcium; the amplitude of the calcium release diminishes as the myocyte continues to hypertrophy. This results in a significant increase in calcium release during diastole, which leads to diastolic dysfunction. Calcineurin, a calcium-regulated phosphatase, has been shown to play a role in the progression of cardiac myocyte hypertrophy and heart failure in the transgenic mouse and human heart. Applying this knowledge, calcineurin inhibitors may have a future role in managing HCM.

Metabolic disorders have been identified as a cause of HCM, primarily mitochondrial fatty acid oxidation and oxidative phosphorylation. The inheritance pattern of genetic mutations accounting for errors in fatty acid oxidation is autosomal recessive. The pathogenesis of HCM in these patients is not clearly understood. One proposed mechanism is myocyte damage secondary to inadequate myocardial energy supply and arrhythmias secondary to toxic effects of elevated intracellular intermediate fatty acid metabolites. Defects in oxidative phosphorylation are maternally inherited (i.e., mitochondrial inheritance) and also arise from spontaneous mitochondrial DNA mutations. Mitochondrial mutations are commonly associated with HCM.

There are additional syndromes that have been associated with HCM, such as Wolff-Parkinson-White syndrome. In one family, a link to chromosome 7 was seen in all of the affected family members. Some noncardiac syndromes associated with HCM are Noonan's syndrome, Beckwith-Wiedemann syndrome, infiltrative disorders (i.e., Hurler's syndrome, Hunter's syndrome), storage diseases (i.e., Fabry's disease, Pompe's disease), and other metabolic derangements.

Making the diagnosis of HCM requires an accurate and precise history and physical exam. Once there is suspicion of HCM, further evaluation of the anatomy and hemodynamics is necessary. The echocardiogram is the gold standard for diagnosing HCM. Depending on the results of the evaluation, appropriate management can be tailored.

The electrocardiogram is abnormal in most patients with HCM. Left ventricular hypertrophy is the most common finding (Fig. 5-4). ST segment changes and T-wave inversion, left atrial enlargement, abnormal Q waves, and diminished or absent R waves in the lateral leads have been seen. In the apical form of HCM, there are characteristic "giant" negative T waves. In some patients, preexcitation may be present.

On echocardiogram, the three principal features of HCM are left ventricular hypertrophy, an intraventricular pressure gradient, and systolic anterior motion of the mitral valve. The criterion used to determine hypertrophy has been a ratio greater than 1.5 when comparing the interventricular septal wall thickness to the posterior wall thickness in diastole (Fig. 5-5). The most precise way to demonstrate the intraventricular pressure gradient is to use continuous-wave Doppler measurements in the left ventricular outflow tract. Systolic anterior motion of the anterior leaflet of the mitral valve is abnormal. Its anterior motion during systole obstructs the left ventricular outflow tract (Fig. 5-6). In addition to these cardinal findings on echocardiogram, there is often a small left ventricular cavity, reduced septal wall motion, mitral valve prolapse, reduced rate of mitral valve closure secondary to decreased left ventricular compliance, abnormal mitral inflow pattern, and partial or coarse systolic closure of the aortic valve, caused by turbulent flow.

Although cardiac catheterization is not typically used as a diagnostic tool in HCM, it can be useful to evaluate diastolic dysfunction and monitor hemodynamics. Because of the intraventricular pressure gradient, higher left ventricular end diastolic pressures are required to maintain left ventricular filling. As the pressure in the left ventricle increases, left atrial and pulmonary capillary wedge pressures rise concomitantly. Diastolic dysfunction alters the manner in which the left ventricle fills. The rapid filling phase is prolonged and occurs mainly during atrial contraction. This is seen as accentuated "a" waves on the left atrial or pulmonary capillary wedge pressure recordings. During a cardiac catheterization, provocative tests are performed to evaluate the severity of the left ventricular outflow obstruction. This can be done by decreasing afterload or preload, or both, or increasing contractility. Because the obstruction is dynamic, the waveform that is seen has a characteristic "spike and dome" morphology. The spike is caused by the initial rapid increase in aortic pressure, which is then followed by a slight decrease in pressure and finally a dome, which represents a secondary peak pressure. In children, right ventricular outflow tract obstruction can be seen, depending on the severity of the hypertrophy. In some cases, it may be even more severe than the left ventricular outflow tract obstruction.

The primary aim in treating HCM is improving ventricular compliance and minimizing the risk of life-threatening

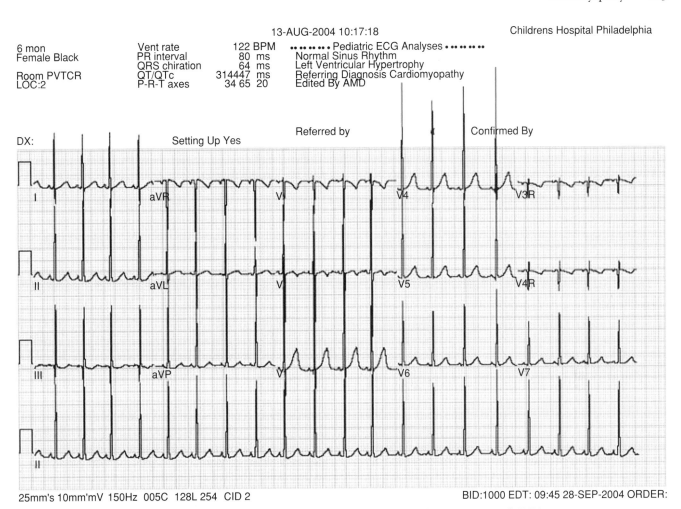

13-AUG-2004 10:17:18

Figure 5-4   ECG demonstrating left ventricular hypertrophy in a patient with HCM.

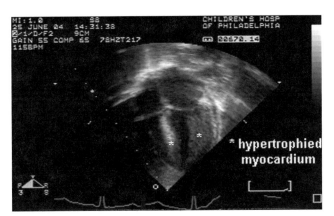

Figure 5-5   Echocardiogram shows hypertrophied myocardium (*) on both the free and septal walls of the left ventricle.

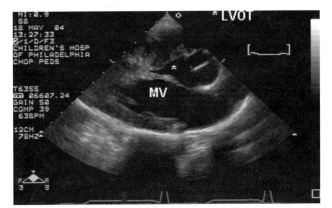

Figure 5-6   During systole, the anterior motion of the mitral valve *(MV)* obliterates the left ventricular outflow tract *(LVOT)* in patients with HCM.

arrhythmias and sudden death. Treating asymptomatic patients remains a controversial topic. There is no evidence that prophylactic treatment will reduce the risk of sudden death. β-blockers, calcium-channel blockers, or disopyramide, or a combination thereof, remains the first-line medical therapy in treating symptomatic patients. β-blockers have been shown to improve diastolic function by reducing the heart rate and isovolumic relaxation time. It is theorized that there is improvement in late diastolic filling and in coronary reserve by minimizing coronary fibrosis and enhancing distal coronary perfusion. In addition, β-blockers improve symptoms of exertional angina and dyspnea by inhibiting the sympathetic stimulation of the heart, which then decreases the catecholamine-sensitive obstruction of the left ventricular outflow tract. β-blockers are thought to diminish myocardial oxygen demand by reducing heart rate, left ventricular contractility, and myocardial wall stress during systole. Calcium-channel blockers have been shown to improve symptoms and exercise capacity in patients with HCM, regardless of whether obstruction is present or not. These agents reduce cytosolic calcium concentrations and improve diastolic function by lessening abnormalities of myocardial relaxation. Calcium-channel blockers decrease myocardial oxygen demand and improve regions of subendocardial coronary underperfusion.

There have been some studies that refute the role of calcium-channel blockers in the management of HCM. These studies state that even though calcium-channel blockers do normalize diastolic filling, there is a commensurate rise in left ventricular end-diastolic pressure and a lengthening of the diastolic relaxation time. They argue that improved diastolic filling does not indicate improved ventricular relaxation and compliance. Disopyramide is used in treating HCM for its potential to decrease subaortic obstruction by acting as a negative inotrope. Patients report improved exercise capacity. Although not its primary use, disopyramide also has antiarrhythmic effects and can be used to manage both atrial and ventricular arrhythmias associated with HCM.

Because of the high risk of malignant ventricular dysrhythmias, antiarrhythmics are a mainstay in the medical management of HCM. Amiodarone is considered the drug of choice in the treatment of ventricular ectopy and nonsustained ventricular tachycardia in this patient population. It has been shown that amiodarone decreases QT dispersion and protects against life-threatening arrhythmias. In some studies, sudden death has occurred despite the use of a therapeutic dose. In addition, amiodarone reduces atrial arrhythmias, which is important in patients who depend on atrial contraction for ventricular filling. Sotalol has been used as an agent to treat both atrial and ventricular ectopy and has been shown to decreases QT dispersion.

For patients who remain symptomatic despite maximal medical therapy, placement of a dual-chamber pacemaker may provide some relief of the left ventricular outflow tract obstruction. Dual-chamber atrioventricular pacing is speculated to induce paradoxical interventricular septal wall motion, which increases the left ventricular outflow tract dimension and, in turn, reduces the blood velocity leaving the ventricle. This reduction in velocity reduces the systolic anterior motion of the mitral valve and lessens the mitral regurgitation. Patients with severe obstruction receive the most symptomatic

relief. In one study, symptoms were cured in 33% of the patients and reduced in 56% of the patients. Patients report improved exercise capacity and lack of symptoms on exertion. At rest, the degree of left ventricular outflow tract obstruction is significantly less. Dual-chamber atrioventricular pacing also appears to affect the left ventricle on a cellular level. In some patients, the left ventricle remodels and wall thickness is reduced. In follow-up studies, after dual-chamber pacing had been discontinued, the reduction in left ventricular outflow tract obstruction and the improvement in hemodynamic indices persisted. Although data from these early studies provided hope, subsequent studies from different investigators have not reproduced the same degree of improvement as previously cited.

Consensus guidelines have recently been developed for caring for patients with hypertrophic cardiomyopathy. The indications for use of an implantable cardioverter/defibrillator (ICD) include patients who are at high risk for sudden cardiac death. Most HCM patients at high risk for sudden cardiac death are young, asymptomatic or with few symptoms, and have preserved systolic function. Prevention of sudden death could offer these patients a normal or near-normal life expectancy. A previous episode of resuscitated sudden death, spontaneously occurring and sustained ventricular tachycardia, a strong family history of sudden death, identification of a high-risk mutant gene, and extreme left ventricular hypertrophy are strong indications for ICD implantation. Its prophylactic role in asymptomatic pediatric patients should be strongly considered as the incidence of sudden death is greatest during adolescence. It is worthwhile to note that implantable defibrillators are often quiescent for up to 9 years; this underscores the unpredictable timing of sudden death events, the life-long risk, and the need for long-term follow-up.

For patients who fail or cannot tolerate medical management, surgical myectomy or myotomy has been recommended. Once again, the indication for surgical intervention is unclear. Many studies have reported using a left ventricular outflow tract gradient of 50 mmHg or greater, regardless of symptomatology as an indication. The 10-year survival rate was reported at 86% in one study. Although the removal of the muscular obstruction reduces symptoms, the risk of life-threatening arrhythmias and sudden death does not change. For asymptomatic patients, surgical myectomy or myotomy is not recommended. The prophylactic use of this procedure in patients with a strong family history of sudden death is still controversial.

Ultimately, many patients with HCM will need a cardiac transplantation. The prognosis is variable, but the onset of systolic dysfunction and the development of congestive heart failure are associated with poor outcome. Early referral for cardiac transplantation prior to significant deterioration from a low-cardiac output state improves long-term outcome.

RESTRICTIVE CARDIOMYOPATHY

Restrictive cardiomyopathy is defined as myocardial disease in which ventricular filling is impaired. This impairment is due to increased stiffness (i.e., decreased compliance) of the ventricle causing abrupt elevation of the ventricular pressure with small changes in volume. The left upward shift of the pressure-volume curve is reflected by increased early filling and decreased late filling during diastole. The restrictive physiology behind this disease is classically characterized by four hemodynamic findings: normal systolic function, equalization of the right ventricular and left ventricular end-diastolic pressures, an increase in mean atrial and ventricular end-diastolic pressures, and a dip–plateau pattern of ventricular filling.

Although most cases of restrictive cardiomyopathy are idiopathic, it is important to fully evaluate the patient for possible systemic disease that can cause restrictive myocardial disease. Constrictive pericarditis should be considered in the differential and can cause similar signs and symptoms. The differential should include systemic lupus erythematosus, sarcoidosis, amyloidosis, infiltrative diseases (e.g., Gaucher's disease or Hurler's syndrome) and storage diseases (e.g., Fabry's disease or hemochromatosis). Thorough investigation should be undertaken to rule out constrictive pericarditis, because it is typically a remediable process.

Restrictive cardiomyopathy can affect either ventricle and symptoms of right or left ventricular dysfunction, or both, can be manifest. "Right-sided" symptoms include elevated jugular venous pressure, hepatomegaly, ascites, and peripheral edema, all of which reflect diminished right ventricular compliance and elevated systemic venous pressure. As a clinical sign, jugular venous pulsation may estimate disease severity: the jugular venous pulse fails to fall during inspiration and may actually rise (Kussmaul's sign). Long-standing or advanced disease is demonstrated by a pulsatile and enlarged liver, ascites, and peripheral edema. Patients with left-sided failure can have signs and symptoms representative of pulmonary edema, including dyspnea on exertion, paroxysmal nocturnal dyspnea, orthopnea, exercise intolerance, breathlessness, and resting tachypnea. Although these symptoms are not specific to this disease process, restrictive cardiomyopathy should be on the differential diagnosis for any patient presenting with these symptoms (Box 5-3).

To further evaluate a patient with these symptoms and determine the etiology, both screening tests and specific studies must be ordered. On chest x-ray, the size of the heart, in contrast to patients with dilated cardiomyopathy, is usually normal. Interstitial edema, Kerley B lines, and other signs of pulmonary congestion are usually present. When atrioventricular valve regurgitation is severe, there may be atrial enlargement.

An electrocardiogram in restrictive cardiomyopathy is nonspecific. There may be abnormalities in depolarization, repolarization, and conduction. Some patients may have a bundle branch block pattern or ventricular hypertrophy. Intraventricular conduction delay and varying degrees of atrioventricular block may be present. There may be ST-segment or T-wave abnormalities, or both, and these may represent ongoing subendocardial ischemia. It is not unusual for patients with restrictive cardiomyopathy to have atypical chest pain syndromes, which should be evaluated for ischemia using the electrocardiogram and cardiac enzymes [i.e., troponin and creatine phosphokinase (CPK)].

The characteristic finding on echocardiogram is an increased early diastolic filling velocity (*e wave*) and decreased atrial filling velocity (*a wave*) for the mitral valve inflow pattern (Fig. 5-7). Both of these findings on Doppler echocardiography are caused by premature cessation of ventricular filling. As the myocardium becomes more restrictive and stiff, the disparity in these velocities becomes more pronounced. On two-dimensional imaging, the heart may have a characteristic "ice cream cone" appearance with hugely dilated atria and small conical ventricles (Fig. 5-8). Mitral and tricuspid valve insufficiency may be apparent. Estimates of pulmonary arterial hypertension may be gained from echocardiogram. Pericardial echogenicity or brightness is sometimes noted and may be read as pericardial

---

Box 5-3   Clinical Findings in Restrictive Cardiomyopathy

SIGNS AND SYMPTOMS

- Dyspnea on exertion
- Paroxysmal nocturnal dyspnea
- Orthopnea
- Exercise intolerance
- Breathlessness
- Resting tachypnea
- Chest pain

PHYSICAL EXAM FINDINGS

- Jugular venous distention
- Jugular venous pulse that fails to fall and may rise with inspiration (Kussmaul's sign)
- Hepatomegaly
- Ascites
- Peripheral edema

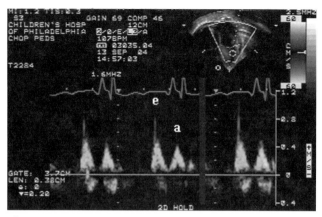

Figure 5-7 Echocardiogram demonstrating an increased early diastolic filling velocity (e wave) and decreased atrial filling velocity (a wave) for the mitral valve inflow pattern.

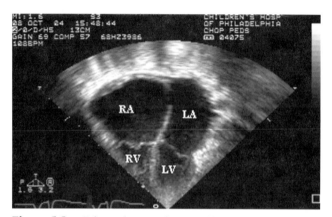

Figure 5-8 Echocardiogram showing dilated right atrium (RA) and left atrium (LA) and conical right ventricle (RV) and left ventricle (LV), which give the characteristic "ice cream cone" appearance.

inflammation, hence constrictive pericarditis. In such cases, cardiac magnetic resonance imaging (MRI) can delineate pericardial from myocardial disease.

Hemodynamic evaluation by cardiac catheterization is an important diagnostic component. During hemodynamic evaluation, rapid decline in ventricular pressure at the onset of diastole followed by a rapid rise to a plateau in early diastole is known as the "dip and plateau" or "square-root sign"; this tracing is associated with restrictive physiology. Another finding in cardiac catheterization is equalization of the left and right ventricular end-diastolic pressures. As pressure rises during ventricular filling because of the restrictive nature of the myocardium, pressure is dissipated between the two ventricles. Endomyocardial biopsy is typically not necessary and usually shows nonspecific interstitial fibrosis and myocyte hypertrophy.

The mainstay of medical therapy for patients with restrictive cardiomyopathy is symptomatic treatment.

Diuretics are used to decrease venous congestion in both systemic and pulmonary circulation but should be used judiciously because reducing the ventricular filling pressure can result in a decrease in cardiac output. Because of the increased risk for atrial arrhythmias from atrial enlargement, some patients are started on antiarrhythmics such as amiodarone to maintain sinus rhythm. The contribution of the "atrial kick" to the ventricular filling is important to preserve cardiac output. In patients with bradyarrhythmias from atrioventricular (AV) node disease, pacemakers are used to maintain an adequate heart rate to prevent hypoperfusion and end-organ damage. Because of the atrial dilation and risk of thrombus formation and embolic events, warfarin or low molecular weight heparin is part of the medical management of these patients. Due to the natural history of this disease and the poor prognosis, patients with restrictive cardiomyopathy often require cardiac transplantation for long-term survival. In patients with systemic disease as the cause of the cardiomyopathy, the extent of the underlying illness and its prognosis must be fully explored before proposing cardiac transplantation as a treatment option.

NONCOMPACTION CARDIOMYOPATHY

Noncompaction or spongiform cardiomyopathy is thought to be due to persistence of embryonal myocardial tissue, represented by a loosely interwoven mesh of immature myocytes. Characteristic echocardiographic findings include prominent trabeculations and deep intertrabecular cavitations. The immature myocardium has abnormal systolic function; low cardiac output may be the first sign of cardiac disease. Infants may present with a picture similar to dilated cardiomyopathy and with diminished cardiac output. With time, some patients improve as the affected myocardium hypertrophies; systolic function improves, and as the process progresses, restrictive physiology may be apparent. Noncompaction is seen most typically in children; however, there are some reports of noncompaction cardiomyopathy found incidentally or as a result of a heart failure evaluation in adults. A diagnosis of noncompaction cardiomyopathy merits a thorough metabolic, neuromuscular, and genetic evaluation; noncompaction is not uncommonly seen with Barth syndrome.

MYOCARDITIS

Myocarditis is defined as inflammation of the heart muscle. In 1897, Emmet Holt described this process in his book, *The Diseases of Infancy and Children*. "Myocarditis may...occur at any age, even in foetal life. As seen in children, it is almost invariably a secondary lesion, usually the result of some infectious process....In many cases in which advanced lesions have been found at autopsy, there have been no symptoms during life, and in others none until the occurrence of sudden death." Over 100 years later, our understanding of the disease process remains limited.

The working etiologic hypothesis favors that myocarditis develops in response to some stimulation that causes the immune system to overexpress components, resulting in inflammation and myocyte damage. These imbalances include an abnormal ratio between helper and killer T cells, inappropriate expression of major histocompatibility complexes (MHCs) on cardiac tissue, and circulating autoantibodies. The potential exists for the autoimmune response to eventually resolve. To some degree, these theories are supported by in vitro and animal studies.

Myocarditis typically is a silent disease until the onset of fulminant heart failure and severe respiratory distress, arrhythmia, shock, cardiogenic collapse, or sudden death. A presumptive diagnosis may be based on patient history, which often includes a viral prodrome; clinical signs and symptoms of congestive cardiac failure; echocardiographic evidence of ventricular dysfunction; and supporting evidence on electrocardiogram such as left bundle branch block pattern, ischemic changes, or low voltage, especially in the lateral precordial leads. Although definitive diagnosis may be elusive, further diagnostic testing provides contributory evidence. Blood testing may reveal elevated C-reactive proteins, erythrocyte sedimentation rates, white blood cell counts, and platelet counts. Elevations in hepatic enzymes suggest an associated hepatitis. Measurement of creatine kinase and cardiac troponin T and troponin I can provide evidence of myocardial cell damage. Peripheral viral culture and serology results are typically slow to obtain, often inconclusive, and rarely helpful during the acute phase. Definitive proof of viral etiology may be provided by polymerase chain reaction (PCR), which can rapidly detect the presence of viral nucleic acid in infected tissues and fluids. This process amplifies viral DNA, making sufficient quantities for virus identification. Adenovirus, enterovirus, parvovirus B19, coxsackie virus, and herpes virus have all been implicated as causative agents of myocarditis. Although potentially useful, PCR testing is not routinely available from commercial laboratories.

Direct tissue examination obtained by endomyocardial biopsy may show histological signs of inflammation (i.e., mononuclear or lymphocytic cellular infiltration and edema) with or without myocyte damage or necrosis. Disparities exist, however, in the reported incidence of myocarditis based on biopsy evidence, and this may be due to differences in patient selection (as myocarditis is more common in children than in adults), diagnostic criteria, and the limitations imposed by light microscopy in detecting inflammatory disease. Nonetheless, positive findings on light microscopy evaluation of myocardial tissue are diagnostic for myocarditis, although negative results do not necessarily eliminate this diagnosis.

Different types of myocarditis include idiopathic giant cell myocarditis, which on biopsy reveals macrophage-derived giant cells. Although more commonly described in adults, this process can occur in infants and children, is rapidly progressive, and often is fatal unless cardiac transplantation is implemented. Hypersensitivity myocarditis occurs after some stimulating exposure, such as to an antibiotic or other medication, which initiates a consequent allergic reaction. This type of myocarditis appears as a predominantly eosinophilic infiltrate on endomyocardial biopsy. Viral myocarditis is the most common etiology of myocardial inflammation in the pediatric age group.

Because most patients afflicted with myocarditis present with symptoms of cardiac failure, the primary line of treatment must be supportive. Intravenous diuresis, inotropic support, and mechanical ventilation for patients with more severe failure may be required during the immediate presentation. Maintenance of cardiac output in the presence of rapidly failing myocardium may require rapid institution of circulatory support with ECMO or another ventricular assist device. Some advocate that supporting the heart through the acute phase of myocarditis will allow for healing to occur and potential full resolution of symptoms. This is one possible outcome for this disease and may occur in up to 45% of patients; fulminant, unremitting progression is also a likely outcome, occurring in about 30%. Cardiac transplantation has been lifesaving in such cases.

The immunologic component of myocarditis has lead many physicians to believe that immunosuppression and anti-inflammatory therapy should be beneficial to patients with this disease. Many uncontrolled clinical trials and case series reports support the use of immunoglobulin, as well as combination therapy including steroids, azathioprine, cyclosporine, cyclophosphamide, and other immunosuppressant medications. When confronted with a progressively failing heart and a diagnosis that strongly suggests myocarditis, it is not inappropriate to use such interventions. The only definitive answer to the application of immunologic manipulation rests in a blinded, multicenter clinical trial. In about 25% of cases, the active myocarditis phase resolves but is followed by a chronic dilated cardiomyopathy. On endomyocardial biopsy, the inflammatory findings are replaced by fibrosis. Some patients are left with stable cardiac dysfunction; ongoing therapy with ACE inhibitors and beta-blocking agents may arrest progression of the chronic phase of this disease. In other patients, dysfunction is progressive and, ultimately, cardiac transplantation is necessary.

SUMMARY

As molecular and genetic research continues to elucidate the etiologies of cardiomyopathy and myocarditis, and new diagnostic tools and therapies are invented, the understanding of the pathophysiology and management of patients with these entities is constantly evolving. Patients will be diagnosed earlier in their disease process. Optimal medical therapy will be instituted earlier, reducing morbidity and mortality. Through early diagnosis and enhanced medical management, patients are living longer. Important lifestyle modifications such as the inclusion of moderate exercise, nutrition, and medical compliance have improved the quality of life for these patients.

MAJOR POINTS

- Cardiomyopathy accounts for only 1% of all pediatric cardiac disease.
- DCM is the most common myocardial disease in childhood (0.4–8.0 cases per 100,000 people, with a prevalence of 36 cases per 100,000 people).
- The hallmark of DCM is systolic dysfunction.
- In children, the etiology of the majority of cases of DCM remains unidentified or idiopathic.
- There are multiple patterns of inheritance in familial DCM, with autosomal dominant being the most common; six genes have been localized.
- In infants with DCM, failure to thrive is often a chief complaint. In older patients, the initial presenting symptom is respiratory distress, secondary to pulmonary edema from congestive heart failure.
- The main goals of treatment for patients with DCM are supportive therapy to improve cardiac function and prevention of complications such as thromboembolic events and significant arrhythmias.
- The prevalence of HCM is estimated to be 10–100 cases per 100,000 people.
- The onset of symptoms usually occurs in early adulthood for most patients with HCM.
- The most severe complication of HCM is sudden death. The incidence of sudden death has been reported at between 4–6% in children and 1–4% in adults.
- The clinical manifestations of HCM can be explained by diastolic dysfunction, outflow tract obstruction, and mitral regurgitation.
- Over 90% of reported cases of HCM are considered to be inherited.
- Some noncardiac syndromes associated with HCM are Noonan's, Beckwith-Wiedemann, Hurler's, Hunter's, as well as Fabry's and Pompe's diseases.
- The primary aim in treating HCM is improving ventricular compliance and minimizing the risk of life-threatening arrhythmias and sudden death.

MAJOR POINTS—CONT'D

- Amiodarone is considered the drug of choice in the treatment of ventricular ectopy and nonsustained ventricular tachycardia in this patient population.
- Most cases of RCM are idiopathic.
- The restrictive physiology is classically characterized by four hemodynamic findings: normal systolic function, equalization of the right ventricular and left ventricular end-diastolic pressures, an increase in mean atrial and ventricular end-diastolic pressures, and a dip-plateau pattern of ventricular filling.
- The mainstay of medical therapy for patients with restrictive cardiomyopathy is symptomatic treatment.
- Noncompaction or spongiform cardiomyopathy is thought to be due to persistence of embryonal myocardial tissue, represented by a loosely interwoven mesh of immature myocytes.
- Cardiac transplantation may be the treatment of choice for many patients with progressive or end-stage cardiomyopathic disease.
- The working etiologic hypothesis favors that myocarditis develops in response to some stimulation that causes the immune system to overexpress components, resulting in inflammation and myocyte damage.
- The immunologic component of myocarditis has guided the treatment regimen to include immunosuppression and anti-inflammatory agents.

REFERENCES

1. Akagi T, Benson LN, Lightfoot NE, et al: Natural history of dilated cardiomyopathy in children. *Am Heart J* 121: 1502–1506, 1991.

2. Ammash NM, Seward JB, Bailey KR, et al: Clinical profile and outcome of idiopathic restrictive cardiomyopathy. *Circulation* 101(21):2490–2496, 2000.

3. Arola A, Tuominen J, Ruuskanen O, Jokinen, E: Idiopathic dilated cardiomyopathy in children: prognostic indicators and outcome. *J Pediatr* 101(3):369–376, 1998.

4. Bruns LA, Chrisant MK, Lamour JM, et al: Carvedilol as therapy in pediatric heart failure: an initial multicenter experience. *J Pediatr* 138(4):505–511, 2001.

5. *Burch M, Blair E:* The inheritance of hypertrophic cardiomyopathy. Pediatr Cardiol 20:313–316, 1999.

6. Chan KY, Iwahara M, Benson LN, et al: Immunosuppressive therapy in the management of acute myocarditis in children: a clinical trial. *J Am Coll Cardiol* 17:458–460, 1991.

7. Charron P, Dubourg O, Desnos M: Diagnostic value of electrocardiography and echocardiography for familial hypertrophic cardiomyopathy in genotyped children. *Eur Heart J* 19:1377–1382, 1998.

8. Drucker NA, Colan SD, Lewis AB, et al: γ-Globulin treatment of acute myocarditis in the pediatric population. *Circulation* 89(1):252–257, 1994.

9. Duncan BW, Bohn DJ, Atz AM, et al: Mechanical circulatory support for the treatment of children with acute fulminant myocarditis. *J Thorac Cardiovasc Surg* 122(3):440-448, 2001.

10. Fananapazir L: Advances in molecular genetics and management of hypertrophic cardiomyopathy. *JAMA* 281(18):1746-1752, 1999.

11. Feldman AM, McNamara D: Myocarditis. *N Engl J Med* 343(19):1388-1398, 2000.

12. Gajarski RJ, Towbin JA: Recent advances in the etiology, diagnosis, and treatment of myocarditis and cardiomyopathies in children. *Curr Opin* 7:587-594, 1995.

13. Kelly DP, Strauss AW: Mechanisms of disease: Inherited cardiomyopathies. *N Engl J Med* 330(13):913-919, 1994.

14. Kleinert S, Weintraub RG, Wilkinson JL, Chow CW: Myocarditis in children with dilated cardiomyopathy: incidence and outcome after dual therapy immunosuppression. *J Heart Lung Transplant* 16(12):1248-1254, 1997.

15. Kushwaha SS, Fallon JT, Fuster V: Restrictive cardiomyopathy. *N Engl J Med* 336(4):267-276, 1997.

16. Lauer B, Neiderau C, Kuhl U, et al: Cardiac troponin T in patients with clinically suspected myocarditis. *J Am Coll Cardiol* 30(5):1354-1359, 1997.

17. Leiden JM: The genetics of dilated cardiomyopathy—emerging clues to the puzzle. *N Engl J Med* 337(15):1080-1081, 1997.

18. Lewis AB, Chabot M: Outcome of infants and children with dilated cardiomyopathy. *Am J Cardiol* 68:365-369, 1991.

19. Lipshultz SE, Sleeper LA, Towbin JA, et al: The incidence of pediatric cardiomyopathy in two regions of the United States. *N Engl J Med* 348(17):1647-1655, 2003.

20. Maron BJ: Sudden death in young athletes. *N Engl J Med* 349:1064-1075, 2003.

21. Maron BJ, McKenna WJ, Danielson GK, et al: American College of Cardiology/European Society of Cardiology clinical expert consensus document on hypertrophic cardiomyopathy: A report of the American College of Cardiology Foundation Task Force on Clinical Expert Consensus Documents and the European Society of Cardiology Committee for Practice Guidelines. *J Am Coll Cardiol* 42:1687-1713, 2003.

22. Martin AB, Webber S, Fricker J, et al: Acute Myocarditis: Rapid diagnosis by PCR in children. *Circulation* 90(1):330-339, 1994.

23. McNamara DM, Rosenblum WD, Janosko KM, et al: Intravenous immune globulin in the therapy of myocarditis and acute cardiomyopathy. *Circulation* 95(11):2476-2478, 1997.

24. Nishimura RA, Holmes Jr DR: Hypertrophic Obstructive Cardiomyopathy. *N Engl J Med* 350(13):1320-1327, 2004.

25. Packer M, Colucci WS, Sackner-Bernstein JD, et al: Double-blind, placebo-controlled study of the effects of carvedilol in patients with moderate to severe heart failure: the PRECISE Trial (Prospective Randomized Evaluation of Carvedilol on Symptoms and Exercise). *Circulation* 94(11):2793-2799, 1996.

26. Runge MS, Sheahan RG, Stouffer GA (eds): Hypertrophic cardiomyopathy: Presentation and pathophysiology. Cardiology grand rounds from the University of Texas Medical Branch. *Am J Med Sci* 314(5):324-329, 1997.

27. Seidman CE, Seidman JG: Molecular genetic studies of familial hypertrophic cardiomyopathy. *Basic Res Cardiol* 93:Suppl 3, 13-16, 1998.

28. Spirito P, Seidman CE, McKenna WJ, Maron BJ: The management of hypertrophic cardiomyopathy. *N Engl J Med* 336(11):775-785, 1997.

29. Towbin JA: Pediatric myocardial disease. *Pediatr Clin North Am* 46(2):289-312, 1999.

30. Towbin JA, Bowles KR, Bowles NE: Etiologies of cardiomyopathy and heart failure. *Nat Med* 5(3):266-267, 1999.

31. Yetman AT, Hamilton RM, Benson LN, McCrindle BW: Long-term outcome and prognostic determinants in children with hypertrophic cardiomyopathy. *J Am Coll Cardiol* 32(7):1943-1950, 1998.

Acquired Heart Disease

STEPHEN PARIDON

INFECTIOUS ENDOCARDITIS

Infectious endocarditis (IE) is a condition that results primarily from bacterial and fungal infection of those structures in the heart lined by endocardium. The clinical and laboratory spectrum of IE's presentation in children has evolved considerably over the last three decades. This has occurred as a consequence of changes in the makeup of this population, changes in medical technology and practice, and the evolution of the organisms responsible for IE in children. Fortunately, despite a growing frequency of IE, the morbidity and mortality continues to decrease as a consequence of improved diagnostic and therapeutic techniques.

Epidemiology

The overall incidence of IE in developed countries is uncertain. Among adults in the United States, the overall number of new cases are in the range of 15,000–20,000 yearly.[1] A study of a medium-sized urban area in Sweden found an overall yearly incidence of the entire population of 6.2 per 100,000. The incidence in children appears to be less than in adults, and the overall incidence of IE appears to increase with the age of the population.[2,3]

Nonetheless, IE accounts for approximately 1 in 1280 pediatric admissions per year, according to a study by Van Hare *et al.* from the mid 1980s.[4]

There is little doubt that the epidemiology of IE in children has changed significantly in the last 30 years. Prior to the 1970s, rheumatic heart disease accounted for anywhere between 30% and 50% of the cases of IE. With the dramatic decrease in acute rheumatic fever in the developed countries, rheumatic heart disease has become rare and is no longer a significant source of new cases of IE.

At the same time, the overall incidence of IE in children has been increasing, and the age at presentation has become older.[3-6] The average age of presentation has increased from about 5 years of age in the 1950s to 10 years of age in the current era.[4,5] This trend appears to be due to congenital heart disease now accounting for most of the cases of IE. As the rate of survival of congenital heart disease continues to improve, this population increases both in size and age. This results in both the increasing incidence and the older age of the patients at presentation.

Despite the overall increase in the age of the patients, IE in neonates has also risen dramatically.[3,4] This is due primarily to the rapid advances in neonatal life support over the past 30 years. The majority of these patients are infants with structurally normal hearts in which IE develops as a consequence of infected indwelling central catheters.[3,4,7]

Incidence in Congenital Heart Disease

It is clear that the incidence of IE is not uniform throughout the spectrum of congenital heart lesions. Those most at risk appear to be patients with lesions that result in high-velocity jets, such as semilunar valve stenosis and ventricular septal defects (VSD). In the second natural history study, the incidences of IE for aortic stenosis and VSD were 27.1 and 14.5 per 10,000 patient-years, respectively.[8] This represents a 35-fold increase in IE from the First Natural History Study.

The proportion of IE occurring after cardiac surgery is also much higher in the current era. In recent studies, postoperative patients accounted for between 50% and 70% of subjects in these series.[3,5,8,9] This increase in IE after surgery may result from several factors, including an increase in the number of surgeries performed, a longer survival of patients with complex diseases, and the more severe nature of the cardiac defects undergoing surgery. In the Second Natural History Study, the severity of aortic stenosis was a more significant predictor of IE than surgery.[8] Complex cyanotic defects, especially those involving aorta to pulmonary shunts, are at the highest risk for postsurgical IE.[3,10] The use of prosthetic material and valves also increases the risk of early postsurgically acquired IE.[4]

Pathophysiology

Infective endocarditis occurs at sites of damage to the endothelium. In congenital heart defects, these usually occur at the sites of high shear forces and would be most commonly on the low-pressure side of high-velocity, high-turbulence lesions. For this reason, IE is most common in aortic stenosis and in VSDs in unoperated children.[3,8] In operated patients, complex defects with turbulent shunts or conduits appear to be the most at risk.[10]

The damage to the endocardium increases thrombogenesis at the site of damage. This results in the formation of a nonbacterial thrombotic vegetation. In the presence of a bacteremia, this sterile vegetation may become colonized, resulting in an infected vegetation. The ability of different types of organisms to colonize sterile vegetations is quite variable. Surface structures of various organisms, especially streptococci, may influence their ability to colonize a vegetation. These organisms also include dextran and fibronectin.[3,4,11]

Once colonized, the vegetation grows both by an increase in organisms and a continued thrombus formation. The organisms that are imbedded in the thrombus are relatively isolated from the body's immune defense responses.[4,12,13] Growth of the vegetation into the surrounding myocardial tissue may result in disruption and destruction of the affected structure, such as valvular apparatus. Extension into the myocardium can result in abscess formation and damage to the conduction system (especially in VSDs). Hemodynamic compromise may result from damaged or disrupted valves. More rarely, a large vegetation can itself compromise cardiac function by obstructing blood flow.

Large or friable vegetations are more prone to embolization. The site of embolization will depend on the location of the vegetations. Lesions on the right side of the heart and in shunts will tend to embolize to the pulmonary bed. Left-sided vegetations will embolize into the systemic bed. The renal arteries are the most common site of embolization, but embolization to the brain and spleen are also commonly seen.[4,14]

The immune response to chronic infection also plays an important role in the disease process of IE. Circulating immune complexes appear to be associated with glomerulonephritis, commonly seen with IE.[15] The presence of autoantibodies have also been reported in cases of IE, suggesting an elevated nonspecific immune response to IE.[4]

Clinical Presentation

The clinical presentation of IE is extremely variable and depends on the underlying cardiac condition, the causative organism, and the patient's immunologic response. The acute fulminant IE is rare in children. When present, it may mimic acute overwhelming septicemia and shock. Cardiovascular collapse due to destruction of the cardiac valves may occur. A more acute course is commonly seen in neonatal presentation.[3,4,7,16] These infants often have no underlying structural heart disease. In the intensive care setting, this IE is often associated with placement of central indwelling catheters.[3,4,10,17]

More typically, IE is an indolent disease that progresses over days to months. The presentation is often one of prolonged low-grade fever, malaise, fatigue, and weight loss. Diaphoresis and rigors are also seen.[1,3,4,14,18] Arthralgias and gastrointestinal complaints, including persistent vomiting and nonspecific chest pain, may also occur at lower frequencies. Although none of these symptoms are specific for IE, the grouping of any number of these complaints in a child with an underlying heart disease should suggest IE.

The physical findings of IE are also quite variable and reflect the ongoing damage to the heart as well as the systemic effects of infection and the body's immune response. The finding of a heart murmur is often not helpful in diagnosing IE in the presence of a preexisting congenital defect. Changes in a previously heard murmur may be useful, especially when appreciated by a physician who is familiar with the patient's baseline auscultatory findings. Hemodynamic changes due to progressive valve destruction are uncommon but should strongly suggest IE.

The classic noncardiac physical findings of IE are due to the embolic events and the immune response of the body to infection. Although they all may occur in children, they do so at a significantly lower frequency than in adults with IE.[3,4,14,18] Petechial rash and splenomegaly are the most common of these findings, occurring in up to half of the patients. The classic findings of Osler's nodes, Janeway lesions, splinter hemorrhages, and Roth's spots generally occur in less than 10% of children with IE.

Laboratory Findings

Blood Cultures
Only about 5–7% of definitely proven IE will have persistently negative blood cultures.[1,3,14,18,19] These cases often involve very uncommon and fastidious organisms that are rarely seen in children. Blood cultures can be drawn at any time for IE because bacteriemia is usually constant. Three cultures from separate vena puncture sites should be obtained initially (5–7 mL each for children; 1–3 mL each for infants). Two more cultures should be obtained the next day if the initial cultures remain negative.[3] More than five cultures are not necessary unless the patient has had previous antibiotic treatment. The blood cultures should be held for at least 2 weeks to allow time for growth of fastidious organisms.

Acute-Phase Reactants
Erythrocytes sedimentation rate (ESR) and C-reactive protein are elevated in a large majority of children with IE.[3,4] These are nonspecific markers of infection and are seen in many other disease processes besides IE. Elevated rheumatoid factor and hypergammaglobulinemia are also seen in a significant percentage of patients.

Hematuria
Hematuria may result from glomerular damage secondary to immune complex deposits in the kidneys. Like other laboratory data, it is not specific to IE, but its presence should increase clinical suspicion.

Echocardiography
Echocardiography is an extremely important diagnostic test for IE, both for adults and children. Its use remains controversial. Data from studies of IE in adults show that standard transthoracic echocardiograms (TTE) have excellent specificity (98%) but poor sensitivity (less than 60%) in the detection of vegetations.[1] This is particularly true for small vegetations (i.e., less than 2 mL). Left-sided vegetations and vegetations with prosthetic valves were also poorly visualized. Transesophageal echocardiography (TEE) has significantly better sensitivity than TTE for both left-sided and difficult to image lesions.[1,3,4] The sensitivity of TEE for left-sided lesions, perivulvar leaks and abscesses, and infective prosthetic valves in adults ranges from 75–100% in various studies.[1,20,21] TEE has become the diagnostic method of choice for adults with moderate or high clinical suspicion of IE.[1] Figure 6-1 shows an algorithm for echocardiographic evaluation from the recent American Heart Association (AHA) statement on management of IE in adults.[1]

The role of echocardiography in diagnosing IE in children is clearly of increasing importance, but its indications are even more controversial than they are in diagnosing adults. As a screening tool for IE, data seem clear that echocardiography has a low yield. Recent studies on the use of TTE to screen for vegetations in low- to moderate-risk patients have shown poor sensitivity in diagnosing IE.[20,22,23] Earlier studies report better sensitivity and suggest that TTE is superior for diagnosing IE in children, compared with diagnosing in adults.[24] Differences in these studies no doubt reflect methodology and subject selection.

Increasingly, TEE has been used in children with suspected IE. Data are not currently available regarding the specificity and sensitivity in this modality in the diagnoses of vegetations. It would appear likely that TEE should be useful in diagnosis of vegetations associated with complex defects, especially those with artificial conduits, patches, and valves. The current AHA scientific statement on IE in childhood would support the use of TTE as a first screen tool, but use of TEE whenever the imaging is inadequate or the diagnosis remains unclear.[3]

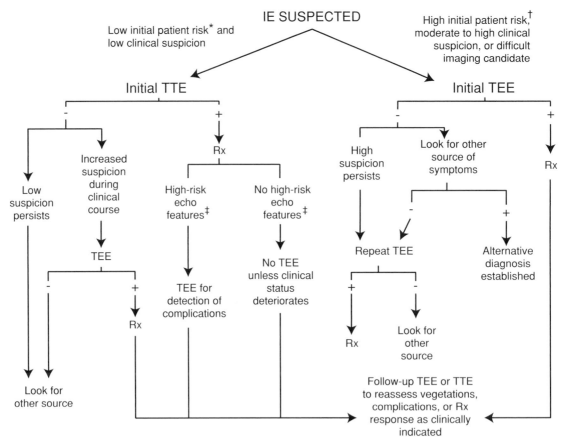

Figure 6-1 Algorithm for the diagnostic use of echocardiography. *For example, a patient with fever and a previously known heart murmur and no other stigmata of IE. †High initial patient risks include prosthetic heart valves, many congenital heart diseases, previous endocarditis, new murmur, heart failure, or other stigmata of endocarditis. ‡High-risk echocardiographic features include large and/or mobile vegetations, valvular insufficiency, suggestion of perivalvular extension, or secondary ventricular dysfunction. "Rx" indicates antibiotic treatment for endocarditis. (Adapted from Bayer AS, Bolger AF, Taubert KA, et al: Diagnosis and management of infective endocarditis and its complications. Circulation 98:2936–2948, 1998.)

Diagnosis

Diagnosis of IE may often be challenging in the absence of classical clinical and laboratory findings. In 1994, when attempting to improve diagnostic criteria, Durack et al.[25] proposed the Duke criteria for diagnosis of IE in adults. Multiple studies in adult patients have shown the Duke criteria to be superior to previous diagnostic criteria.[1] Far less data are available in children. Stockheim *et al.*[19] showed a clear superiority of the Duke criteria over the older Beth Israel criteria when retrospectively applied to 111 cases of IE in children.

Boxes 6-1 and 6-2 show the Duke criteria. The criteria are divided into major and minor criteria. Definitive IE is defined as two major criteria, one major and three minor criteria, or five minor criteria. Possible IE and rejected IE are also defined (Box 6-1). The Duke criteria are weighted heavily for the findings of blood cultures and cardiovascular manifestations. The embolic and immunologic findings, classically described in IE but now rarely seen, are all listed under minor criteria (Box 6-2).

Causative Organisms

Gram-positive cocci remain by far the largest group of causative organisms for IE in children. Within this group, there has been a change in the percentage of various types of organisms found in IE over the past several decades. A recent review by the AHA shows that the alpha-hemolytic viridans group streptococcus account for approximately 32–43% of IE in childhood.[3] Staphylococcus aureus has increased significantly as a causative agent, representing 27–33% of the cases of IE.[3] Coagulase-negative staphylococci usually make up less than 10% of cases. Gram-negative endocarditis is rare, making up less than 5% of the cases.[3,4,19] Gram-negative rods such as

Box 6-1 Criteria for Definite and Possible Infective Endocarditis, Based on the Duke Criteria

Definite Infective Endocarditis
  Pathologic criteria
    Microorganisms: demonstrated by culture
      or histology in a vegetation, or in a vegetation that
      has embolized, *or* in an intracardiac abscess, *or*
    Pathologic lesions: vegetation or intracardiac
      abscess present, confirmed by histology showing
      active endocarditis
  Clinical criteria, using specific definitions listed
    in Box 6-2
      2 major criteria, *or*
      1 major and 3 minor criteria, *or*
      5 minor criteria
Possible Infective Endocarditis
  Findings consistent with infective endocarditis that
    fall short of "definite," but not "rejected"
Rejected
  Firm alternate diagnosis for manifestations of
    endocarditis, *or*
  Resolution of manifestations of endocarditis, with
    antibiotic therapy for 4 days or less, *or*
  No pathologic evidence of infective endocarditis
    at surgery or autopsy, after antibiotic therapy for
    4 days or less

Adapted from Durack DT, Lukes AS, Bright DK. Am J Med 96:200–209, 1994.

Box 6-2 Definitions of Major and Minor Duke Criteria

MAJOR CRITERIA

Positive blood culture for infective endocarditis
  Typical microorganism for infective endocarditis from
    two separate blood cultures
    (i)   Viridans streptococci,* *Streptococcus bovis*,
          HACEK group, *or*
    (ii) Community-acquired *Staphyloccus aureus or*
          enterococci, in the absence of a primary focus, *or*
  Persistently positive blood culture, defined as
    recovery of a microorganism consistent with
    infective endocarditis from:
    (i)   Blood cultures drawn more than 12 hours
          apart, *or*
    (ii) All of three or a majority of four or more
          separate blood cultures, with first and last
          drawn at least 1 hour apart
Evidence of endocardial involvement
  Positive echocardiogram for infective endocarditis
    (i)   Oscillating intracardiac mass, on valve or
          supporting structures, *or* in the path of
          regurgitant jets, *or* on implanted material, in
          the absence of an alternative anatomic
          explanation, *or*
    (ii) Abscess, *or*
    (iii) New partial dehiscence of prosthetic valve, *or*
  New valvular regurgitation (increase or change in
    pre-existing murmur not sufficient)

MINOR CRITERIA

Predisposition: predisposing heart condition *or*
  intravenous drug use
Fever: ≥ 38.0°C (100.4°F)
Vascular phenomena: major arterial emboli, septic
  pulmonary infarcts, mycotic aneurysm, intracranial
  hemorrhage, conjunctival hemorrhages, Janeway
  lesions
Immunologic phenomena: glomerulonephritis, Osler's
  nodes, Roth spots, rheumatoid factor
Microbiologic evidence: positive blood culture but
  not meeting major criterion as noted previously *or*
  serologic evidence of active infection with
  organism consistent with infective endocarditis
Echocardiogram: consistent with infective
  endocarditis but not meeting major criterion
  as noted previously

Adapted From Durack DT, Lukes AS, Bright DK. Am J Med 96:200–209, 1994.
HACEK = *Haemophilus* spp., *Actinobacillus actinomycetemcomitans*,
Cardiobacterium hominis, *Eikenella* spp., and *Kingella kingae*.
*Including nutritional variant strains.
† Excluding single positive cultures for coagulase-negative staphylococci and
organisms that do not cause endocarditis

Pseudomonas are sometimes seen in burn and immunologically compromised patients, often in a hospital setting. The *Haemophilus, Actinobacillus, Cardiobacterium, Eikenella, Kingella* (HACEK) group include gram-negative coccobacilli, primarily *Haemophilus* species, as well as *Actinobacillus* species and *Eikenella* species. These rarely cause IE in adults and are extremely rare in children.[1,3,4,14]

The changing nature of the gram-positive cocci infection reflects the changing settings in which IE now occurs. In older children who have acquired IE in a community setting and have not undergone a recent surgery, viridans streptococcus is the most likely organism; in about 5% of patients, enterococcus is the cause.[3,4,19] *Staphylococcus aureus* and coagulase-negative staphylococcus are primarily organisms seen following surgery and in neonatal IE. These cases usually present within the first 60 days after surgery or are associated with catheter placement in infants.[3,7,16,17]

Fungal endocarditis in children is most commonly seen in infants.[7,19] *Candida* species are the most commonly isolated organisms. Of the filamentous fungus, Aspergillus may also cause IE. In a recent series of adults and children from Brazil, *Candida* species accounted for 95 of 152 cases, and *Aspergillus* caused another

28 cases.[26] In this series, predisposing factors, in addition to cardiac lesions, included immunosuppression from chemotherapy or following either bone marrow transplantation or solid organ transplantation, as well as intravenous hyperalimentation. Thirty percent had central venous catheters.

Culture-negative endocarditis accounts for about 5% of cases.[1,3,14,19] This occurs most commonly in a setting of prior recent antibiotic therapy or when a very fastidious organism is responsible for IE. *Aspergillus* and other filamentous fungi will often have negative blood cultures but may be evident as abscesses in other body structures. The negative blood cultures in these cases may be as high as 70%.[26]

Therapy

Antimicrobial Therapy

The use of antimicrobial agents has changed over the past several decades to reflect the changing pattern of microbial sensitivity to various antibiotics. It is often necessary to consult an infectious disease specialist to determine the type of antibiotics, dosage, and duration of therapy for any individual case.[1,3] This may be particularly important when considering outpatient administration of antibiotics or when dealing with less common organisms such as gram-negative bacteria and fungal IE.

Tables 6-1 and 6-2 show the current AHA regimens for treatment of streptococci in patients who are and are not able to tolerate β-lactam antibiotics.[3] Dosages should be adjusted in individual cases to achieve appropriate levels based on the treating hospital's laboratory values. These recommendations are for patients without prosthetic material.

In the presence of prosthetic material, a 6-week course of therapy is recommended.[1,3,4] In β-lactam-sensitive cases, antibiotic therapy as listed in Table 6-2 for 6 weeks' duration is acceptable. If the minimal inhibitory concentration of penicillin is greater than 0.1 μg/mL, gentamicin should be added for 6 weeks.[3] For patients intolerant of β-lactams, vancomycin for 6 weeks plus gentamicin for the first 2 weeks is the suggested therapy.[3]

Table 6-1   Regimens for Therapy of Native Valve IE Caused by *viridans* Group Streptococci, *Streptococcus bovis*, or Enterococci

Organism	Antimicrobial Agent	Dosage (kg/24 hr)	Frequency of Administration	Duration (wk)
Penicillin-susceptible streptococci (MIC ≤0.1 μg/mL)*	Penicillin G[†] or	200,000 U IV	q 4-6 hr	4
	ceftriaxone	100 mg IV	q 24 hr	4
	Penicillin G[†] or	200,000 U IV	q 4-6 hr	2
	ceftriaxone plus	100 mg IV	q 24 hr	2
	gentamicin	3 mg IM or IV	q 8 hr*	2
Streptococci relatively resistant to penicillin (MIC >0.1-0.5 μg/mL)	Penicillin G[†] or	300,000 IV	q 4-6 hr	4
	ceftriaxone plus	100 mg IV	q 24 hr	4
	gentamicin	3 mg IM or IV	q 8 hr[‡]	2
Enterococci,[‡] nutritionally variant viridans streptococci or high-level penicillin-resistant streptococci (MIC >0.5 μg/mL)	Penicillin G[†] plus	300,000 U IV	q 4-6 hr	4-6[ǁ]
	gentamicin	3 mg IM or IV	q 8 hr[§]	4-6[ǁ]

Adapted from Ferrieri P, Gewitz MH, Gerber MA. Circulation 105(17): 2115-2126, 2002.

For treatment of patients with prosthetic cardiac valves of other prosthetic materials, see text. MIC indicates minimum inhibitory concentration of penicillin.

Dosages suggested are for patients with normal renal and hepatic function. Maximum dosages per 24 hours: penicillin 18 million units; ampicillin 12 g; ceftriaxone 4 g, gentamicin 240 mg. The 2-week regimens are not recommended for patients with symptoms of infection >3 months in duration, those with extracardiac focus of infection, myocardial abscess, mycotic aneurysm, or infection with nutritionally variant viridans streptococci (*Abiotrophia* sp.).

*Studies in adults suggest gentamicin dosage may be administered in single daily dose. If gentamicin is administered in three equally divided doses per 24 hours, adjust dosage to achieve peak and trough concentrations in serum of ≈3.0 and <1.0 μg of gentamicin per mL, respectively.

[†]Ampicillin 300 mg/kg per 24 hours in 4-6 divided dosages may be used as alternative to penicillin.

[‡]Studies in adults suggest that 4 weeks of therapy is sufficient for patients with enterococcal IE with symptoms of infection of <3 months' duration; 6 weeks of therapy is recommended for patients with symptoms of infection of >3 months' duration.

[§]Adjust gentamicin dosage to achieve peak and trough concentrations in serum of ≈3.0 and <1.0 μg of gentamicin per mL, respectively.

[ǁ]For enterococcal-resistant to penicillins, vancomycin, or aminoglycosides, treatment should be guided by consultation with specialist in infectious diseases (cephalosporins should not be used to treat enterococcal endocarditis regardless of in vitro susceptibility).

Suggested AHA treatment regimens for both coagulase-positive and coagulase-negative staphylococci are listed in Table 6-3.[3] In all cases, duration of therapy is at least 6 weeks.[1,3] Early postsurgical IE is most likely to be *Staphylococcus aureus*. This carries a worse outcome and is associated with higher mortality.[3] As such, a combination of medical and surgical therapy may be indicated (see later discussion).[3]

Treatment of less common forms of IE should be done in conjunction with an infectious disease service. Antibiotic

Table 6-2   Treatment Regimen for Therapy of IE Caused by *Viridans* Group Streptococci, *Streptococcus bovis*, and Enterococci in Patients Unable to Tolerate a β-Lactam

Organism	Antimicrobial Agent	Dosage, per kg per 24 hr	Frequency of Administration	Duration, wk
NATIVE VALVE (NO PROSTHETIC MATERIAL)				
Streptococci	Vancomycin	40 mg IV	q 6–12 hr	4–6
Enterococci* or nutritionally variant viridans streptococci	Vancomycin plus gentamicin	40 mg IV 3 mg IM or IV	q 6–12 hr q 8 hr[†]	6 6
PROSTHETIC DEVICES				
Streptococci	Vancomycin plus gentamicin	40 mg IV 3 mg IM or IV	q 6–12 hr q 8 hr[†]	6 2
Enterococci* or nutritionally variant viridans streptococci	Vancomycin plus gentamicin	40 mg IV 3 mg IM or IV	q 6–12 hr q 8 hr[†]	6 6

Adapted from Ferrieri P, Gewitz MH, Gerber MA. Circulation 105(17): 2115–2126, 2002.
Dosages suggested are for patients with normal renal function. Maximum daily dose per 24 hours of gentamicin is 240 mg.
*For enterococci resistant to vancomycin or aminoglycosides, treatment should be guided by consultation with specialist in infectious diseases.
[†]Dosage of gentamicin should be adjusted to achieve peak and trough concentration in serum of ≈3.0 and <1.0 μg of gentamicin per mL, respectively.

Table 6-3   Treatment Regimen for IE Caused by Staphylococci

Organism	Antimicrobial Agent	Dosage, per kg per 24 hr	Frequency of Administration	Duration, wk
NATIVE VALVE (NO PROSTHETIC MATERIALS)				
Methicillin susceptible	Nafcillin or oxacillin with or without gentamicin*	200 mg IV 3 mg IM or IV[†]	q 4–6 hr q 8 hr	6 wk 3–5 day
β-Lactam allergic	Cefazolin[‡] with or without gentamicin*	100 mg IV 3 mg IM or IV[†]	q 6–8 hr q 8 hr	6 wk 3–5 day
	or			
	vancomycin	40 mg IV	q 6–12 hr	6 wk
Methicillin resistant	Vancomycin	40 mg IV	q 6–12 hr	6 wk
PROSTHETIC DEVICE OR OTHER PROSTHETIC MATERIALS				
Methicillin susceptible	Nafcillin or oxacillin	200 mg IV	q 4–6 hr	≥6 wk
	or			
	cefazolin[‡]	100 mg IV	q 6–8 hr	≥6 wk
	plus rifampin[§]	20 mg po	q 8 hr	≥6 wk
	plus gentamicin*	3 mg IM or IV[†]	q 8 hr	2 wk
Methicillin resistant	Vancomycin	40 mg IV	q 6–12 hr	≥6 wk
	plus rifampin[§]	20 mg po	q 8 hr	≥6 wk
	plus gentamicin*	3 mg IM or IV[†]	q 8 hr	2 wk

Adapted from Ferrieri P, Gewitz MH, Gerber MA. Circulation 105(17): 2115–2126, 2002.
Dosages suggested are for patients with normal renal and hepatic function. Maximum daily doses per 24 hours: oxacillin or nafcillin 12 g; cefazolin 6 g; gentamicin 240 mg; rifampin 900 mg.
*Gentamicin therapy should be used only with gentamicin-susceptible strains.
[†]Dosage of gentamicin should be adjusted to achieve peak and trough concentrations in serum of ~3.0 and <1.0 μg of gentamicin per mL, respectively.
[‡]Cefazolin or other first-generation cephalosporin in equivalent dosages may be used in patients who do not have a history of immediate type hypersensitivity (urticaria, angioedema, anaphylaxis) to penicillin or ampicillin.
[§]Dosages suggested for rifampin are based on results of studies conducted in adults and should be used only with rifampin-susceptible strains.

selection for various gram-negative organisms will depend on the local sensitivities of these bacteria, especially because they are usually acquired in the hospital setting. Treatment for fungal IE remains unsatisfactory. Amphotericin B continues to be the main antifungal agent used in IE. Addition of fluconazole or 5-fluorocytosine has also been used in combination with amphotericin B.[3]

Surgical Therapy

The decision for surgical intervention must be made on an individual basis, with careful weighing of the risks involved in the therapeutic choice. There are clearly certain organisms and circumstances that predispose to the need for surgical intervention in IE.[1,3,4,26] IE with *S. aureus* is such a case. This is especially true in perioperative states in which prosthetic material is involved.[1,3] Medical therapy alone is usually unsuccessful in treating fungal infections.[1,3] This is especially true in nonyeast infections.[26]

Clinical symptoms may also dictate the need for surgical intervention. The presence of congestive heart failure is associated with the high need for surgical intervention when it occurs as a consequence of valve dysfunction or dehiscence of prosthetic material.[1,3] Other findings that may indicate the need for surgery include embolization of the vegetations or persistent or growing vegetations.[1,3] Perivalvular extension or myocardial abscess may also require surgical intervention. Myocardial abscess may be complicated by heart block when the abscess occurs near the conduction system.[1]

Prophylactic Therapy

Prophylaxis for IE has been recommended for certain populations and circumstances.[27] There obviously remain many situations in which bacteremia occurs but is not readily identifiable or treatable. Box 6-3 lists the current AHA classification for risk of IE based on heart lesions.[27] Dental procedures are a common concern for prophylaxis. Box 6-4 lists the common dental procedures that may or may not require prophylaxis.[27] Other common nondental medical procedures are listed in Box 6-5.[27]

The choice of antibiotic for prophylaxis depends on the individual patient's tolerance and the procedure requiring prophylaxis. Tables 6-4 and 6-5 show the current AHA antibiotic choices and dosages for various situations that require prophylaxis.[27]

Outcomes

Morbidity and mortality for IE in children varies greatly depending on the clinical situation. The presence of prosthetic material, perioperative infections, and infection under 2 years of age are all associated with poor outcome and higher risks of complication.[1,3-5,9,10,26] *S. aureus* infections are more likely to have poor outcomes, as are fungal infections.[3,26]

Box 6-3   Cardiac Conditions Associated with Endocarditis

ENDOCARDITIS PROPHYLAXIS RECOMMENDED

High-risk category
    Prosthetic cardiac valves, including bioprosthetic and homograft valves
    Previous bacterial endocarditis
    Complex cyanotic congenital heart disease (e.g., single ventricle states, transposition of the great arteries, tetralogy of Fallot)
    Surgically constructed systemic pulmonary shunts or conduits
Moderate-risk category
    Most other congenital cardiac malformations (other than above and below)
    Acquired valvar dysfunction (e.g., rheumatic heart disease)
    Hypertrophic cardiomyopathy
    Mitral valve prolapse with valvar regurgitation and/or thickened leaflets

ENDOCARDITIS PROPHYLAXIS NOT RECOMMENDED

Negligible-risk category (no greater risk than the general population)
    Isolated secundum atrial septal defect
    Surgical repair of atrial septal defect, ventricular septal defect, or patent ductus arteriosus (without residua beyond 6 mo)
    Previous coronary artery bypass graft surgery
    Mitral valve prolapse without valvar regurgitation
    Physiologic, functional, or innocent heart murmurs
    Previous Kawasaki disease without valvar dysfunction
    Previous rheumatic fever without valvar dysfunction
    Cardiac pacemakers (intravascular and epicardial) and implanted defibrillators

Adapted from Dajani AS, Taubert KA, Wilson W, et al. Circulation 96:358–366, 1997.

For the past decade, in series involving children and congenital heart defects, the overall mortality has ranged from 10% to 27%.[5,9,10] Mortality for fungal infection is significantly higher, approaching 50% or greater.[10,26] These outcomes represent a great improvement over earlier eras.[6] This is encouraging in view of the growing incidence of IE and the growing population of patients with congenital heart defects who are at risk for acquiring IE.

RHEUMATIC FEVER

Acute rheumatic fever (RF) has been a scourge of children and young adults for centuries. In the United States, prior to the later half of the 20th century, it remained the leading cause of cardiac disability in the young.[28-30] It remains the leading cause of heart disease in this population in much

Box 6-4 Dental Procedures and Endocarditis Prophylaxis

ENDOCARDITIS PROPHYLAXIS RECOMMENDED*

Dental extractions

Periodontal procedures including surgery, scaling and root planing, probing, and recall maintenance

Dental implant placement and reimplantation of avulsed teeth

Endodontic (root canal) instrumentation or surgery only beyond the apex

Subgingival placement of antibiotic fibers or strips

Initial placement of orthodontic bands but not brackets

Intraligamentary local anesthetic injections

Prophylactic cleaning of teeth or implants where bleeding is anticipated

ENDOCARDITIS PROPHYLAXIS NOT RECOMMENDED

Restorative dentistry[†] (operative and prosthodontic) with or without retraction cord[‡]

Local anesthetic injections (nonintraligamentary)

Intracanal endodontic treatment; postplacement and buildup

Placement of rubber dams

Postoperative suture removal

Placement of removable prosthodontic or orthodontic appliances

Taking of oral impressions

Fluoride treatments

Taking of oral radiographs

Orthodontic appliance adjustment

Shedding of primary teeth

Adapted from Dajani AS, Taubert KA, Wilson W, et al. Circulation 96:358–366, 1997.
*Prophylaxis is recommended for patients with high- and moderate-risk cardiac conditions.
[†]This includes restoration of decayed teeth (filling cavities) and replacement of missing teeth.
[‡]Clinical judgment may indicate antibiotic use in selected circumstances that may create significant bleeding.

Box 6-5 Other Procedures and Endocarditis Prophylaxis

ENDOCARDITIS PROPHYLAXIS RECOMMENDED

Respiratory tract
  Tonsillectomy and/or adenoidectomy
  Surgical operations that involve respiratory mucosa
  Bronchoscopy with a rigid bronchoscope
Gastrointestinal tract*
  Sclerotherapy for esophageal varices
  Esophageal stricture dilation
  Endoscopic retrograde cholangiography with biliary obstruction
  Biliary tract surgery
  Surgical operations that involve intestinal mucosa
Genitourinary tract
  Prostatic surgery
  Cystoscopy
  Urethral dilation

ENDOCARDITIS PROPHYLAXIS NOT RECOMMENDED

Respiratory tract
  Endotracheal intubation
  Bronchoscopy with a flexible bronchoscope, with or without biopsy[†]
  Tympanostomy tube insertion
Gastrointestinal tract
  Transesophageal echocardiography[†]
  Endoscopy with or without gastrointestinal biopsy[†]
Genitourinary tract
  Vaginal hysterectomy[†]
  Vaginal delivery[†]
  Cesarean section
  In uninfected tissue:
    Urethral catheterization
    Uterine dilatation and curettage
    Therapeutic abortion
    Sterilization procedures
    Insertion or removal of intrauterine devices
Other
  Cardiac catheterization, including balloon angioplasty
  Implanted cardiac pacemakers implanted defibrillators, and coronary stents
  Incision or biopsy of surgically scrubbed skin
  Circumcision

Adapted from Dajani AS, Taubert KA, Wilson W, et al. Circulation 96:358–366, 1997.
*Prophylaxis is recommended for high-risk patients; it is optional for medium-risk patients.
[†]Prophylaxis is optional for high-risk patients.

of the developing world.[31] In recent decades, RF has made resurgence in the United States and in other developed countries.[29] For this reason, it remains an important health problem in most areas of the world.

Etiology

It has been recognized for many decades that there is a clear association of RF with group A β-hemolytic streptococcal (GABHS) infections. As early as the 1930s, certain strains of GABHS and routes of infection were noted to result in RF. Only those strains resulting in pharyngeal infections were associated with RF. Streptococcal infections of the skin are not associated with RF but may result in poststreptococcal glomerulonephritis (PSG).[32-34]

Strains of GABHS are identified by their M proteins. These are found in the cell wall of the organism. Certain M-types are associated with RF, whereas others are associated with PSG.[27,32-34] The M-types responsible for RF

Table 6-4 Prophylactic Regimen for Dental, Oral, Respiratory Tract, and Esophageal Procedures

Situation	Agent	Regimen*
Standard general prophylaxis	Amoxicillin	Adults: 2.0 g; children: 50 mg/kg orally 1 hr before procedure
Unable to take oral medications	Ampicillin	Adults: 2.0 g IM or IV; children: 50 mg/kg IM or IV within 30 min before procedure
Allergic to penicillin	Clindamycin *or*	Adults: 600 mg; children: 20 mg/kg orally 1 hr before procedure
	Cephalexin[†] or cefadroxil[†] *or*	Adults: 2.0 g; children; 50 mg/kg orally 1 hr before procedure
	Azithromycin or clarithromycin	Adults: 500 mg; children: 15 mg/kg orally 1 hr before procedure
Allergic to penicillin and unable to take oral medications	Clindamycin *or*	Adults: 600 mg; children: 20 mg/kg IV within 30 min before procedure
	Cefazolin[†]	Adults: 1.0 g; children: 25 mg/kg IM or IV within 30 min before procedure

Adapted From Dajani AS, Taubert KA, Wilson W, et al. Circulation 96:358–366, 1997.

IM, Intramuscularly; *IV*, Intravenously.

*Total children's dose should not exceed adult dose.

[†]Cephalosporins should not be used in individuals with immediate-type hypersensitivity reaction (urticaria, angioedema, or anaphylaxis) to penicillins.

Table 6-5 Prophylactic Regimens for Genitourinary-Gastrointestinal Procedures (Excluding Esophageal Procedures)

Situation	Agents*	Regimen[†]
High-risk patients	Ampicillin plus gentamicin	Adults: ampicillin 2.0 g IM or IV plus gentamicin 1.5 mg/kg (not to exceed 120 mg) within 30 min of starting procedure; 6 hr later, ampicillin 1 g IM/IV or amoxicillin 1 g orally
		Children: ampicillin 50 mg/kg IM or IV (not to exceed 2.0 g) plus gentamicin 1.5 mg/kg within 30 min of starting the procedure; 6 hr later, ampicillin 25 mg/kg IM/IV or amoxicillin 25 mg/kg orally
High-risk patients allergic to ampicillin/amoxicillin	Vancomycin plus gentamicin	Adults: vancomycin 1.0 g IV over 1-2 hr plus gentamicin 1.5 mg/kg IV/IM (not to exceed 120 mg); complete injection/infusion within 30 min of starting procedure
		Children; vancomycin 20 mg/kg IV over 1-2 hr plus gentamicin 1.5 mg/kg IV/IM; complete injection/infusion within 30 min of starting procedure
Moderate-risk patients	Amoxicillin or ampicillin	Adults: amoxicillin 2.0 g orally 1 hr before procedure, or ampicillin 2.0 g IM/IV within 30 min of starting procedure
		Children: amoxicillin 50 mg/kg orally 1 hr before procedure, or ampicillin 50 mg/kg IM/IV within 30 min of starting procedure
Moderate-risk patients allergic to ampicillin/amoxicillin	Vancomycin	Adults: vancomycin 1.0 g IV over 1-2 hr complete infusion within 30 min of starting procedure
		Children: vancomycin 20 mg/kg IV over 1-2 hr; complete infusion within 30 min of starting procedure

Adapted from Dajani AS, Taubert KA, Wilson W, et al. Circulation 96:358–366, 1997.

IM, Intramuscularly; *IV*, Intravenously.

*Total children's dose should not exceed adult dose.

[†]No second dose of vancomycin or gentamicin is recommended.

are heavily encapsulated due to larger production of hyaluronic acid. This results in the typical mucoid appearance are seen when these organisms are cultured on blood agar. The presence of this thick capsule appears to result in much of the organism's virulence and may be lost by repeated cultures in blood agar.[29,30]

Although the precise mechanism remains unknown, it appears clear that M proteins and the virulence of these highly encapsulated strains are essential in the development of RF. This larger antigen burden results in antigens that cross-react with the infected host, setting up a breakdown in the immune tolerance. The result of this action is the body forming cross-reactive antibodies to skin, heart tissue, synovial tissue, and the basal ganglia, which are in turn responsible for the pathology seen in RF.[29,35]

Host factors are also important, both for susceptibility and for clinical expression. An immune competent host is necessary, but it is unclear whether there is a specific genetic predisposition. Attempts to date to isolate specific human haplotypes have been inconclusive.[35-37] Clinical presentation may vary with age and sex (chorea is almost never seen in adult males).[28,29]

Epidemiology

The epidemiology of RF is that of the GABHS and, more specifically, those M-types that are associated with RF. In much of the world, RF remains a disease of poverty and overcrowding. Data from developing countries are often incomplete and conflicting, but certain trends appear to be consistent. High prevalence of RF occurs in areas of increased population density, low socioeconomic status, and rapid urbanization. Access to medical care and nutrition may also be factors.[31]

In the developed countries, the epidemiology of RF is quite different. RF declined dramatically in the United States over most of the past century. This was associated with improved living conditions as well as public health measures to treat GABHS pharyngitis.[28-30] Interestingly, the prevalence of GABHS cultured from the pharynx has not decreased dramatically, compared with the fall in RF. Rather, it is the elimination of the M-types responsible for RF from the population that has resulted in this decline.[29]

This was shown clearly in the 1980s and 1990s with new outbreaks of RF in the West and among military personnel.[38-40] The mucoid strains that had previously been eliminated in these areas were again cultured from the affected individuals. These recent clustered outbreaks also occurred predominately in middle-class patients. The usual environmental factors still seen in developing countries do not appear to be significant in the recent cases in the United States and other developed countries.

Clinical Presentation

There is typically a latent period between GABHS pharyngitis and the onset of RF. This usually is 2–3 weeks but may be as short as a week and as long as 6 months. A prolonged latent phase is more commonly seen in cases presenting with Sydenham's chorea.[28-30]

The modified Jones criteria remained a diagnostic standard now, as they have over the last century. Promulgated by TD Jones in the 1950s, these criteria are still the mainstay for clinical diagnosis for RF. This was reaffirmed in 2002 by the American Heart Association.[41] They did note that these criteria should not be adhered to rigidly, and that clinical cases may occur that will not fulfill the criteria. This may be the case where there is a long latent phase or an indolent course of the disease. This results in the patient being assessed for RF perhaps months after the onset of the disease process.

The modified Jones criteria are shown in Box 6-6. The diagnosis of RF requires evidence of a recent GABHS injection plus either one major and two minor criteria or two major criteria. Evidence of a recent GABHS infection is obtained by serologic studies. The most common antibody is antistreptolysin O. Others used included antideoxyribonuclease-B, antidiphosphopyridine nucleotidase, and antihyaluronidase.[28,29]

Major Criteria

Arthritis

The arthritis of RF is usually of the large joints: knees, elbows, ankles, and wrists. The joints are hot, erythematous in appearance, and tender to palpation. The arthritis is typically migratory. It will usually diminish over several days to a week in an affected joint and will reoccur in unaffected joints. It is one of the more common major criteria, occurring in upward of 80% of patients.[1] In some patients, the initial pattern may be one of increasing multiple joint involvement rather than the typical migratory pattern.[30]

The arthritis of RF responds well to treatment with either nonsteroidal anti-inflammatory agents (NSAIDs) or corticosteroids. The joints heal without significant sequelae or deformation. Relapses of the arthritis after initial therapy may occur, requiring repeated courses of anti-inflammatory agents.[28]

Erythema Marginatum

Erythema marginatum is a serpiginous, blanching, and nonindurated rash. It begins as an area of erythema that spreads with central clearing. It will blanch to pressure and the leading edges will be pinkish or salmon in color. The rash may be difficult to observe in any but lightly

---

Box 6-6 Modified Jones Criteria

MAJOR CRITERIA

Carditis
Arthritis
Sydenham's chorea
Subcutaneous nodules
Erythema marginatum

MINOR CRITERIA

Fever
Arthralgia
Elevated acute-phrase reactants
First-degree AV block
Previous rheumatic fever

pigmented individuals. The size and shape of the rash as well as its intensity may change very rapidly.[28-30] Erythema marginatum is seldom seen in the current era. It usually occurs on the trunk when present. Although a major criterion, it is not exclusive to RF and may occur in other clinical settings, notably drug reactions.

Subcutaneous Nodules

Like erythema marginatum, subcutaneous nodules are rarely seen in the current era.[29] They are small (usually less than 2 cm). They are usually found over the bony prominences and in tendon sheaths.[28,29] Areas to palpate for subcutaneous nodules include the extensor surfaces of joints, the spinous processes of the vertebrae, the mastoid process, and the scapulae.

Sydenham's Chorea

Chorea is often a late finding in RF, with a latent period of up to 6 months. As such, evidence of a recent GABHS infection may be absent by the time it presents. Nonetheless, patients should receive treatment for GABHS infection upon its diagnosis.[29,41]

Sydenham's chorea is characterized by uncoordinated, purposeless, involuntary movements of the body and extremities. This motion is usually jerky in nature. It is usually preceded or accompanied by various degrees of emotional lability. As stated earlier, chorea does not appear in adult men for unknown reasons.[29] It appears to affect both sexes equally in preadolescent children.[28] The chorea is self-limiting. It usually lasts several months but may persist as long as a year.

Carditis

Carditis is the most serious of the clinical presentations of RF, both in its presentation as well as in its long-term consequences. Cardiac involvement as rheumatic heart disease is the only significant longterm sequela of RF. The incidence of carditis in first cases of RF is variable and depends on several factors. It appears to be more common in younger patients and may be as high as 90% in very young children. It decreases steadily throughout childhood and adolescence. The overall incidence for all first cases approaches 50%.[28] Carditis is more common in cases of recurrent RF. This is particularly true if carditis had occurred in the primary episode. Residual rheumatic heart disease is the rule after carditis and is more likely and more severe with each subsequent reoccurrence.[28,30]

The presentation and the extent of carditis in RF may vary from none to life-threatening heart failure. The degree of symptomatology will vary depending on the intensity of the carditis, the type of cardiac involvement, and whether there is already underlying rheumatic heart disease. The carditis is a pancardiac inflammation but may be primarily limited to valvulitis, myocarditis, or pericarditis in individual cases.

Valvulitis is commonly seen in RF carditis. It is also the cause of most long-term sequelae of rheumatic heart disease. The mitral valve is the most commonly affected valve, followed by the aortic valve. The pulmonary and tricuspid valves are rarely involved. The mitral is affected approximately three times more commonly than the aortic valve. Both valves may be affected, but isolated aortic involvement is more rare.[28]

In the case of both the aortic and the mitral valve, the primary clinical finding is that of valvular insufficiency. In the mitral valve, this will result in an apical, high-frequency, holosystolic murmur of mitral insufficiency. In severe cases, a mid-diastolic murmur may also be appreciated at the apex. This is due to relative mitral stenosis secondary to leaflet edema and to high flow across the valve as a consequence of mitral insufficiency.

Aortic insufficiency will result in the high-frequency, decrescendo diastolic murmur. This is usually best heard at the left midsternal border in the sitting position. It will usually radiate along the left ventricular outflow tract from the apex to the right upper sternal border. A widened pulse pressure and accentuated pulses by palpation will be present in moderate to severe cases of aortic insufficiency.

Diagnosis of valvulitis can usually be made by careful precordial auscultation.[29] Echocardiography has become extremely useful in assessing the cardiac function both acutely and as surveillance of long-term rheumatic heart disease.[28-30] Care must be taken when using echocardiography to diagnose valvulitis, especially in young children. Current echocardiography machines can detect very trivial amounts of mitral and aortic insufficiency in young children. These are often seen as normal physiologic findings. They should not be confused as valvulitis in an otherwise normal-appearing heart.

Myocarditis and pericarditis rarely occur without some evidence of valvulitis. When they do occur as isolated findings, nonrheumatic origins should be considered.[29] The findings of myocarditis include tachycardia and gallop rhythm. Echocardiography can diagnose evidence of decreased systolic shortening and dilation of the left ventricle. The dilation may occur as a consequence of either poor myocardial function or increased stroke volume from concomitant mitral insufficiency, or a combination of both factors.

Pericarditis may result in a friction rub on precordial auscultation. A pericardial effusion is easily seen by echocardiography but may or may not be present. Electrocardiogram will show the characteristic diffuse ST segment elevations of pericarditis.

Minor Criteria

The minor criteria for RF occur quite commonly. They are nonspecific and so are not highly diagnostic of RF.

Fever

Fever in RF is classically described as initially high-grade and than becoming a chronic low-grade fever after approximately the first week. The initial fever may be as high as 40°C. Low-grade fever from onset of the disease is now more frequently seen.[28,29]

Elevated Acute-Phase Reactants

The most commonly used acute phase reactants are the erythrocyte sedimentation rate (ESR) and the C-reactive protein (CRP). Both ESR and CRP are indicators of an acute and flammatory response. However, both are non-specific and seen in many disease processes.

Prolonged PR interval

Prolonged PR interval may be found in patients with RF. But, like other minor criteria, it is nonspecific. It may occur as an incidental finding. It is also associated with other diseases that cause inflammation of the cardiac conduction system, such as Lyme disease.[42]

Differential Diagnosis

The diagnosis of RF can be very difficult except in the rare classic presentation. Each of the major and minor Jones criteria (with the exception of Sydenham's chorea) may have a large list of causes if it presents as an isolated finding.

Polyarthritis and fever have a long list of causes in children and adolescents. These include infectious etiology such as Lyme disease, rubella, and meningococcal and staphylococcal infections.[28,29,41,43] Various autoimmune diseases may present with fever and arthritis, including juvenile rheumatoid arthritis, lupus, and ankylosing spondylitis. The presence of a recent GABHS infection may be helpful in the differentiation from other types of arthritis. Arthritis usually occurs early in the course of RF, when serology titers for GABHS are often high. In the absence of serologic evidence of GABHS infection, other causes of arthritis need to be considered.[29]

The nature of poststreptococcal reactive arthritis (PSRA) and its relationship with RF remains uncertain.[29,41] This entity consists of a prolonged polyarthritis, beginning 3–14 days after GABHS pharyngitis. Unlike RF, it does not respond promptly to NSAIDs or steroids. Patients generally do not fulfill the Jones criteria. There is a tendency for this entity to be more common in female adults. Long-term follow-up of children has shown development of rheumatic heart disease in up to 7% of the population.[29,41] This would suggest either a misdiagnosed RF or a continuity of the disease process of RF and PSRA. The use of secondary prophylaxis in this population remains controversial, but many patients receive such prophylaxis.[29,41,43]

There are multiple causes of carditis (i.e., myocarditis, pericarditis, and endocarditis), which should be considered when evaluating a patient with possible RF. In most cases, the clinical courses of these diseases will allow them to be differentiated from RF. Most cases of myocarditis and pericarditis fail to meet the necessary diagnostic Jones criteria. They may be confused in the early presentation, especially if they are secondary manifestations of an autoimmune process such as lupus. Endocarditis may present with fever and evidence of mitral or aortic valvulitis, but the clinical course usually allows for the exclusion of RF. This includes positive blood cultures and evidence of embolic and immune complex seeding of other organ systems.

Treatment

Antibiotics

All patients diagnosed with RF (either primary or recurrent) should receive a course of anti-GABHS antibiotics.[28,29,30,43] Intramuscular penicillin G benzathine, given as a single dose, has been shown to be effective. Oral penicillin V, given in 2–3 divided doses for 10 days, is also effective if compliance with therapy is assured. Patients allergic to penicillin may receive a 10-day course of erythromycin. A 10-day course of a first-generation cephalosporin is also an acceptable alternative to penicillin.[29,43]

Anti-Inflammatory Agents

Even after more than 50 years of evaluation, the role of anti-inflammatory agents in the treatment of RF remains controversial.[28-30,44,45,46] Most evidence suggests that these agents do little or nothing to alter the long-term outcome of RF and the subsequent development of rheumatic heart disease.[28-30] These drugs do generally control symptoms, resulting in a rapid improvement in the patient's clinical course. However, premature use can mask the disease presentation, complicating the diagnosis.

The choice of corticosteroids versus NSAIDs in the treatment of RF also remains controversial. Despite the more potent anti-inflammatory properties, evidence suggests that steroids do not alter the course of valvular damage in RF. Recent meta-analysis of steroids versus salicylates showed no difference in the prevention of rheumatic heart disease 1 year after therapy.[44] Therefore. it would appear that steroids should be reserved for cases of severe carditis and fever, in which their potent anti-inflammatory effects may be useful in the management of patients with overt heart failure.[28,29]

Aspirin remains the most commonly used NSAID and is usually very well-tolerated in children. Dosage is usually 60–120 mg/kg/day in six divided doses. This therapy is usually continued until clinical and laboratory evidence of acute inflammation subsides.[28] This may take 1–3 months. The dosage can then be tapered. Abrupt discontinuation may cause a rebound of symptoms.

Prednisone at 2 mg/kg/day can be used in those cases in which steroid therapy is warranted. This treatment should be given for 3–4 weeks and than tapered.[28] As with aspirin, rebound may occur on cessation of therapy.

The ineffectiveness of either NSAIDs or steroids in altering the incidence of rheumatic heart disease following RF have led investigators to assess the usefulness of intravenous gamma globulin (IVIG) therapy in the treatment of RF. Data are limited but do not show a compelling response. In a recent randomized study from New Zealand of 59 children, there was no difference in rheumatic valve disease at 1-year follow-up.[46]

Activity Restriction

Bed rest and activity restriction have been mainstays of RF therapy for decades. Restriction of physical activity appears to be prudent, especially in the presence of active carditis. Patients should have bed rest until the acute febrile symptoms resolve. Light activity, including school, should be permitted once laboratory evidence and clinical signs of carditis resolve. This may take 1–2 months. Vigorous activity should not be allowed for at least 2 months and not until all signs of carditis are completely resolved.[28]

Treatment of Chorea

Chorea with RF is self-limiting but frequently requires treatment for symptom relief. Haloperidol is often used to help control involuntary movements of chorea. Sedation may occasionally be necessary. Although these therapies may improve symptoms, there is no evidence that they alter the time course of the chorea.[28,29]

Prophylaxis

The purpose of prophylaxis is to prevent either the primary occurrence or the reoccurrence of RF. The goal is to eliminate those strains of GABHS that predispose to RF from the patient. Prophylaxis will not eliminate the carrier state, which in a population may range from 15% to 50%.[29,43] The risk of transmission or the development of RF with the asymptomatic carrier state appears to be minimal.[30]

Primary Prophylaxis

Primary prophylaxis should be given to patients with GABHS pharyngitis. This is uncommon before 3 years of age, except in rare outbreaks sometimes seen in a daycare setting. Treatment should be the same as that listed above following the diagnosis of an acute episode of RF.[43]

Secondary Prophylaxis

The goal of secondary prophylaxis is the prevention of subsequent reoccurrence of RF in a patient following the initial episode of RF. The type and length of prophylaxis continues to be debated. The age of the patient, the likelihood of compliance with medical therapy, and the prevalence of RF in the patient's community all appear to be relevant to determining the type and length of therapy.[29,30] As a rule, the worse the cardiac involvement in the initial episode, the lower the patient's age, and the higher the prevalence of RF in the community, the longer the period of secondary prophylaxis. Tables 6-6 and 6-7 show the current recommendations from the American Heart Association for the United States.[47]

Clinical Course

The clinical course of RF is determined primarily by the presence and severity of carditis. The incidence of carditis in initial attack decreases with the age of the patient. Approximately 50% of school-age children will have carditis with the first attack, but carditis is rare in adults with an initial episode. In the very young, the incidence of carditis is even higher.[28–30]

In those patients who have no clinical evidence of carditis, the longterm outcome is excellent. The incidence of development of rheumatic disease is very low.

Table 6-6 Duration of Secondary Rheumatic Fever Prophylaxis	
Category	**Duration**
Rheumatic fever with carditis and residual heart disease (persistent valvar disease*)	At least 10 yr since last episode and at least until age 40 yr, sometimes lifelong prophylaxis
Rheumatic fever with carditis but no residual heart disease (no valvar disease*)	10 yr or well into adulthood, whichever is longer
Rheumatic fever without carditis	5 yr or until age 21 yr, whichever is longer

Adapted from Dajani A, Taubert K, Ferrieri P, et al. Pediatrics 96: 758–764, 1995.
*Clinical or echocardiographic evidence.

Table 6-7	Prophylaxis for Secondary Prevention of Rheumatic Fever	
Agent	**Dose**	**Mode**
Benzathine penicillin G	1,200,000 U every 4 wk*	Intramuscular
	or	
Penicillin V	250 mg twice daily	Oral
	or	
Sulfadiazine	0.5 g once daily for patients ≤27 kg (60 lb)	
	1.0 g once daily for patients >27 kg (60 lb)	Oral
FOR INDIVIDUALS ALLERGIC TO PENICILLIN AND SULFADIAZINE		
Erythromycin	250 mg twice daily	Oral

Adapted from Dajani A, Taubert K, Ferrieri P, et al. Pediatrics 96: 758–764, 1995.
*In high-risk situations, administration every 3 weeks is justified and recommended.

Their risk of reoccurrence is also lower. This is reflected in the AHA prophylaxis recommendations (Table 6-6).

Most patients with carditis as part of their initial attack will develop some degree of rheumatic heart disease. The severity of residual abnormalities increases with the-severity of the carditis. The presence of carditis in the first attack is associated with an increased risk of carditis in any subsequent reoccurrence.[28] The presence of residual rheumatic heart disease also increases the risk that subsequent GABHS infection will result in recurrent RF. For these reasons, those patients with a history of carditis should have more prolonged periods of secondary prophylaxis. Even more stringent prophylaxis should be given to the group of patients with rheumatic heart disease (see Table 6-6).[47]

LYME DISEASE

Lyme disease is a multiorgan system disease caused by the treponema-like spirochete *Borrelia burgdorferi*. The disease takes its name from Lyme, Conn., where the disease was first described in an epidemic form by Steere *et al.*[48] It is an uncommon but increasing cause of acquired cardiac illness in children.[42,49-52]

Etiology and Epidemiology

B. burgdorferi is the etiologic agent of Lyme disease. This spirochete is carried by hard-bodied ticks of the genus *Ixodes*, which act as its vector. The distribution of Lyme disease in the United States reflects the distribution of these ticks.[42,52,53] Most cases occur in the northeastern United States, from southern Maine to northern Virginia. The primary tick vector in the region is *Ixodes scapularis*.[53] The disease is seen with less frequency in the northwestern United States, where the primary vector is

Ixodes pacificus.[53] Small clusters of cases also occur in Minnesota and Wisconsin.

The primary hosts for *B. burgdorferi* in the Northeast are white-footed mice and white-tailed deer.[43] Human exposure occurs as a result of being bitten by an infected tick. For this reason, there is a seasonal distribution for Lyme disease. Approximately 90% of cases will occur between May and September, when tick exposure is at its highest.[42,52,53] Lyme disease has now been recognized in Canada as well as in parts of Europe, Russia, and eastern Asia.[53]

Clinical Presentation

In the United States, there appears to be a bimodal age distribution for Lyme disease, with most cases clustering between 5-9 years of age and 45-54 years of age.[53] There does not appear to be a sexual difference in infection rates.[51] In a study by Asch *et al.*,[51] the average number of hours spent outdoors per affected patient averaged 23 hours per week.

The clinical manifestations are divided into three stages, beginning with the tick bite. The first stage is the early localized stage and usually occurs within 3-7 days of the tick bite but may occur as late as several weeks.[42,50,52,53] The initial finding is the characteristic rash of erythema migrans. This rash starts as an annular erythematous lesion occurring at the site of the tick bite. It may be macular or papular.[53] It will expand over the next several days up to a week, to an average size of 15 cm.[51] There is frequently central clearing and induration as the lesion expands.[53] Erythema migrans occurs in 60-80% of cases.[42,50,51,53] The incidence is probably higher since tick bites often occur in areas of the body that are not easily observed, such as the groin and axillae. The incidence of erythema migrans may be somewhat lower in children, at about 50%.[51]

Systemic symptoms usually occur within days of the rash making its presentation. Early-stage symptoms are flu-like and include fever, headache, malaise, arthralgia, and myalgia.[42,50,51,53] These symptoms are present in approximately 80% of infected patients.[42,51]

Stage 2 of Lyme disease is the early disseminated stage. This is characterized by hematogenous spread of the spirochete. The onset of stage 2 is usually 1–5 months after the tick bite.[53] The most prominent manifestation of stage 2 is the appearance of multiple erythema migrans-like lesions. These occur in up to 50% of pediatric cases.[50] Arthritis is also commonly seen in this stage, affecting 40–50% of the patients.[50,51] It is usually an oligoarthritis that is asymmetrical and involves the large joints.[50]

Neurologic involvement may occur in 10–20% of patients during the second stage.[42,50–52] Neurologic findings may include various cranial nerve palsies, especially the facial nerve. Encephalitis and aseptic meningitis are also seen. An aseptic lymphocytic meningitis is the most common neurologic finding in children.[50]

Cardiac findings are present in about 10% of stage 2 patients. These will be discussed in detail in the next section.

Late-stage Lyme disease may occur anywhere from 5 months to years after infection.[42] Arthritis may persist or may develop as a new finding during this stage. Late neurologic findings include chronic encephalomyelitis, memory loss, and severe fatigue.[42,50]

Cardiac Manifestations

Lyme disease results in cardiac manifestations in approximately 10% of patients.[42,49,51,52] Although Lyme carditis has been documented to involve the entire myocardium as well as the pericardium, the conduction system appears to be most commonly affected.[42,52] As stated above, this usually occurs during the second stage of the disease.

The most common manifestation of the carditis is varying degrees of atrioventricular (AV) block.[42,53] This may include first-degree AV block, second-degree AV block (usually Wenckebach) and complete AV block.[53] Symptoms generally only occur in the presence of complete block. These may include dizziness, presyncope, and syncope. Chest pain and easy fatigability are also reported.[42,49,53]

Electrophysiologic studies of patients with complete AV block have shown that the block is usually above the bundle of His.[49,53] Escape rhythms are usually narrow complex. Occasionally, wide complex escape rhythms and long pauses have been seen in patients with complete AV block.[49] Patients with complete AV block need continuous monitoring to ensure that they maintain

adequate backup rhythm. Insertion of a temporary transvenous pacemaker is required in some cases. Atropine and isoproterenol have also been used to augment heart rate.[43,49,53] Conduction generally normalizes in response to treatment. This usually occurs over a period of several days to weeks and may represent resolving inflammation of the conduction system.[42] There is often a progression from complete AV block to Wenckebach and then to first-degree AV block. There is then a gradual shortening of the P-R interval.[42,49,53] Permanent AV block is rarely seen but may occur.[49,53] Under these unusual circumstances, placement of a permanent pacemaker system may rarely be necessary.

More global myocarditis and pericarditis are less commonly seen in Lyme disease. Biopsies of acute Lyme carditis have shown transmural lymphoplasmacytic infiltrate, neutrophil and macrophage nodules, and myocyte necrosis. Spirochetes may also be seen in the myocardium.[42] Diffuse ST segments flattening and inversion may be seen up to 65% of cases.[42] Signs and symptoms of congestive heart failure are rare but have been reported.[42]

Laboratory Findings

In Stage 1, laboratory tests are of little use and the diagnosis is made by clinical appearance.[53] immunoglobulin M (IgM) specific antibodies do not peak until 3–6 weeks into the infection and immunoglobulin G (IgG) antibodies do not peak often for months. For these reasons, serologic testing is not recommended for children with a clinical course that suggests early Lyme disease.[53]

Most patients with Stage 2 and nearly all patients with Stage 3 disease will have elevated antibodies titers. Enzyme immunoassay (EIA) is the initial screening test for the later stages of Lyme disease. There is some cross-reaction with other spirochete and viral infections so that false-positive results will occur. Western immunoblot tests can be used to confirm a positive in equivocal EIA tests. Current recommendations are for screening with EIA and confirming as needed with Western blot testing.[53]

Treatment

Antibiotic treatment should be given at the time of diagnosis. The type of antibiotics and the duration of therapy depend on several factors. Oral therapy for 2–4 weeks is usually adequate for most stage 1 and 2 infections. Persistent or recurrent cases and those cases with carditis will require a more aggressive intravenous therapy. Current American Academy of Pediatrics recommendations are shown in Table 6-8.[53]

Table 6-8   Recommended Treatment for Lyme Disease in Children

Disease Category	Drug(s) and Dose*
EARLY LOCALIZED DISEASE*	
8 yr of age or older	Doxycyline, 100 mg, orally, twice a day for 14–21 days
All ages	Amoxicillin, 25–50 mg/kg/day, orally, divided into 2 doses (maximum 2 g/day) for 14–21 days
EARLY DISSEMINATED AND LATE DISEASE	
Multiple erythema migrans	Same oral regimen as for early disease but for 21 days
Isolated facial palsy	Same oral regimen as for early disease but for 21–28 days[†,‡]
Arthritis	Same oral regimen as for early disease but for 28 days
Persistent or recurrent arthritis[§]	Ceftriaxone sodium, 75–100 mg/kg, IV or IM, once a day (maximum 2 g/day), for 14–21 days: or penicillin, 300,000 U/kg/day, IV, given in divided doses every 4 hr (maximum 20 million U/day) for 14–28 days *or* same oral regimen as for early disease
Carditis	Ceftriaxone or penicillin: see persistent or recurrent arthritis
Meningitis or encephalitis	Ceftriaxone or penicillin: see persistent or recurrent arthritis, but for 30–60 days

Adapted from Committee on Infectious Diseases, American Academy of Pediatrics. RED BOOK 2003 Report of the Committee on Infectious Diseases, 2003.
IV, intravenously; *IM*, intramuscularly.
*For patients who are allergic to penicillin, cefuroxime axeril, and erythromycin are alternative drugs.
[†]Corticosteroids should not be given.
[‡]Treatment has no effect on the resolution of facial nerve palsy; its purpose is to prevent late disease.
[§]Arthritis is not considered persistent or recurrent unless objective evidence of synovitis exists at least 2 months after treatment is initiated. Some experts administer a second course of an oral agent before using an IV-administered antimicrobial agent.

MAJOR POINTS

- Acute rheumatic fever remains common in much of the developing world and is reappearing in certain developed areas.
- The epidemiology of acute rheumatic fever is linked to the re-emergence of certain streptococcal strains in geographic areas.
- The Jones criteria remain a useful guideline to the diagnosis of acute rheumatic fever.
- Infective endocarditis has continued to increase in frequency over the past 30 years.
- The changing patterns of infectious organisms and the frequency of infections in infective endocarditis are due to the changing patterns of congenital heat surgery and intensive care management, especially in the neonatal setting.
- Lyme disease is a growing cause of myocarditis affecting the conduction system in the school-age and adolescent population.

REFERENCES

1. Bayer AS, Bolger AF, Taubert KA, et al: Diagnosis and management of infective endocarditis and its complications. Circulation 98:2936–2948, 1998.
2. Hogevik H, Olaison L, Andersson R, et al: Epidemiologic aspects of infective endocarditis in an urban population. A 5-year prospective study. Medicine 74(6):324–339, 1995.
3. Ferrieri P, Gewitz MH, Gerber MA, et al: Unique features of infective endocarditis in childhood. Circulation 105(17): 2115–2126, 2002.
4. Friedman RA, Starke JR: Infective endocarditis. In Garson A, Bricker JT, Fisher DJ, Neish SR (eds): The Science and Practice of Pediatric Cardiology, 2nd ed. Baltimore: Lippincott Williams & Wilkins, 1998, pp 1759–1775.
5. Martin JM, Neches WH, Wald ER: Infective endocarditis: 35 years of experience at a children's hospital. Clin Infect Dis April 24(4):669–675, 1997.
6. Johnson DH, Rosenthal A, Nadas AS: A forty-year review of bacterial endocarditis in infancy and childhood. Circulation 51(4):581–588, 1975.
7. Millard DD, Shulman ST: The changing spectrum of neonatal endocarditis. Clin Perinatol 15:587–608, 1988.
8. Gersony WM, Hayes CJ, Driscoll DJ, et al: Bacterial endocarditis in patients with aortic stenosis, pulmonary stenosis, or ventricular septal defect. Circulation 87(2 Suppl): I121–I126, 1993.
9. Awadallah SM, Kavey RE, Byrum CJ, et al: The changing pattern of infective endocarditis in childhood. Am J Cardiol 68(1):90–94, 1991.
10. Saiman L, Prince A, Gersony WM: Pediatric infective endocarditis in the modern era. J Pediatr 122(6):847–853, 1993.

11. Baddour LM, Sullam PM, Bayer AS: The pathogenesis of infective endocarditis. In Sussman M (ed): Molecular Medical Microbiology. San Diego, CA: Academic Press, 2001, pp 999–1020.

12. Durack DT, Beeson PB: Experimental bacterial endocarditis. II. Survival of bacteria in endocardial vegetations. Br J Exp Pathol 53(1):50–53, 1972.

13. Tunkel AR, Scheld WM: Experimental models of endocarditis. In Kaye D (ed): Infective Endocarditis, 2nd ed. New York: Raven Press, 1992, pp 37–56.

14. Mylonakis E, Calderwood ST: Infective endocarditis in adults. N Engl J Med 345(18):1318–1330, 2001.

15. Bayer AS, Theofilopoulos DB, Tillman DB, et al: Use of circulating immune complex levels in the serodifferentiation of endocarditic and nonendocarditic septicemias. Am J Med 66(1):58–62, 1979.

16. Oelberg DG, Fisher DJ, Gross DM, et al: Endocarditis in high-risk neonates. Pediatrics 71(3):392–397, 1983.

17. Symchych PS, Krauss AN, Winchester P: Endocarditis following intracardiac placement of umbilical venous catheters in neonates. J Pediatr 90:287–289, 1977.

18. Eykyn SJ: Endocarditis: basics. Heart 86(4):476–480, 2001.

19. Stockheim JA, Chadwick EG, Dessler S, et al: Are the Duke criteria superior to the Beth Israel criteria for the diagnosis of infective endocarditis in children? Clin Infect Dis 27(6):1451–1456, 1998.

20. Daniel WG, Mugge A, Grote J, et al: Comparison of transthoracic and transesophageal echocardiography for detection of abnormalities of prosthetic and bioprosthetic valves in the mitral and aortic positions. Am J Cardiol 71:210–215, 1993.

21. Daniel WG, Erbel R, Kasper W, et al: Safety of transesophageal echocardiography: A multicenter survey of 10,419 examinations. Circulation 83:817–821, 1991.

22. Aly AM, Simpson PM, Humes RA: The role of transthoracic echocardiography in the diagnosis of infective endocarditis in children. Arch Pediatr Adolesc Med 153(9):950–954, 1999.

23. Sable CA, Rome JJ, Martin GR, et al: Indications for echocardiography in the diagnosis of infective endocarditis in children. Am J Cardiol 75(12):801–804, 1995.

24. Kavey RE, Frank DM, Byrum CJ, et al: Two-dimensional echocardiographic assessment of infective endocarditis in children. Am J Dis Child 137:851–856, 1983.

25. Durack DT, Lukes AS, Bright DK: New criteria for diagnosis of infective endocarditis: utilization of specific echocardiographic findings. Duke endocarditis service. Am J Med 96:200–209, 1994.

26. Pierrotti LC, Baddour LM: Fungal endocarditis, 1995–2000. Chest 122:302–310, 2002.

27. Dajani AS, Taubert KA, Wilson W, et al: Prevention of bacterial endocarditis: Recommendations by the American Heart Association. Circulation 96:358–366, 1997.

28. El-Said GM, El-Refaee MM, Sorour KA, El-Said, HG: Rheumatic fever and rheumatic heart disease. In Garson A, Bricker JT, Fisher DJ, Neish SR (eds): The Science and Practice of Pediatric Cardiology, 2nd ed.

Baltimore: Lippincott Williams & Wilkins, 1998, pp 1691–1724.

29. Stollerman GH: Rheumatic fever in the 21st century. Clin Infect Dis 33:806–814, 2001.

30. Stollerman GH: Rheumatic fever. Lancet 349(9056): 935–942, 1997.

31. Steer AC, Carapetis JR, Nolan TM, Shann F: Systematic review of rheumatic heart disease prevalence in children in developing countries: The role of environmental factors. J Ped & Child Health 38(3)229–234, 2002.

32. Stollerman GH, Siegel AC, Johnson EE: Variable epidemiology of streptococcal disease and the changing pattern of rheumatic fever. Mod Concepts Cardiovascul Dis 34:45–48, 1965.

33. Wannamaker LW: Differences between streptococcal infections of the throat and of the skin. N Engl J Med 282(1): 23–31, 1970.

34. Bisno AL, Pearce IA, Wall HP, et al: Contrasting epidemiology of acute rheumatic fever and acute glomerulonephritis: Nature of the antecedent streptococcal infection. N Engl J Med 283:561–565, 1970.

35. Cunningham MW: Pathogenesis of group A streptococcal infections. Clin Microbiol Rev 13:470–511, 2000.

36. Carreno-Manjarrez R, Visvanathan K, Zibriskie JB: Immunogenic and genetic factors in rheumatic fever. Curr Infect Dis Rep 2:302–307, 2000.

37. Khanna AK, Buskirk DR, Williams RC Jr, et al: Presence of a non-HLA B cell antigen in rheumatic fever patients and their families as defined by a monoclonal antibody. J Clin Invest 83:1710–1716, 1989.

38. Veasy LG, Wiedmeier SE, Garth SO, et al: Resurgence of acute rheumatic fever in the intermountain area of the United States. N Engl J Med 316:421–427, 1987.

39. Kaplan EL: Global assessment of rheumatic fever and rheumatic heart disease at the close of the century. Circulation 88:1964–1672, 1993.

40. Centers for Disease Control: Acute rheumatic fever: Utah. Morb Mortal Wkly Rep 36:108–110, 115, 1987.

41. Ferrieri P: Proceedings of the Jones Criteria Workshop. Circulation 106:2521–2523, 2002.

42. Cox J, Krajden M: Cardiovascular manifestations of Lyme disease. Am Heart J 122(5):1449–1455, 1991.

43. Committee on Infectious Diseases, The American Academy of Pediatrics: Group A Streptococcal Infections. RED BOOK 2003 Report of the Committee on Infectious Diseases, 26th ed, pp 573–591.

44. Albert DA, Harel L, Karrison T: The treatment of rheumatic carditis: A review and meta-analysis. Medicine 74(1):1–12, 1995.

45. Cilliers AM, Manyemba J, Saloojee H: Anti-inflammatory treatment for carditis in acute rheumatic fever. Cochrane Database Syst Rev. (2):CD003167, 2003.

46. Voss LM, Wilson NJ, Neutze JM, et al: Intravenous immunoglobulin in acute rheumatic fever: A randomized controlled trial. Circulation 103(3):401–406, 2001.

47. Dajani A, Taubert K, Ferrieri P, et al: Treatment of acute streptococcal pharyngitis and prevention of rheumatic fever: A statement for health professionals. Committee on Rheumatic Fever, Endocarditis, and Kawasaki Disease of the Council on Cardiovascular Disease in the Young, The American Heart Association. Pediatrics 96:758-764, 1995.

48. Steere AC, Malawista SE, Snydwan DR, et al: Lyme arthritis: An epidemic of oligoarticular arthritis in children and adults in three Connecticut communities. Arthritis Rheum 20:7-17, 1977.

49. McAlister HF, Klementowicz, PT, Andrews C, et al: Lyme carditis: An important cause of reversible heart block. Ann Intern Med 110:339-345, 1989.

50. Prose NS, Abson KG, Berg D: Lyme disease in children: Diagnosis, treatment, and prevention. Semin Dermatol 11(1):31-36, 1992.

51. Asch ES, Bujak DI, Weiss M, et al: Lyme disease: An infectious and postinfectious syndrome. J Rheumatol 21:454-461, 1994.

52. Barron KS: Cardiovascular manifestations of connective tissue diseases. Lyme disease. In The Science and Practice of Pediatric Cardiology, 2nd ed. Baltimore: Lippincott Williams & Wilkins, 1998, pp 1725-1740.

53. Committee on Infectious Diseases, American Academy of Pediatrics: Lyme disease (*Borrelia burgdorferi* infection). RED BOOK 2003 Report of the Committee on Infectious Diseases, 26th ed, 2003, pp 407-413.

Kawasaki Disease

VICTORIA L. VETTER

Kawasaki disease (KD) was first described in 1967 in 50 Japanese children with fever, rash, conjunctival injection, erythema and swelling of the hands and feet, and cervical lymphadenopathy; the disease was then labeled mucocutaneous lymph node syndrome. KD is a self-limited vasculitis with an unclear etiology affecting infants and children. It is complicated by coronary and peripheral arterial aneurysms and myocardial infarction in some patients. The diagnosis is made by the combination of a number of clinical characteristics associated with fever. It is now the most common cause of acquired heart disease in children in the United States, having surpassed rheumatic fever. It is the second most common vasculitic illness of childhood, with Henoch-Schönlein purpura being the most common.

EPIDEMIOLOGY

KD occurs in all races of children but is most common in Japan and in children of Japanese ancestry. In the United States, KD is most common in Asians and Pacific Islanders, followed by African Americans and then Hispanics. It is seen less commonly in Caucasians. Other factors indicating a genetic component are a positive family history in some cases, with an occurrence rate of 2.1% in siblings, and a history of the disease during childhood in parents of children with the disease. There is a predisposition of males over females, with a ratio of 1.5–1.7 to 1. KD most commonly affects young children, with 76% of those affected being less than 5 years of age.

When affected, very young or children older than 8 are more likely to have complications of the disease. Factors reported to be associated with KD include preceding respiratory illness, exposure to carpet cleaning, eczema, humidifier use, and residence near a standing body of water. KD is most likely to occur during the winter and spring.

The mortality rate is around 0.17%, with most deaths associated with early cardiac sequelae, peaking at 15 to 45 days after the onset of fever. Sudden death has been reported years after the initial episode in those who have developed coronary aneurysms.

DIAGNOSIS

The diagnosis of KD is based on a constellation of clinical findings in association with at least 5 days of fever (Box 7-1). Four of the following five clinical features must be present to make the diagnosis, or three of the five if coronary artery aneurysms are present by echocardiography. Although the criteria require fever for 5 days, some have suggested that, in the presence of four or more criteria, the diagnosis may be made on day 4. It is important to note that these findings do not appear simultaneously and that the history may be the only indication that some of these fleeting signs have been present.

The first feature involves acute changes in the extremities, especially edema and erythema, notably of the palms and soles. Subsequent findings 2 to 3 weeks after the onset of the illness include peeling of the fingers and toes. The second set of clinical signs involves the conjunctivae with bilateral nonexudative conjunctivitis that is limbic sparing (Fig. 7-1). Third, there are changes in the lips and oral cavity, including erythema and cracking of

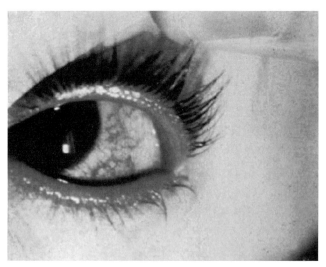

Figure 7-1 Note limbic sparing conjunctivitis, typical of Kawasaki disease. (Image courtesy of Jane W. Newburger, MD, Professor of Pediatrics, Harvard Medical School.)

the lips, strawberry tongue, and injection of the oral and pharyngeal mucosae. Cervical lymphadenopathy (typically > 1.5 cm) is the fourth criterion for diagnosis. The cervical adenopathy often is unilateral and more likely to be present in older children. The fifth feature is rash, which appears during the first week of the illness, covers the body, is nonspecific, and may be maculopapular, urticarial, scarlatiniform, erythema multiforme-like or micropustular, bullous, or vesicular. In young children, the rash may be accentuated in the diaper region with associated peeling.

In addition to these features is the aforementioned fever; it is typically 39–40° C and lasts, on average, over 10 days in untreated patients, with some reports of over 2 months of fever. With appropriate treatment, the majority of cases have resolution of the fever within 2 days after treatment.

Conjunctivitis appears shortly after onset of the fever and may only last a day or two. Eye pain is generally not present, although photophobia may be. The cracked red lips are seen in most patients at the time of presentation, often accompanied by the strawberry tongue, which is identical to that seen with scarlet fever. The parent is usually the first to notice the extremity edema, which can be confused with the normal pudginess of the toddler as it is nonpitting. Although at least one large (i.e., >1.5 cm) lymph node is required to meet one of the diagnostic criteria, smaller nodes may be present. The large node is generally tender and may be mistaken for a suppurative adenitis.

Multiple organ systems can be involved. The most significant involvement is that of the cardiovascular system, which is the leading cause of long-term morbidity and mortality. Inflammation of the pericardium,

---

> **Box 7-1 Diagnostic Clinical Criteria of Kawasaki Disease**
>
> Fever persisting at least 5 days*†
> Presence of at least four of the following features:
> - Changes in the extremities: Erythema of palms and soles, edema of hands and feet, periungual peeling of fingers and toes in second and third week
> - Bilateral bulbar conjunctival injection without exudate (limbic sparing)
> - Injection of oral pharyngeal mucosae, including injected pharynx, erythema and cracking of lips, and strawberry tongue
> - Cervical lymphadenopathy (>1.5 cm in diameter), usually unilateral
> - Polymorphous exanthema
>
> Exclusion of other diseases with similar findings (see Table 7-3)

*In the presence of four or more criteria, the diagnosis of Kawasaki disease can be made on day 4 of illness.
†Patients with fever for at least 5 days and fewer than four criteria can be diagnosed as having Kawasaki disease when coronary artery abnormalities are detected by two-dimensional echocardiography or angiography.

myocardium, endocardium, valves, and coronary arteries occurs in the acute phase of the illness. This can result in myocarditis and congestive heart failure or pericarditis that may result in cardiac tamponade, or all three. Valvular regurgitation, especially of the mitral valve, can occur. The most significant involvement is that of the coronary arteries, with aneurysms that may rupture or thrombose acutely. In addition, aneurysms can occur in noncoronary arteries, especially the axillary and iliofemoral areas. A peripheral vasculitis can result in gangrene of the extremities. Physical findings in the cardiovascular system can include tachycardia, a hyperdynamic precordium, a gallop, and a flow murmur or a systolic regurgitant murmur.

Other systems involved include the musculoskeletal with arthritis and arthralgia of multiple large weight-bearing or small interphalangeal joints, resulting in an inability to stand or walk and severe pain in the joints. Gastrointestinal involvement can result in diarrhea, vomiting, and abdominal pain. Hepatitis with liver enlargement and jaundice and gallbladder hydrops are reported. Respiratory involvement includes pneumonia and pleural effusion. These children have extreme irritability, a finding that often has been attributed to aseptic meningitis, found in up to 50% of patients. The genitourinary system may be involved with urethritis, meatitis, testicular swelling, and sterile pyuria. Otitis and uveitis may occur.

Positive laboratory findings are shown in Box 7-2. Over half of the patients have white blood counts at over 15,000/mm^3. An elevated erythrocyte sedimentation rate and C-reactive protein (CRP) is common and frequently elevated for 6 to 8 or more weeks after the illness. Elevated platelet counts are characteristic of KD and are often as high as 500,000–1,000,000/mm^3 by the second week of the illness. These elevated counts may not return to normal for 4 to 8 weeks. Plasma cholesterol, high-density lipoprotein (HDL) cholesterol, and apolipoprotein A (APOA) may be decreased. Liver enzymes are elevated in 40% to 67% of patients. Low serum albumin is associated with more severe and prolonged episodes. One third of the patients have sterile pyuria, and, in those with spinal taps, half have an aseptic meningitis profile.[1] Other diseases with similar clinical findings must be excluded. The most common are shown in Box 7-3.

Atypical (Incomplete) Kawasaki Disease

Some cases subsequently shown to have KD by echocardiography (i.e., development of coronary artery aneurysms) will present with fewer than the required number of clinical findings to diagnose KD, especially in younger children.[2] Thus, KD must be considered in a child with a febrile exanthematous illness persisting longer than 5 days, especially if 2 to 3 of the characteristic findings, such as rash, oral changes, conjunctivitis, or lymphadenopathy, are present. The laboratory findings may be helpful in supporting the diagnosis of KD.

ETIOLOGY

Over three decades since its first description, the etiology of KD remains unclear. It is debated whether a specific conventional bacterial or viral agent, resulting in an exaggerated immune response in a genetically susceptible individual, or a superantigen-induced immune response is the initial trigger for KD. Multiple agents, including Staphylococcus, Streptococcus, and Rickettsia viruses and environmental chemicals, have been implicated.[3,4] Because of the seasonal outbreaks, the rareness of cases in children younger than 6 months old (who would be protected by maternal antibodies), and the lack of disease in adults who may be immune to the disease, an infectious etiology is thought to be likely. It has been noted that an exaggerated immunoglobulin immune

---

Box 7-2 Laboratory Findings in Kawasaki Disease

- Leukocytosis with neutrophilia and immature forms
- Elevated erythrocyte sedimentation rate
- Elevated C-reactive protein
- Thrombocytosis after first week
- Anemia
- Abnormal plasma lipids
- Hypoalbuminemia
- Hyponatremia
- Elevated serum transaminases
- Elevated serum gammaglutamyl transpeptidase
- Sterile pyuria
- Pleocytosis of cerebrospinal fluid

Box 7-3 Differential Diagnosis of Kawasaki Disease

Viral infections (i.e., adenovirus, measles)
Staphylococcal scalded skin syndrome
Scarlet fever
Toxic shock syndrome
Stevens–Johnson syndrome
Drug hypersensitivity reactions
Rocky Mountain spotted fever
Leptospirosis
Juvenile rheumatoid arthritis
Cervical lymphadenitis

response in association with plasma cell infiltration of the vascular wall, as well as other tissues such as myocardium, respiratory tract, kidney, and pancreas, occurs in patients with KD. Investigators suggest a mucosal portal of entry, especially of the respiratory tract of a conventional antigen.[5-8]

Because the clinical symptoms of KD are similar to toxin-mediated disease, the role of superantigens in mediating the disease has been suggested.[1,9] Superantigens result in polyclonal B-cell activation, extensive proinflammatory cytokine production, and changes in the number of circulating T lymphocytes that bear a specific surface receptor. These findings have been described in patients with KD.[3] Thus far, no consistent toxin-producing strain of bacteria has been isolated from patients with KD.[10]

It is possible that KD results from an immunologic response that may be triggered by several different infectious agents.

PATHOGENESIS

KD is an acute vasculitis, affecting small- and medium-sized arteries such as coronary arteries. It is considered an immune-mediated disorder with cytokine cascade activation and endothelial cell activation.[11] Coronary artery aneurysms are thought to be secondary to the combined action of several cytokines on the vascular endothelial cells.[12] Coronary artery inflammation has been reported to be associated with endothelial cell activation and IgA plasma cells.[13]

Pathology

KD is a generalized systemic vasculitis involving multiple blood vessels in the body. Although coronary artery aneurysms are the most common, aneurysms occur in other muscular arteries such as the mesenteric, femoral, iliac, renal, axillary, and brachial arteries. Within the coronary arteries, the earliest inflammatory response is in the media, with an influx of neutrophils, mononuclear cells and lymphocytes, and eventually immunoglobulin A (IgA) plasma cells.[13] Enzymes, including matrix metalloproteinases, vascular endothelial growth factor (VEGF), monocyte chemotactic and activating factor (MCAF or MCP-1), tumor necrosis factor alpha (TNF-α), and interleukins, are involved in the vasculitic process.[14] Eventually, the internal elastic lamina is destroyed and fibrosis occurs. Remodeling or revascularization of the coronary arteries may occur at times, leading to stenosis, thrombosis, or both.

Risks of Aneurysm

Risk scores have been developed to predict the likelihood of coronary artery aneurysm development.[15-17]

Fever duration is one of the most significant predictors, along with male gender and age $\leq$ 12 months. Other laboratory criteria are associated with coronary artery aneurysm development and include elevated neutrophils and band counts, low hemoglobin, and low platelet counts.

Coronary Aneurysm

Approximately 25% (20% to 40%) of untreated KD patients develop coronary artery abnormalities. Approximately 50% of these lesions regress within 5 years, with mild coronary artery aneurysms (i.e., 3 to 4 mm) regressing within 2 years. Giant aneurysms (i.e., > 8 mm) are unlikely to resolve. Of the 50% with persistent moderate-sized aneurysms, half become smaller, one third develop stenoses, and the remainder have irregularities of the coronaries without stenosis.[11] Stenosis, coronary thrombosis, myocardial infarctions, and death may complicate giant coronary artery aneurysms.

The Japanese Ministry of Health provided the original criteria for coronary artery aneurysms. In patients < 5 years of age, an internal lumen diameter > 3 mm is considered abnormal. By 5 years of age, > 4 mm is abnormal. A segment that measures (in internal diameter) at least 1.5 times that of an adjacent segment or an irregular lumen is another criterion for abnormality.[18]

The coronary arteries involved, in order of decreasing frequency, are the proximal left anterior descending and proximal right coronary arteries, the left main coronary artery, the left circumflex, and the distal right coronary artery and the junction between the right coronary artery and posterior descending coronary artery.

Aneurysms are classified as saccular (i.e., axial and lateral diameters equal), fusiform (i.e., symmetric dilation with gradual proximal and distal tapering), and ectatic coronary artery aneurysms (i.e., larger than normal without a segmental aneurysm) (Fig. 7-2).

In the past, a classification system by size was utilized: small aneurysms are < 5 mm, medium are 5 to 8 mm, and giant are > 8 mm.[19] Current United States echocardiographic measurements consider the body surface area and consider abnormal values those with a z score for a particular coronary artery of $\geq$ 2.5. Figure 7-3 shows an echocardiogram of a fusiform coronary artery aneurysm.

The incidence of patients developing giant aneurysms is 0.5% to 1%. Factors affecting the development of giant coronary aneurysms are an age of less than 1 year, male gender (1.99, compared with females), a hospital visit on days 1 to 3 of illness, an elevated leukocyte count, elevated neutrophils, low hemoglobin, a low platelet count, CRP over 3, elevated alanine aminotransferase (ALT), low albumin, or a low serum sodium level (i.e., < 135 mEq/L).[20]

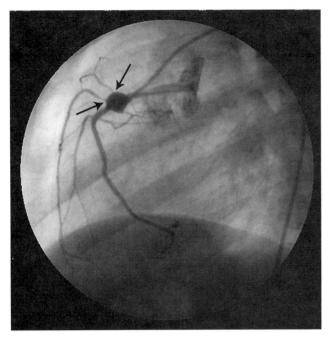

Figure 7-2   Coronary angiogram in lateral view showing right coronary artery with saccular aneurysm. Note stenotic take-off of coronary artery branches (*arrows*).

NATURAL HISTORY

Regression of Coronary Artery Aneurysms

Approximately one half to two thirds of patients with coronary artery aneurysms will have angiographic resolution of the lesions 1 to 2 years after onset of KD.[21] Regression occurs most of the time by myointimal proliferation but may occur by organization and recanalization of a thrombus. On pathologic examination, fibrous intimal thickening is seen often with a normal coronary artery lumen diameter.[22] Regressed coronary artery aneurysms show reduced vascular reactivity, indicating endothelial dysfunction.[23] Larger aneurysms are much less likely to resolve than smaller ones.[22] Patients who are less than 1 year of age and develop coronary artery aneurysms have a greater chance of resolution of the coronary artery aneurysms, as do those with fusiform rather than saccular aneurysms and those with aneurysm location in a distal coronary segment.[24] Rupture of coronary arteries is rare and usually occurs in the first few months of the disease.

Persistent Coronary Artery Aneurysms

Coronary artery aneurysms that do not resolve may develop stenosis or occlusion. Half of the patients with coronary artery aneurysm stenosis will have this

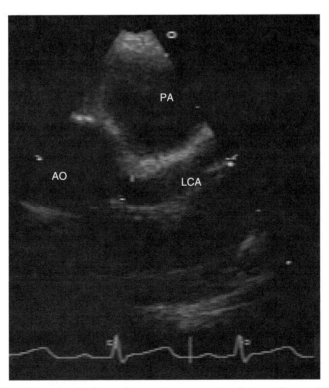

Figure 7-3   Two-dimensional echocardiogram in cross-sectional view. *AO*, aorta; *PA*, pulmonary artery; *LCA*, left coronary artery. Note dilated fusiform aneurysm of LCA.

development within 2 years of the disease onset, with the rest occurring over time.[21] Large aneurysms are more likely to progress. Giant aneurysms (i.e., > 8 mm) are most likely to develop thromboses, as shown in Figure 7-4.

Myocardial Infarction

Myocardial infarction is the most common cause of death in these patients. Figure 7-5 is an electrocardiogram showing an inferior infarction in a 12-year-old with a stenotic distal right coronary artery. Most fatal myocardial infarctions occur in association with obstruction of the left main coronary artery or the right main and left anterior descending coronary arteries. The highest risk of myocardial infarction occurs in the first year after disease onset.[25] The incidence of serious coronary sequelae is 2% to 3%, but mortality is as high as 22% in high-risk patients.[26]

Course in Kawasaki Disease with No Detected Coronary Artery Aneurysms

Even in patients who never appear to develop coronary artery aneurysms, there is evidence of endothelial dysfunction.[27] Lipid metabolism remains abnormal after resolution of the clinical disease.[28] Studies have shown lower myocardial flow reserve and higher total coronary resistance, compared with normal controls.[29] The effect of with these changes on long-term coronary artery disease is yet to be determined.

Myocarditis

Myocarditis is present in most patients with KD but rarely causes decreased ventricular function. Evidence of myocarditis may be seen with left atrial or left ventricular dilation and decreased shortening fraction or ejection fraction on echocardiography. Electrocardiographic findings include tachycardia beyond that expected for fever, or PR and/or QTc interval prolongation. These findings regress soon after intravenous immunoglobulin (IVIG) administration, but late biopsy studies have shown myocardial changes, including fibrosis and abnormalities in the myocytes.[30]

Valvular Regurgitation

The mitral valve is the most commonly involved. Early regurgitation has been associated with papillary muscle dysfunction, but late valvulitis has been reported. Aortic regurgitation and aortic root dilation are less common but have been reported.[31]

EVALUATION

Echocardiography

The initial echocardiogram should be obtained once the diagnosis is entertained. If there are sufficient criteria to treat, the IVIG treatment should not be withheld to obtain

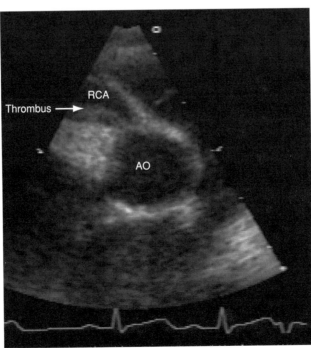

Figure 7-4   Two-dimensional echocardiogram, cross-sectional view. Note fusiform giant aneurysm of RCA with thrombus in coronary artery. *AO*, aorta; *RCA*, right coronary artery.

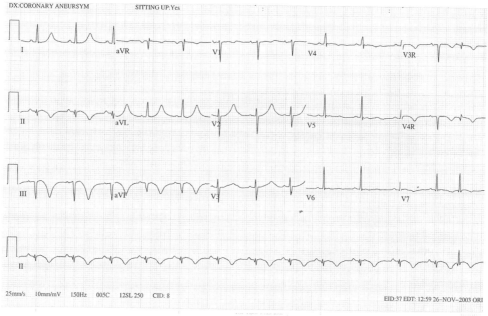

Figure 7-5   A 15-lead electrocardiogram in a 12-year-old girl with a stenotic right coronary artery after Kawasaki disease. Note Q waves in leads III and aVF and T wave inversion in leads II, III, and aVF, indicating an inferior myocardial infarction.

the echocardiogram, but it should be obtained as soon as possible. The echocardiogram may require sedation in young or very irritable children, as it is essential to obtain clear views of all coronary arteries. A high-frequency transducer should be used, even in older children, to obtain better resolution of the coronary arteries. Measurements should be made of the internal diameters of the coronary arteries, and these should be compared with normal values. Observation for thrombi should be part of the evaluation. In addition to evaluating the coronary arteries, assessment should be made of the left ventricular chamber dimensions and ventricular function, as well as of the aortic root diameter. Doppler interrogation of the valves for regurgitation should be performed, especially the mitral and aortic valves. As pericarditis may occur, observation for a pericardial effusion should be made. Follow-up echocardiography is recommended at 2 and 6 weeks after the onset of the illness. For those in whom early abnormalities are found, more frequent echocardiograms should be obtained (weekly or more frequently) depending on the clinical findings. Repeat follow-up echocardiograms should be at 6- to12-month intervals in those with stable coronary artery aneurysms or regression and from 1 to 5 years in those with no early aneurysms.

Magnetic Resonance Imaging

Magnetic resonance imaging or magnetic resonance angiography may identify coronary artery aneurysms in the proximal coronary artery segments and may provide flow data.

Cardiac Stress Testing

Evidence of myocardial ischemia or abnormal coronary perfusion may be evaluated with a variety of exercise and pharmacologic stress tests, including technetium (Tc) 99m, single photon emission computed tomography (SPECT) studies, nuclear perfusion scans, exercise stress echocardiography, dobutamine, dipyridamole, and adenosine stress echocardiography. Abnormal stress results may result in progression to more invasive imaging, such as coronary angiography.

Cardiac Catheterization and Angiography

Cardiac catheterization is rarely indicated acutely but may be used to evaluate the details of stenotic vessels in patients being considered for catheter intervention or coronary surgical revascularization surgery, especially those with giant coronary aneurysms. Patients who have had these interventions may require catheterization for evaluation of efficacy of the therapy. Intravascular ultrasound may show abnormal intimal and media thickening in those who appear by echocardiography or angiography to have had regression of the coronary aneurysms.

TREATMENT

Treatment is aimed at decreasing inflammation and preventing coronary artery aneurysms with subsequent thrombosis and stenosis, which could result in myocardial infarction (Table 7-1).

Treatment with IVIG and aspirin has been shown to decrease the incidence of coronary artery aneurysms to 5% to 6%.[32] In the 12% of patients who required retreatment for recurrent fever, the incidence of coronary aneurysms was 50%.[33] Persistent fever, possibly related to elevated cytokines, is thought to be an indicator of persistent vasculitis and is associated with a higher incidence of coronary artery involvement.[15] An occasional patient will require a third dose of IVIG, with an overall incidence of resistance to immunoglobulin of 2%.

Aspirin

Aspirin is given in the acute phase of the illness in "anti-inflammatory doses" of 80 to 100 mg/kg/day in four divided doses. After the fever abates, the dose of aspirin should be decreased to a low antiplatelet dose of 2 to 5 mg/kg once daily. Some choose to use high-dose aspirin for up to 2 weeks, regardless of the fever duration. In the presence of coronary artery aneurysms, the low dose of aspirin may be continued indefinitely or may be replaced by other anticoagulant medications. Use of ibuprofen should be avoided because of the potential to interfere with the antiplatelet effects of aspirin. Aspirin has not been shown to decrease the frequency of coronary artery aneurysms.[32] Because of the risk of Reye's syndrome in patients with varicella or influenza, children on long-term aspirin should receive an influenza vaccine yearly; aspirin should be held during the course of these illnesses.

Intravenous Immunoglobulin (IVIG)

In 1984, Furusho[34] reported the beneficial use of IVIG in KD. Several studies have shown that a dose of 2 gm/kg of intravenous gamma globulin is more effective in treating KD and preventing coronary aneurysms than lower-dose regimens.[35] Although the exact mechanism of its effect is unclear, possible mechanisms include crystallizable fragment (Fc) receptor blockade, neutralization of causative agents or of a toxin produced by an infectious

Table 7-1 Current Recommended Therapy		
	Medication	**Dosage**
Acute	IVIG	2 gm/kg
	Aspirin	80-100 mg/kg in 4 divided doses until afebrile × 48 hours
		3-5 mg/kg once daily once afebrile for 6 weeks
Chronic With coronary artery abnormalities < 8 mm	Aspirin	3-5 mg/kg/day
With coronary artery abnormalities ≥ 8 mm	Aspirin ±	3-5 mg/kg
	Clopidogrel +	1 mg/kg/day (Max: 75 mg/day)
	Warfarin or	0.1 mg/kg/day to INR 2-2.5
	LMW Heparin SC	
Acute Thrombosis **Use in all:**	Aspirin	3-5 mg/kg
	+ Heparin or	*Heparin*
		Load: 50 U/kg
		Infusion: 20 U/kg/hr
	+ LMW Heparin	LMW *Heparin*:
		Infants < 12 mo
		Treatment: 3 mg/kg/day, divided every 12 hours
		Prophylaxis: 1.5 mg/kg/day, divided every 12 hours
		Children and adolescents
		Treatment: 2 mg/kg/day, divided every 12 hours
		Prophylaxis: 1 mg/kg/day, divided every 12 hours
Add one:	Streptokinase IV	Bolus: 1000-4000 U/kg over 30 min
		Infusion: 1000-1500 U/kg/h
	Urokinase IV	Bolus: 4400 U/kg over 10 minutes
		Infusion: 4400 U/kg/h
	Tissue plasminogen activator IV	Bolus: 1.25 mg/kg
		Infusion: 0.1-0.5 mg/kg/h for 6 hours, then reassess
	Abciximab IV	Bolus: 0.25 mg/kg
		Infusion: 0.125 mcg/kg/min for 12 hours

SC, Subcutaneous; *IV,* intravenous; *LMW,* low molecular weight.

agent, down regulation of cytokine production, or a direct immunomodulating effect and induction of suppressor activity.[36] Up to 10% to 20% require retreatment for persistent (i.e., > 48 hours after IVIG dose completion) or recurrent (i.e., 2 to 7 days after treatment) fever, as persistent fever has been correlated with a higher risk of coronary artery ectasia or aneurysm formation.[37-39] Factors associated with retreatment include low hemoglobin (i.e., < 10 gm/dL), low albumin, and high white blood count and high neutophil count (i.e., > 75%). These factors are predictive of coronary artery abnormalities. In those with a higher C-reactive protein, bilirubin and aspartate aminotransferase (AST) levels are more likely to be IVIG resistant.[40] Measles and varicella immunizations should not be given for 5 to 6 months after a patient has received high-dose IVIG.

Steroids

Recent interest has focused on the use of steroids in treatment. An early study by Kato suggested an increased incidence of coronary artery aneurysms (65% of 17 patients) in patients who received prednisolone without other treatment, and, for many years, steroids were not used. Steroids had been reserved for those resistant to IVIG or with severe manifestations such as gangrene. Cremer and Rieger[41] reported that oral steroids with aspirin helps prevent coronary artery aneurysms. In 1999, Shinohara[42] reported that steroids (oral and IV) in 300 patients reduced the incidence of coronary artery aneurysms. In a study of pulsed intravenous methylprednisolone (IVMP) of 30 mg/kg, patients had decreased fever duration and no increase in coronary artery aneurysms.[43]

A multi-center, randomized, double-blind placebo controlled trial was conducted by the Pediatric Heart Network supported by the National Heart, Lung, and Blood Institute (NHLBI) to determine whether addition of IV methylprednisolone (IVMP) to conventional therapy improves coronary outcomes.[44] It was found that the use of IVMP when added to IVIG therapy does not improve the coronary outcome. Thus the conclusion was that the addition of pulse IVMP to IVIG is not indicated for primary treatment of KD.

To determine the efficacy of primary steroid treatment for Kawasaki disease, Wooditch and colleagues[45] recently performed a meta-analysis. Among the eight studies that met these criteria and were included in the meta-analysis, only one had blinded reading of echocardiography, only two were prospective, and five studies used no IVIG. Although the meta-analyses concluded that primary treatment with corticosteroids was associated with a lower risk of coronary artery aneurysm, these conclusions are limited by the quality and design of the studies included in the meta-analysis. A few studies using oral prednisolone therapy or combining dexamethasone

with IVIG have been reported with no effect on coronary artery abnormalities[46] Okada[47] found that steroids decrease symptoms by reducing cytokine levels.

Sundel[48] reported a prospective randomized trial of IVMP with aspirin/IVIG versus aspirin/IVIG alone. Those with IVMP had faster resolution of fever, more rapid improvement in markers of inflammation, and shorter length of hospitalization.[48] This effect has been shown to decrease cellular adhesion molecules, to suppress cytokines, and to decrease TNF-α expression in inflamed tissues.[49]

It is recommended by some that a pulse of methylprednisolone be considered if there is no response to two to three standard doses of IVIG.[5]

Other Treatments

Treatment of gangrene and peripheral ischemia has included thrombolytic agents, anticoagulants, and intravenous prostacyclin.[11] Pentoxifylline inhibits TNF-α messenger ribonucleic acid (mRNA) transcriptions. One clinical trial suggested a beneficial effect.[50] Ulinastatin, available in Japan, is a urinary trypsin inhibitor that inhibits neutrophil elastase activity. Plasma exchange has been reported in an uncontrolled clinical trial to be effective in patients refractory to IVIG. Abciximab, a glycoprotein IIb/IIIa receptor inhibitor, has been used in patients with giant coronary artery aneurysms. One study suggested that greater regression of the coronary artery aneurysms occurred when abciximab was used with IVIG, compared with IVIG alone.[51] Infliximab is a monoclonal antibody against TNF-α and has been suggested as a therapy for IVIG-resistant patients. Cyclophosphamide has been suggested as a potential agent. Little data are available on these newer therapies.

Early Treatment

In a study by Fong et al,[33] treatment before day 5 of the illness was associated with persistent or recrudescent fever, requiring retreatment in 33%, compared with a control group treated after 5 days of illness who had 8% retreatment. Despite retreatment, there was no significant increase in the prevalence of coronary artery aneurysms. Early treatment on day 4 did not affect the incidence of coronary artery aneurysms, but more patients required retreatment.[52] Sugahara[53] reported a decrease in the overall duration of fever in those treated early.

Thrombosis Prevention

Various regimens have been suggested, depending on the presence, regression, or absence of coronary artery aneurysms and the presence of giant coronary artery aneurysms. Most regimens include aspirin alone for small aneurysms. In the presence of larger aneurysms, aspirin with dipyridamole or clopidogrel is recommended. An additional regimen for higher-risk patients is warfarin or low-molecular-weight heparin, with or without aspirin, or a combination of warfarin and heparin (see Table 7-1).

Patients with giant coronary aneurysms with or without stenosis are at relatively high risk for thrombosis development and generally should receive both aspirin and warfarin. The desired INR range is 2 to 2.5.

Thrombosis Treatment

The main goal is to reestablish perfusion of the myocardium. Many agents have been used, including streptokinase, urokinase, and tissue plasminogen activator (tPA) (see Table 7-1). In addition, warfarin and aspirin should be used in these patients. Another agent that has been used is abciximab. Angioplasty and stent placement have been reported to be successful.

Surgical Treatment

Coronary artery bypass for stenotic or occluded coronary arteries has been reported to be successful.[54] The internal mammary arteries are most commonly used. After 10 years, 70% of patients having coronary artery bypass grafting (CABG) have had no cardiac events. Longer follow-up data are not available. The indications for CABG in children have not been established, they but follow adult indications with regard to occlusion and ischemia. CABG after myocardial infarction in children has been successful.[25]

Catheter Interventions

Catheter interventions, including balloon angioplasty, rotational ablation, and stent placement, have been performed in small numbers of children with coronary artery lesions after KD (Fig. 7-6).[55]

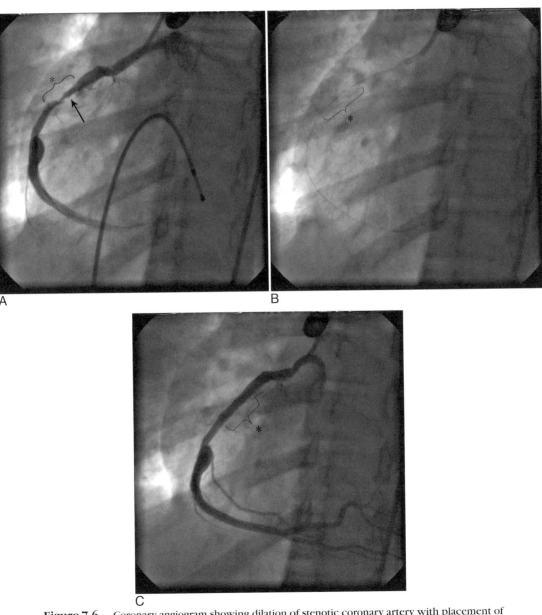

Figure 7-6   Coronary angiogram showing dilation of stenotic coronary artery with placement of stent. **A,** Note 90% narrowing of mid right coronary artery. **B,** Wire in coronary artery. **C,** Stent placed in dilated coronary artery, relieving obstructed area.

Transplant

Transplant from weeks to years after disease onset has been utilized in KD patients with severe myocardial dysfunction, intractable ventricular arrhythmias, severe coronary artery lesions unresponsive to interventional catheterization, or coronary artery bypass grafts, or those with coronary artery rupture.[22,56]

Other Miscellaneous Issues

It is recommended that any live vaccination be delayed for > 3 to 6 months after an episode of KD due to the potential of the disease to flare with the vaccination and the likelihood that the IVIG can block replication of live viral vaccines with suppression of acquired immunity.[57] Those patients on chronic aspirin therapy should receive a yearly influenza immunization. Limitation of strenuous activity is recommended for those with coronary stenosis and giant coronary aneurysms. Avoidance of contact sports is suggested in those on long-term anticoagulant therapy.

Early Follow-Up

Echocardiography should be performed at diagnosis, 2 weeks later, and at 6 to 8 weeks after onset of KD. If the initial echocardiogram is abnormal, it should be repeated within 1 week and at appropriate intervals thereafter.

Long-Term Follow-Up

Patients with giant coronary artery aneurysms should have yearly stress testing and possible periodic coronary angiography to identify stenotic lesions. Warfarin should be added to prevent thrombosis. Clopidogrel or aspirin may be added to warfarin.

RISK STRATIFICATION

Risk for Premature Atherosclerosis

It has been postulated that patients who have had KD are at a higher risk for the development of atherosclerosis.[58] Cheung found an adverse cardiovascular risk profile with proatherogenic alteration of the lipid profile and increased arterial stiffness.[59] Those with coronary artery aneurysms had the highest-risk profile with low HDL cholesterol, low apoA-I levels, high apoB levels and increased peripheral arterial stiffness. Others have reported low HDL cholesterol levels up to 3 years after the initial illness.[28]

Recommendations for Follow-Up

Risk categories have been determined by the American Heart Association (AHA) Committee on Rheumatic Fever, Endocarditis, and Kawasaki Disease of the Council on Cardiovascular Disease in the Young and are described in Table 7-2, with recommendations for therapy, physical activity, follow-up and diagnostic testing, and invasive testing.

MAJOR POINTS

- KD is most common in the United States in Asians and Pacific Islanders, followed by African-Americans and Hispanics.
- Diagnosis of KD is based on at least 5 days of fever and presence of at least four of five clinical features, including conjunctivitis, rash, cracked red lips or strawberry tongue, extremity swelling or redness of palms or soles, and cervical lymphadenopathy. If coronary artery aneurysms are present, only three clinical criteria are required.
- Multiple organ systems are involved, but cardiovascular system involvement is the most significant long-term sequellae.
- Other diseases with similar clinical findings, such as viral infections, scarlet fever, staphylococcal scaled skin syndrome, or toxic shock syndrome, should be eliminated.
- Atypical KD can occur with fewer than the required number of clinical findings for diagnosis.
- Cardiovascular involvement includes the pericardium (pericarditis), myocardium (myocarditis), valves (valvulitis) and, most importantly, the coronary arteries (coronary artery aneurysms).
- Others systems frequently involved include the joints (arthralgia or arthritis), the gastrointestinal system (hepatitis or gall bladder hydrops), and the central nervous system (irritability, meningitis).
- Positive laboratory findings include an elevation of white blood counts, platelet counts, erythrocyte sedimentation rate, and C-reactive protein.
- The etiology of KD is unclear but is most likely an immunologic response to an infectious agent in a genetically susceptible individual.
- KD is a vasculitis that affects small and medium-sized arteries, especially coronary arteries.
- Coronary artery aneurysms (CAAs) are more common in young patients, those with prolonged fever, and those with high neutrophil and band counts, low hemoglobin, and low platelet counts.
- CAAs occur in 25% of untreated KD patients.
- 50% of CAAs regress in 5 years, with small CAAs most likely to regress.
- CAAs occur most commonly in the proximal left anterior descending and proximal right coronary arteries.

(Continued)

Table 7-2   Risk Stratification

Risk Level	Pharmacological Therapy	Physical Activity	Follow-Up and Diagnostic Testing	Invasive Testing
I (no coronary artery changes at any stage of illness)	None beyond first 6-8 weeks	No restrictions beyond first 6-8 weeks	Cardiovascular risk assessment, counseling at 5-yr intervals	None recommended
II (transient coronary artery ectasia disappears within 1st 6-8 weeks)	None beyond first 6-8 weeks	No restrictions beyond first 6-8 weeks	Cardiovascular risk assessment, counseling at 3- to 5-yr intervals	None recommended
III (1 small-medium coronary artery aneurysm/major coronary artery)	Low-dose aspirin (3-6 mg/kg aspirin/d), at least until aneurysm regression documented	For patients <11 yr old, no restriction beyond 1st 6-8 weeks; patients 11-20 yr old, physical activity guided by biennial stress test, evaluation of myocardial perfusion scan; contact or high-impact sports discouraged for patients taking antiplatelet agents	Annual cardiology follow-up with echocardiogram + ECG, combined with cardiovascular risk assessment, counseling; biennial stress test/evaluation of myocardial perfusion scan	Angiography, if noninvasive test suggests ischemia
IV (≥1 large or giant coronary artery aneurysm, or multiple or complex aneurysms in same coronary artery, without obstruction)	Long-term antiplatelet therapy and warfarin (target INR 2.0-2.5) or low-molecular-weight heparin (target: antifactor Xa level 0.5-1.0 U/mL) should be combined in giant aneurysms	Contact or high-impact sports should be avoided because of risk of bleeding; other physical activity recommendations guided by stress test/evaluation of myocardial perfusion scan outcome	Biannual follow-up with echocardiogram + ECG; annual stress test/evaluation of myocardial perfusion scan	1st angiography at 6-12 mo or sooner if clinically indicated; repeated angiography if noninvasive test, clinical, or laboratory findings suggest ischemia; elective repeat angiography under some circumstances (see text)
V (coronary artery obstruction)	Long-term low-dose aspirin; warfarin or low-molecular-weight heparin if giant aneurysm persists; consider use of β-blockers to reduce myocardial O₂ consumption	Contact or high-impact sports should be avoided because of risk of bleeding; other physical activity recommendations guided by stress test/myocardial perfusion scan outcome	Biannual follow-up with echocardiogram and ECG; annual stress test/evaluation of myocardial perfusion scan	Angiography recommended to address therapeutic options

Adapted from Newburger JW, Takahashi M, Gerber MA, et al: Diagnosis, Treatment, and Long-Term Management of Kawasaki Disease. American Heart Association Scientific Statement. Circulation 2004;110:2747-2771. © 2004 American Heart Association, Inc.

MAJOR POINTS—CONT'D

- Giant aneurysms are > 8 mm and occur most often in male patients < 1 year of age.
- CAAs that do not regress can develop thrombosis, stenosis, or occlusion, and result in myocardial infarction.
- Early evaluation should be by echocardiography, which should be repeated, even if there is no initial CAA, at 2 and 6 weeks.
- Initial treatment is with aspirin and IVIG.
- IVIG treatment reduces CAA from 25% to 5-6%.
- Retreatment with IVIG is required in 10% to 20%.
- Antithrombosis treatment is used, especially in those with giant CAA.
- Catheter intervention or coronary artery surgery is required in a small number of patients.
- Long-term follow-up is necessary in many patients.
- Most patients with KD do well in the long term.

REFERENCES

1. Dengler LD, Capparelli EV, Bastian JF, et al: Cerebrospinal fluid profile in patients with acute Kawasaki disease. Pediatr Infect Dis J 17:478-481, 1998.

2. Witt MT, Minich LL, Bohnsack JF, Young PC: Kawasaki disease: More patients are being diagnosed who do not meet American Heart Association criteria. Pediatrics 104(1): e10, 1999.

3. Curtis N, Chan B, Levin M: Toxic shock syndrome toxin-secreting staphylococcus-aureus in Kawasaki syndrome. Lancet 343:299, 1994.

4. Burns JC, Mason WH, Glode MP, et al: Clinical and epidemiologic characteristics of patients referred for evaluation of possible Kawasaki disease. J Pediatr 118:680-686, 1991.

5. Hung JJ, Chiu CH: Pulse methylprednisolone therapy in the treatment of immune globulin-resistant Kawasaki disease: Case report and review of the literature. Ann Trop Paediatr 24:89-93, 2004.

6. Rowley AH, Shulman ST, Mask CA, et al: IgA plasma cell infiltration of proximal respiratory tract, pancreas, kidney, and coronary artery in acute Kawasaki disease. J Infect Dis 182:1183-1191, 2000.

7. Rowley AH, Shulman ST, Mask CA, Baker SC: Oligoclonal IgA response in the vascular wall in acute Kawasaki disease. J Immunol 166(2):1334-1343, 2000.

8. Shulman ST, Rowley AH: Advances in Kawasaki disease. Eur J Pediatr 163:285-291, 2004.

9. Leung DYM, Meissner C, Fulton D, Schlievert PM: The potential role of bacterial superantigens in the pathogenesis of Kawasaki syndrome. J Clin Immunol 15:S11-S17, 1995.

10. Leung DYM, Meissner HC, Shulman ST, et al: Prevalence of superantigen-secreting bacteria in patients with Kawasaki disease. J Pediatr 140:742-746, 2002.

11. Shulman ST, Deinocencio J, Hirsch R: Kawasaki disease. Pediatr Clin North Am 42:1205-1222, 1995.

12. Leung DYM, Geha RS, Newburger JW, et al: Two monokines, interleukin-1 and tumor necrosis factor, render cultured vascular endothelial cells susceptible to lysis by antibodies circulating during Kawasaki syndrome. J Ex Med 164:1958-1972, 1986.

13. Rowley AH, Shulman ST, Spike BT, et al: Oligoclonal IgA response in the vascular wall in acute Kawasaki disease. J Immunol 166:1334-1343, 2001.

14. Yasukawa K, Terai M, Shulman ST, et al: Systemic production of vascular endothelial growth factor and fms-like tyrosine kinase-1 receptor in acute Kawasaki disease. Circulation 105:766-769, 2002.

15. Koren G, Lavi S, Rose V, Rowe R: Kawasaki disease: Review of risk-factors for coronary aneurysms. J Pediatr 108:388-392, 1986.

16. Daniels SR, Specker B, Capannari TE, et al: Correlates of coronary artery aneurysm formation in patients with Kawasaki disease. Am J Dis Child 141:205-207, 1987.

17. Harada K, Yamaguchi H, Kato H, et al: Indication for intravenous gamma globulin treatment for Kawasaki. In Takahashi M, Taubert K (eds): Proceedings of the Fourth International Symposium on Kawasaki Disease. Dallas: American Heart Association, 1993, pp 459-462.

18. Research Committee on Kawaski Disease: Report of subcommittee on standardization of diagnostic criteria and reporting of coronary artery lesions in Kawasaki disease. Tokyo, Japan: Ministry of Health and Welfare, 1984.

19. Dajani AS, Taubert KA, Gerber MA, et al: Diagnosis and therapy of Kawasaki disease in children. Circulation 87: 1776-1780, 1993.

20. Nakamura Y, Yashiro M, Uehara R, et al: Use of laboratory data to identify risk factors of giant coronary aneurysms due to Kawasaki disease. Pediatr Int 46:33-38, 2004.

21. Kato H, Sugimura T, Akagi T, et al: Long-term consequences of Kawasaki disease. A 10- to 21-year follow-up study of 594 patients. Circulation 94:1379-1385, 1996.

22. Fijiwara T, Fujiwara H, Hamashima Y: Size of coronary aneurysm as a determining factor of the prognosis in Kawasaki disease in stage IV. Jpn Circ J Engl Ed 50:709, 1986.

23. Iemura M, Ishii M, Sugimura T, et al:. Long term consequences of regressed coronary aneurysms after Kawasaki disease: Vascular wall morphology and function. Heart 83:307-311, 2000.

24. Takahashi M, Mason W, Lewis AB: Regression of coronary aneurysms in patients with Kawasaki syndrome. Circulation 75:387-394, 1987.

25. Kato H, Ichinose E, Kawasaki T: Myocardial infarction in Kawasaki disease: Clinical analyses in 195 cases. J Pediatr 108:923-927, 1986.

26. Kitamura S: The role of coronary bypass operation on children with Kawasaki disease. Coron Artery Dis 14:95, 2002.

27. Fulton DR, Meissner C, Peterson MB: Effects of current therapy of Kawasaki disease on eicosanoid metabolism. Am J Cardiol 61:1323-1327, 1988.

28. Newburger JW, Burns JC, Beiser AS, Loscalzo J: Altered lipid profile after Kawasaki syndrome. Circulation 84:625–631, 1991.

29. Muzik O, Paridon SM, Singh TP, et al: Quantification of myocardial blood flow and flow reserve in children with a history of Kawasaki disease and normal coronary arteries using positron emission tomography. J Am Coll Cardiol 28:757–762, 1996.

30. Yutani C, Go S, Kamiya T, et al: Cardiac Biopsy of Kawasaki Disease. Arch Pathol Lab Med 105:470–473, 1981.

31. Ravekes WJ, Colan SD, Gauvreau K, et al: Aortic root dilation in Kawasaki disease. Am J Cardiol 87:919–922, 2001.

32. Durongpisitkul K, Gururaj VJ, Park JM, Martin CF: The prevention of coronary artery aneurysm in Kawasaki disease: A meta-analysis on the efficacy of aspirin and immunoglobulin treatment. Pediatrics 96:1057–1061, 1995.

33. Fong NC, Hui YW, Li CK, Chin MC: Evaluation of the efficacy of treatment of Kawasaki disease before day 5 of illness. Pediatr Cardiol 25:31–34, 2004.

34. Furusho K, Nakano H, Shinomiya K, et al: High-dose intravenous gammaglobulin for Kawasaki disease. Lancet 2:1055–1058, 1984.

35. Newburger JW, Takahashi M, Beiser AS, et al: A single intravenous infusion of gamma globulin as compared with four infusions in the treatment of acute Kawasaki syndrome. N Engl J Med 324:1633–1639, 1991.

36. Shulman ST. Ivgg therapy in Kawasaki disease: Mechanism(s) of action. Clin Immunol Immunopathol 53:S141–S146, 1989.

37. Durongpisitkul K, Soongswang J, Laohaprasitiporn D, et al: Immunoglobulin failure and retreatment in Kawasaki disease. Pediatr Cardiol 24:145–148, 2003.

38. Wright DA, Newburger JW, Baker A, Sundel RP: Treatment of immune globulin-resistant Kawasaki disease with pulsed doses of corticosteroids. J Pediatr 128:146–149, 1996.

39. Burns JC, Capparelli EV, Brown JA, et al: Intravenous gamma-globulin treatment and retreatment in Kawasaki disease. Pediatr Infect Dis J 17:1144–1148, 1998.

40. Sano T, Nagai T, Maki I, et al: Prediction of resistance to two intravenous infusions of high-dose gamma-globulin in patients with Kawasaki disease before treatment. Pediatr Res 53:180, 2003.

41. Cremer H and Rieger C: Epidemiology of Kawasaki syndrome in Germany (FGR). Prog Clin Biol Res 250:61–65, 1987.

42. Shinohara M, Sone K, Tomomasa T, Morikawa A: Corticosteroids in the treatment of the acute phase of Kawasaki disease. J Pediatr 135:465–469, 1999.

43. Kang SM, In SM, Moon EK, Kil HR: Corticosteroids add-on therapy in the acute phase of Kawasaki disease. Pediatr Res 53:164, 2003.

44. Newberger JW, Sleeper LA, McCrindle BW, et al: Randomized trial of pulse steroid therapy in Kawasaki disease. Circulation 112 (Suppl II): 419, 2005.

45. Wooditch AC, Aronoff SC: Effect of initial corticosteroid therapy on coronary artery aneurysm formation in Kawasaki disease: a meta-analysis of 862 children. Pediatr 116(4):989–995, 2005.

46. Okada Y, Shinohara M, Kobayashi T, et al: Effect of corticosteroids in addition to intravenous gamma globulin therapy on serum cytokine levels in the acute phase of Kawasaki disease in children. J Pediatr 143:363–367, 2003.

47. Okada Y, Shinohara M, Kobayashi T, et al: Effect of corticosteroids in addition to intravenous gamma globulin therapy on serum cytokine levels in the acute phase of Kawasaki disease in children. J Pediatr 143:363–367, 2003.

48. Sundel RP, Baker AL, Fulton DR, Newburger JW. Corticosteroids in the initial treatment of Kawasaki disease: Report of a randomized trial. J Pediatr 142:611–616, 2003.

49. Youssef PP, Haynes DR, Triantafillou S, et al: Effects of pulse methylprednisolone on inflammatory mediators in peripheral blood, synovial fluid, and synovial membrane in rheumatoid arthritis. Arthritis Rheum 40:1400–1408, 1997.

50. Furukawa S, Matsubara T, Umezawa Y, et al: Pentoxifylline and intravenous gamma globulin combination therapy for acute Kawasaki disease. Eur J Pediatr 153:663–667, 1994.

51. Williams RV, Wilke VM, Tani LY, Minich LL: Does Abciximab enhance regression of coronary aneurysms resulting from Kawasaki disease? Pediatrics 109(1):E4, 2002.

52. Muta H, Ishii M, Egami K, et al. Early intravenous gamma-globulin treatment for Kawasaki disease: The nationwide surveys in Japan. J Pediatr 144:496–469, 2004.

53. Sugahara Y, Ishii M, Muta H, et al: The effectiveness and safety of early intravenous immune globulin treatment for Kawasaki disease. Pediatr Res 53:179, 2003.

54. Yoshikawa Y, Yagihara T, Kameda Y, et al: Result of surgical treatments in patients with coronary-arterial obstructive disease after Kawasaki disease. Eur J Cardiothorac Surg 17:515–519, 2000.

55. Ishii M, Ueno T, Akagi T, et al: Guidelines for catheter intervention in coronary artery lesion in Kawasaki disease. Pediatr Int 43:558–562, 2001.

56. Checchia PA, Pahl E, Shaddy RE, Shulman ST: Cardiac transplantation for Kawasaki disease. Pediatrics 100:695–699, 1997.

57. Siber GR, Werner BG, Halsey NA, et al: Interference of immune globulin with measles and rubella immunization. J Pediatr 122:204–211, 1993.

58. Burns JC, Shike H, Gordon JB, et al: Sequelae of Kawasaki disease in adolescents and young adults. J Am Coll Cardiol 28:253–257, 1996.

59. Cheung YF, Yung TC, Tam SCF, et al: Novel and traditional cardiovascular risk factors in children after Kawasaki disease: Implications for premature atherosclerosis. J Am Coll Cardiol 43:120–124, 2004.

CHAPTER 8

The Genetics of Congenital Heart Disease

HEIKE E. SCHNEIDER

ELIZABETH GOLDMUNTZ

Major Chromosomal Anomalies

Trisomy 21 (Down Syndrome)

Trisomy 18 (Edwards' Syndrome)

Trisomy 13 (Patau's Syndrome)

Monosomy X (Turner's Syndrome)

Gene Deletion Syndromes

The 22q11 Deletion Syndrome

Single Gene Defects

Alagille Syndrome

Holt–Oram Syndrome

Ellis–van Creveld Syndrome

Char Syndrome

Noonan Syndrome

Familial ASD and Atrioventricular Conduction Disturbance

Heterotaxy Syndrome

Vasculopathies

Marfan Syndrome

Williams–Beuren Syndrome

Familial Supravalvar Stenoses

Ehlers–Danlos Syndrome

Evaluation of the Patient with CHD for a Genetic Etiology

Congenital heart malformations are the most common type of major birth defect, occurring in 4–8/1000 live births.[1] The prevalence of congenital heart disease (CHD) may increase substantially (to 75/1000 live births) if mild defects ascertained after 1 year of age are included. Tremendous progress has been made toward the successful medical and surgical management of CHD. In the past decade, substantial progress has been made toward understanding the etiology of these common disorders.

Early studies identified a few environmental factors and maternal diseases that increased the risk that an infant would be born with a malformed heart.[1] For example, infants of a diabetic mother were found to be at higher risk for CHD. However, infants exposed to a teratogen did not necessarily develop CHD, and most cases could not be explained by environmental exposure. Additional factors must contribute to the etiology.

Evidence now clearly points to a genetic contribution to the etiology of CHD. First, at least 25% of children with CHD will have a chromosomal anomaly, heritable genetic syndrome, or additional organ system malformation. Certain recurrent chromosomal anomalies are frequently associated with CHD, such as trisomy 21. Second, reports of kindred with several affected members suggest an inherited basis for CHD, as does an observed increase in recurrence risk among first-degree relatives. In certain cases, the genetic contribution follows simple Mendelian patterns of inheritance consistent with a single gene disorder, but, in other cases, complex patterns of inheritance suggest a more complex etiology. Theories of multifactorial or complex inheritance, whereby several genetic and environmental factors combine to cause CHD, have been suggested.

Efforts to identify the genetic contribution to CHD have increased substantially in the last decade. Linkage analyses of rare large kindred with multiple affected members and the molecular analysis of recurrent associated chromosomal anomalies have identified disease-related genes and loci, lending insight into the etiology of these disorders. Additional studies have used animal models to identify candidate genes for human disease. In the future, association studies correlating genetic variants with the risk of disease may identify which are disease-related.

The overall purpose of identifying the genetic factors contributing to CHD is to assess the impact of genotype on clinical outcome in order to improve clinical management. Although progress has been made, much about the genetic contribution to CHD remains to be defined. An enormous variety of chromosomal alterations and genetic syndromes have been reported in association with CHD. Studies report that at least 11% of all children with CHD have an abnormal karyotype. The online version of

Mendelian Inheritance of Man (OMIM)[2] lists over 300 syndromes with CHD. Because a description of every known genetic association is beyond the scope of this chapter, highlights of the most common syndromes and recent findings will be addressed.

MAJOR CHROMOSOMAL ANOMALIES

Aneuploidy, defined as a change in chromosome number, is the most common human chromosomal disorder. A change in chromosome number can be identified by routine karyotype analysis. Although most combinations are lethal prior to birth, several aneuploidy syndromes are found in live births (Table 8-1). The most common one, trisomy 21, now has a life expectancy well into adulthood. Because there is either an extra copy or a loss of an entire or a large part of a chromosome with hundreds of genes, it is not surprising that all major chromosomal abnormalities involve multiple organ systems. The cardiovascular system is frequently affected

(see Table 8-1) and contributes significantly to morbidity and mortality.

Trisomy 21 (Down Syndrome)

Trisomy 21 (OMIM #190685) is the most common aneuploidy, with a prevalence of 1 in 660 newborns (see Table 8-1). In nearly 95% of cases, there are three complete copies of chromosome 21 due to nondysjunction of chromosomes at meiosis; this mechanism is strongly associated with advanced maternal age. In the remaining cases, chromosomal mosaicism (1-2%) results in three copies of chromosome 21 found in a proportion of the cells, and translocations between two or more chromosomes (1-4%) can lead to three copies of a part of chromosome 21, so-called partial trisomy 21.

Trisomy 21 carries a high risk of CHD; approximately 40-50% of the patients are affected. Atrioventricular canal type defects, also called endocardial cushion defects, occur in 60% of patients with trisomy 21 and CHD. Conversely, approximately 60% of liveborn infants

---

Table 8-1 Congenital Heart Defects in Aneuploidy Syndromes

Karyotype	Syndrome (prevalence)	Most Common CHD	Frequency of CHD	Most Common Noncardiac Features
47,+21	Down (1 in 660 births)	CCAVC VSD/ASD/PDA TOF TOF/CAVC	40-50%	Dysmorphic facies Hypotonia Short, webbed neck Limb anomalies Gastrointestinal anomalies Mental retardation
47,+18	Edwards' (1 in 4000-5000 births)	VSD/ASD/PDA CAVC Valvular disease COA	90%	Craniofacial anomalies Limb anomalies Dysmorphic facies (small face) Omphalocele
47,+13	Patau's (1 in 5000-8000 births)	VSD/ASD/PDA Valvular disease Left-sided lesions (HLHS)	80%	Cleft palate Microphthalmia Holoprosencephaly Postaxial polydactyly
45,XO	Turner's (1 in 2000-2500 liveborn females)	BAV, AS, COA TAPVR MVP Aortic dissection HLHS Hypertension	20%	Congenital lymphedema of extremeties Broad, shield-like chest Low posterior hairline Webbed neck Skeletal anomalies Renal anomalies (horseshoe kidney) Short stature Gonadal dysgenesis Dysmoprhic facies

AS, Aortic stenosis; *ASD*, atrial septal defect; *BAV*, bicuspid aortic valve; *COA*, coarctation of the aorta; *CAVC*, common atrioventricular canal (i.e., endocardial cushion defect); *HLHS*, hypoplastic left heart syndrome; *MVP*, mitral valve prolapse; *PDA*, patent ductus arteriosus; *TAPVR*, total anomalous pulmonary venous return; *TOF*, tetralogy of Fallot; *VSD*, ventricular septal defect.

with a complete common atrioventricular canal defect have Down syndrome.[3] Other cardiac septation defects are described in approximately 30% of patients with trisomy 21 and CHD, including, in decreasing order of frequency, ventricular septal defects, atrial septal defects, and patent ductus arteriosus. Less common cardiac defects include tetralogy of Fallot and the rare combination of tetralogy of Fallot with complete common atrioventricular canal. In addition to cardiac defects, patients with trisomy 21 have multiple other anomalies, including mental retardation, characteristic facial features, gastrointestinal and skeletal anomalies, and hypotonia, to name a few.

The relationship of the chromosomal anomaly to the pathogenesis of CHD is not clear. Mouse models, including a murine trisomy 16 (the murine chromosome 16 is partially syntenic with the human chromosome 21) and a chimeric mouse containing the human chromosome 21, have been developed to try to recapitulate the chromosomal alteration and clinical phenotype. Although both models exhibit several typical features of Down syndrome, such as neurodevelopmental and gastrointestinal anomalies, neither model displays the common defects of the atrioventricular canal. Instead, other major cardiac defects, such as conotruncal malformations and atrioventricular valve dysplasia, are observed. Investigators have also tried to define which piece of human chromosome 21 confers CHD by analyzing the cohort with partial trisomy. A specific region on chromosome 21 proposed to be critical to cardiovascular disease has been reported.[4] A candidate gene mapping into this region, DSCAM (Down syndrome cell adhesion molecule), is currently under investigation since it is expressed in the heart during development.

Trisomy 18 (Edwards' Syndrome)

Trisomy 18 (or Edwards' syndrome) is the second most common aneuploidy syndrome, with a prevalence of approximately 1/3000 live births (see Table 8-1). Most fetuses with this chromosomal anomaly do not survive to term. CHD is diagnosed in nearly 90% of patients and most commonly includes one or more of the following anomalies: ventricular septal defect, patent ductus arteriosus, or atrial septal defect. Other cardiac malformations include bicuspid aortic and pulmonary valves, pulmonic stenosis, coarctation of the aorta, and, rarely, tetralogy of Fallot or transposition of the great vessels. Multiple organ systems are affected, including the neurologic, skeletal, gastrointestinal, genitourinary, and pulmonary. Characteristic facial features and anomalies are also found. The life expectancy is low, with only half of the affected patients surviving the first week of life without intervention. Only 5–10% of patients survive their first year, although case reports describe children older than 10 years of age. Those with partial trisomy 18 may have a less severe phenotype.

Trisomy 13 (Patau's Syndrome)

Trisomy 13 was first described by Patau in the 1960s. The prevalence is approximately 1 in 5000–8000 live births (see Table 8-1). CHD is diagnosed in approximately 80% of affected patients; the most common defects include ventricular septal defect, atrial septal defect, patent ductus arteriosus, and semilunar valvar abnormalities. The prognosis is poor for these children: 65% of infants succumb before 6 months of age, and only 18% survive the first year; survival beyond 3 years is described in rare case reports. The severity of the cardiac defect is usually not the cause of demise. Additional abnormalities include severe mental retardation, seizures, apnea, hypotonia, cleft lip or palate, skeletal anomalies, cryptorchidism, and hernia.

Monosomy X (Turner's Syndrome)

Turner's syndrome results from monosomy of chromosome X [45 (XO)] with a prevalence of 1 in 2000–2500 liveborn females (see Table 8-1).[5] Cardiac lesions are noted in 25–35% of affected patients and most commonly involve the left side of the heart.[6] Some hypothesize that the abnormal lymphatic flow seen in Turner's syndrome alters blood flow in the developing aortic arches and causes the associated left-sided cardiac defects. The most common malformations include coarctation of the aorta or bicuspid aortic valve, or both, whereas hypoplastic left heart syndrome is rare. Other important cardiovascular features that are rare but are often overlooked include the late occurrence of hypertension and aortic dilation resulting in death secondary to aortic dissection. These late risks suggest that even patients without overt CHD should be followed regularly by examination and echocardiography. Turner's syndrome is also characterized by lymphedema of the hands and feet as a neonate, webbed neck, widely spaced nipples, short stature, and primary amenorrhea, as well as renal, skeletal, and thyroid anomalies.

GENE DELETION SYNDROMES

With advanced cytogenetic techniques, consistent deletions or duplications of parts of chromosomes are now detected by karyotype using high-resolution banding, fluorescence *in situ* hybridization, or both. These techniques have helped identify new disease-related loci and define genetic syndromes (Table 8-2). Most recently, techniques to detect rearrangements in the gene-rich subtelomeric regions have been developed, but their

Table 8-2   Congenital Heart Defects in Select Chromosome Deletion/Duplication Syndromes

Chromosome	Syndrome	Cardiovascular Defect	Frequency of CHD	Most Common Noncardiac Features
22q11 deletion	DiGeorge, velocardiofacial, and conotruncal face anomaly	TOF, TOF/PA, IAA, truncus arteriosus, VSD, aortic arch anomalies	75–80%	Hypocalcemia Immunodeficiency Palate anomaly Delayed/hypernasal speech Learning disabilities Behavioral/psychiatric disorders Renal anomalies Skeletal anomalies Dysmorphic facies
Partial duplication 22	Cat-eye	TAPVR, TOF, VSD	30–40%	Ocular coloboma Anal atresia Ear pit/tag
7q11 deletion	Williams–Beuren	Supravalvar AS and PS	50–85%	Growth delay Mental retardation Elfin facies Locacious personality Hypercalcemia (infancy)
5p deletion	Cri du chat	VSD, ASD, PDA	30–60%	Cat cry (infancy) Simian crease Dysmorphic facies
4p deletion	Wolf-Hirschhorn	ASD, VSD, PDA, LSVC	50%	Cleft lip Hypospadias Seizures Scalp defect Dysmorphic facies

AS, Aortic stenosis; *ASD,* atrial septal defect; *IAA,* interrupted aortic arch; *LSVC,* left-sided superior vena cava; *PDA,* patent ductus arteriosus; *PS,* pulmonary stenosis; *TAPVR,* total anomalous pulmonary venous return; *TOF,* tetralogy of Fallot; *TOF/PA,* tetralogy of Fallot with pulmonary atresia; *VSD,* ventricular septal defect.

specific application to CHD remains to be defined. The sections below describe the most common deletion syndrome, the 22q11 deletion syndrome, characterized in part by CHD. Williams–Beuren syndrome, a deletion syndrome of 7q11, is discussed in the section on vasculopathies.

The 22q11 Deletion Syndrome

Deletions of a segment of chromosome 22, or 22q11 deletions, have recently been identified in a significant number of patients with a variety of congenital heart defects (Tables 8-2, 8-3). This discovery has increased our ability to identify the genetic cause for a substantial number of patients and has led to the early identification of associated noncardiac anomalies (OMIM #188400).[7] In particular, DiGeorge syndrome was originally considered to be a rare developmental field defect characterized by conotruncal cardiac defects, hypocalcemia from hypoparathyroidism, immunodeficiency from aplasia or hypoplasia of the thymus, and distinct facial features. Chromosomal anomalies that resulted in the loss of the proximal long arm of chromosome 22 were identified in

10–15% of patients. Subsequent molecular analyses demonstrated that approximately 90% of patients with DiGeorge syndrome had a deletion of one segment of chromosome 22 in the region of 22q11. Investigators subsequently demonstrated that the vast majority of patients with velocardiofacial (i.e., Shprintzen's) and conotruncal anomaly face syndromes, whose clinical features overlapped with those of DiGeorge syndrome, also had a 22q11 deletion. Thus, the majority of patients meeting the clinical diagnosis of DiGeorge, velocardiofacial, or conotruncal anomaly face syndromes share a common genetic etiology, namely a 22q11 deletion. (The collection of these syndromes was given the acronym of CATCH 22, with CATCH standing for cardiac, abnormal facies, thymic hypoplasia, cleft palate, and hypocalcemia, but more recently it is referred to as the 22q11 deletion syndrome.) The 22q11 deletion syndrome is the most common deletion syndrome and occurs with an estimated frequency of 1 in 4000 live births. The frequency is likely to be higher due to a large number of unidentified adults with a subtle phenotype. Approximately 10% of cases result from autosomal dominant inheritance of a 22q11 deletion.

Patients with a chromosome 22q11 deletion have a wide spectrum of clinical features that are characteristic of the syndrome but highly variable between affected individuals. The most common features include cardiovascular defects, palatal anomalies, feeding disorders, learning and speech disabilities, hypocalcemia, immunodeficiency, and specific facial features (Box 8-1, Fig. 8-1). In particular, approximately 75% of patients have a cardiovascular anomaly, of which the most common include conotruncal defects (truncus arteriosus, tetralogy of Fallot, or interrupted aortic arch type B), aortic arch anomalies (such as right aortic arch, double aortic arch, or aberrant subclavian artery), and ventricular septal defects (perimembranous, malalignment types and conoseptal hypoplasia). The most common palate defects include velopharyngeal insufficiency resulting in hypernasal speech, as well as cleft palate. Feeding disorders result not only from palate anomalies but also from nasopharyngeal insufficiency during infancy, gastroesophageal reflux, esophageal dysmotility, and gastrointestinal structural anomalies. Hypoplasia or aplasia of the parathyroid gland results in transient, long-term, and/or late-onset hypocalcemia. Thymic hypoplasia (ectopic location) or aplasia results in varying degrees of immunodeficiency that can be severe enough to require a thymic transplant (occurring in < 1% cases). However, most patients with a 22q11 deletion have a mild immunodeficiency resulting in frequent, lengthy infections that continue into adulthood. Other anomalies include renal and skeletal findings. The majority of patients experience delayed emergence of speech, as well as learning and behavioral disabilities. Typical facial features are usually notable in the school-age child but may be difficult to

Box 8-1   Most Common Features of the 22q11 Deletion Syndrome

Cardiovascular anomalies
    Intracardiac malformations
    Aortic arch anomalies
Palate abnormalities
    Overt cleft palate
    Submucosal cleft palate
    Velopharyngeal insufficiency
Immunodeficiency
    Sinusitis/otitis media
Hypocalcemia
Feeding disorders
    Nasopharyngeal reflux
    Gastroesophageal reflux
Speech disabilities
Neurocognitive deficits
    Learning disabilities
Behavioral and psychiatric disorders
    Schizophrenia
Renal anomalies
Skeletal anomalies
Facial dysmorphia

identify in the newborn (see Fig. 8-1). The clinical phenotype is highly variable. Some patients with a 22q11 deletion have a very mild phenotype, characterized, for example, by mild learning disabilities or hypernasal speech whereas others, even within the same family, have a much more severe phenotype with multiple anomalies.

Because cardiovascular defects of a particular type are such a common feature of the 22q11 deletion syndrome,

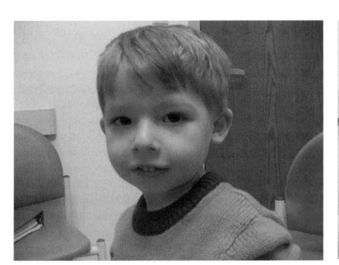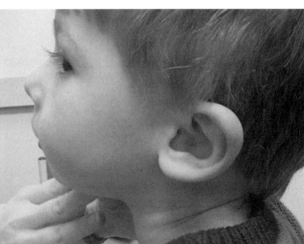

Figure 8-1   Full face and profile of a 3-year-old boy with the 22q11 deletion syndrome demonstrating dysmorphic features consistent with the diagnosis, including hooding of the eyelids, apparent hypertelorism versus telecanthus, small cupped and protuberant ears with mildly thick and overfolded helices, malar flatness, a bulbous nasal tip with minimally hypoplastic alae nasae, and micrognathia. (Images courtesy of Elaine Zackai, MD, and Donna McDonald-McGinn, M.S., Division of Human Genetics, The Children's Hospital of Philadelphia.)

investigators have conversely studied the frequency of a 22q11 deletion in the cardiac population.[8] As detailed in Table 8-3, a 22q11 deletion is frequently found in patients with interrupted aortic arch (particularly type B), truncus arteriosus, tetralogy of Fallot, isolated aortic arch anomalies, and certain types of ventricular septal defects. In contrast, relatively few patients with double outlet right ventricle and even rarer cases of transposition of the great arteries are found to have a 22q11 deletion. Studies further demonstrate that the subset of patients with an aortic arch anomaly (such as a right-sided or cervical arch), regardless of the type of intracardiac abnormality, is at a higher risk of having a 22q11 deletion.

Ideally, the diagnosis of the 22q11 deletion syndrome should be made in the neonate or infant, given the associated features and implications for the family. Although all patients with a 22q11 deletion will eventually manifest additional syndromic features beyond cardiac defects, identifying the at-risk newborn with CHD may be difficult, given the challenge of identifying the characteristic facial or other syndromic features in this age group. Therefore, when a physician is caring for a patient with one of these cardiac defects, careful consideration must be given to whether the patient should be tested for a 22q11 deletion. Although controversial, most investigators would recommend testing all infants with interrupted aortic arch, truncus arteriosus, isolated aortic arch anomalies, and tetralogy of Fallot. All infants with a ventricular septal defect and concurrent aortic arch anomaly also warrant testing for a 22q11 deletion, whereas those with a ventricular septal defect and normal aortic arch warrant careful observation for other syndromic features and possible testing. Of note, a 22q11 deletion has been diagnosed in patients with a wide range of CHD even though it is most commonly observed in a subset of lesions.

A 22q11 deletion is now easily detected from a sample of whole blood using a clinically available molecular cytogenetic technique called fluorescence *in situ* hybridization. Identifying the cardiac patient with a 22q11 deletion allows for the early detection of and intervention for associated noncardiac features. Such testing also allows for appropriate family counseling. Approximately 10% of parents have been found to carry a 22q11 deletion but may have only mild features of the disorder, such as learning or speech disabilities. Given that the offspring of a parent carrying a 22q11 deletion has a 50% chance of inheriting the deletion baring chromosome, recognition of the familial cases and appropriate counseling is critical. Identification of the cardiac patient with a 22q11 deletion warrants referral to a geneticist, as well as other subspecialists, and testing of both parents (Box 8-2).

For many years, several laboratories have attempted to identify which gene or genes mapping into the deleted segment causes the symptoms associated with the 22q11 deletion syndrome. Approximately 30 genes have been identified in the deleted segment and their role in the development of involved organs has been evaluated. One gene, *TBX1*, has come to be of particular interest because of its pattern of expression in the mouse embryo.[9] Several mouse models lacking partial or complete expression of this gene have been engineered and have demonstrated features consistent with but not completely identical to the human 22q11 deletion syndrome. In one report, three human subjects with the clinical features of the 22q11 deletion syndrome but without a chromosomal 22q11 deletion were found to have presumably disease-causing mutations. Thus, the role of *TBX1* and the other genes from the region remains under investigation. It is likely that other genetic and environmental factors modulate the expression of the deletion to result in the highly variable clinical features seen in this syndrome.

Table 8-3 Frequency of a 22q11 Deletion in Patients with Conotruncal Cardiac Defects

Cardiac Defect	Frequency* (%)
Tetralogy of Fallot	16
Truncus arteriosus	35
Interrupted aortic arch	50
Ventricular septal defect[†]	10
with aortic arch anomaly	40
with normal aortic arch	3
Isolated aortic arch anomaly	24
Double outlet right ventricle	<5
Transposition of the great arteries (S,D,D)	<1
Total	**18**

*The frequencies increase in the face of concurrent arch anomalies such as right sided or cervical locations or abnormal branching patterns.
[†]Perimembranous, malalignment, or conoseptal hypoplasia ventricular septal defects.

Box 8-2 Initial Evaluation of the Cardiac Patient Diagnosed with a 22q11 Deletion

Test parents for 22q11 deletion
Refer for clinical genetics consultation
Evaluate for hypocalcemia
Check white blood count to identify severely immunodeficient newborns
Order abdominal ultrasound to evaluate renal anatomy
Refer for the evaluation of the following:
  Cardiovascular status (if not already known)
  Palate anatomy and function
  Immunologic status
  Feeding and speech skills
  Developmental/neurocognitive status

SINGLE GENE DEFECTS

Alagille Syndrome

Alagille syndrome is an autosomal dominant disorder characterized by cardiac, hepatic, ocular, skeletal, craniofacial, and renal abnormalities (Table 8-4) (OMIM #118450). By the initial definition, the diagnosis of this syndrome required biopsy-proven paucity of intralobular bile ducts, along with three of five of the following features: chronic cholestasis, cardiovascular abnormalities, vertebral abnormalities, ocular abnormalities, and characteristic facial features (Fig. 8-2). Cardiovascular anomalies of the right side of the heart were predominantly described. A recent study of a large cohort demonstrated that 93% of patients with Alagille syndrome had some cardiovascular anomaly, ranging from a murmur consistent with peripheral pulmonary stenosis (i.e., mild changes) to tetralogy of Fallot with pulmonary atresia (i.e., severe defects).[10] Overall, 76% of the cohort had peripheral pulmonary stenosis; 35% of the cohort had peripheral pulmonary stenosis in isolation, whereas the rest (41%) had peripheral pulmonary stenosis in conjunction with other cardiac anomalies. Right-sided cardiac defects were most common (55% of entire cohort), but left-sided cardiac abnormalities were also seen (7%). Multiple other anomalies (14%) including septal defects (10%) were identified as well. Of note, recent studies of a large Alagille cohort demonstrate that 9% of patients have additional extracardiac vascular abnormalities that contribute significantly to their morbidity and mortality.

Approximately 5% to 10% of the patients with Alagille syndrome were noted to have chromosomal abnormalities involving chromosomal region 20p11. Additional molecular genetic studies identified disease-related mutations in a candidate gene named *JAG1*, which mapped into the most commonly deleted region of 20p11, thereby establishing *JAG1* as the disease gene for Alagille syndrome.[11] *JAG1* encodes the Jagged1 protein, a cell surface protein that functions as one of five ligands for the four human Notch receptors. The Notch signaling pathway has been implicated in several human diseases and is critical to developmental cell fate decisions.

Currently, nearly 90% of patients with the classic features of Alagille syndrome are found to have a *JAG1* alteration. The mutations in *JAG1* include total gene deletions (3–7% of mutations) and intragenic mutations. The intragenic mutations are protein truncating (frameshifts and nonsense account for ~70% of mutations), splicing (~10%) and missense (~10%). Thus, Alagille syndrome appears to result from haploinsufficiency, or half the amount, of Jagged1 protein. The mutations are distributed across the entire gene, with no specific mutation "hotspots."

Subsequent evaluations have demonstrated that patients with a subset of clinical features of Alagille

---

Table 8-4 Single-Gene Defects and Congenital Heart Disease

Syndrome	Gene	Cardiac Anomaly	Most Common Noncardiac Features
Alagille	*JAG1*	Right-sided defects (55%), left-sided lesions (7%)	Paucity of intrahepatic bile ducts Ocular (posterior embryotoxin) Skeletal (butterfly vertebrae) Typical facial features
Holt–Oram	*TBX5*	ASD, VSD, CAVC, HLHS, dysrhythmias	Upper limb defects Triphalangeal, absent, or hypoplastic thumb
Familial ASD/AVB	*NKX2.5*	AVB, secundum ASD, other CHD	None
Ellis–van Creveld	*EVC* *EVC2*	Common atrium, other ASD ASD	Short limbs and ribs Postaxial polydactyly Dysplastic nails and teeth
Char	*TFAP2B*	PDA	Facial dysmorphia Abnormal fifth digits
Noonan	*PTPN11*	Valvar PS, HCM	Short neck with webbing or redundant skin Unusual shape of chest Developmental delay Cryptorchidism Bleeding diathesis Short stature Typical facies

ASD, Atrial septal defect; *AVB*, atrioventricular block; *CAVC*, common atrioventricular canal (endocardial cushion defect); *HCM*, hypertrophic cardiomyopathy; *HLHS*, hypoplastic left heart syndrome; *PDA*, patent ductus arteriosus; *PS*, pulmonary stenosis; *VSD*, ventricular septal defect.

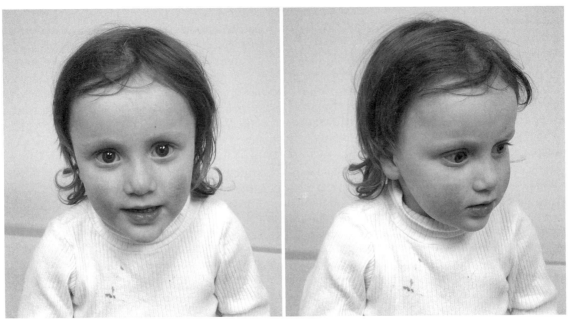

Figure 8-2 Full face and profile of a 28-month-old girl with Alagille syndrome. Note the broad forehead, deep-set eyes, long nose with rounded tip, and pointed chin, giving the appearance to the face of an inverted triangle. (Images courtesy of Ian Krantz, MD, Division of Human Genetics, The Children's Hospital of Philadelphia.)

syndrome (or a "microform" of Alagille syndrome) can have a *Jag1* mutation in the absence of clinically apparent hepatic disease. In particular, several patients with CHD in the absence of overt hepatic disease have been found to have a *Jag1* mutation.[12,13] The frequency with which patients with apparently isolated right-sided cardiac defects have a *Jag1* mutation is currently under investigation.

Expression studies in the mouse embryo demonstrate that *Jag1* is expressed in tissues affected in Alagille syndrome. A mouse model lacking *Jag1* expression failed to recapitulate features of the human disease. However, a mouse model lacking *Jag1* expression and a low level of Notch2 expression exhibits most developmental abnormalities observed in Alagille syndrome. This model demonstrates that gene interactions may play a role in the variable phenotypic expression of Alagille syndrome.

Holt–Oram Syndrome

Holt–Oram syndrome is one of several so-called heart-hand syndromes, characterized by cardiac and limb defects (OMIM #142900). A rare disorder, the prevalence of Holt–Oram syndrome is estimated to be approximately 1 per 100,000 live births. An autosomal dominant disorder, it is fully penetrant with highly variable expression. Linkage analysis of several large families with typical cardiac and skeletal findings identified a candidate disease locus on 12q2. Subsequent analyses demonstrated that the T-box gene, *TBX5*, is the cause of

Holt–Oram syndrome.[14-16] The majority of cases (50–85%) are attributed to new mutations of *TBX5*. Approximately 90% of patients with Holt–Oram syndrome have heart defects, which are typically defects in septation, including atrial and ventricular septal defects. Both secundum and atrioventricular canal types of atrial septal defects are seen. Additional defects include those of the left side of the heart, conduction defects, sinus bradycardia, and progressive AV block. The radial deformities can be subtle and only detectable by radiography, or they can be severe, such as phocomelia. Typical skeletal defects include triphalangeal thumbs and upper limb preaxial radial ray defects.

Ellis–van Creveld Syndrome

Ellis–van Creveld (EVC) syndrome, or chondroectodermal dysplasia, is an autosomal recessive disorder also characterized by skeletal and cardiac anomalies (OMIM #225500). Skeletal anomalies include short limbs, short ribs, narrow thorax, postaxial polydactyly, and dysplastic nails and teeth. Congenital heart disease occurs in 60% of individuals and manifests typically as a common atrium, followed by other defects of the atrial septum. Linkage analysis mapped the EVC phenotype to genetic markers on chromosome 4p16. Positional cloning revealed a novel gene at this locus, EVC, mutated in individuals with the classic phenotype. However, only 20% to 25% of patients with the clinical features of EVC were found to have a mutation of EVC, suggesting genetic heterogeneity.

Further examination of other pedigrees with indistinguishable phenotypes led to the identification of a second disease-related gene, *EVC2*, in the same region of chromosome 4p16.

Char Syndrome

Char syndrome, also known as syndromic patent ductus arteriosus, is an autosomal dominant disorder characterized by patent ductus arteriosus, facial dysmorphism, and an abnormal fifth digit of the hand (OMIM #169100). Linkage analysis mapped the Char critical region to the chromosomal region 6p12–p21 and led to the characterization of the first genetic mutations in humans thought to be involved in persistence of the ductus arteriosus. Further molecular studies identified mutations in the transcription factor, TFAP2B, which exerted a dominant negative effect on protein function.

Noonan Syndrome

Noonan syndrome is a relatively common autosomal dominant disease with a prevalence of 1 in 1000–2500 live births (OMIM #163950). More than one third of cases are thought to be inherited. Typical features include facial dysmorphism, short stature, and CHD (Fig. 8-3). Nearly two-thirds of affected patients have heart disease, of which nearly 50% have pulmonary valve stenosis due to a dysplastic pulmonary valve. Hypertrophic cardiomyopathy is the next most common cardiac anomaly, although other types of CHD have been reported.

Identification of multiple affected kindred allowed for linkage analysis to identify a disease-associated region at 12q24. Subsequent analysis of a candidate gene in the disease locus identified missense mutations in *Ptpn11*, which encodes the protein tyrosine phosphatase SHP-2.[17] In the mouse model, *Ptpn11* is essential for semilunar valvulogenesis, and in functional assays, the missense mutations resulted in a gain-of-function change in the protein. Of note, mutations of *Ptpn11* were found in only 50% of the cases studied, implying genetic heterogeneity of this clinical syndrome.[18] Genotype-phenotype analysis revealed that pulmonary valve stenosis was more prevalent in the group with *Ptpn11* mutations, whereas hypertrophic cardiomyopathy was less prevalent. There was no genotype/phenotype correlation noted for the other features.

Familial ASD and Atrioventricular Conduction Disturbance

Secundum atrial septal defects account for 10% of isolated congenital heart defects. Different inheritance patterns behave been observed for familial, nonsyndromic cases of atrial septal defects. The genetic basis for one of these disorders came from a recent analysis of four nonsyndromic kindred, characterized by secundum atrial septal defects, atrioventricular conduction delay, or both. Linkage analyses of these four kindred identified a disease locus at 5q35, wherein mapped a transcription factor, *NKX2.5*, known to be critical to cardiovascular development (Table 8-4). Further analysis identified disease-related mutations of *NKX2.5* in affected family members and demonstrated that familial atrial septal defects and atrioventricular conduction delay was, in some cases, a single gene disorder inherited as an autosomal dominant trait.[19] Subsequent studies identified sporadic cases with atrioventricular conduction delay,

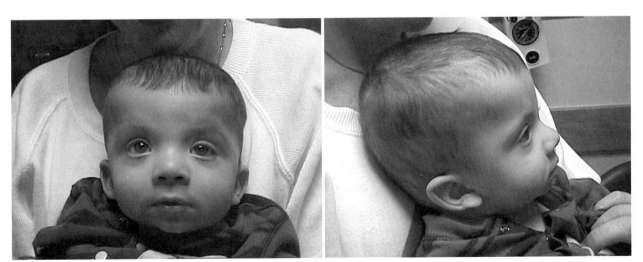

Figure 8-3   Full face and profile of an 11-month-old boy with Noonan syndrome. Note characteristic facial appearance, including a tall and boxy forehead, a down slant of the palpebral fissures, epicanthal folds, mild ptosis on the left, low-set ears, and a small chin. (Images courtesy of Ian Krantz, MD, Division of Human Genetics, The Children's Hospital of Philadelphia.)

secundum atrial septal defect, or both, with similar mutations.[20] The majority of mutations identified in this cohort caused protein truncation or changed critical amino acids in the DNA binding domain.

Careful inspection of the affected pedigrees demonstrated that some family members with *NKX2.5* mutations had different types of CHD, including ventricular septal defects, tetralogy of Fallot, or tricuspid valve anomalies. Investigators have since examined large cohorts of patients with different types of CHD without atrioventricular conduction delay to identify the affected cohort. Mutations have been identified in a small number of nonsyndromic patients, predominantly those with tetralogy of Fallot or other related conotruncal defects.[21,22] However, the types of mutations are different than those identified in the original pedigrees or those with atrioventricular delay in that they are missense mutations. The role that these alterations play in disease is still under investigation.

A mouse model lacking *Nkx2.5* expression (i.e., a "null" mouse) had been developed before the pedigree analysis was completed. The mouse lacking *Nkx2.5* expression was noted to have severe developmental disorders including cessation of cardiac development soon after looping. The mouse heterozygous for *Nkx2.5* expression had not been carefully examined until after the pedigree analysis was performed. The heterozygous mouse with some *Nkx2.5* expression was subsequently demonstrated to have subtle atrial anatomic abnormalities in conjunction with conduction abnormalities. Thus, concordant findings between the mouse phenotype and human disease were eventually described.

Heterotaxy Syndrome

Although vertebrates appear to be symmetric, their internal organs are asymmetric along the left-right axis. The positioning of abdominal and thoracic organs is vital for proper organ function, especially in the heart. When the left-right axis is disrupted, then heterotaxy (a Greek word meaning "different arrangement") results, which is frequently associated with significant intracardiac and venous anomalies. To date, heterotaxy syndromes carry the highest mortality among complex CHD.

Linkage analysis followed by physical mapping in large pedigrees with X-linked inheritance of heterotaxy syndrome identified the first disease-related gene on the X-chromosome, *ZIC3* (Table 8-4) (OMIM #306955).[23] The gene *ZIC3* is the homologue to a murine transcription factor, which is expressed in embryonic development at the time the first markers of left-right asymmetry are detected. The mutations found to date are in highly conserved domains of the gene, and most affected male humans who carry a mutation have complex heart disease with other manifestations of abnormal situs. Animal

models have identified a number of additional genes that participate in establishing left-right asymmetry in the developing embryo. These genes are candidate genes for human heterotaxy syndromes and are under further investigation.[24]

VASCULOPATHIES

Vasculopathies represent a subtype of CHD wherein alterations in connective tissue cause abnormalities of the vessels. Other organ systems with connective tissue, such as the skeleton, may be affected. The genetic etiology of many of these disorders has been defined because large kindred with multiple affected members have been available for linkage analysis and subsequent disease-gene identification. Most represent single gene disorders, although Williams–Beuren syndrome is a contiguous gene deletion syndrome.

Marfan Syndrome

Marfan syndrome is an autosomal dominant disorder characterized by aortic root dilation, mitral valve prolapse, tall and disproportionate stature, thoracic cage deformity, joint laxity, dislocation of the ocular lens, abnormal skin stretch marks, and pneumothorax[25] (OMIM #154700). Biochemical studies followed by linkage and mutation analyses demonstrated that mutations of the FBN1 gene cause Marfan syndrome. FBN1 encodes the protein fibrillin-1, which is a component of the extracellular microfibril. Most families harbor unique mutations in this large gene, making genetic testing particularly difficult. The clinical features are highly variable, even among family members sharing the same mutation. Affected individuals require repeated cardiovascular assessments for aortic root dilation and mitral valve regurgitation. Although genetic testing is available, it is of limited use given the expense and the ability to arrive at the diagnosis by clinical evaluation. However, it may be useful to demonstrate that a family member is not carrying the disease-related mutation in order to avoid ongoing cardiovascular testing or exercise limitation.

Williams–Beuren Syndrome

Williams–Beuren syndrome (OMIM #194050) is an autosomal dominant disorder characterized by specific cardiovascular defects, infantile hypercalcemia, skeletal and renal anomalies, cognitive deficits, "social personality," and elfin facies (Fig. 8-4).[26] As with other deletion syndromes (see the 22q11 deletion syndrome above), Williams–Beuren syndrome has a variable clinical phenotype. Typical cardiovascular anomalies include supravalvar aortic stenosis, often in conjunction with

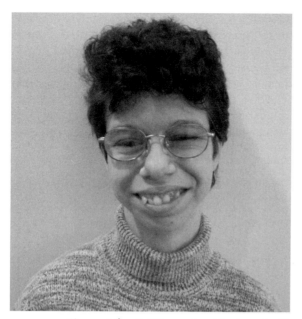 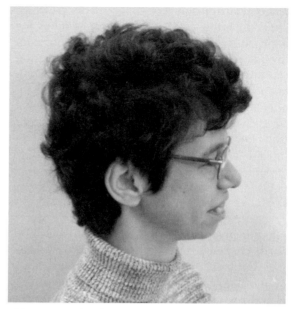

Figure 8-4   Full face and profile view of a 23-year-old woman with Williams–Beuren syndrome. Note the periorbital fullness, narrow nasal root with bulbous nasal tip, full lips with wide mouth, full cheeks, dental malocclusion, and long neck. (Images courtesy of Ian Krantz, MD, Division of Human Genetics, The Children's Hospital of Philadelphia.)

supravalvar pulmonary stenosis. The degree of cardiovascular involvement and the involvement of the pulmonic or aortic vessels varies widely. The supravalvar aortic stenosis has been shown to progress in most cases, whereas the supravalvar pulmonary stenosis usually regresses with time.

Approximately 90% of individuals with a clinical diagnosis of Williams–Beuren syndrome have been found to have a deletion at chromosome 7q11.23 on one homologue. This deletion is not usually apparent on a routine karyotype but can be detected by fluorescent *in situ* hybridization in the cytogenetic laboratory. Molecular analyses comparing clinical phenotype to genotype have demonstrated that this syndrome is a contiguous gene deletion syndrome: deletion or alteration of specific genes in the deleted region corresponds with specific clinical features in a one-to-one correlation. For example, the elastin gene maps into the deleted region. Deletion of one copy of the elastin gene causes the cardiovascular manifestations of this disorder, namely supravalvar aortic and pulmonic stenosis. Deletion of different genes in the region accounts for different manifestations of the disorder. Molecular diagnostic testing for a deletion at 7q11.23 in subjects suspected clinically of having Williams-Beuren syndrome is clinically available. Given the phenotypic variability of Williams–Beuren syndrome, it is appropriate to consider testing all patients with supravalvar aortic or pulmonic stenosis for a 7q11.23 deletion at the time of diagnosis.

Familial Supravalvar Stenoses

Familial supravalvar aortic stenosis and pulmonic stenosis (OMIM #185500) can result from genetic rearrangement, deletion, or mutation of the elastin gene.[27] As such, these patients have only cardiovascular manifestations with no other features of Williams–Beuren syndrome. Additional genetic etiologies of supravalvar aortic stenosis and pulmonic stenosis likely exist but have not been identified to date. Clinical genetic testing for elastin mutations is not currently available.

Ehlers–Danlos Syndrome

Ehlers–Danlos syndrome (EDS) comprises a collection of connective tissue disorders caused by abnormalities of the different types of collagen. Although typical features, such as fragility of the skin and blood vessels, easy bruising, poor wound healing, joint hypermobility, and skin hyperelasticity are frequently observed, no one feature is common to all types. EDS type IV, the vascular type, is the most severe form, associated with significant morbidity and mortality from severe fragility of connective tissues (OMIM #130050). Typically, children present with easy bruising and adults have characteristic facial features, easy bruising, and translucent skin with visible veins and rupture of vessels. The fragility of connective tissues allows for arterial and gastrointestinal rupture spontaneously or after minor trauma, often with catastrophic consequences.

Inherited in an autosomal dominant pattern, EDS IV results from mutations in the *COL3A1* gene coding for type III procollagen. The diagnosis is typically confirmed by cultured skin fibroblast assays demonstrating abnormal collagen III metabolism or by the identification of a mutation in *COL3A1*. Genetic testing is complicated, however, by the finding that most mutations appear to be unique to each family, or "private." There is no apparent correlation between genotype and phenotype.

EVALUATION OF THE PATIENT WITH CHD FOR A GENETIC ETIOLOGY

Identifying the genetic basis of CHD has proven to be particularly challenging given the paucity of large affected kindred and the evidence for decreased penetrance. For example, even with an entire extra chromosome 21 in Down syndrome, only 40–50% of patients have CHD. Thus, additional factors must impact upon the risk of disease. Nonetheless, the previous discussion demonstrates that substantial progress has been made in the elucidation of the genetic basis of congenital cardiovascular disorders by linkage analysis of rare kindred and molecular analysis of recurrent chromosomal alterations associated with genetic syndromes. The application of these findings to the nonsyndromic child with CHD is still under investigation, but these discoveries have certainly provided insight into the basic mechanisms of these disorders. Studies will continue to identify new genetic etiologies and will evaluate the impact of genotype upon clinical outcome. To date, only limited genetic testing is available, but as technology progresses, clinical testing for disease-related mutations will become available. Given the clinical and family counseling implications, it is critical to assess the child with CHD for genetic alterations using currently available tools.

In particular, a detailed family medical history to identify inherited disease should be taken upon the diagnosis of CHD in a child. Furthermore, all infants and children with CHD should be carefully examined for noncardiac anomalies, including neurocognitive deficiencies. The latter should no longer be considered a consequence of congenital heart surgery, but instead a potential manifestation of a multisystem disorder. Any patient with additional anomalies warrants a clinical genetic evaluation and, at a minimum, a karyotype. Additional cytogenetic studies, such as fluorescence *in situ* hybridization for a 22q11 or sub-telomere deletion, should be based upon specific clinical profiles. Molecular testing for single gene disorders is becoming increasingly available and changes on a daily basis (see http://www.genetests.org), but it remains costly, is not necessarily covered by insurance, and is incomplete. In most cases, the diagnosis of specific syndromes such as Holt–Oram syndrome is still made on a clinical basis. As the molecular tests become more automated, less expensive, and more available, genetic testing may assist in the diagnosis and assessment of prognosis. Such testing, as with all genetic testing, will raise new medical and ethical questions, such as the counseling provided to the so-called silent carrier of a disease-related mutation. However, the opportunity for premorbid evaluation and early intervention will likely improve clinical outcome in certain cases.

MAJOR POINTS

- Chromosome anomalies and genetic syndromes are common in patients with CHD.
- Significant progress has been made recently to define the genetic basis of CHD by linkage analysis of rare large kindred with CHD and the molecular analysis of recurrent chromosomal anomalies. Animal models have also identified candidate genes.
- Several aneuploidy syndromes (e.g., trisomy 21 or Down syndrome) are associated with CHD. They are suspected clinically and are confirmed by standard karyotype.
- Advanced cytogenetic techniques including fluorescent *in situ* hybridization (FISH) detect smaller chromosomal deletions. FISH is now commonly clinically used to test for smaller chromosome deletions.
- The 22q11 deletion syndrome is the most common deletion syndrome and is present in a large proportion of patients with conotruncal and related defects. The 22q11 deletion syndrome is characterized by multiple highly variable findings.
- Single gene disorders characterized in part by CHD have been identified, including Alagille and Noonan syndromes. Genetic testing is variably available and useful in these disorders.
- Care should be taken to identify the genetic basis of CHD clinically, given the counseling and clinical implications. A detailed family history for birth defects and a detailed assessment of the cardiac patient for other organ system involvement is important. Any patient with other organ system involvement, facial dysmorphia, or family history of birth defects should undergo clinical genetic evaluation with at least a karyotype. Other cytogenetic tests may be warranted.

REFERENCES

1. Loffredo CA: Epidemiology of cardiovascular malformations: Prevalence and risk factors. Am J Med Genet 97:319–325, 2000.

2. Online Mendelian Inheritance in Man (OMIM). Available online at *http://www.ncbi.nlm.nih.gov/entrez/query.fcgi?db=OMIM*.

3. Ferencz C, Correa-Villasenor A, Loffredo CA, Wilson PD: Atrioventricular septal defects with and without Down

syndrome. In Genetic and Environmental Risk Factors of Major Cardiovascular Malformations: The Baltimore-Washington Infant Study: 1981-1989, vol. 5. Armonk, NY: Futura Publishing Company, Inc., 1997, pp 103-122.

4. Barlow GM, Chen XN, Shi ZY, et al: Down syndrome congenital heart disease: A narrowed region and a candidate gene. Genet Med 3:91-101, 2001.

5. Frias JL, Davenport ML: Health supervision for children with Turner syndrome. Pediatrics 111:692-702, 2003.

6. Prandstraller D, Mazzanti L, Picchio FM, et al: Turner's syndrome: Cardiologic profile according to the different chromosomal patterns and long-term clinical follow-up of 136 nonpreselected patients. Pediatr Cardiol 20:108-112, 1999.

7. Emanuel BS, McDonald-McGinn D, Saitta SC, Zackai EH: The 22q11.2 deletion syndrome. Adv Pediatr 48:39-73, 2001.

8. Goldmuntz E, Clark BJ, Mitchell LE, et al: Frequency of 22q11 deletions in patients with conotruncal defects. J Am Coll Cardiol 32:492-498, 1998.

9. Epstein JA: Developing models of DiGeorge syndrome. Trends Genet 17:S13-S17, 2001.

10. McElhinney DB, Krantz ID, Bason L, et al: Analysis of cardiovascular phenotype and genotype-phenotype correlation in individuals with a JAG1 mutation and/or Alagille syndrome. Circulation 106:2567-2574, 2002.

11. Krantz ID, Piccoli DA, Spinner NB: Clinical and molecular genetics of Alagille syndrome. Curr Opin Pediatr 11:558-564, 1999.

12. Eldadah ZA, Hamosh A, Biery NJ, et al: Familial tetralogy of Fallot caused by mutation in the jagged1 gene. Hum Mol Genet 10:163-169, 2001.

13. Krantz ID, Smith R, Colliton RP, et al: Jagged1 mutations in patients ascertained with isolated congenital heart defects. Am J Med Genet 84:56-60, 1999.

14. Basson CT, Bachinsky DR, Lin RC, et al: Mutations in human TBX5 [corrected] cause limb and cardiac malformation in Holt-Oram syndrome. Nat Genet 15:30-35, 1997.

15. Li QY, Newbury-Ecob RA, Terrett JA, et al: Holt-Oram syndrome is caused by mutations in TBX5, a member of the Brachyury (T) gene family. Nat Genet 15:21-29, 1997.

16. Mori AD, Bruneau BG: TBX5 mutations and congenital heart disease: Holt-Oram syndrome revealed. Curr Opin Cardiol 19:211-215, 2004.

17. Tartaglia M, Mehler EL, Goldberg R, et al: Mutations in PTPN11, encoding the protein tyrosine phosphatase SHP-2, cause Noonan syndrome. Nat Genet 29:465-468, 2001.

18. Tartaglia M, Kalidas K, Shaw A, et al: PTPN11 mutations in Noonan syndrome: Molecular spectrum, genotype-phenotype correlation, and phenotypic heterogeneity. Am J Hum Genet 70:1555-1563, 2002.

19. Schott JJ, Benson DW, Basson CT, et al: Congenital heart disease caused by mutations in the transcription factor NKX2-5. Science 281:108-111, 1998.

20. Benson DW, Silberbach GM, Kavanaugh-McHugh A, et al: Mutations in the cardiac transcription factor NKX2.5 affect diverse cardiac developmental pathways. J Clin Invest 104:1567-1573, 1999.

21. Goldmuntz E, Geiger E, Benson DW: NKX2.5 mutations in patients with tetralogy of Fallot. Circulation 104:2565-2568, 2001.

22. McElhinney DB, Geiger E, Blinder J, et al: NKX2.5 mutations in patients with congenital heart disease. J Am Coll Cardiol 42:1650-1655, 2003.

23. Gebbia M, Ferrero GB, Pilia G, et al: X-linked situs abnormalities result from mutations in ZIC3. Nat Genet 17:305-308, 1997.

24. Belmont JW, Mohapatra B, Towbin JA, Ware SM: Molecular genetics of heterotaxy syndromes. Curr Opin Cardiol 19:216-220, 2004.

25. Pyeritz RE: The Marfan syndrome. Annu Rev Med 51:481-510, 2000.

26. Tassabehji M: Williams-Beuren syndrome: A challenge for genotype-phenotype correlations. Hum Mol Genet 12 Spec No 2:R229-237, 2003.

27. Metcalfe K, Rucka AK, Smoot L, et al: Elastin: Mutational spectrum in supravalvular aortic stenosis. Eur J Hum Genet 8:955-963, 2000.

CHAPTER 9

Heart Failure in Pediatrics

JONDAVID MENTEER

ALEXA N. HOGARTY

MARYANNE R.K. CHRISANT

Heart failure refers to any state in which the heart is unable to deliver forward output commensurate with the metabolic demands of the body, including oxygen and nutrient delivery and waste removal. Decreased cardiac output sets in motion compensatory cascades within the heart, the vasculature, and the neurohormonal systems of the body.[1] Myocardial adaptations occur, including alterations in gene expression, metabolic changes, hypertrophy, and apoptosis (programmed cell death), the end result of which is deleterious ventricular remodeling. In the short term, these mechanisms are important for maintaining cardiac output and perfusing the vital organs of the body; sustained activation of these cascades results in adverse long-term consequences. Ideally, optimized pharmacotherapy targets these compensatory systems by reversing some of their ill effects, by augmenting positive effects, and by slowing the progression of heart failure.

Heart failure does occur in children, although it is more typically described in the adult population; in the pediatric population, the etiologies are different and more varied. In adult patients, the leading causes of heart failure are ischemic heart disease and idiopathic dilated cardiomyopathy. In pediatric patients, heart failure can occur in a setting of structural congenital heart disease (such as ventricular septal defects), primary diseases of the cardiac muscle (such as dilated cardiomyopathy or myocarditis), or genetic and metabolic diseases (such as Duchenne type muscular dystrophy, mitochondrial cytopathies, and carnitine deficiency).

PHYSIOLOGY AND PATHOPHYSIOLOGY

In discussing heart failure, it is important to recall the following fundamental concepts that describe normal physiology, and to understand how the physical principles represented by these concepts are altered in response to the failing myocardium.

Cardiac Output

First, it is useful to consider cardiac output (CO) as the volume pumped by one cardiac cycle (stroke volume [SV]), in liters or milliliters, times the heart rate (HR) in beats per minute: $CO = SV \times HR$. This simple equation describes a basic relationship that, when referenced, assists in solving diagnostic and management problems. SV and HR act in concert to improve cardiac output as needed. In heart failure syndrome, resting heart rate is typically elevated to help maintain cardiac output, as the poorly functioning ventricle is unable to increase stroke volume (Fig. 9-1).

The second important concept is the Frank–Starling mechanism, which describes the heart's ability to increase the force of contraction and, therefore, the stroke volume in response to an increase in venous return. That is, increased venous return increases ventricular filling and, thus, the end-diastolic volume or preload. This stretches or increases the myocyte fiber (the sarcomere length), which results in an increased force

159

Fetal/Neonatal Myocardium
Response to Increasing Heart Rate

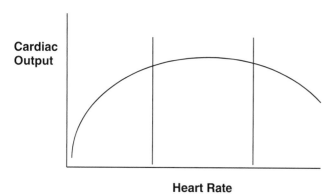

Figure 9-1   Effect of heart rate on cardiac output. Cardiac output is determined by the body's needs, and ventricular stroke volume varies inversely with heart rate. Cardiac output is decreased at very slow heart rates in which stroke volume is limited by maximal ventricular dilatation. Conversely, at fast heart rates, ventricular filling (i.e., stroke volume) is limited by short diastole.

Fetal/Neonatal Myocardium
Response to Increasing Preload

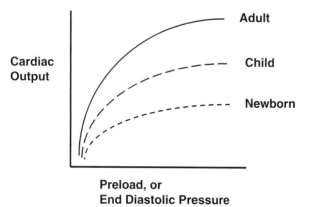

Figure 9-2   Frank–Starling curves for neonatal, child, and mature myocardium. Neonatal myocardium is less able to increase cardiac output with increasing filling pressure (preload or end diastolic pressure).

of contraction and leads to an increased stroke volume or cardiac output. (See Fig. 9-2.)

When a sarcomere is too short, as would be the case in an under-filled ventricle, the thin filaments of the sarcomere overlap, preventing optimal coupling of myosin to actin and reducing the amount of force produced. Increases in the length of the sarcomere lead to more efficient actin–myosin interaction, with increases in the amount of force generated, and an increase in contractility; this progresses until actin and myosin chains are separated to the point at which fewer myosin heads overlap onto the actin chains, and the sarcomere is overstretched. In a volume-overloaded ventricle, the overstretched sarcomeres cannot generate adequate force to shorten effectively, a process that is reversed by diuresis and the consequent reduction in preload and ventricular distension. In heart failure syndrome, the basic sarcomere must function near the peak of its Frank–Starling curve at all times, with limited reserve to increase stroke volume with increased metabolic demand. Maintaining ideal preload conditions to allow the heart to function optimally is often problematic, and even modest increases in intravascular volume may result in decompensation, or "falling off the Starling curve."

The third fundamental concept is that, on a cellular level, physiologic differences exist between immature and mature myocardium that influence the heart's response to pathophysiologic processes. The immature or infant myocardium is not as compliant as that of an adult (compliance is the change in volume that accompanies a change in pressure). In the less compliant infant myocardium, a small increase in volume generates a relatively large increase in pressure compared with mature myocardium. In part, this is due to inefficient uptake of calcium by the immature sarcoplasmic reticulum. An immature heart that is volume-loaded and maximally stretched pushes the myocardium onto the down-slope of its Starling curve, resulting in diminished cardiac output. These characteristics lead to a limited ability for the infant heart to increase stroke volume. In the infant heart, processes that require increased cardiac output typically begin by increasing heart rate (remember the above equation, CO = SV × HR). In contrast, older children and adults have more compliant myocardium, responding efficiently to increases in filling volume with better maximal contractility: stroke volume is increased, as is heart rate, to maintain adequate cardiac output.

Neurohormonal Compensatory Mechanisms

When cardiac output falls, decreased renal perfusion results in the production of renin, which in turn increases conversion of angiotensin I to angiotensin II, with a subsequent increase in production of aldosterone. Aldosterone causes the kidneys to retain sodium and water in an attempt to increase blood volume and to improve perfusion; in the heart, aldosterone stimulates apoptosis and adverse ventricular remodeling. Angiotensin II increases systemic vascular resistance, shunting blood away from cutaneous tissues and toward central organs.[2] Although these events may initially restore perfusion in part, intravascular fluid retention overfills the heart, maximally increases preload, and eventually leads to extravasation and congestion (i.e., pulmonary edema, organomegaly, ascites, or peripheral edema). The increase in vascular resistance (i.e., afterload) caused by angiotensin II, compounded by the fluid-heavy tissues, makes it more difficult for the struggling heart to maintain forward flow, further diminishing cardiac output. Defining the role of the renin-angiotensin system (RAS) has provided improved targets for heart failure therapy.

In addition to stimulating the RAS, low cardiac output activates the sympathetic (i.e., adrenergic) nervous system in both adults and children. The catecholamines, epinephrine and norepinephrine, increase heart rate, improve myocardial contractility, and increase vascular tone to maintain blood pressure.[1] The net effect is improved cardiac output. The cost of this effect, however, is increased myocardial oxygen consumption, enhanced predisposition to ectopy, and potentiation of the RAS. Long-term exposure to norepinephrine contributes to the induction of myocyte apoptosis and hypertrophy. Chronic adrenergic stimulation results in desensitization and down-regulation of cardiac β receptors; this blunts the response of the failing heart to further adrenergic stimulation, which may be beneficial inasmuch as it is deleterious. Adrenergic agents are often the first line of therapy for heart failure.

Natriuretic peptides are a group of related molecules that are secreted by various organs in response to heart failure and may offset some of the effects mediated by other neurohumoral systems. Atrial (or A-type) natriuretic peptide (ANP) is secreted in substantial amounts by the atria in response to chamber distension; brain (or B-type) natriuretic peptide (BNP) is secreted from the brain, the atria, and the ventricles. Both peptides stimulate ANP-receptors found in the kidney and result in natriuresis, or enhanced excretion of sodium, and diuresis by increasing glomerular filtration. Atrial natriuretic peptide also decreases renin production and inhibits the actions of angiotensin II and aldosterone. Laboratory measurement of circulating BNP levels has become a common adjunct in determining the severity of heart failure. Increased BNP levels correlate with decreased ventricular ejection fraction, increased preload, and worsening heart failure symptoms. Trends in BNP blood levels are helpful in assessing the heart failure (HF) patient acutely and chronically. Manipulation of the natriuretic peptide system has shown potential as a heart failure therapy.

C-type natriuretic peptide is released from endothelial cells and acts as a local endothelin antagonist and vasodilator. It differs from ANP and BNP in that it has little natriuretic activity and does not significantly attenuate the RAS. Endothelin represents a family of peptides (ET-1, ET-2, and ET-3) that possess similar activity. Endothelin is a potent vasoconstrictor that is increased in certain states such as heart failure and pulmonary hypertension. In adult heart failure patients, plasma levels of endothelin have correlated with severity of heart failure symptoms (as determined by New York Heart Association functional classification), and with right and left heart filling pressures, pulmonary vascular resistance, and mean systemic arterial pressure.

All of these systems interact in complex ways, and major advances in the treatment of heart failure have resulted from our improved understanding of these principal systems.

ETIOLOGIES

The etiologies of heart failure in the pediatric population are numerous and varied. Box 9-1, which is by no means exhaustive, contains a list of conditions that should aid the physician in evaluating a patient with symptomatic heart failure. Consideration must be given to the patient's age, presentation, prior history, and laboratory findings. In infants, heart failure may be a presenting sign of structural congenital heart disease. Defects such as hypoplastic left heart syndrome and aortic stenosis often present with signs and symptoms of low cardiac output; mitral stenosis and total anomalous pulmonary venous return may present with pulmonary congestion and low output, and Ebstein's anomaly may present with right heart failure symptoms and low systemic output. In older children, ventricular septal defects (VSDs) and patent ductus arteriosus (PDA), which result in left-to-right shunting, may present with pulmonary congestion and failure. Pediatric patients must be closely assessed to determine if structural congenital heart disease is present and causing the heart failure. Other causes of heart failure include primary diseases of the heart muscle (i.e., cardiomyopathies) and cardiac dysfunction, secondary to genetic, metabolic, or neuromuscular diseases.

Acute causes of heart failure can result from mechanical issues, such as pericardial effusion related to pericarditis or postoperative fluid collection, and resultant tamponade. Tamponade limits venous return and diminishes preload, severely limiting stroke volume. The body compensates by increasing adrenergic output to increase heart rate and to maintain cardiac output. Heart failure can be caused by tachyarrhythmia that persists for a long duration; the resultant myocardial failure is usually, but not always, reversible when the arrhythmia is controlled. Such arrhythmias may include atrial flutter, supraventricular tachycardia, or ventricular tachycardia. Noncardiovascular causes of high-output heart failure include hypermetabolic states such as anemia, fever, sepsis, and hyperthyroidism.

Box 9-1   Etiologies of Heart Failure in the Pediatric Population

I.   Diseases of the heart muscle: Resulting in systolic dysfunction, diastolic dysfunction, or both
  A.   Primary cardiomyopathy (CM): As we are better defining precise etiologies, the following types may be regarded as descriptive features rather than absolute diagnoses:
    1.   Dilated
    2.   Noncompacted
    3.   Restrictive
    4.   Hypertrophic
  B.   Secondary cardiomyopathy: These have structural features of the above types; however, their etiologies are diverse and may be grouped as follows:
    1.   Metabolic and genetic disorders
      a.   Carnitine deficiency
      b.   Mitochondrial cytopathies
      c.   Syndromes that include CM (e.g., Barth, Williams, MELAS, MIDAS)
      d.   Thyroid disease/hypothyroidism
    2.   Storage diseases
      a.   Pompe's disease
      b.   Amyloidosis
    3.   Mucopolysaccharidoses
    4.   Neuromuscular diseases
      a.   Muscular dystrophies
        i.   Duchenne
        ii.   Becker's
        iii. Emery Dreifuss
    5.   Toxic exposure
      a.   Adriamycin and other anthracyclines
      b.   Cocaine
      c.   Alcohol
    6.   Malnutrition
  7.   Infectious diseases
    a.   Myocarditis
    b.   Sepsis
    c.   Bacterial endocarditis
      i.   Pancarditis
      ii. Acute valvar insufficiency
II. Coronary disease: Although rare in children, ischemia should be considered when evaluating for myocardial dysfunction.
  A.   Ischemia
    1.   Kawasaki disease: Giant aneurysms
    2.   Structural coronary anomalies
      a.   Anomalous origin of the left coronary artery from the pulmonary artery (ALCAPA)
      b.   Right ventricular dependent coronary circulation
      c.   Coronary-cameral fistula
    3.   Hypercholesterolemia
    4.   Infantile coronary calcinosis
    5.   Intramural large coronary arteries
III. Structural congenital heart disease
  A.   Shunt lesions
  B.   Valvular disease
  C.   Outflow tract obstructive lesions
IV. Mechanical causes
  A.   Arrhythmia
  B.   Cardiac tamponade
  C.   Restrictive pericardial disease
  D.   Acute onset of AV valve insufficiency
  E.   Intracardiac tumor
V.   High output failure
  A.   Anemia
  B.   Arteriovenous malformations
  C.   Thyrotoxicosis

EVALUATION OF HEART FAILURE

History and Physical Examination

Evaluation of a patient with heart failure poses many challenges; the primary challenge is to properly diagnose the patient as *having* heart failure. Infants, children, and adolescents may have profound respiratory or gastrointestinal symptoms that can masquerade as primarily GI or pulmonary disorders and can mislead the treating physician into adopting an erroneous diagnosis and subsequent management. Respiratory symptoms such as chronic productive cough, fever, shortness of breath, and general malaise may encourage a diagnosis of pneumonia. Abdominal pain, vomiting, anorexia, and nausea may lead to a diagnosis of gastroenteritis or appendicitis. However, both these groups of symptoms can represent heart failure.

The key to evaluating any patient and arriving at a correct diagnosis is two-fold: first, a complete history must be obtained, and second, the patient must be thoroughly examined. When heart failure is suspected, the parents and patient (if of an appropriate age) should be queried with questions directed toward solidifying (or disproving) the diagnosis and unmasking a possible etiology. Essential topics to explore include past medical history, recent illnesses, current symptoms, duration of symptoms, feeding history (how much, how often, and whether there is early satiety or postprandial vomiting), sleep history (orthopnea, sudden awakening, increased sleeping, or insomnia), respiratory complaints (shortness of breath or chronic cough), GI complaints (abdominal pain, nausea, vomiting, or loss of appetite), muscular complaints (muscle fatigue or cramping), fluid retention (edema of the hands and feet, periorbital edema, abdominal swelling, or decreased urination), weight loss or gain, loss of developmental milestones or prior abilities (stair climbing or running), change in activity level (wanting to stay indoors and watch television as opposed to playing outside), school attendance, medications, and drug exposures. A pertinent family history should be taken, including questions about first- and second-degree relatives with heart failure, congenital heart disease, cardiomyopathy, sudden death, or death at a young age.

Once the history-taking is complete, the child should be examined. The patient should be assessed for overall level of activity: is the child irritable, listless, or in distress, or is the child alert, interactive, and comfortable? Does the child have facial features or a body habitus suggestive of a syndrome, such as Williams–Beuren syndrome, a neuromuscular disorder, or storage disease? Does the patient have age-appropriate motor skills and development? Height and weight parameters should be assessed for growth failure. The vital signs will reveal tachypnea, tachycardia at rest, and hypotension. Can the child lie flat on the exam table, or does the child experience respiratory distress? When flat, does the child have jugular venous distension? On examination of the lungs, are the breath sounds clear bilaterally or is there evidence of pleural effusion with diminished sounds and rales? Is the PMI displaced laterally and inferiorly; is the precordium hyperdynamic? Are the heart tones crisp and audible or distant and muffled? Is the heart rate elevated or slow? Is the rhythm regular or irregular? Is there a third heart sound? Is there a murmur? Is the abdomen flat or distended? If distended, is there a fluid wave? Is the abdomen tender, diffusely or focally? Is the liver palpable, and on what side (some patients have heterotaxy)? How far down does the liver extend below the costal margin? Is the spleen enlarged? Is edema present in the extremities? Are the central and peripheral pulses easily palpable? Is the perfusion diminished or good? Is the child pink, mottled, pale, gray, or blue? Are the extremities warm or cold? Clammy and wet or dry?

All aspects of the physical examination provide essential information for the diagnosis and management of heart failure. An elevated resting heart rate may be the first clue to a physician that a patient is unwell and may be the earliest manifestation of myocardial dysfunction. Blood pressure is usually not compromised early in HF because a number of autoregulatory mechanisms counteract minor decreases in cardiac output, such as vasoconstriction in the splanchnic circulation from activation of the sympathetic nervous system early in HF.

Respiratory rate may be increased, but the pattern of respiratory distress is important in differentiating cardiac from respiratory symptoms. In infants, mild resting tachypnea can be due to a number of pulmonary, cardiac, infectious, or metabolic processes; mild resting tachyp-

nea associated with diaphoresis and more profound distress during feeding is consistent with heart failure. In children beyond infancy, "cardiac asthma" can occur, with exertional wheezing and shortness of breath. In addition to tachypnea, basilar rales may be present.

Evaluation of pulses, perfusion, palpation of the precordium, and auscultation of the heart tones may reveal weak pulses, cool extremities, and distant heart tones. Bounding pulses, present in the face of hypotension and low cardiac output, are secondary to decreased vascular tone (e.g., "warm shock") from sepsis or arteriovenous connections such as an arteriovenous fistula. In patients without structural CHD, the presence of a mitral insufficiency murmur indicates left ventricular dilatation and stretching of the mitral annulus.

Abdominal examination may reveal a tender and enlarged liver, occasionally accompanied by splenomegaly. Examination of the extremities is helpful for assessment of pulses, perfusion, temperature, color, and fluid retention. Dependent edema (of the extremities or sacrum) is an infrequent finding in young children, but older children and teenagers may develop significant pitting edema secondary to heart failure. Periorbital edema is sometimes noted in infants and children, especially upon awakening.

Functional Classification

Heart failure signs and symptoms can vary with the age of the patient. Infants outside the newborn period may present with emesis after feeding, decreased oral intake, growth failure, irritability, and decreased activity. Teenagers with dyspnea on exertion, vomiting after eating, anorexia, cough, or fatigue should be evaluated for heart failure. The New York Heart Association devised a basic classification system for adult patients with heart failure (the NYHA Classification). Decreasing activity level, increasing symptoms, and anginal chest pain objectively define a patient's functional class and help predict timing of intervention. This schema has been modified for use in infants and children (Table 9-1). The Ross Classification was developed for grading HF in infants and younger children, and this system is currently used by the Canadian Cardiovascular Society as its official system for grading HF in children; it also is used in the Pediatric Cardiomyopathy Registry. Importantly, this classification system includes growth failure as a measure of heart failure in children.

Laboratory Evaluation of Heart Failure

A chest radiograph is a mandatory component of the heart failure evaluation to assess cardiac size, pulmonary blood flow, and the presence of pulmonary edema and effusions. Chest x-rays are readily obtainable and results

Table 9-1   Functional Classification of Heart Failure: NYHA Class and Ross Classification for Children

	NYHA Functional Classification	Ross Classification for Children
I	Heart disease with no limitation of physical activity. Ordinary activities do not cause undue fatigue, palpitations, dyspnea, or angina.	Heart disease with no limitation of physical activity. School-aged children take gym class and keep up with peers.
II	Slight limitation of physical activity. Comfortable at rest, but ordinary activity can result in fatigue, palpitations, dyspnea, and/or angina.	Mild tachypnea or diaphoresis with feeding in infants. Secondary growth failure may be present. Dyspnea on exertion in older children.
III	Marked limitation of physical activity. Comfortable at rest, but less than ordinary activity results in fatigue, palpitations, dyspnea, or angina.	Marked tachypnea or diaphoresis with feeding in infants; prolonged feeding times; growth failure. In older children, marked dyspnea on exertion.
IV	Inability to carry on any physical activity. Fatigue, palpitations, dyspnea, or angina may be present at rest. Any attempt at physical activity increases symptoms.	Symptoms such as tachypnea, retractions, grunting, or diaphoresis are present at rest in infants and older children. Growth failure likely.

are virtually immediate. Provided that the film was taken with adequate inspiration, a cardiothoracic ratio of greater than 0.5 suggests cardiomegaly (> 0.55 in infants). As a heart fails and the left ventricle dilates and loses its cylindrical contour, the cardiac silhouette becomes more globular. Right ventricular dilatation may contribute to this and may further widen the silhouette. Significant pericardial effusions can also cause the heart to have a globular appearance.

Electrocardiography (ECG) is an important and inexpensive screening tool. In the patient with HF, the ECG can be used to assess for acute ischemia, arrhythmias, ventricular hypertrophy, atrial dilation, heart block, or more complex patterns that can lend clues to the diagnosis of complex congenital heart disease. In the patient with myocarditis, diffuse ST elevations may lend an early clue to the diagnosis. An assessment of the rhythm is important since an elevated heart rate is almost always present, and the distinction between sinus tachycardia and other tachyarrhythmias is important to determine early therapy.

Echocardiography allows excellent visualization of cardiac anatomy and gives qualitative and quantitative measures of ventricular function, chamber size, and regional wall motion. Doppler interrogation of flow identifies myocardial performance, especially regarding the restriction to inflow, which can occur in diastolic dysfunction. M-mode imaging is used routinely for the assessment of standard measurements useful in describing the failing heart, such as left ventricular end-diastolic dimension, end-systolic dimension, wall thickness, and shortening fraction. More advanced techniques can be used, such as tissue Doppler imaging (TDI). TDI is a Doppler ultrasound method used to detect wall motion abnormalities during systole and diastole and to detect and quantify diastolic dysfunction.

Over the past two decades, cardiac catheterization has been used less frequently for anatomic and functional

diagnosis, owing to advances in noninvasive imaging. In the patient with HF, catheterization is generally reserved for patients in whom suspicion of coronary pathology exists, and in whom endomyocardial biopsy must be obtained, or in whom questions or discrepant data exist regarding heart structure or function. Diagnostic cardiac catheterization will generally be performed after the patient has been stabilized and treated medically to some extent. This approach decreases the risk of the procedure and improves the quality of hemodynamic measurements, as stable, steady-state conditions provide the most reliable information. Endomyocardial biopsy of the right ventricle may aid in diagnosing viral myocarditis, eosinophilic myocarditis, or primary cardiomyopathies. Cardiac catheterization with electrophysiologic study may occasionally be necessary to diagnose or treat a patient with HF and refractory arrhythmia. Interventional procedures have limited applicability for treating HF; however, patients with failure due to persistent patent ductus arteriosus benefit from closure at the time of catheterization.

Exercise testing is useful for assessing and following patients with chronic heart failure. Exercise testing generally involves a graduated treadmill or stationary bicycle workload with concomitant monitoring of the patient's heart rate, blood pressure, ECG, oxygen saturation, oxygen consumption, carbon dioxide production, and symptoms. This test requires that the patient be cooperative with the protocol and motivated to perform at maximal effort. Medications, such as β-blockers, can affect the results. A second type of exercise assessment is the 6-minute walk. The patient is asked to walk, usually back and forth along a premeasured distance, as far as he or she is able within a 6-minute time period. The patient may stop for rest at any time. The measurements made are the total distance, the maximal heart rate attained, and, if indicated, the transcutaneous oxygen saturation. Both of these exercise assessments provide useful information about a patient's functional capacity and "real-world" limitations during day-to-day activities.

Laboratory blood chemistry analysis is a useful adjunct in determining the severity of heart failure and the extent of other organ dysfunction. Electrolyte levels, lactic acid production, arterial blood gas (in patients with respiratory distress), and a complete blood count should be checked at the time of presentation. In severe HF, a metabolic acidosis results with elevated lactate levels, and bicarbonate is consumed quickly. Elevated lactate in a patient with less than severe presentation may indicate the presence of a metabolic disease (such as lactate dehydrogenase deficiency) and possible etiology for the myocardial dysfunction. Electrolyte abnormalities are often found in the patient with decompensated HF. Hyponatremia is a classic finding, resulting from total body water overload with normal or low (after chronic diuretic therapy and sodium loss) total body sodium. A complete blood count will identify anemia or infection. Creatinine and BUN (blood urea nitrogen) levels assess renal function and nitrogen balance. Liver function tests, such as serum transaminase levels and bilirubin, may be elevated in HF, reflecting hepatic congestion from right sided heart failure or chronic "cardiac cirrhosis." Erythrocyte sedimentation rate (ESR) and C-reactive protein level can lend clues to inflammatory processes, such as rheumatic heart disease or Kawasaki disease, that have cardiovascular effects.

The identification of cardiomyopathy or myocarditis is more important in the acute phase of evaluation than in discovering the exact infectious or metabolic etiology. In patients with newly diagnosed cardiomyopathy, a metabolic evaluation should be undertaken. Thyroid function testing can be useful in some clinical settings, but hypo- and hyperthyroidism are infrequent causes of cardiomyopathy in the pediatric age group.

Specific to heart failure, the plasma BNP level is a useful marker of disease, disease progression, and efficacy of treatment. BNP is elevated in proportion to heart failure symptom severity and typically improves in response to heart failure therapy.

MANAGEMENT OF HEART FAILURE

Pharmacology

The first documented uses of digitalis in treating heart failure were described by William Withering in *An Account of the Foxglove*, published in 1785. Although we continue to rely on digitalis derivatives as a component of heart failure therapy, our pharmacopoeia now encompasses diuretics, angiotensin-converting enzyme (ACE) inhibitors, aldosterone inhibitors, β-blockers, adrenergic sympathomimetics, phosphodiesterase inhibitors, and other drugs. As we have better defined the cascade of events initiated by low cardiac output, available targets for therapy have presented themselves. Advances in heart failure therapy mainly result from the treatment of adults with ischemic and nonischemic cardiomyopathies.

Although the etiologies may differ, the principles of heart failure management in children are similar. Medications are typically used in combination to improve a patient's hemodynamic status by one or more of the following processes: increasing cardiac contractility, decreasing afterload, optimizing preload, and decreasing compensatory neurohormonal activation. Although pharmacology is more completely addressed elsewhere in this volume, several medications commonly used to treat heart failure are noted below.

Digoxin, a digitalis glycoside, functions at several levels: (1) inhibition of the sodium pump (sodium-potassium ATPase), which in turn promotes calcium influx by the sodium-calcium exchange mechanism; the end result is increased cytosolic calcium and improved cardiac contractility, (2) decreased activity of the renal sodium pump, resulting in depressed renin release and enhanced natriuresis, and (3) inhibition of the sympathetic autonomic system, which acts to decrease sinoatrial (SA) nodal and atrioventricular (AV) nodal conduction times, and activation of the parasympathetic system, which results in sinus slowing and AV nodal inhibition; this dual autonomic inhibition-activation results in slowing the heart rate and prolonging the P-R interval.

Digoxin is a mild inotrope and is useful in controlling atrial arrhythmias. It is typically used in conjunction with other medications. In patients with heart failure, digoxin is typically well-tolerated, but levels should be followed and patients should be closely monitored; drug interactions are not uncommon, electrolyte abnormalities may enhance proarrhythmic effects, and deteriorating renal function may alter digoxin metabolism.

Diuretics were the next group of medications to be applied to the treatment of heart failure. The principal use of diuretics is to promote excretion of water from the body, alleviating the negative effects of volume overload, including cardiac congestion, ventricular overfilling, organomegaly, ascites, and peripheral edema. Furosemide and bumetanide are commonly used diuretics. Called "loop diuretics," they act by blocking the $NaKCl_2$ ATPase in the thick ascending limb of the loop of Henle, resulting in loss of water and ions with the potential side effects of hyponatremia, hypokalemia, hypochloremia, and alkalosis. These agents are potent in both induction and maintenance phases of diuresis.

Thiazides are sometimes employed when treating children with heart failure and act synergistically with loop diuretics. Their site of action is in the distal nephron, limiting sodium and chloride reabsorption. Spironolactone and eplerenone are competitive antagonists of aldosterone in the distal collecting tubule, inhibiting Na^+ to K^+ exchange. These drugs are typically used as second agents with a loop diuretic. The main benefits of these drugs may stem from their effects on the aldosterone system, which is chronically activated in heart failure syndrome. In vitro and in adult patients, aldosterone-blockers act at the level of the myocardium to prevent myocyte apoptosis and to inhibit the development of myocardial fibrosis, slowing deleterious ventricular remodeling.

ACE inhibitors block the action of ACEs and prevent the conversion of angiotensin I to angiotensin II, as well as the breakdown of bradykinin by the same enzyme, alternatively named "kininase." Angiotensin-converting enzyme activity is found in the vascular endothelium of all vascular beds, including the lungs and coronary arteries. Their net clinical effect is to affect vasodilatation, decreasing systemic vascular resistance, thereby decreasing afterload and lowering blood pressure. Neurohormonal benefits of ACE inhibitors include reduction of aldosterone production, resulting in natriuresis and potassium retention. Captopril and enalapril are the main ACE inhibitors used in pediatrics (Captopril's action was first described in 1977). In addition to their important role in treating heart failure syndrome, ACE inhibitors have desirable effects in patients with structural heart disease, such as in patients with mitral regurgitation, in which reduced afterload improves forward flow, reducing the regurgitant fraction and the volume load on the ventricle. Common side effects of ACE inhibitors include cough, hyperkalemia, and worsening renal function.

Angiotensin II receptor blockers are a relatively new class of agents; the first, losartan, was approved by the FDA in 1995. These drugs are now considered an acceptable alternative for patients who suffer from cough and renal toxicity due to ACE inhibitors.

Beta-adrenergic receptor blockers were first used in heart failure therapy nearly 30 years ago, resulting in some clinical improvement in the small numbers of patients tested. Not until the early 1990s was the true survival benefit from β-blockade demonstrated in a large group of adults with moderate heart failure from ischemic or dilated cardiomyopathy. β-blockers act to reverse the compensatory adrenergic stimulation caused by heart failure; the results of β-blocker therapy are slower heart rate, decreased myocardial oxygen consumption, and reverse ventricular remodeling. β-blockers decrease renin production, which positively impacts on the renin-angiotensin system activated in heart failure syndrome. To date, large studies testing β-adrenergic receptor blockade for the treatment of heart failure have not been published in the pediatric population, although there is presently an ongoing multicenter trial testing the safety and efficacy of carvedilol in children with heart failure.

Carvedilol is a nonselective β-1 and β-2 antagonist with α-1 blocking properties and mild antioxidant properties. Because of its combined α and β inhibition, carvedilol affords more immediate afterload reduction. In adult patients, carvedilol improves markers for heart failure, such as ejection fraction and exercise performance; importantly, carvedilol has been shown to improve survival in patients with moderate heart failure.

The most current drug added to the heart failure pharmacopoeia is nesiritide, or brain natriuretic peptide. Nesiritide is now available as an intravenous infusion and is under investigation in adult trials for use in acute heart failure. This drug reduces filling pressures by increasing diuresis and causing systemic vasodilation, thereby improving cardiac output.

Acute heart failure management typically is directed toward urgently maintaining cardiac output. The medications used to effect this are administered intravenously. The term *inotrope* refers to any drug that improves myocardial contractility; a *pressor* refers to drugs that primarily increase systemic vascular resistance, raising systemic blood pressure. In mild and moderate conditions, dopamine and dobutamine are usual first-line inotropes, although at high doses, dopamine functions as a pressor. In severe cases in which blood pressure must be rapidly supported, norepinephrine or epinephrine are commonly used. Phosphodiesterase (PDE) inhibitors, including milrinone and amrinone, inhibit phosphodiesterase-III, preventing the breakdown of cyclic-AMP in cardiac and smooth muscle, leading to an increase in intracellular c-AMP activity and increased intracellular calcium. The net result is augmented cardiac contractility and peripheral venous and arterial vasodilation. The inotropic and vasodilatory effects of these medications are mediated principally through inhibition of PDE-3. In the intensive care setting, these drugs provide a potent combination of inotropic effects and afterload reduction, leading to substantial improvements in cardiac output.

Biventricular Pacing

Children and adolescents with severe left ventricular dysfunction and delayed depolarization of the left ventricle secondary to a left bundle branch block or nonspecific interventricular conduction delay may benefit from biventricular pacing or cardiac resynchronization therapy. This makes use of conventional transvenous pacemaker technology, adding an additional or second ventricular lead, which results in resynchronizing the depolarization of the both ventricles. Specially designed pacemakers control each ventricular pacing lead and can be programmed to synchronize ventricular depolarization in a more uniform fashion than is possible with a single (right) ventricular lead. The goal of biventricular pacing is to provide more uniform ventricular depolarization than that afforded by a patient's native conduction system, resulting in enhanced coordinated contractility and improved cardiac output. Pediatric experience with resynchronization therapy is limited and reported only in several small or multi-center retrospectively correct case series.

Surgical Treatment for End-Stage Heart Failure

Recent technology has advanced the design and production of ventricular assist devices (VADs) that are of small enough size to support children (weighing more than roughly 20 kg or with a body surface area of at least 1.0 square meter) and adolescents. These devices are pumps that fill from blood flow through the systemic ventricular inflow cannula and return blood to the circulation through an outflow cannula into the aorta. Pulmonary or right ventricular assist to the lungs may also be accomplished in children who are of large enough body size to accommodate two devices and biventricular support. In children, these devices may serve as a "bridge" to transplantation and are being used more frequently as rescue for medication-refractory HF; they are also used in patients with end-stage failure and structural congenital heart disease. Some patients recover, such as those with myocarditis or other potentially reversible processes, and device explantation is possible.

Major complications of VAD therapy include infection, bleeding, thrombus formation, stroke, arrhythmia, and (rarely) mechanical malfunction. Patients' post-device implantation are typically extubated and ambulatory within a relatively short time after surgery. The goal of VAD support is to reverse end-stage heart failure and to allow for improved nutritional and physical rehabilitation, thus making the patient a better candidate for transplantation and, in some cases, full recovery.

Devices may be implanted internally, with the pump implanted between the muscle layers of the abdominal wall, and an external power supply and controller electrically coupled to the machine through the intact skin. These devices are too large in size to be implanted into children less than about 1.3 square meters in body surface area. Some devices, such as the Thoratec, are paracorporeal; that is, there is a partially internalized pump with an external pneumatic actuator. The power supply is a large but mobile unit that provides positive pressure to a blood-filled bladder that ejects the blood. The advantage of the Thoratec device is that it can fit into children as small as about 20 kg or 1.0 m^2.

For infants with refractory or severe acute heart failure, the mainstay of circulatory support remains ECMO (extracorporeal membrane oxygenation). This necessitates intubation, paralysis, and sedation for the duration of therapy. Cannulation is either through the internal jugular and carotid vessels or directly through the open chest into the heart. Infants receiving ECMO support are often listed for cardiac transplantation; ECMO is not infrequently used to support failing patients with congenital heart disease after surgery and recovery is possible.

A fourth type of device, a continuous axial flow pump, is presently under development for use in infants and small children. The advantage of this device is its small size.

Cardiac transplantation may be considered for the patient in whom other treatments have failed. The long-term outcome of heart transplantation is improving. At most transplant centers, 1-year survival for patients transplanted at less than 18 years of age is about 90%, and 5-year survival is about 70%. Transplant candidates are carefully evaluated for infections, anatomy, prior surgeries, associated multiorgan disease, and psychosocial complications that may affect treatment after the transplant and overall success.

SUMMARY

The pediatric population with HF is heterogeneous. Various congenital heart defects, acquired heart disease, and genetic syndromes that lead to different pathophysiologic states can make the evaluation of a patient with evidence of HF challenging. A mastery of certain key skills, including history taking and physical examination (including cardiac auscultation), along with experience at evaluating several key tests (including chest x-ray, ECG, and routine blood tests) can provide enough clinical information in most cases to formulate a plan for initial stabilization and subsequent referral to a hospital or outpatient cardiology setting.

MAJOR POINTS

- Heart failure can be simply defined as the inability of the heart to keep up with the body's needs.
- Cardiac Output = Stroke Volume × Heart Rate (CO = SV × HR)
- The Frank–Starling curve describes the heart's ability to increase the force of contraction, increasing the stroke volume in response to an increase in venous return. In heart failure, the sarcomere must function near the peak of its Frank–Starling curve at all times, with limited reserve to increase stroke volume with increased metabolic demand.

Continued

MAJOR POINTS—CONT'D

- The immature myocardium responds poorly to volume loading because it is less compliant than mature myocardium. The immature myocardium responds to the need for increased CO by increasing heart rate.
- Causes of heart failure in children are varied and can include cardiomyopathy, myocarditis, and end stage structural congenital heart disease. A careful history and physical examination reveal signs and symptoms of heart failure syndrome.
- Poor cardiac output results in stimulation of humoral systems within the body in an attempt to increase CO.
- The adrenergic and renin-aldosterone-angiotensin systems work overtime to compensate for diminished cardiac function.
- Digitalis was the first heart failure medication employed in the 18th century and is still in use today.
- Diuretics benefit the failing heart by "unloading" the ventricle and decreasing circulating volume.
- ACE inhibitors block the conversion of angiotensin I (A-I) to angiotensin II (A-II), thereby diminishing the amount of A-II in circulation. A-II is a potent vasoconstrictor; by decreasing this chemical, afterload is effectively reduced and the failing heart may more easily effect forward flow.
- Medications such as spironolactone and eplerenone block aldosterone receptors, further decreasing sodium and water retention.
- β-receptor blockers slow the tachycardia associated with heart failure and improve cardiac filling. They also act centrally to cause peripheral vasodilation and to reduce afterload.
- The net effect of these medications, when administered together as "optimized" heart failure therapy, is to abrogate the effects of poor cardiac output on stimulating compensatory mechanisms that eventually perpetuate heart failure syndrome.
- The use of β-receptor blockers to effectively treat chronic heart failure is well described in the adult population.
- Mechanical ventricular assist devices scaled for use in children are being developed in the United States and Europe. These devices would improve longevity while awaiting transplantation in children with end-stage heart failure and may provide a "bridge to recovery" for some patients.
- Cardiac transplantation remains the ultimate therapy for children with end-stage heart failure due to primary myocardial disease or severe, irreparable congenital heart disease.

REFERENCES

1. Hirsch AT, Creager MA: The peripheral circulation in heart failure. In Hosenpud JD, Greenberg BH (eds): Congestive Heart Failure: Pathophysiology, diagnosis, and comprehensive approach to management. New York: Springer-Verlag, 1996.

2. Pieruzzi F, Abassi ZA, Keiser HR: Expression of renin-angiotensin system components in the heart, kidneys, and lungs of rats with experimental heart failure. Circulation 92(10):3105-3112, 1995.

3. Bigger Jr JT: Why patients with congestive heart failure die: Arrhythmias and sudden cardiac death. Circulation 75(Suppl IV):IV28-IV35, 1987.

4. Bristow MR: Beta-adrenergic receptor blockade in chronic heart failure. Circulation 101:558-569, 2000.

5. Cohn JN: The management of chronic heart failure. N Engl J Med 335(7):490-498, 1996.

6. DeiCas L, Metra M, Leier CV: Electrolyte disturbances in chronic heart failure: Metabolic and clinical aspects. Clin Cardiol 18:370-376, 1995.

7. Frishman WH: Carvedilol. N Engl J Med 339(24):1759-1765, 1998.

8. Grossman W: Diastolic dysfunction in congestive heart failure. N Engl J Med 325(22):1557-1564, 1991.

9. Kumpati GS, McCarthy PM, Hoercher KJ: Surgical treatments for heart failure. Cardiol Clinics 19(4):669-682, 2001.

10. Maisel A: B-type natriuretic peptide in the diagnosis and management of congestive heart failure. Cardiol Clinics 19(4):557-572, 2001.

11. Morgan JP: Abnormal intracellular modulation of calcium as a major cause of cardiac contractile dysfunction. N Engl J Med 325(9):625-632, 1991.

12. Pai RG, Buech GC: New Doppler measurements of left ventricular diastolic function. Clin Cardiol 19:277-288, 1996.

13. Parmley WW: Neuroendocrine changes in heart failure and their clinical relevance. Clin Cardiol 18:440-445, 1995.

14. Pavia SV, Wilkoff BL: Biventricular pacing for heart failure. Cardiol Clinics 19(4):637-652, 2001.

15. Reinhartz O, Keith FM, El-Banayosy A, et al: Multicenter experience with the Thoratec ventricular assist device in children and adolescents. J Heart Lung Transplant 20(4):439-448, 2001.

16. Rosenthal D, Chrisant MR, Edens E, et al: International Society for Heart and Lung Transplant practice guidelines for the management of heart failure in children. J Heart Lung Transplant Accepted for publication, February, 2004. Paper endorsed by International Society of Heart and Lung Transplantation, August 2004.

17. Rowland T, Potts J, Potts D, et al: Cardiovascular responses to exercise in children and adolescents with myocardial dysfunction. Am Heart J 137(1):126-133, 1999.

18. Shaddy RE: Optimizing treatment for chronic congestive heart failure in children. Crit Care Med 29(Suppl 10):S237-S240, 2001.

19. Towbin JA, Bowles JA: The failing heart. Nature 415(10): 227-233, 2002.

20. Wessel DL: Managing low cardiac output syndrome after congenital heart surgery. Crit Care Med 29(Suppl 10):S220-S230, 2001.

CHAPTER 10

Arrhythmias and Sudden Cardiac Death

JONATHAN R. KALTMAN

NANDINI MADAN

VICTORIA L. VETTER

LARRY A. RHODES

Common arrhythmias found in the pediatric population, including tachyarrhythmias and bradyarrhythmias, and sudden death will be discussed in this chapter. Although the causes of sudden death are quite diverse in the pediatric population, their final common pathway is arrhythmia.

TACHYARRHYTHMIAS

Pathophysiology

An understanding of the pathophysiology of tachyarrhythmias is crucial to their correct diagnosis and proper treatment. There are three main electrophysiologic mechanisms for abnormally fast rhythms: reentry, increased automaticity, and triggered automaticity. Reentry, the most common mechanism, describes the phenomenon of an electrical wavefront reentering cardiac tissue through which it has already traveled. There are three essential elements required for the existence of a reentrant circuit. These are (1) two parallel pathways, (2) a unidirectional block in one pathway (signifying different refractory properties of the two pathways), and (3) slow conduction in the other pathway (Fig. 10-1). An electrical impulse will enter the circuit and will begin to pass down the two pathways. If that impulse arrives in one limb of the pathway at such a time that the pathway with the longer refractory period has not recovered from the previous impulse, a block will occur in that pathway. If the second pathway has recovered (because of a shorter refractory period), the impulse will propagate down that pathway. Propagation down that pathway may be slow enough to allow for the recovery of the first pathway, thus allowing the electrical impulse to travel in a retrograde fashion up the first pathway. This will return it to the original entry site, into the circuit, and will establish a reentry circuit.

Reentrant arrhythmias behave in a predictable manner. They typically have a very regular rate with a sudden onset and termination. In addition, these tachycardias can be provoked by an electrical stimulus such as a premature atrial or ventricular contraction or by pacing maneuvers, and they can be terminated by both pacing and direct current (DC) cardioversion.

The second tachycardia mechanism is increased or enhanced automaticity. Automaticity refers to a cell's or a group of cells' ability to spontaneously depolarize.

When cells outside of the dominant pacemakers of the heart (i.e., the sinus node and the atrioventricular [AV] node) develop increased automaticity, they have the potential for overdriving or suppressing the sinus node if their rate of depolarization is greater than that of the sinus node. If these pathologic cells fire in a repetitive fashion, they result in a tachycardia.

Automatic tachycardias have relatively predictable behavior. This includes an irregular rate that is sensitive to the body's catecholamine state. They typically have warm-up and cool-down phases. Finally, pacing or DC cardioversion does not convert these arrhythmias.

The third mechanism, triggered automaticity, results from small oscillations of a cell's membrane potential during or after repolarization. If these oscillations are of sufficient amplitude to reach threshold, then depolarization will occur. There has been no direct evidence implicating triggered activity as a mechanism of clinically observed arrhythmias. However, in vitro models of triggered activity clearly emulate certain clinical entities such as torsades de pointes of long QT syndrome and arrhythmias seen in digoxin toxicity.

Tachycardias derived from triggered activity share characteristics of both reentrant and automatic arrhythmias. Like automatic tachycardias, these abnormal rhythms are catecholamine sensitive and have warm-up and cool-down phases. Like reentrant tachycardias, they can be induced by rapid pacing and can be terminated by pacing and DC cardioversion.

The next level of pathophysiologic classification involves the location in the heart in which these different mechanisms originate. Reentrant circuits may involve only atrial tissue, giving rise to atrial flutter and atrial fibrillation. In the setting of palliated congenital heart disease, reentrant pathways within the atrium may exist around surgical scars. This type of atrial flutter has been termed intra-atrial reentrant tachycardia or incisional tachycardia. Reentry may involve pathways within or leading to the AV node, resulting in atrioventricular node reentry tachycardia (AVNRT). In addition, reentry may involve ventricular tissue. In fact, the majority of ventricular tachycardia involves reentrant circuits around areas of infarction, surgical scars, or anatomic obstacles.

The last group of the reentrant tachycardias, and the most common in the pediatric population, are those involving an accessory pathway. An accessory pathway is an anomalous electrical connection between atrial and ventricular myocardium across the AV groove. These tachycardias, called atrioventricular reentrant tachycardias (AVRTs), use the accessory pathway (usually the pathway with the longer refractory period) and the AV node (usually the pathway with the slow conduction) as the two limbs of the reentrant circuit. Accessory pathways have different properties. For example, the

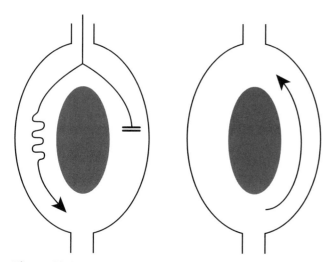

Figure 10-1 Schematic diagram representing a reentrant circuit. Requirements for reentry include two pathways, a unidirectional block in one pathway (=), and slow conduction in the other pathway (~).

Wolff–Parkinson–White (WPW) syndrome involves an accessory pathway that supports both antegrade and retrograde-conduction. Concealed bypass tracts can only support retrograde conduction.

Automatic tachycardias may originate in any of the cardiac segments. Ectopic atrial tachycardia (EAT), or automatic atrial tachycardia (AAT), is derived from a single focus of increased automaticity within the atrium, whereas multifocal atrial tachycardia (MAT), or chaotic atrial tachycardia, is derived from multiple atrial foci firing during the same time interval. Increased automaticity near the AV node gives rise to junctional ectopic tachycardia (JET). Finally, some rare types of ventricular tachycardias may arise from isolated foci within the Purkinje fibers in the ventricle.

Diagnostic Approach

The diagnostic approach to tachyarrhythmias should begin with a 12-lead electrocardiogram (ECG) (Fig. 10-2). If the tachycardia cannot be captured on an ECG, longer-term evaluation with Holter monitoring or transtelephonic monitors may be required. The tachycardias can then be divided into two general groups:

narrow complex and wide complex. Narrow complex tachycardias imply conduction through the normal AV node and the His-Purkinje system. These tachycardias are supraventricular in origin (Fig. 10-3). In children and adolescents, wide complex tachycardias are, for the most part, ventricular in origin, with certain exceptions. These exceptions include supraventricular tachycardias in which there is preexisting bundle branch block or rate-dependent aberrancy. Another exception is antidromic reciprocating tachycardia. In reentrant tachycardias involving an accessory pathway, conduction around the circuit can occur in two different ways. The first involves conduction antegrade (i.e., atria to ventricles) down the AV node and retrograde (i.e., ventricles to atria) up the accessory pathway; this is called orthodromic reciprocating tachycardia and is narrow complex. The second type involves antegrade conduction down the accessory pathway with retrograde conduction up the AV node; this is called antidromic reciprocating tachycardia and is wide complex.

The next diagnostic step is to determine the relationship of atrial to ventricular activation.[1] If the ratio of atrial-to-ventricular activation (i.e., the number of

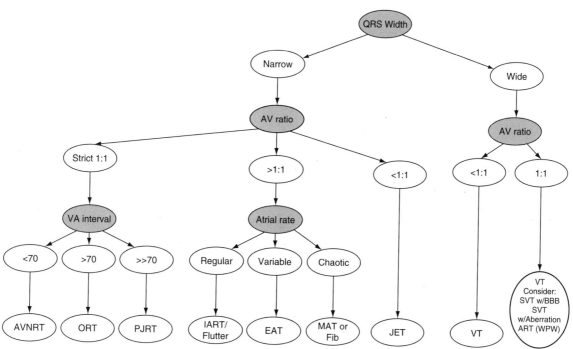

Figure 10-2   Diagnostic approach for determining tachycardia mechanism. *ART,* Antidromic reciprocating tachycardia; *AV,* atrioventricular; *AVNRT,* atrioventricular nodal reentrant tachycardia; *BBB,* bundle branch block; *EAT,* ectopic atrial tachycardia; fib, atrial fibrillation; *IART,* intra-atrial reentrant tachycardia; *JET,* junctional ectopic tachycardia; *MAT,* multifocal atrial tachycardia; *ORT,* orthodromic reciprocating tachycardia; *PJRT,* permanent junctional reciprocating tachycardia; *SVT,* supraventricular tachycardia; *VA,* ventriculoatrial; *VT,* ventricular tachycardia; *WPW,* Wolff–Parkinson–White. (Modified from Walsh EP, Saul JP, Triedman JK (eds): Cardiac Arrhythmias in Children and Young Adults with Congenital Heart Disease. Philadelphia: Lippincott Williams & Wilkins, 2001, p 103.)

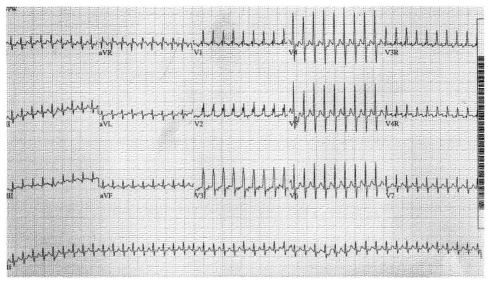

Figure 10-3   ECG showing supraventricular tachycardia in an infant.

P waves to the number of QRS complexes) is 1, then AVNRT or AVRT is the likely cause. To differentiate between these two, the retrograde ventriculoatrial (VA) conduction time (i.e., the time interval from the beginning of the QRS complex to the beginning of the retrograde P wave, or the R-P interval) should be determined. If the VA time is less than 70 ms, then AVNRT is likely. If the VA time is greater than 70 ms, then AVRT is the probable etiology. One should note that sinus tachycardia will have a narrow complex tachycardia with an A:V ratio of 1. However, the P-wave axis in sinus tachycardia will be 0 to +90 degrees, and the P-wave axis in AVNRT or AVRT will be negative.

An A:V ratio > 1 is diagnostic of a primary atrial tachycardia, although 1:1 AV conduction can occur with a primary atrial tachycardia. If the atrial rate is very regular, then atrial flutter or intra-atrial reentrant tachycardia (IART) is likely. An irregular atrial rate with a single P-wave morphology different from the normal sinus P-wave morphology and with an axis outside of the 0- to +90-degree range suggests ectopic atrial tachycardia. Finally, an irregular atrial rate with three or more P-wave morphologies suggests multifocal atrial tachycardia.

Junctional ectopic tachycardia may have 1:1 VA conduction or a VA dissociation with occasional sinus capture and a ventricular rate greater than the atrial rate.

Wide complex tachycardias should be assumed to be ventricular, especially in the emergent setting, until proven otherwise. A wide complex tachycardia with AV dissociation (i.e., no relationship between atrial and ventricular activation) and a ventricular rate greater than the atrial rate is nearly diagnostic of ventricular tachycardia (Fig. 10-4). A wide complex tachycardia with an A:V ratio of 1 can be ventricular tachycardia with retrograde atrial

conduction or supraventricular tachycardia (SVT) with aberrancy, SVT with bundle branch block, or antidromic SVT (Fig. 10-5).

The above is a general framework with which to approach the diagnosis of tachyarrhythmias. Further details will be supplied in the discussion of the individual arrhythmias.

SUPRAVENTRICULAR ARRHYTHMIAS

Single premature atrial contractions (PACs) are not uncommon in infants and children. Rarely is intervention required. Closely coupled PACs may block in the AV node. If a neonate has frequent blocked PACs, then bradycardia may result. Frequent blocked PACs are one of the most common causes of bradycardia in the newborn. If the infant is otherwise well and without hemodynamic compromise, therapy is often not needed.

Sinus arrhythmia is not an abnormal rhythm but deserves mention as it is a common finding in pediatrics. Sinus arrhythmia refers to the normal reflex-derived changes in heart rate in response to the respiratory cycle. During inspiration, the heart rate accelerates, and, during expiration, the heart rate decelerates. Sinus arrhythmia is typically more pronounced in school-aged children and adolescents. It should be considered in the differential diagnosis of an otherwise well child with an irregular heart rhythm.

Reentrant Supraventricular Tachycardia

SVT is the most common tachycardia seen in the pediatric population, with a reported incidence of 1 in 250–1000.[2]

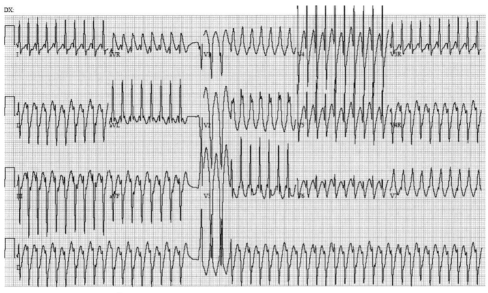

Figure 10-4   ECG showing idiopathic ventricular tachycardia in a 2-year-old.

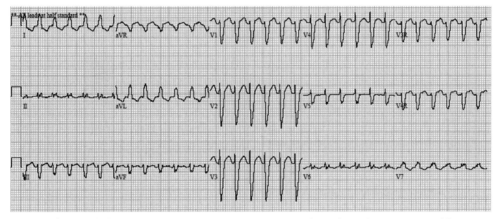

Figure 10-5   ECG showing antidromic supraventricular tachycardia in a 10-year-old.

Mechanisms of SVT include reentry and enhanced automaticity. The most common mechanism of childhood SVT is reentry.[3]

Presentation

Reentrant SVT may present at any age in infancy and childhood and even in the fetus. Accessory pathway-mediated tachycardias are more common in infants and young children, whereas AVNRT is more common in adolescence. Clinical presentation is often dependent on age. Fetal tachycardia may be detected by auscultation of the fetal heart rate or by fetal echocardiography. Prolonged fetal tachycardia is one cause of nonimmune fetal hydrops. Infants frequently will have symptoms of irritability and poor feeding. If the SVT is longstanding (i.e., over 24–48 hours), congestive heart failure may develop. Manifestations of heart failure in the infant include tachypnea, diaphoresis, pallor, and lethargy. Older children will complain of palpitations or flutter-

ing in their chest, chest pain, abdominal pain, and dizziness. Syncope may occur if the tachycardia rate is sufficiently fast to impede diastolic filling, resulting in hypotension and cerebral hypoperfusion. Children old enough to describe their symptoms may relate a sudden onset or termination of the tachycardia as well as an ability to self-terminate the arrhythmia with a Valsalva maneuver or other vagal maneuvers such as standing on their head.

Types of Reentrant Supraventricular Tachycardia
Wolff–Parkinson–White Syndrome
WPW anomaly is diagnosed when an ECG in sinus rhythm has a short P-R interval and a delta wave, which represents ventricular pre-excitation (Fig. 10-6). Ventricular pre-excitation is defined as activation of ventricular muscle earlier than would be expected for normal conduction through the AV node and down the His-Purkinje system. WPW syndrome requires an

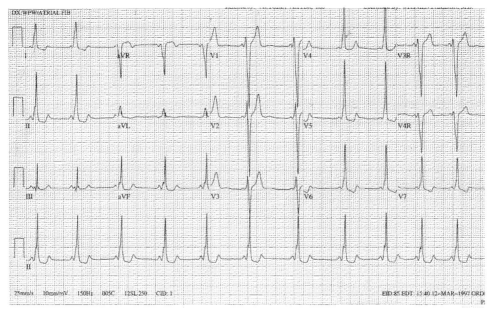

Figure 10-6   ECG of infant from Figure 10-3 during sinus rhythm. The infant has Wolff–Parkinson–White syndrome with a short PR interval and a delta wave.

accessory pathway that supports both antegrade and retrograde conduction. The SVT seen in WPW may be either orthodromic tachycardia (down the AV node) or antidromic tachycardia (down the accessory pathway) with the significant majority being orthodromic. Patients with WPW have a high risk of having atrial flutter or atrial fibrillation. If the accessory pathway supports rapid conduction of the atrial arrhythmia, sudden death may result. In patients with WPW, the risk of sudden death is 1% every 10 years.[4]

The incidence of WPW in childhood is approximately 1 in 1000.[5] Congenital heart disease occurs in approximately 20% of patients with WPW, with Ebstein's anomaly and L-transposition of the great arteries being the most common. Although the SVT seen in WPW frequently presents in early infancy, presentation may occur at any age. Of those who present in infancy, only about one third continue to experience episodes of SVT after 1 year of age.[6] Conversely, later age of SVT presentation indicates a greater chance for recurrence. A subgroup of patients with WPW is asymptomatic, and their diagnoses are made incidentally. This group of patients provides a clinical dilemma, because their risk of sudden death is unknown. Some studies suggest that assessment of the conduction properties of the accessory pathway may be the best means for risk-stratifying this group of patients. This has not been clearly defined in the pediatric population.

Concealed Bypass-Tract Tachycardia
Concealed bypass tracts only support retrograde conduction and orthodromic tachycardia. The orthodromic tachycardias found with WPW and concealed bypass tracts are virtually indistinguishable during the tachycardia. The only way to differentiate between these arrhythmias is by ECG when the patient is no longer having SVT. In normal sinus rhythm, the ECG of a patient with a concealed bypass tract appears normal, with a normal PR interval and no evidence of pre-excitation. Although the differences between these two entities may seem subtle, they in fact have significant ramifications when choosing between therapeutic options. Like WPW, patients with concealed bypass tracts can present with SVT at any age from infancy through adolescence and into adulthood. Caution should be advised in definitively ruling out WPW by the resting ECG in the infant because some pathways that can conduct antegrade may be subtle or latent and difficult to see on the initial ECG. As the child grows and the heart rate slows, pre-excitation may become manifest on the resting ECG.

An unusual type of SVT involving a concealed bypass tract is the permanent junctional reciprocating tachycardia (PJRT). PJRT has a concealed bypass tract that has a slow retrograde conduction. Therefore, the RP interval during tachycardia is quite long. The descriptor "permanent" is used because the arrhythmia is often quite difficult to convert, medically or electrically, to sinus rhythm. Many of these bypass tracts insert into the atria at the posterior septum, which is near the AV node, also called the AV junction. More recently, electrophysiology studies have suggested that these tracts may insert anywhere along either the left or the right AV groove, although the posterior septum remains a common location.

Atrioventricular Nodal Reentrant Tachycardia

The pathways used as substrate for the reentrant circuit in AVNRT are electrical approaches to the AV node located in the atrium. Two such pathways have been described. The "slow" pathway has slower conduction and longer refractoriness and is anatomically located in the mid- to posteroseptal region of the AV groove. The "fast" pathway has faster conduction and shorter refractory periods and is located in the anteroseptal aspect of the AV groove. Typical AVNRT involves conduction antegrade down the slow pathway and retrograde up the fast pathway. Atypical AVNRT involves the opposite sequence. Interestingly, in some patients with AVNRT, dual AV node pathways are not manifest during electrophysiology testing. In addition, many individuals who do not have AVNRT may have dual AV node physiology on electrophysiology testing.

The incidence of AVNRT increases with age. In fact, AVNRT represents the most common type of reentrant SVT in adults. In the pediatric population, it is most commonly seen during adolescence. A possible explanation for this is that the AV node undergoes electrophysiologic alterations with age. In one study, dual AV node pathways were found in 15% of children younger than 13 years of age and in 44% of children older than 13 years of age.[7]

Atrial Flutter

Atrial flutter is observed in two distinct groups in the pediatric population: newborns and patients with congenital heart disease, especially following atrial surgery for congenital heart defects.

The reentrant circuit of atrial flutter of infancy is generally confined to the right atrium. Similar to typical adult atrial flutter, it may utilize the isthmus between the tricuspid valve and the inferior vena cava as the area of slow conduction. Characteristic flutter waves may be present in leads II, III, and aVF (Fig. 10-7). Atrial rates may reach over 400 beats per minute (bpm). There is frequently 2:1 or greater AV block, which results in a ventricular response rate of $\geq$ 200 beats per minute.

Atrial flutter of infancy is rare. It may present in utero or in the newborn period. Congenital heart defects may coexist with the arrhythmia, so echocardiography is recommended as part of the workup. Typical associated defects include atrial septal defect, aneurysm of atrial septum, and Ebstein's anomaly. Conversion to normal sinus rhythm is often spontaneous. If it persists, the arrhythmia is generally quite responsive to therapy. The prognosis for atrial flutter in infancy with a structurally normal heart is promising, with recurrences infrequent after the initial conversion.

Atrial flutter is also seen in patients who have undergone surgical correction of congenital heart disease. Atrial flutter seen in this setting is usually referred to as intraatrial reentrant tachycardia (IART) or as incisional atrial tachycardias to highlight its differences from typical atrial flutter. The surgical procedures that predispose patients to IART generally involve surgery in the atria, the most common being repair of an atrial septal defect, atrial baffling procedures (i.e., the Senning or the Mustard

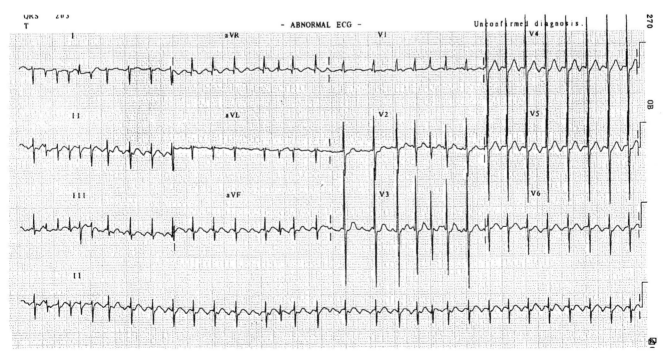

Figure 10-7   ECG showing atrial flutter with variable 1:1, 2:1, and 3:1 conduction in a newborn. Note the typical flutter waves in leads II, III, and aVF.

operation) for D-transposition of the great arteries, and Fontan procedures for single ventricle physiology (Fig. 10-8). Older age at surgery is an important risk factor for the development of atrial arrhythmias following a repair of an atrial septal defect.[8] The reentrant circuit of IART may occur anywhere within the atria and frequently incorporates an anatomic barrier or a surgical scar. During electrophysiology testing, more than one reentrant circuit may be defined. On surface EGGs, the typical saw-tooth flutter waves are absent. In fact, noninvasive monitoring may reveal multiple flutter wave morphologies, indicative of multiple reentrant circuits.

The incidence of IART following congenital heart surgery increases with age. Possible predisposing factors include surgical scars within the atrium, elevated atrial pressure, abnormal atrial anatomy associated with the primary lesion, and sinus node dysfunction.[9] Atrial rates in IART range considerably, from 150 to 450 bpm with variable conduction to the ventricle. Symptomatology is related to the ventricular response rate and myocardial function. A fast ventricular response may result in palpitations, syncope, or sudden death. A slower ventricular response rate may result in fatigue or exercise intolerance, especially in the Fontan patient in whom maintenance of AV synchrony may be crucial for adequate cardiac output. If the ventricular response rate is slow enough, patients may not even perceive the arrhythmia. Long-standing IART in a patient after a Fontan procedure may result in sluggish blood flow in the Fontan baffle and the potential for clot formation.

Treatment of Reentrant Supraventricular Tachycardia

Treatment of reentrant SVT can be divided into acute and chronic therapy. Acute therapy seeks to interrupt the reentrant circuit and to restore sinus rhythm immediately. The selection of the type of acute therapy depends upon the clinical situation. A patient who presents in shock as a result of SVT should be treated differently from someone who has SVT but is in stable condition. In the emergent setting, the ABCs of resuscitation must be followed. (Once the Airway is secured and Breathing is assured, attention can be paid to Circulation.) Chronic therapy attempts to prevent recurrence of SVT and depends significantly upon the type of SVT.

AVRT and AVNRT

For AVRT and AVNRT, adenosine is a rapid pharmacologic means of interrupting the reentrant circuit at the AV node. Adenosine requires that intravenous access is swiftly achieved. Its effectiveness needs a sufficient bolus to reach the heart quickly because it has a very short half-life. If IV access cannot readily be obtained, if the patient is in extremis, or both, then electrical direct current cardioversion is the preferred next option. Cardioversion should be performed with an energy output of 0.5–1 J/kg. The output can be doubled to a maximum of 5–6 J/kg until the treatment is effective.

In the acute but stable patient with AVRT or AVNRT, the first-line therapy is adenosine. Digoxin is effective and especially useful in the patient with decreased myocardial function, but it may require several hours for conversion. More rapid digitalization can be performed with careful

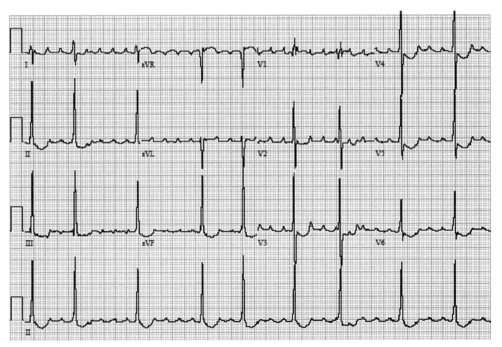

Figure 10-8   ECG showing intra-atrial reentrant tachycardia with variable conduction in a 4-year-old with hypoplastic left heart syndrome status post Fontan operation.

intravenous administration of digoxin. Other pharmacologic therapies used in the acute setting include intravenous β-blockers such as esmolol, intravenous procainamide, and intravenous amiodarone. These medications should be used with caution as they all have negative inotropic effects. Other therapeutic modalities include transesophageal pacing and vagal maneuvers. Vagal maneuvers for adolescents and older children include the Valsalva maneuver and the headstand. In infants, a bag of ice to the center of the face elicits the diving reflex and often is successful in terminating the SVT. Although IV calcium-channel blockers are an important therapy for SVT in adults, they are contraindicated in children, especially in those under 1–3 years of age. There have been reports of hemodynamic decompensation and sudden death in infants who were given verapamil.[10]

Chronic therapy for AVRT and AVNRT is similar. Digoxin and β-blockers are first-line oral therapy agents. Digoxin and calcium-channel blockers are contraindicated in patients with WPW. The reason is that these medicines slow AV nodal conduction and can enhance antegrade conduction down the accessory pathway, allowing for a more rapid ventricular response during atrial flutter or fibrillation. For AVRT or AVNRT refractory to first-line therapy, other agents such as flecainide, procainamide, sotalol, amiodarone, and verapamil can be employed. Generally, during initiation of anti-arrhythmics, children are admitted to the hospital for at least five half-lives of the medicine, which is the amount of time required to achieve steady-state pharmacologic levels. During this time, the families are educated about the signs and symptoms of SVT, and they learn how appropriately to dose the medication. Young children must be monitored for hypoglycemia and hypotension when β-blockers are started.

An increasingly popular therapeutic modality for recurrent SVT is catheter ablation. Radiofrequency ablation involves application of radiofrequency energy by a steerable electrode catheter to the arrhythmia substrate or location (e.g., an accessory pathway or an AV nodal slow pathway). Radiofrequency energy causes tissue heating and necrosis. Radiofrequency catheter ablation has been used successfully to cure various types of arrhythmias in pediatric patients. Success rates for AVRT have been reported between 86% and 97%, depending on the location of the accessory pathway, and at greater than 95% for AVNRT. Complication rates are low, at 3–4%. The most common serious complications are AV block, catheter perforation, pericardial effusion, and thrombi or emboli.[11] Common indications for radiofrequency ablation of AVRT and AVNRT include life-threatening arrhythmias, medically resistant tachycardias, adverse drug reactions, tachycardia-induced cardiomyopathy, impending cardiac surgery, and patient choice. Recently, cryoenergy has also been used to ablate arrhythmia substrates, especially when they are located close to the AV node.

Atrial Flutter

Atrial flutter in the newborn is generally converted to sinus rhythm with medications, transesophageal pacing, or cardioversion. Medications include intravenous preparations of digoxin, procainamide, amiodarone, and sotalol. Procainamide should be used in conjunction with digoxin, which will increase the degree of AV block as procainamide may slow the flutter rate, resulting in more rapid AV conduction. Once atrial flutter in the newborn period is converted to sinus rhythm, recurrence is uncommon.

Treatment of IART in the postoperative heart can be divided into acute and chronic therapy. Prior to any attempts at converting IART to sinus rhythm, the presence of an atrial thrombus must be ruled out. This usually requires transesophageal echocardiography, especially in older children and adolescents, as transthoracic windows may not be adequate to visualize an intra-atrial thrombus. Acute therapy includes medications, transesophageal pacing, and cardioversion. Medications that have been proven successful in this setting include procainamide, propafenone, amiodarone, and sotalol. An agent to slow AV nodal conduction, such as digoxin, should be used in conjunction with Class IA antiarrhythmics such as procainamide.

Chronic therapy for IART is often quite difficult, necessitating multiple medications and modalities. Digoxin is usually the first-line therapy. Because it may have little direct effect on the arrhythmia substrate, it often must be supplemented with a second agent. Second-line medications include procainamide, disopyramide, flecainide, propafenone, amiodarone, and sotalol. Other modalities include overdrive pacing techniques and radiofrequency ablation. Antibradycardia pacing has proven useful in those patients who have a significant bradycardia component to their disease (i.e., bradycardia-tachycardia syndrome). Antitachycardia pacing devices have recently been reintroduced into the market and have shown some modest benefit.[12] Radiofrequency ablation has been used to interrupt the reentrant circuits of IART. Due to various complicating factors—multiple reentrant circuits, complex atrial anatomy, or thick atrial muscle—success rates have been in the range of 70–80%, with recurrence rates as high as 50%.[9] New technologies, such as improved mapping systems and cooled catheter tips, may help to improve success rates and to decrease postablation recurrence.

Automatic Supraventricular Tachycardia

Presentation

Automatic SVT results from a focus or foci of cells that have increased automaticity. Atrial automatic tachycardias tend to present in children less than 6 years of age; they are not uncommon in older children and adolescents. Automatic tachycardias arising from the region of the AV node, or junctional ectopic tachycardia, present in two distinct settings. The first is during infancy and childhood in a familial form and the second is in patients immediately following intracardiac surgery.

Automatic tachycardias initiate with a gradual increase in heart rate (the warm-up phase) until they reach their maximum heart rate. Termination involves a gradual decrease in heart rate (the cool-down phase). The heart rate is inappropriately high for the patient's activity level. The rate of the tachycardia is catecholamine-sensitive. During sleep or under the influence of sedation, the rate will be slower or the tachycardia may even be suppressed by the normal sinus node activity. During times of stress, the tachycardia rate is faster. These tachycardias tend to be chronic and incessant. Because of the warm-up phase and their incessant nature, these arrhythmias are often not perceived by the patient. Persistence of the tachycardia may eventually lead to myocardial dysfunction. Presentation for many patients includes signs and symptoms of congestive heart failure.

Types of Automatic Supraventricular Tachycardia
Ectopic Atrial Tachycardia
EAT, or AAT, represents between 10% and 20% of the SVT seen in the pediatric population. Ectopic atrial tachycardia arises from a single focus of increased automaticity located within the atria. The firing rate of the ectopic focus is faster than that of the sinus node and overrides the normal sinus node activity. Heart rates can range from 130–210 bpm in children and adolescents but can reach 300 bpm in infants (Fig 10-9). The location of the ectopic focus can be in either atria, with the right slightly

more common than the left. Usual sites include the atrial appendages and the orifices of the pulmonary veins. AV block may occur during the tachycardia but will not interrupt the arrhythmia.

Although EAT is not specifically associated with a certain type of congenital heart disease, it is associated with conditions that result in atrial dilation such as AV valve regurgitation and postoperative atrial surgery (e.g., atrial-level baffling for transposition of the great arteries or Fontan repair for single ventricles). In addition, the arrhythmia has been associated with chronic cardiomyopathy and myocarditis.

In some patients, the tachycardia will spontaneously resolve without need for prolonged therapy. The majority require chronic therapy.

Multifocal Atrial Tachycardia
MAT, or chaotic atrial tachycardia, is a very rare type of SVT that arises from multiple foci of increased automaticity located within the atria. The tachycardia is defined by the presence of three or more P-wave morphologies (Fig. 10-10). Multifocal atrial tachycardia is frequently confused with atrial fibrillation because of the irregular rate and the variable P-wave morphologies and P-R intervals. The most common presentation is in the newborn period, with one third to one half of patients having an associated cardiac defect or other medical condition. Frequently, this type of tachycardia will spontaneously resolve during the first year of life.

Junctional Ectopic Tachycardia
JET occurs as a result of enhanced automaticity in the region of the AV node. JET is characterized on ECG by a narrow complex tachycardia, with the ventricular

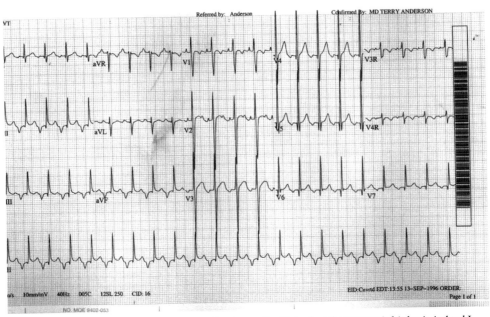

Figure 10-9 ECG showing ectopic atrial tachycardia. Note that the P wave is biphasic in lead I and negative in leads II and aVF.

rate greater than the atrial rate, and by AV dissociation (although 1:1 VA conduction can be seen in newborns and infants) (*see* Fig. 10-11). In the pediatric population, JET is seen in two settings. The first is a familial form and is often called congenital JET. These patients present in infancy, with some cases detected in utero. Congestive heart failure is frequently the presenting sign and is significantly associated with higher heart rates.[13] Early papers reported 50% of the cases to have an associated congenital heart defect.[14] The majority of these patients require therapy. After several months to years, some of these patients can be weaned off their medications. In a follow-up study of congenital JET, of those patients who were weaned from their medications, all were either entirely in sinus rhythm or mostly in sinus rhythm with intermittent episodes of a slow junctional ectopic rhythm. Sudden death has been reported in this population.[13]

The second form of JET occurs in the immediate postoperative period following surgery for congenital heart disease. Postoperative JET usually is transient and self-limiting, lasting from 24 to 72 hours. Despite its transient nature, postoperative JET can cause significant hemodynamic instability and can be fatal. The simultaneous occurrence of depressed myocardial function following bypass surgery, tachycardia to rates as high as 250 bpm (or higher), and loss of AV synchrony will significantly impede cardiac output in the postoperative setting. This arrhythmia needs to be aggressively treated. If the ventricular rate can be slowed and the patient supported for 24–72 hours, JET typically will resolve with restoration of normal sinus rhythm. Postoperative JET has been observed after most types of congenital heart surgery, but it is most commonly seen after repairs that include VSD closure.[15]

Treatment of Automatic Supraventricular Tachycardia
EAT and MAT

Treatment of automatic SVT may be difficult. There are two strategies to address this arrhythmia. The first involves decreasing the ventricular response rate by slowing AV conduction. Digoxin is the most common agent utilized for this strategy. Calcium-channel blockers will also slow conduction through the AV node, but they should be used with caution as they also have negative inotropic properties, and they should never be used in children under 1 year of age and rarely under 3 years of age.

The second strategy attempts to decrease the automaticity of the abnormal focus or foci. Commonly used medications include β-blockers, which oppose adrenergic stimulation of the focus; class IA agents, such as procainamide, and class IC agents, such as flecainide and propafenone, which decrease automaticity and prolong refractoriness; and class III agents, such as amiodarone

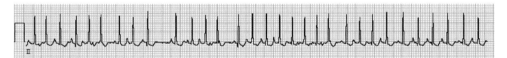

Figure 10-10   ECG of a 3-month-old with multifocal atrial tachycardia. Note the multiple P-wave morphologies.

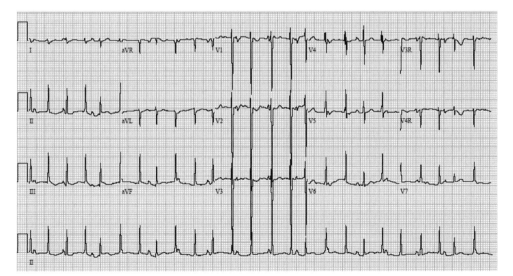

Figure 10-11   ECG showing congenital junctional ectopic tachycardia in a 3-day-old. Note the narrow QRS complexes and the AV dissociation, with the ventricular rate faster than the atrial rate.

and sotalol, which slow conduction throughout the myocardium. These agents should be used with caution in the patient with depressed myocardial function as they all have negative inotropic properties.

Radiofrequency ablation of the ectopic focus has become an effective means of curing EAT and is the treatment of choice for medically refractory arrhythmia. New mapping systems have increased the success rate of the procedure. Technical difficulties arise because the arrhythmia is catecholamine-sensitive and, under sedation, the focus may be suppressed.

Overdrive pacing and cardioversion will not be successful in treating these automatic tachycardias.

JET

For the congenital form of JET, first-line therapy is with digoxin to slow the tachycardia rate and to support cardiac function. Often a second-line agent is required. In this case, a class IA, class IC, or class III agent may be added. Amiodarone has proven to be the most successful agent in controlling the arrhythmia in this population. If a significant amount of antiarrhythmic medication is required to control the JET, sinus node dysfunction may occur, warranting the need for a pacemaker. Radiofrequency ablation has been used to cure JET. This modality is reserved for the most resistant cases because the focus is located near the AV node and His-Purkinje system and ablation within this region carries a high risk for the development of complete AV block.

Various measures have been used to treat postoperative JET. Pharmacologic agents have included digoxin, intravenous procainamide, and intravenous or oral amiodarone. In our experience, intravenous amiodarone has been most effective. Other measures have included controlling fever, hypothermia with core temperatures reduced to 33–35°C, and sedation. Several pacing protocols have also been used in the treatment of postoperative JET. These include AV sequential pacing to restore AV synchrony and paired ventricular pacing to decrease the effective heart rate and the augment cardiac output. In one study of various therapeutic options for treating postoperative JET, a combination of hypothermia and procainamide was found to be the most reliable.[15]

VENTRICULAR ARRHYTHMIAS

Types of Ventricular Arrhythmias

Ventricular arrhythmias include premature ventricular contractions (PVCs), couplets, nonsustained ventricular tachycardia (VT) (3–30 bpm), sustained ventricular tachycardia (>30 bpm) and ventricular fibrillation (VF). Ventricular arrhythmias are further distinguished by the morphology of the QRS complexes, with similar-appearing complexes being described as monomorphic

and complexes with multiple QRS morphologies being described as polymorphic. Examples of polymorphic VT include torsades de pointes, which is seen in the long QT syndrome, and bidirectional VT, which can be seen in digoxin toxicity.

PVCs are not uncommon in normal infants and adolescents. The reported incidence of isolated PVCs in infants is 10–15% and in adolescents is 20–35%.[16] If a thorough workup reveals no identifiable cause, then the diagnosis of idiopathic PVCs is given. Idiopathic PVCs are generally benign. Characteristically, benign PVCs are monomorphic and are easily suppressed with exercise. The prognosis is quite favorable and treatment is often not warranted.

Accelerated ventricular rhythm of the newborn is a VT in which the rate is no faster than 10% of the sinus rate, which can be as high as 200 bpm but is usually <150 bpm.[16] Typically, no therapy is required, and the arrhythmia resolves by early childhood.

Presentation

The presentation of ventricular arrhythmias depends on the etiology, the clinical setting, and the presence of structural heart disease. Ventricular arrhythmias can present at any age. In one study of children with ventricular tachycardia without underlying heart disease, the mean age of presentation was 5.4 years, with 27% of the patients presenting in infancy.[17]

Clinical findings depend upon the rate of the arrhythmia and the age of the patient. Arrhythmia rates just above normal sinus rates may cause no symptoms. However, significantly elevated rates may cause the patient to complain of palpitations, chest or abdominal pain, shortness of breath, fatigue, dizziness, or syncope. Infants may display poor feeding, irritability, or fatigue. Older patients will report a sudden onset of the palpitations; less frequently, they may describe a gradual onset of the symptoms. Signs will include tachypnea, hypotension, pallor, and other signs of heart failure. Sudden death can occur with a ventricular arrhythmia.

Etiology

An attempt to determine the cause of the ventricular arrhythmia is crucial as different etiologies may carry widely divergent prognoses. The presentation and clinical situation will guide the workup. Testing may include a 12-lead ECG, serum electrolytes, a serum drug screen, a Holter monitor, an echocardiogram, an exercise stress test with or without radionuclide perfusion scans, a cardiac magnetic resonance imaging (MRI), cardiac catheterization with or without endomyocardial biopsy, and electrophysiology testing.

Although there are various classification schemes for the etiologies of ventricular arrhythmias, we will classify the causes as acute or chronic.

Acute Causes

The acute causes of ventricular arrhythmias are listed in Box 10-1. Ventricular arrhythmias due to acute etiologies generally will resolve once the offending abnormality has been corrected.

Chronic Causes

The chronic etiologies of ventricular arrhythmias are listed in Box 10-2. Several of these associated conditions are discussed in further detail.

Postoperative Congenital Heart Disease

Patients who undergo surgical repair of congenital heart disease are at risk for ventricular arrhythmias. The mechanism of VT in this population is usually reentrant, with the circuit developing around an area of scar or ischemia. Generally recognized risk factors for the development of ventricular arrhythmias after congenital heart surgery include the presence of a ventriculotomy scar or pressure load or volume load on the affected ventricle.

Although VT can occur following the repair of any type of congenital heart defect, the most commonly associated defect and the one most widely studied is tetralogy of Fallot. Ventricular arrhythmias are thought to be responsible for sudden death in this population. Risk factors for the development of VT and sudden death following tetralogy repair include older age at repair, longer interval after surgery, residual pressure overload of the right ventricle, right ventricular volume overload with severe pulmonary regurgitation, and other significant abnormal hemodynamic factors. A QRS duration of greater than 180 ms on a 12-lead electrocardiogram has been positively correlated with the development of ventricular arrhythmias.

The incidence of ventricular arrhythmias is as high as 15% after tetralogy of Fallot repair and is even higher if provocative testing is included. Determining who of this population is at risk for sudden death and whom to treat has been difficult. Using invasive electrophysiology testing and noninvasive tests to risk-stratify these patients has proven inconclusive. Our general approach has been to treat patients with complex ventricular arrhythmias (i.e., rapid ventricular rates or polymorphic VT), clinically significant VT, VT with symptoms, or VT with abnormal hemodynamics. Treatment can include surgical revision of residual anatomic defects, pharmacologic agents, radiofrequency ablation, and implantation of an internal cardiac defibrillator (ICD). Commonly used medications are β-blockers, mexiletine, procainamide, and amiodarone. Radiofrequency ablation has become a more frequently used modality, with success rates enhanced if the ventricular arrhythmia is sustained and does not cause significant hemodynamic instability.

Automatic ICDs have become an important therapeutic option in preventing sudden death in the postoperative congenital heart disease population. Indications for ICD implantation in the patient following tetralogy of Fallot repair include syncope, aborted sudden death, and unstable VT or VF induced in the electrophysiology laboratory.

Cardiomyopathy/Myocarditis

Ventricular arrhythmias may be observed in various types of cardiomyopathies. Ventricular arrhythmias may indicate worsening function in dilated cardiomyopathy. The presence of nonsustained VT in adult populations with dilated cardiomyopathy and poor function suggests poorer prognosis. Novel pacing techniques, such as biventricular pacing, have provided therapeutic benefit in the adult dilated cardiomyopathy population. Ventricular

---

Box 10-1 Etiologies of Acute Ventricular Arrhythmias

METABOLIC

Hypoxia
Acidosis
Hypokalemia
Hypocalcemia
Hypomagnesemia
Hypoglycemia
Hyperkalemia

TRAUMATIC

Blunt trauma: cardiac contusion
Cardiac catheters
Thoracic surgery

MYOCARDIAL ISCHEMIA

Myocardial infarction
Anomalous coronary artery
Kawasaki disease

INFECTIOUS

Myocarditis
Pericarditis
Rheumatic fever

DRUGS/TOXINS

Antiarrhythmics
Sympathomimetics or catecholamine infusions
General anesthetics
Caffeine
Nicotine
Cocaine or other illicit drugs
Psychotropic agents: tricyclic antidepressants
    or phenothiazines

IDIOPATHIC

Box 10-2 Etiologies of Chronic Ventricular Arrhythmias

CONGENITAL HEART DISEASE

Aortic valve disease
Mitral valve prolapse
Anomalous coronary artery
Ebstein's anomaly
Eisenmenger's syndrome

POSTOPERATIVE CONGENITAL HEART DISEASE

Tetralogy of Fallot
Ventricular septal defects
Common AV canal
Single ventricle after Fontan operation
Transposition of the great arteries after intra-atrial repair

CARDIOMYOPATHY

Hypertrophic cardiomyopathy
Right ventricular dysplasia
Muscular dystrophy

ACQUIRED HEART DISEASE

Rheumatic heart disease
Lyme disease
Myocarditis
Kawasaki disease

TUMORS/INFILTRATES

Rhabdomyoma
Myocardial hamartomas
Hemosiderosis
Oncocytic cardiomyopathy
Leukemia

PRIMARY ELECTRICAL ABNORMALITIES

Long QT syndrome
Brugada syndrome
Catecholaminergic polymorphic VT
Familial ventricular fibrillation

IDIOPATHIC

Right ventricular outflow tract VT
Left ventricular septal VT

---

arrhythmias in hypertrophic cardiomyopathy are relatively common and clearly associated with syncope and sudden death. Treatment options for these populations include antiarrhythmic medications and ICD.

Right ventricular dysplasia is a rare familial cardiomyopathy characterized by fibrous or fatty tissue replacement, or both, of the right ventricular wall. It is an autosomal dominant genetic condition that predisposes

affected patients to VT with a left bundle branch pattern and sudden death. Diagnosis is most reliably made by cardiac MRI. Treatment is with β-blockers or sotalol and ICDs.

A range of ventricular arrhythmias may also be observed in patients with myocarditis, from PVCs and nonsustained runs of monomorphic VT to more complex ventricular arrhythmias, including ventricular fibrillation. Treatment of the underlying condition—the inflammation and myocardial dysfunction—is primary. Care must be taken when using inotropic agents as they can exacerbate the ventricular arrhythmias. Treatment of the ventricular arrhythmia can range from observation to aggressive use of antiarrhythmic agents.

Primary Electrical Abnormalities

There are several rare inherited arrhythmogenic syndromes associated with structurally normal hearts that predispose patients to ventricular arrhythmias and sudden death. These diverse conditions have been shown to have mutations in genes that form ion channels responsible for cardiac excitability.

Long QT syndrome is caused by various genetic mutations in genes that encode ion channel proteins. These genetic alterations prolong cardiac repolarization and increase the risk for ventricular arrhythmias and sudden death. The characteristic VT observed in long QT syndrome is described as torsades de pointes (twisting around a point) (Fig. 10-12).

Brugada syndrome is caused by a mutation in a sodium channel protein. The syndrome is defined by the association of sudden death, presumably due to ventricular fibrillation and the ECG findings of right bundle branch block and ST elevation in the right precordial leads.

Catecholaminergic polymorphic ventricular tachycardia describes a phenotype of stress- or emotion-induced polymorphic ventricular arrhythmia, often with a pattern of bidirectional VT, presenting in the absence of structural heart disease. In some cases, this syndrome has been found to be caused by a mutation in the ryanodine receptor gene, which encodes for a calcium channel in the sarcoplasmic reticulum.[18]

Idiopathic Causes

VT in the absence of structural heart disease and known genetic syndrome is uncommon in pediatrics. There are two patterns of repetitive monomorphic VT frequently observed. The first, called right ventricular outflow tract VT, has a typical left bundle branch block pattern with an inferior axis. Other possible etiologies of VT must be ruled out before this diagnosis can be made. The VT may be induced with pacing techniques in the electrophysiology laboratory. Patients with this type of VT are often asymptomatic, although they can have palpitations or, rarely, syncope and sudden death.

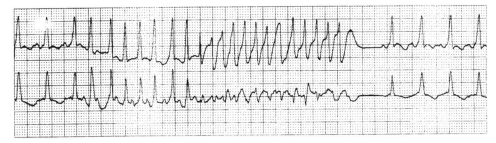

Figure 10-12   ECG showing torsades de pointes in a patient with long QT syndrome.

Treatment can be observation as some of these cases will resolve with time, β-blockers, mexiletine, or radiofrequency ablation.

The second form of repetitive monomorphic VT in patients without underlying heart disease is idiopathic left ventricular VT. The VT originates from the left ventricular side of the septum, giving an electrocardiographic appearance of right bundle branch block with left axis deviation. This type of VT can be initiated and terminated with atrial or ventricular pacing. It is typically sensitive to verapamil, and radiofrequency ablation can be curative.

Treatment

Although therapeutic options have been discussed with the individual conditions, some general points are salient.

VT should be treated as an emergency unless the rate is slow and the patient is hemodynamically stable. The ABCs of resuscitation should be followed. Any acute and reversible causes of the VT, such as electrolyte abnormalities or acidosis, should be sought and addressed. If the patient is hemodynamically stable, intravenous lidocaine should be administered at a dose of 1 mg/kg. If successful, a lidocaine infusion should be started. If the patient is in extremis, the lidocaine was not successful in converting the rhythm to sinus, or no intravenous access is readily available, then synchronized cardioversion at 1–2 J/kg should be performed. Other medications that have proven effective in the emergent setting include intravenous procainamide and intravenous amiodarone.

Chronic therapy is important for maintaining the stability of the patient and for preventing future cardiac events. If the patient initially responded to lidocaine, then mexiletine may prove to be effective as a chronic agent. β-blockers, such as propanolol and nadolol, are effective for catecholamine-sensitive arrhythmias such as the VT of long QT syndrome. Class I agents and amiodarone are second-line medications for other forms of VT. With newer technologies,

radiofrequency ablation has become a more successful treatment option for VT. Difficulties arise if the VT has greater than one morphology, is not sustained, or causes hemodynamic instability.

SUDDEN CARDIAC DEATH

Incidence of Sudden Cardiac Death

Sudden death is a natural unexpected fatal event occurring within 1 hour of the beginning of symptoms in an apparently healthy subject or in one whose disease was not severe enough to predict such an abrupt outcome.[19] Sudden death (excluding that caused by the sudden infant death syndrome) accounts for approximately 5% of all deaths in children with a reported incidence varying between 1.5 and 8 per 100,000 patient-years.[20] An estimated 5000–7000 asymptomatic children die suddenly in the United States each year, compared with the adult incidence of sudden cardiac death (SCD) of 300,000–400,000 per year. In addition, SCD in competitive athletes (up to 35 years of age) has been estimated to occur in 1 in 50,000–100,000 population.[21]

Pathophysiology and Causes of Sudden Death

Cardiac arrest may be mechanical when the heart and circulatory functions are suddenly impeded by mechanical factors (i.e., aortic rupture or pericardial tamponade) or, more commonly, arrhythmic. Evaluation of electrocardiograms recorded in adult patients suffering cardiac arrest show three possible rhythm disturbances associated with this event: VF, asystole, and electromechanical dissociation (EMD). Most studies in adults suggest that up to 90% of sudden deaths are caused by ventricular tachyarrhythmias, whereas 10–20% are caused by primary bradyarrhythmias.[22] There is a subset of patients with rapidly conducting accessory pathways (i.e., WPW syndrome) in whom atrial fibrillation can conduct rapidly to the ventricles and can degenerate into ventricular tachycardia or fibrillation, or both. Unlike adults in whom ventricular arrhythmias associated with coronary artery disease are the overwhelming cause of SCD, the etiology in children is much more diverse. A systematic classification of the common causes of SCD in children is described in Box 10-3. A brief description of the more important entities follows. A more detailed description can be found in the suggested reading and references section.

Congenital Heart Disease

Patients with congenital heart disease at the highest risk for SCD are those with structural abnormalities that result in residual hemodynamic abnormalities. These lead to pressure or volume overload of the affected ventricle, which in turn increases the risk of developing ventricular arrhythmias. The highest-risk patients are those with pulmonary hypertension. Sinus node dysfunction, which is often seen after the atrial repair of transposition of the great vessels and the Fontan operation but may be seen after any cardiac surgical procedure, increases the risk of developing atrial arrhythmias. These are poorly tolerated in compromised hearts that are dependent on the "atrial kick" to achieve adequate cardiac output. The atrial arrhythmias may also conduct rapidly to the ventricles, leading to ventricular fibrillation.

Congenital abnormalities of the coronary arteries associated with sudden cardiac death include entities such as origin of the left coronary artery from the right sinus of Valsalva with the left coronary artery passing between the aorta and the pulmonary artery, origin of a coronary artery from the pulmonary artery, a right coronary artery arising from the left sinus, and coronary ostial stenosis. Apart from the last mentioned variant, these entities are generally asymptomatic and are discovered incidentally either during an echocardiogram or during investigation of syncope or a sudden death event. The mechanisms for ischemia include compression between the two great arteries, kinking, and competitive flow into a low-pressure circuit. Treatment involves surgical rerouting of the coronary blood flow.

Hypertrophic Cardiomyopathy

This disease is more common than previously recognized, with a prevalence of 1 in 500 in the U.S. population. Sudden death is a well-known complication, with an annual incidence of 6% reported in large referral centers, although the true risk in an unselected population may be closer to 1%.[23] Hypertrophic cardiomyopathy is the most common cause of SCD in the adolescent population.

Factors that increase the risk of SCD include a family history of sudden death, young age, a severe left ventricular outflow tract obstruction and ventricular hypertrophy, a history of syncope and presyncope, and documented ventricular arrhythmias. Close follow-up and careful risk stratification are useful in preventing sudden death. Patients may be treated with a combination of procedures aimed at relieving outflow obstruction, anti-arrhythmic drugs, and implantable cardioverter defibrillators.

Other Cardiomyopathies

Dilated cardiomyopathy is a genetically and clinically heterogeneous disease that can affect all age groups. Many deaths are due to progressive pump failure, but a large proportion of patients die suddenly, most secondary to a ventricular arrhythmia and a smaller proportion secondary to a bradyarrhythmia.[24] Risk stratification is difficult, although syncope, spontaneous ventricular arrhythmias, and severe left ventricular dysfunction are generally considered poor prognostic signs.[25] It is not clear if any form of invasive or noninvasive testing is sensitive or specific in estimating risk in these patients.

Arrhythmogenic right ventricular dysplasia is one of the leading causes of sudden death in athletes.[26] It is a heart muscle disease of unknown etiology, often familial, that is characterized pathologically by fibrous fatty infiltration of the right ventricular myocardium. This

---

Box 10-3   Causes of Sudden Cardiac Death in Childhood

WITH STRUCTURAL HEART DISEASE

Congenital heart disease
  Tetralogy of Fallot
  Transposition of the great arteries
  Post Fontan operation for univentricular heart
  Aortic stenosis
  Eisenmenger's syndrome
  Marfan syndrome
  Congenital coronary artery abnormalities
  Hypertrophic cardiomyopathy
  Arrhythmogenic right ventricular dysplasia
Acquired heart disease
  Myocarditis
  Dilated cardiomyopathy
  Kawasaki disease

WITHOUT STRUCTURAL HEART DISEASE

Long QT syndrome
Wolff–Parkinson–White syndrome
Brugada syndrome
Primary ventricular tachycardia and ventricular
  fibrillation
Primary pulmonary hypertension
Commotio cordis
Drug toxicity
Electrolyte imbalance

forms the substrate for electrical instability, which results in the clinical manifestation of this condition: ventricular arrhythmia with a left bundle branch morphology, indicating a right ventricular origin. Left ventricular involvement occurs late in the course of the disease. The natural history of this disease is a function of both the electrical instability, which can precipitate arrhythmic cardiac arrest at any time during the disease course, and the progressive myocardial loss, which results in heart failure. Prevention of sudden death depends on early recognition, familial screening, exercise restrictions, and follow-up using noninvasive methods such as cardiac MRI and Holter monitoring. Ventricular arrhythmias may be amenable to anti-arrhythmic drug therapy. Sudden death may be prevented by ICD implantation or cardiac transplantation.

Myocarditis

Myocarditis is an inflammatory heart muscle disease associated with cardiac dysfunction and is an often underestimated cause of sudden death. Reviews of major series of sudden cardiac deaths in young patients revealed that myocarditis accounts for up to 44% of fatal events.[27] Subclinical myocarditis with subtle or no signs of heart failure may be the cause of "idiopathic" ventricular fibrillation in as many as 42% of patients.[28]

The disease is characterized by an unstable myocardial substrate with inflammation, edema, myocardial necrosis, and fibrosis. This can precipitate life-threatening ventricular arrhythmias and sudden death in the active and healed phases. These arrhythmias may be precipitated by exertion, and a convalescence period of 6 months is recommended after the onset of symptoms.[29] The risk of dangerous ventricular arrhythmias persists long after the initiating event, and risk stratification of these patients is undefined. Athletic participation depends on ventricular function, the absence of clinical arrhythmias, and sufficient time period for recovery following the acute episode.

Kawasaki Disease

This is the most common cause of acquired coronary artery disease in infants and young children. Approximately 20–25% of untreated Kawasaki disease patients develop coronary abnormalities, which can lead to sudden death due to massive myocardial infarction secondary to coronary thrombosis in areas of coronary artery aneurysms. The institution of therapy with intravenous gamma globulin within the first 10 days of disease onset reduces the prevalence of coronary abnormalities to 2–4%.[30] In a long-term study by Kato et al.,[31] 10–21 years after acute Kawasaki disease, progressive coronary artery stenosis was seen in patients with aneurysms, which leads to a persistent risk for myocardial infarction and lethal arrhythmias. Myocardial

infarction occurred in 39% of these patients, and overall mortality was 0.8%.

Patients with coronary artery abnormalities should be closely followed. Activity restrictions, chronic anticoagulation and intermittent evaluation of myocardial perfusion, dobutamine stress echocardiography, and coronary angiography are recommended. Patients with symptoms, arrhythmias, or ischemia should receive intervention in the form of coronary bypass surgery.

Long QT Syndrome

The long QT syndromes are an established cause of ventricular arrhythmias and exercise- or stress-related syncope and cardiac arrest in young patients. Hereditary syndromes of QT prolongation associated with polymorphic ventricular tachycardia and sudden death were first described by Jerville and Lange-Nielsen (associated with congenital deafness) and Romano-Ward (autosomal dominant without deafness).

Patients have diverse clinical features and the diagnosis must be considered in any child with syncope or resuscitated sudden death who has a corrected QT interval of > 440 ms. Some of the salient clinical and electrocardiographic features are presented in Box 10-4. Criteria for the diagnosis of long QT syndrome were updated in 1993.[32] The clinical course and treatment strategies for young patients were reviewed in a collaborative study published in 1993.[33] In the study, 9% of the study population presented with cardiac arrest, and the risk of sudden death during follow-up was related to the degree of prolongation of the QT interval.

Treatment with β-blockers eliminates symptoms as well as ventricular arrhythmias in a large proportion of

---

Box 10-4   Clinical and Electrocardiographic Features of Long QT Syndrome

ECG FINDINGS

QTc > 450 ms
Torsades de pointes
Abnormal T-wave morphology
Bradycardia for age

CLINICAL FEATURES

Syncope
Seizures
Congenital deafness
Sudden death

FAMILY HISTORY

Family members with definite long QT syndrome
Unexpected sudden death in young family members

the patients. In patients in whom β-blocker therapy is not totally effective, mexiletine, pacemaker therapy, left cervicothoracic sympathectomy, and implantable cardioverter defibrillators may be helpful in preventing or aborting life-threatening arrhythmias.[34]

Prevention of Sudden Death

Studies conducted on adults with sudden death have demonstrated that less than 20% will survive a cardiac arrest and be discharged alive from the hospital; of the survivors, 50% will be dead in 3 years. In addition, less than 1% of patients have a history of sustained ventricular arrhythmias preceding the cardiac arrest. Pediatric patients have different substrates underlying the cardiac arrest; the results are equally dismal. Primary prevention and risk stratification, especially in the competitive athlete, is important and will be the focus of the next section.

Preparticipation Screening

Sudden cardiac death in young athletes is a devastating but rather infrequent event, and only a small percentage of participants in organized sports events are at risk. Currently, universally accepted standards for screening of high school and college athletes are not available, nor are there are approved certification procedures for the individuals who perform these screening exams, although such standards were suggested by a 1996 American Heart Association consensus panel.[42] A retrospective analysis of 134 young athletes who died from various cardiovascular causes demonstrated that only 3% of these patients exposed to standard preparticipation screening were suspected of having cardiac disease, and less than 1% ultimately received an accurate diagnosis.[36]

The standard history and the physical examination screening are of value by virtue of identifying cardiovascular abnormalities in some at-risk athletes. Genetic diseases such as hypertropic cardiomyopathy, Brugada syndrome, and long QT syndrome may be suspected because of transient symptoms or a detailed family history. A detailed physical examination may raise the suspicion of other lesions, such as those associated with left ventricular outflow tract obstruction, Marfan syndrome, or coarctation of the aorta. The addition of noninvasive diagnostic tests to the screening process has the potential to enhance the detection of certain cardiovascular abnormalities. Although echocardiography has the potential to detect structural lesions, cost-efficiency issues have precluded the application of this test to large populations. The 12-lead ECG has been proposed as a practical and cost-effective alterative to echocardiography for population-based screening.[37] Finally, it is important to recognize that some of the lesions considered potentially responsible for sudden death in young patients may be difficult or impossible to detect, even if routine noninvasive testing is incorporated into the standard screening process, specifically those lesions involving coronary artery anomalies.

BRADYARRHYTHMIAS

Bradyarrhythmias can occur secondary to a wide variety of normal physiological and abnormal pathological condition (Box 10-5). In fact, in both pediatric and adult populations, the large majority of symptomatic bradyarrhythmias are due to causes extrinsic to the specialized conduction system, including relatively common conditions such as severe sepsis, drug overdose, intracranial lesions, or hypoxia. Consequently, optimum management of a patient with symptomatic bradyarrhythmia should include a complete evaluation of the patient to exclude the presence of extrinsic factors or underlying medical conditions that may be responsible for the condition. Strategies to treat symptomatic bradyarrhythmias are outlined in Box 10-6.

Sinus Node Dysfunction

The clinical manifestations of sinus node dysfunction (SND) consist of pronounced sinus bradycardia, exercise-induced chronotropic incompetence, and sinus pauses (> 2.5–3 seconds while awake, dependent on age). These episodes of bradycardia are often interspersed with SVT or atrial flutter or fibrillation constituting the "tachy-brady" syndrome. There are intrinsic causes

---

Box 10-5 Causes of Bradycardia

INTRINSIC (PRIMARY)

Sinus node dysfunction
Congenital heart block
Calcification and fibrotic degeneration of the conduction system

EXTRINSIC (SECONDARY)

Metabolic (hypoxia, hypocalcemia)
Pharmacological (digoxin overdose, calcium-channel blockers, β-blockers)
Hypothyroidism
Infectious (typhoid fever, Q fever, Chagas disease)
Neurological (increased intracranial pressure, meningitis)
Ischemic
Autonomic (increased vagal tone)

Box 10-6   Treatment of Symptomatic Bradycardia

REVERSE TRENDELENBURG POSITION

VOLUME EXPANSION

PHARMACOLOGICAL INTERVENTIONS

Anticholinergic agents
    Atropine: 0.02–0.04 mg/kg (maximum 1–2 mg)
β-adrenergic agonists and activators of adenyl cyclase
    Isoproterenol infusion: 0.01–2.0 μg/kg/min
    Epinephrine: 0.01–0.5 mg/kg (IV bolus)
            0.1–2.0 μg/kg/min (infusion)
    Glucagon
    Methyl xanthines
    Digoxin-specific antibody Fab fragments for digoxin
        toxicity
    Temporary transvenous or transcutaneous pacing

of SND, including cardiomyopathy, myocarditis, trauma, ischemia, and infarction. A common cause of symptomatic SND in pediatric patients is repair of congenital heart disease, especially following atrial switch operations, Fontan procedures, and repair of atrial septal defects (especially sinus venosus-type ASDs). Extrinsic sinoatrial dysfunction usually results from autonomic influences (e.g., neurally mediated syncope or carotid sinus hypersensitivity) or cardioactive drugs.

A complete assessment of sinoatrial (SA) node function involves a battery of noninvasive and invasive testing, including exercise stress testing, Holter monitoring, pharmacological challenge, and the invasive electrophysiology test. The decision to pursue aggressive testing is based on the symptomatology and the presence of associated heart disease. The only reliable means to treat symptomatic sinus node dysfunction is an atrial pacemaker.

Abnormalities of AV Conduction

Abnormalities of the atrioventricular conduction system can be classified either on the level of the specialized conduction tissue in which the AV block develops (i.e., on the His bundle or AV node) or based on the surface ECG morphology (Table 10-1). Clinically, it is useful to discuss these disorders based on the surface ECG morphology.

First-Degree AV Block

First-degree AV block occurs most commonly at the level of the AV node and occasionally within the atrium or the His-Purkinje system. On the ECG, it is represented by a prolongation of the PR interval (Fig. 10-13). Common causes of first-degree block are enumerated in Box 10-7. It is usually benign when it occurs as an isolated prolongation of the PR interval, representing an increase in vagal tone. If PR prolongation occurs along with bundle branch block, it may occasionally signify serious His-Purkinje disease. First-degree AV block may occur secondary to inflammatory diseases such as myocarditis, Lyme disease, or rheumatic fever, or it may be due to effects of antiarrhythmic therapy.

First-degree block as an isolated phenomenon does not require investigation or treatment. The importance of first-degree block lies as a manifestation of an underlying disease or conduction disturbance. Prolonged electrocardiographic recordings and an exercise test to exclude high-grade block constitute an adequate investigative protocol for isolated first-degree AV block.

Second-Degree AV Block

Second-degree AV block is the failure of some atrial impulses to traverse the AV node and the infranodal conduction system and to elicit a ventricular response. Two forms are identified: Mobitz Type I and Mobitz Type II.

Table 10-1   Classification of AV Block

Type of AV Block	ECG Features	Usual Site(s) of Block
First-degree AV block	1:1 AV conduction with PR interval prolongation	AV node, His-Purkinje system
Second-degree AV block, Mobitz Type I	Intermittent failure of AV conduction with progressive PR prolongation followed by a nonconducted P wave	AV node
Second-degree AV block, Mobitz Type II	Intermittent failure of AV conduction without any detectable change in PR intervals before or after the nonconducted P wave	His-Purkinje system
Third-degree AV block	Complete absence of AV conduction with AV dissociation	AV node, His-Purkinje system

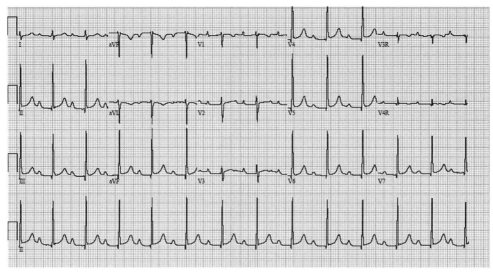

Figure 10-13   ECG showing first-degree AV block in an 11-year-old.

Box 10-7   Causes of First-Degree AV Block

Rheumatic fever
Lyme disease
Diphtheria
Chagas disease
Hypothermia
Increased parasympathetic tone
Electrolyte abnormalities
    Hypokalemia
    Hyperkalemia
    Hypocalcemia
    Hypercalcemia

CONGENITAL HEART DISEASE

    Ebstein's anomaly
    Patent ductus arteriosus
    Atrial septal defect

Mobitz Type I Block (Wenckebach Block)
This type of conduction abnormality is characterized by progressive PR prolongation followed by a P wave that is not associated with a QRS complex (Fig. 10-14). Studies have determined that the site of block lies in the AV node most of the time. The reported incidence depends on the study design and is much higher in Holter studies than in electrocardiograms. In healthy children, Wenckebach periodicity is found mainly in sleep in situations of parasympathetic dominance and is common in adolescents and highly trained athletes. Although this conduction abnormality is considered benign and not requiring treatment, it may be associated with digitalis intoxication, Lyme disease, cardiomyopathy, and myocardial infarction.

Mobitz Type II Block
Mobitz type II second-degree AV block is defined as the intermittent loss of AV conduction without a preceding lengthening of the PR interval. This is uncommon and usually implies a structurally abnormal conduction system and may progress to complete heart block. High-grade second-degree heart block (frequent nonconducted P waves) can be associated with hemodynamic compromise and is treated with pacemaker implantation.

Type II AV Block and Congenital Long Q-T Syndrome
A rare but frequently lethal cause of 2:1 AV block in young children is congenital long QT syndrome. In affected children, the QT interval is so long that the ventricle does not repolarize before the next arriving atrial impulse. Most patients present early, and 80% are diagnosed by the first week of life. The most common presentation is asymptomatic bradycardia. Mortality of untreated patients is high and may reach 50% in the first few months of life.[38] The cause of death is not related to bradycardia and is usually

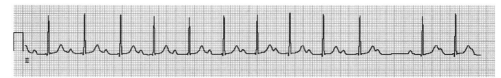

Figure 10-14   ECG showing second-degree AV block, Mobitz Type I, in a 10-year-old. Note the progressive prolongation of the PR interval with block of the 11th P wave.

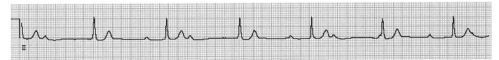

Figure 10-15 ECG showing complete AV block in a 15-year-old. Note the dissociation of the P waves and QRS complexes.

pause-dependent polymorphic ventricular tachycardia. The recommended treatment consists of a combination of β-blocker therapy along with ventricular pacing.

Complete Heart Block (Third-Degree AV Block)

Complete AV block is the inability of an atrial impulse to be propagated to the ventricles. The ECG demonstrates complete AV dissociation (Fig. 10-15). The atrial rate is faster than the ventricular rate (unlike other forms of atrioventricular disassociation such as junctional or ventricular tachycardia). Complete heart block may be congenital or acquired (Box 10-8).

Congenital Complete AV Block

The incidence of congenital complete AV block has been estimated to be between 1/15,000 and 1/25,000 live births, with most estimates at about 1/22,000 live births.[39] Approximately 25–35% of these patients have associated heart disease. There is an association of maternal collagen vascular abnormalities, overt or subclinical, with fetal and postnatal complete AV block. The maternal immunoglobulin G (IgG) antibodies involved are SS-A/Ro or SS-B/La, which can cross the placenta as early as the 16th week of pregnancy In over 60% of cases of congenital complete heart block, diagnosed in utero or at birth, detectable autoantibodies can be found in the mother.[40]

Clinical Features
The spectrum of clinical symptoms depends on the ability of the ventricular rate to meet the patient's metabolic needs. The condition may first manifest in fetal life as persistent bradycardia and, in severe cases, as fetal hydrops. Postnatally, complete heart block may present with symptoms of reduced cardiac output and impaired exercise tolerance. A subset of patients may be at high risk for sudden death due to pause-dependent ventricular arrhythmias.

Treatment
Complete heart block is often diagnosed in the intrauterine period. In the setting of an autoimmune disease in the mother, maternal treatment with steroids and immunoglobulins has been attempted with varying degrees of success. Infants with intrauterine hydrops should be delivered if they are of a viable gestational age. Asymptomatic neonates and infants are usually paced if ventricular rates are <55 bpm, if they have evidence of ventricular dysfunction, or if ventricular rates are <70 bpm and there is associated congenital heart disease. Severe bradycardia may be emergently treated with isoproterenol and temporary pacing.

Older patients may be followed until they are symptomatic, until they develop ventricular rates <40 bpm when awake, or until they have evidence of a wide complex escape rhythm and ventricular ectopy. Some patients may have ventricular dilatation and a cardiomyopathy-like picture that may respond to pacing.

Infants with congenital heart disease and complete heart block all require pacing, because the incidence of death in this group is as high as 29%.[41] Patients with surgically acquired complete heart block are usually paced if the condition persists beyond the 7th postoperative day.

DEVICE THERAPY IN PEDIATRIC PATIENTS

Pacemakers

Permanent pacemakers were first used in children in the early 1960s. Progressive miniaturization, improvements in lead and generator longevity, and multiprogrammability have led to increasing use in children and even infants. The general indications for pacemaker implantation in children fall into the following categories:
1. Congenital, postoperative, or acquired heart block
2. Sinus node dysfunction, either congenital or acquired
3. Symptomatic hypervagal state
4. Long QT syndrome with severe bradycardia, uncontrolled ventricular arrhythmias, or both

Guidelines for pacemaker implantation in adults and children have been set by the joint American College of

---

Box 10-8 Causes of Complete Heart Block

CONGENITAL
Associated with maternal connective tissue disease
Familial
Idiopathic

ASSOCIATED WITH CONGENITAL HEART DISEASE
L-transposition of the great vessels
Heterotaxy syndrome (i.e., left atrial isomerism)

LYME DISEASE
CARDIOMYOPATHY
POSTOPERATIVE

Cardiology/American Heart Asssociation[42] and are periodically updated, reflecting the current consensus opinion. Pacemaker technology has evolved over the last few decades and pacemakers are now versatile tools that can be programmed in different ways to achieve rhythm and rate management in an individual patient. Pacemakers are available in both single and dual chamber systems. In order to minimize confusion, regulatory bodies have adopted a standard nomenclature to describe pacemaker programming. Briefly, the first letter describes the chamber paced; the second, the chamber sensed; the third, the pacemaker's response to the sensed event, which is either inhibition or triggering; and the fourth and fifth refer to advanced programmability options. For instance, a VVIR pacemaker paces the ventricle, senses the ventricle, inhibits in response to a sensed event, and has rate-responsive capabilities.

Technical Issues

Pacemaker leads can be either epicardial, surgically implanted on the surface of the heart, or transvenous, implanted by a percutaneous technique. Initial lead systems were epicardial, and these were associated with high thresholds leading to premature battery depletion. The advent of transvenous leads enabled pacemaker implantation without a thoracotomy. These leads were associated with lower pacing thresholds and a diminished incidence of exit block. Transvenous leads have a higher incidence of dislocation. The newest generation of both epicardial and endocardial leads are steroid eluting and are associated with reduced thresholds and decreased incidence of exit block.

Pacemaker implantation is usually associated with a very low morbidity and mortality. Acute complications include infection, bleeding or cardiac perforation, pneumothorax, and pericardial effusion. Long-term complications include infection, lead insulation fracture and lead dislodgment, and the development of exit block. Long-term lead-related complication rates are similar for endocardial and epicardial leads and approach 35%. There are definite psychological effects, which have not been well studied, of device implantation in children and adolescents.

Device follow-up constitutes an important part of patient management. Many institutions have specialized pacemaker clinics to streamline follow-up of these patients. Patients usually have a wound check 2 weeks post implant and a first follow-up 1 month post implant. If there are no complications, the patients are seen 3 months after implant, when chronic lead thresholds should be achieved. The subsequent follow-up depends on institutional policy but typically is annual or biannual. In addition to clinic visits, patients have regularly scheduled transtelephonic pacemaker function checks. In addition to device checks, patients with endocardial leads require subacute bacterial endocarditis (SBE) prophylaxis before specific surgical procedures, as per current guidelines.

Defibrillators

ICDs are implantable devices that incorporate a defibrillator coil in addition to pacing and sensing leads. This allows internal defibrillation to terminate sustained ventricular arrhythmias using far less energy than external defibrillators. These devices first entered clinical trials in 1980.[43] Subsequently, the clinical use of these devices in children has remained limited due to the rarity of sudden death in young patients and the low salvage rate of young patients who survive cardiovascular collapse.

In 1993, a comprehensive review of the use of these devices in young patients was published.[44] This review and subsequent data have established the fact that the rates of acute implant complications and long-term morbidity were the same in children and adults implanted in the same era. Subsequently technologic improvements that have led to a decrease in device and lead size and an increased ease of implantation have resulted in escalating use of these devices in both adult and pediatric patients. The accumulated experience has led to the publication of clinical guidelines regarding the implantation and follow-up of these devices, the most recent of which were published in 2002. Briefly, three different scenarios representing indications for ICD implantation exist in young patients:

1. Patients resuscitated from sudden cardiac arrest in whom either no arrhythmias are identified or a reliable treatment regimen cannot be established.
2. Patients with recurrent symptomatic ventricular tachycardia at risk for sudden death who are intolerant to antiarrhythmic therapy.
3. Young asymptomatic patients with a strong risk factor for cardiac arrest. This category of primary prevention is the most controversial and includes long QT syndrome with a family history of sudden death, certain patients with Brugada syndrome and other primary electrical diseases, and hypertrophic cardiomyopathy with a family history of sudden death.

The incidence of appropriate shocks following device implant has been estimated to be 50% at a mean follow-up period of 24 months.[44] Device follow-up, usually in device clinics, is an integral part of the management of patients following ICD implant. There are several issues unique to the young ICD recipient, including driving, employment, athletic participation, psychological issues, and concurrent anti-arrhythmic therapy, that require concurrent management with the primary care physician, cardiologist, and pediatric electrophysiologist.

Automated External Defibrillators

The time between the onset of VF and the first defibrillation shock is the most important determinant of patient survival. In order to achieve the earliest possible defibrillation, it is important that, in the prehospital setting, rescuers, often without formal medical training, initiate treatment. The advent of automated external defibrillators (AEDs) with automated rhythm analysis systems allowed first responders to promptly defibrillate victims of cardiac arrest. Under current guidelines, AEDs should only be used in pulseless unconscious patients. The AEDs are attached to patients by two adhesive pads to analyze rhythm and, after analysis, to deliver a shock. The information is relayed by a voice or visual display and the final delivery of the shock is automatic or triggered manually. The specificity of the diagnostic algorithm for VF is between 90% and 100%. The limited literature on the use of AEDs by lay personnel in VF cardiac arrest indicates a survival of between 0% and 54%. The newer generation of AEDs is increasingly available in ambulances, workplaces, airports, schools, and other public places.

MAJOR POINTS

- The three mechanisms of tachyarrhythmias are re-entry, increased automaticity, and triggered activity.
- The most common arrhythmia in children is SVT.
- The presentation of SVT is age dependent. Infants present with irritability, poor feeding, and possibly signs of heart failure, whereas children present with complaints of palpitations, chest pain, nausea, and dizziness.
- Therapy for SVT is medical, with medications such as digoxin or β-blockers or with radiofrequency ablation in appropriate cases.
- WPW syndrome should never be chronically treated with digoxin or calcium-channel blocker because these medicines enhance conduction down the accessory pathway.
- A wide complex tachycardia should be considered ventricular tachycardia until proved otherwise.
- Sudden death accounts for approximately 5% of all deaths in children.
- The majority of symptomatic bradyarrhythmias are due to causes extrinsic to the specialized cardiac conduction system, including relatively common conditions such as severe sepsis, drug overdose, intracranial lesions, or hypoxia.
- The general indications for pacemaker implantation in children include congenital, postoperative, or acquired heart block; sinus node dysfunction, either congenital or acquired; symptomatic hypervagal states; and long Q-T syndrome with severe bradycardia, uncontrolled ventricular arrhythmias, or both.

REFERENCES

1. Walsh EP: Clinical approach to diagnosis and acute management of tachycardias in children. In Walsh EP, Saul JP, Triedman JK (eds): Cardiac Arrhythmias in Children and Young Adults with Congenital Heart Disease. Philadelphia: Lippincott Williams & Wilkins, 2001, pp 95-113.

2. Van Hare GF: Supraventricular tachycardia. In Gillette PC, Garson A (eds): Clinical Pediatric Arrhythmias. Philadelphia: W.B. Saunders, 1999, pp 97-120.

3. Ko JK, Deal BJ, Strasburger JF, Benson AW Jr: Supraventricular tachycardia mechanisms and their age distribution in pediatric patients. Am J Cardiol 69:1028-1032, 1992.

4. Case CL: Diagnosis and treatment of pediatric arrhythmias. Pediatr Clin North Am 46:347-354, 1999.

5. Vetter V: Arrhthmias. In Moller JH, Hoffman JIE (eds): Pediatric Cardiovascular Medicine. Philadelphia: Churchill Livingstone, 2000, pp 833-883.

6. Deal BJ, Keane JF, Gillette PC, Garson A Jr: Wolff-Parkinson-White syndrome and supraventricular tachycardia during infancy: Management and follow-up. J Am Coll Cardiol 5:130-135, 1985.

7. Cohen MI, Wieand TS, Rhodes LA, Vetter VL: Electrophysiologic properties of the atrioventricular node in pediatric patients. J Am Coll Cardiol 29:403-407, 1997.

8. Gatzolulis MA, Freeman MA, Siu SC, et al: Atrial arrhythmia after surgical closure of atrial septal defects in adults. N Engl J Med 340:839-846, 1999.

9. Triedman JK, Saul JP, Weindling SN, Walsh EP: Radiofrequency ablation of intra-atrial reentrant tachycardia after surgical palliation of congenital heart disease. Circulation 91:707-714, 1995.

10. Epstein ML, Kiel EA, Victorica BE: Cardiac decompensation following verapamil therapy in infants with supraventricular tachycardia. Pediatrics 75:737-740, 1985.

11. Kugler JD, Danford DA, Houston KA, et al.: Pediatric radiofrequency catheter ablation registry success, fluoroscopy time, and complication rate for supraventricular tachycardia: Comparison of early and recent eras. J Cardiovasc Electrophysiol 13:336-341, 2002.

12. Stephenson EA, Casavant D, Tuzi J, et al: Efficacy of atrial antitachycardia pacing using the Medtronic AT500 pacemaker in patients with congenital heart disease. Am J Cardiol 92:871-876, 2003.

13. Villian E, Vetter VL, Garcia JM, et al: Evolving concepts in the management of congenital junctional ectopic tachycardia. Circulation 81:1544-1549, 1990.

14. Garson A, Gillette PC: Junctional ectopic tachycardia in children: Electrocardiography, electrophysiology, and pharmacologic response. Am J Cardiol 44:298-302.

15. Walsh EP, Saul JP, Sholler GF, et al: Evaluation of a staged treatment protocol for rapid automatic junctional tachycardia after operation for congenital heart disease. J Am Coll Cardiol 29:1046-1053, 1997.

16. Alexander ME, Berul CI: Ventricular arrhythmias: When to worry. Pediatr Cardiol 21:532-541, 2000.

17. Pfammatter JP, Paul T: Idiopathic ventricular tachycardia in infancy and childhood. J Am Coll Cardiol 33:2067-2072, 1999.

18. Priori SG, Napolitano C, Memmi M, et al: Clinical and molecular characterization of patients with catecholaminergic polymorphic ventricular tachycardia. Circulation 106:69-74, 2002.

19. Goldstein S: The necessity of an uniform definition of sudden coronary death: Witnessed death within 1 hour of onset of acute symptoms. Am Heart J 103:156-159, 1982.

20. Driscoll DJ, Edwards WD: Sudden and unexpected death in children and adolescents. J Am Coll Cardiol 5:B118-B121, 1985.

21. Maron BJ, Roberts WC, McAllister HA, et al: Sudden death in young athletes. Circulation 62:218-229, 1980.

22. Milner P, Platia E, Reid P, Griffith LS: Ambulatory electrocardiographic recordings at the time of fatal cardiac arrest. Am J Cardiol 56:588-592, 1985.

23. Maron BJ, Gardin JM, Flack JM, et al: Prevalence of hypertrophic cardiomyopathy in a general population of young adults. Echocardiographic analysis of 4111 subjects in the CARDIA Study. Coronary Artery Risk Development in (Young) Adults. Circulation 92:758-789, 1995.

24. Wu AH, Das SK: Sudden death in dilated cardiomyopathy. Clin Cardiol 22:267-272, 1999.

25. Burch M, Siddiqui SA, Celermajer DS, et al: Dilated cardiomyopathy in children: Determinants of outcome. Br Heart J 72:246-250, 1994.

26. Thiene G, Nava A, Corrado D, et al: Right ventricular cardiomyopathy and sudden death in young people. N Eng J Med 318:129-133, 1988.

27. Liberthson RR: Sudden death from cardiac causes in children and young adults. N Engl J Med 334:1039-1044, 1996.

28. Phillips M, Robinowitz M, Higgins JR, et al: Sudden cardiac death in Air Force recruits: A 20 year review. JAMA 256:2696-2699, 1986.

29. Maron BJ, Mitchell JH: 26th Bethesda Conference: Recommendations for detecting eligibility for competition in athletes with cardiovascular abnormalities. J Am Coll Cardiol 4:845-899, 1994.

30. Yannagaway H, Nakkamura Y, Yashiro M, et al: Update on the epidemiology of Kawasaki disease in Japan: From the results of the 1993-1994 nationwide survey. J Epidemiol 6:148-157, 1996.

31. Kato H, Ichinose E, Yyoshikowa F, et al: Fate of coronary aneurysms in Kawasaki disease: Serial coronary angiography and long-term follow-up study. Am J Cardiol 49:1758-1766, 1982.

32. Schwartz PJ, Moss AJ, Vincent JM, et al: Diagnostic criteria for the long QT syndrome: An update. Circulation 88:782, 1993.

33. Garson A Jr, Dick M II, Fournier A, et al: The long QT syndrome in children: An international study of 287 patients. Circulation 87:1866-1872, 1993.

34. Eldar M. Griffin JC, Abbot JA, et al: Permanent cardiac pacing in patients with the long QT syndrome: An update. Circulation 88:782, 1993.

35. Maron BJ, Thompson PD, Puffer JC, et al: Cardiovascular preparticipation screening of competitive athletes. Circulation 94:850-856, 1996.

36. Maron BJ, Shirani J, Poliac LC, et al: Sudden death in young competitive athletes: Clinical, demographic and pathological profiles. JAMA 276:199-204, 1996.

37. Maron BJ, Bodison SA, Wesley YE, et al: Results of screening a large group of intercollegiate competitive athletes for cardiovascular disease. J Am Coll Cardiol 10:1214-1222, 1986.

38. Trippel DL, Parsons MK, Gillette PC: Infants with long-QT syndrome and 2:1 AV block. Am Heart J 130(5):1130-1134, 1995.

39. Gochberg SH: Congenital heart block. Am J Obstet Gynecol 88:238-241, 1964.

40. Brucato A, Jonzon A, Friedman D, et al: Proposal for a new definition of congenital complete atrioventricular block. Lupus 12:427-435, 2003.

41. Michaelsson M, Engle MA: Congenital complete heart block: An international study of the natural history. In Brest AN, Engle MA (eds): Cardiovascular Clinics. Philadelphia: FA Davis, 1972, pp 85-101.

42. Gregoratos G, Abrams J, Epstein AE, et al: ACC/AHA/NASPE 2002 guideline update for implantation of cardiac pacemakers and antiarrhythmia devices. Circulation 106:2145-2161, 2002.

43. Mirowski M, Reid PR, Mower MM, et al: Termination of malignant ventricular arrhythmias with an implanted automatic defibrillator in human beings. N Engl J Med 303:322-324, 1980.

44. Silka MJ, Kron J, Dunnigan A, Dick M 2nd: Sudden cardiac death and the use of implantable cardioverter defibrillators in pediatric patients. Circulation 87:800-807, 1993.

The Use of Cardiac Catheterization to Diagnose and Treat Heart Disease in Pediatric Patients

MATTHEW J. GILLESPIE

HEIKE E. SCHNEIDER

JONATHAN ROME

The goal of this chapter is to introduce the reader to the common diagnostic and interventional procedures that occur within the cardiac catheterization laboratory. Upon completion of this chapter, the reader should have an understanding of (1) the indications for diagnostic and interventional cardiac catheterization procedures in pediatric patients, (2) basic hemodynamic measurements and calculations, (3) basic angiography, (4) common interventions in pediatrics, and (5) the risks and complications associated with cardiac catheterization.

A successful diagnostic or interventional procedure depends on the combined skills of the cardiac catheterization lab team. In addition to the cardiologist, any given procedure requires specially trained technicians and nurses to operate the equipment, to ensure adequate sedation, and to monitor the patient. The standard catheterization team makeup is listed in Table 11-1.

In general, pediatric catheterization laboratories are equipped with biplane fluoroscopy (Fig. 11-1). The biplane system allows for multi-angle viewing of the complex three-dimensional anatomy common in congenital cardiac defects. Whereas surgical cutdown was common to achieve vascular access in early years, the approach now is almost always percutaneous, using a modified Seldinger technique. The femoral vein and artery are the most commonly used vessels; in special circumstances, a variety of others may be used, including jugular, subclavian, or transhepatic access to veins, and brachial, axillary, or carotid (by cutdown) access to arteries.

DIAGNOSTIC CATHETERIZATION

The information obtained from diagnostic catheter evaluation falls into two broad categories: (1) anatomy and (2) physiology or hemodynamics. Anatomic data are obtained by angiography, whereas hemodynamics are determined by measuring pressures, oximetry, and by using one or more techniques to determine flow (i.e., Fick or thermodilution methods). Advancements in noninvasive diagnostic modalities (i.e., echocardiography and magnetic resonance imaging [MRI]) over the past 30 years have reduced the number of cardiac catheterizations done solely for attainment of anatomic diagnosis. Cardiac catheterization remains the gold standard for assessment of intracardiac and intravascular physiologic parameters. This is particularly important when noninvasive imaging yields unclear results

Table 11-1   Cardiac Catheterization Team

Team Member	Role in Catheterization Procedure
Interventional pediatric cardiologist	Diagnosis and intervention
Catheterization nurse	Procedural assistant
Circulating nurse	Supplies
Sedation nurse	Patient sedation and monitoring
Radiation technologist	Fluoroscopy operation
Recording nurse	Recording catheterization data

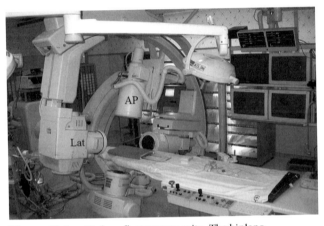

Figure 11-1   Biplane fluoroscopy suite. The biplane fluoroscopy system allows for the multi-angle viewing of complex three-dimensional anatomy. The anteroposterior (AP) and lateral (Lat) image intensifiers are labeled.

or when the assigned cardiac diagnosis is inconsistent with the clinical scenario. Diagnostic catheterization is routinely used for sequential evaluation of patients undergoing staged treatment of complex congenital defects.

Pressure Data

Pressure data are measured with fluid-filled catheters attached to a pressure transducer. Pressure data are reported in millimeters of mercury (mmHg). Waveforms may be recorded on paper or may be converted to digital data and stored for later analysis. The cardiologist positions the catheter tip into a site of interest, and the pressure is recorded. In this way, pressure measurements from all intracardiac chambers and the great vessels are obtained. The data from the individual sites are evaluated in combination to assess function, to identify gradients, and, when combined with flow measurements, to allow calculation of vascular resistances. The synthesis of the pressure data is discussed later in this chapter.

Normal and Abnormal Pressure Tracings

In a normal heart, the right heart and pulmonary arterial pressures are low relative to the left heart and systemic arterial pressures (pulmonary pressure = 1/4 systemic pressure). Within each heart chamber and blood vessel, the pressure changes with each phase of the cardiac cycle (i.e., systole and diastole). There are three characteristic types of pressure tracings: venous and atrial, ventricular, and arterial. Each of these waveforms is influenced by the forces and valves affecting that site. For example, the right atrial pressure waveform is determined by tricuspid opening, atrial contraction, and tricuspid closure. Figure 11-2 shows a characteristic right atrial waveform.

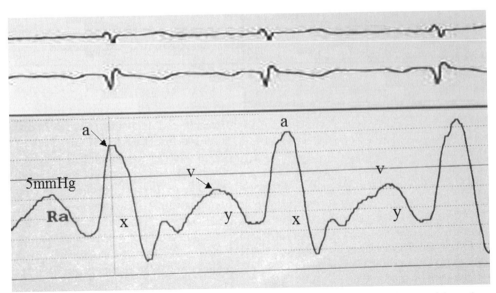

Figure 11-2   Right atrial waveform. The a wave represents intra-atrial pressure during atrial systole. The x descent represents atrial relaxation. The v wave represents atrial filling (i.e,. atrial diastole) and occurs concomitant with tricuspid valve closure. The y descent occurs early in ventricular diastole, as the tricuspid valve opens.

The "a" wave represents the intra-atrial pressure during atrial systole. The fall in pressure after the a wave, called the "x" descent, occurs as a result of atrial relaxation. The "v" wave occurs concomitant with tricuspid valve closure during atrial filling (i.e., atrial diastole). The fall in pressure after the v wave is called the "y" descent. It occurs during the opening of the tricuspid valve in early ventricular diastole. Atrial pressures are reported in terms of the a wave, the v wave, and the mean. In general, right atrial pressure remains low throughout the cardiac cycle. The normal mean right atrial pressure is 1–4 mmHg. The a wave is usually 2–4 mmHg higher than the v wave. There is significant respiratory variation in atrial pressure tracings; in a spontaneously breathing patient, the pressures fall during inspiration and rise on exhalation (the converse occurs during positive pressure ventilation). By convention, pressures are reported at end expiration. Normal ranges for pressures are shown in Table 11-2.

A characteristic right ventricular waveform is shown in Figure 11-3. Early systole is represented by a rapid upstroke. Peak systolic pressure is followed by a brief plateau phase and then by isovolumic relaxation, during which time the pressure falls rapidly. As the ventricle fills during diastole, there is a gradual increase in pressure. The point at which the systolic upstroke begins again is the end diastolic pressure. The peak systolic and end diastolic pressures are typically reported. Normally, the systolic RV pressure ranges from 20 to 30 mmHg and the diastolic pressure ranges from 3–8 mmHg (Table 11-2).

Arterial pressures are reported as peak systolic, diastolic, and mean pressures. In the normal heart, the peak systolic pulmonary artery pressure equals that of the right ventricle (ranging from 20 to 30 mmHg). The pulmonary artery diastolic pressure is usually 8–15

Table 11-2	Range of Normal Pressure Values in Children*
Site	**Pressure**
Right atrium	1–4 mmHg (mean)
Right ventricle	20–30/3–8 mmHg
Pulmonary artery	20–30/8–15 mmHg
Pulmonary capillary wedge	5–10 mmHg (mean)
Left atrium	5–10 mmHg (mean)
Left ventricle	80–120/3–10 mmHg
Aorta	80–120/50–80 mmHg

* In general, pressures increase with age.

mmHg, with a mean of 10–13 mmHg. There usually is no difference between the main and branch PA pressures. A characteristic pulmonary artery pressure waveform is shown in Figure 11-4.

Under normal conditions, the pressure obtained from a catheter wedged into a distal branch of the pulmonary artery accurately reflects the left atrial pressure. The pulmonary veins are valveless, and, if an end hole catheter occludes flow in an artery (usually a balloon-tipped catheter), there is a static column of blood extending from the tip of the catheter through the pulmonary vascular bed to the left atrium (LA). The pressure within the LA throughout the cardiac cycle is reflected back through this static column of blood and may be measured using a transducer. A characteristic wedge waveform is shown in Figure 11-9A. Pulmonary capillary wedge and the left atrial tracings have similar characteristics to those recorded in the right atrium (Fig. 11-2), although they are usually 5–10 mmHg higher, and the v wave is dominant.

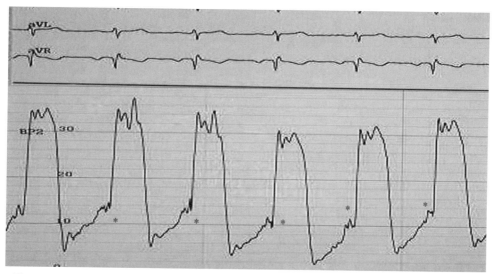

Figure 11-3   Right ventricular waveform. A right ventricular waveform is shown above. Early systole is represented by a rapid upstroke. Peak systole is followed by a brief plateau and then by isovolumic relaxation (rapid downstroke). Early diastole is marked by a gradual increase in pressure as the ventricle fills. The asterisk (*) denotes the right ventricular end-diastolic pressure.

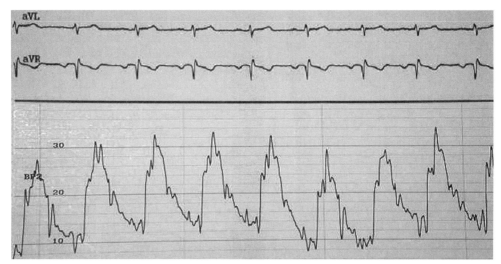

Figure 11-4   Pulmonary arterial waveform. Peak systolic pressure in the pulmonary artery usually equals that of the right ventricle. Diastolic pressure ranges from 8 to 15 mmHg.

Under normal circumstances, the pulmonary capillary wedge waveform accurately reflects left atrial pressure. They may differ in several situations, such as when the wedge pressure is in excess of 20 mmHg, in the presence of pulmonary vascular obstructive disease, or in the case of pulmonary vein stenosis. When there is an elevated wedge pressure and it is discrepant from the left ventricular end-diastolic pressure (LVEDP), direct measurement of the left atrial pressure is necessary. If the atrial septum is intact and a direct measurement is indicated, it can be acquired with the Brockenbrough technique, which involves puncturing the atrial septum with a transseptal needle. A long sheath is passed over the needle and positioned within the left atrium for pressure recording.

The left ventricle is usually accessed in a retrograde fashion through the aorta. Typically, a pigtail catheter is passed over a wire from the femoral artery, around the aortic arch, across the aortic valve, and into the left ventricle. A characteristic left ventricular waveform is shown in Figure 11-5. The features of the left ventricular waveform are similar to those of the right, described above.

Normal pressures vary with age and are listed in Table 11-2. The LVEDP is an important tool in the clinical assessment of left ventricular function. Elevated LVEDP is a sign of poor ventricular compliance and commonly presents with diminished pump function (i.e., cardiomyopathy or myocardial infarction).

Pressure measurements in the aorta are made in both the ascending and descending segments of the vessel. In the absence of aortic valve disease or left ventricular outflow tract obstruction, the peak systolic pressure in the aorta equals that in the left ventricle. In the absence of coarctation, systolic pressure in the ascending and descending aorta should be similar, although that in the descending aorta may be slightly higher due to a reflected wave phenomenon. A characteristic aortic waveform is illustrated in Figure 11-6. The notch seen in diastole (i.e., the dicrotic notch) represents a brief increase in pressure associated with aortic valve closure. The notching is more prominent in the descending aorta and peripheral arteries. Aortic pressure is described in terms of the systolic, diastolic, and mean pressures.

Synthesizing the Pressure Data

In the catheterization lab, simultaneous pressure readings and pullbacks from adjacent or contiguous structures allow for the identification of pressure gradients, which are used to evaluate valvular or vascular stenoses and to determine vascular resistances. Examples of commonly used techniques are described below.

In the normal heart, when the pulmonary capillary wedge and the left ventricular end-diastolic pressures (LVEDP) are simultaneously measured, the wedge tracing a wave should equal the LVEDP (Fig. 11-7A). A gradient between these two values results from obstruction to left ventricular inflow, as seen in mitral valve stenosis (Fig. 11-7B). Another commonly used method for the identification of pressure gradients indicative of structural and functional abnormalities is the pressure pullback. During this maneuver, pressure is continually recorded as the catheter is withdrawn through the vasculature. For example, on the right side of the circulation, the catheter is pulled proximally from the distal pulmonary artery to the proximal, into the main pulmonary artery, across the pulmonary valve, and into the right ventricle. The pullback ends when the catheter tip reaches the right atrium. Examples of normal and abnormal right-sided pressure pullbacks are shown in Figure 11-8. Figure 11-8A shows a normal right-sided pullback. Figure 11-8B shows an example of pulmonary valve stenosis. As the catheter is pulled proximal to the area of stenosis, the pressure increases.

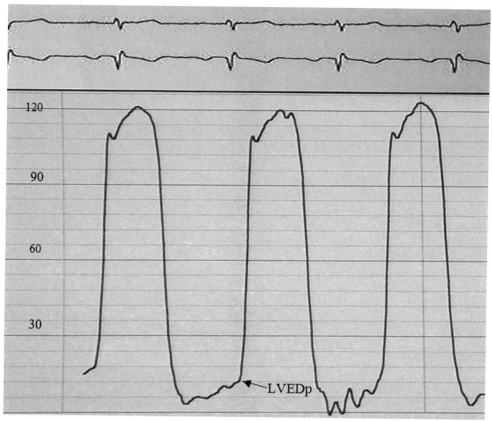

Figure 11-5   Left ventricular waveform. As with the right ventricular waveform, there is a rapid upstroke in early systole followed by a brief plateau phase, isovolumic relaxation (rapid down stroke), and a gradual increase in pressure as the ventricle fills in diastole.

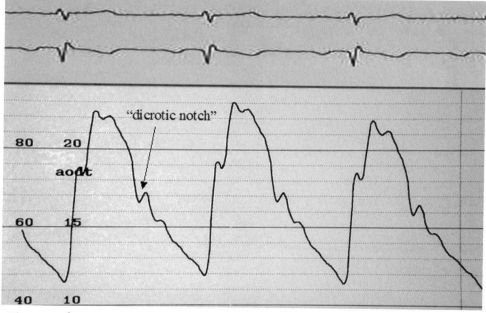

Figure 11-6   Aortic waveform. In normal patients, the peak systolic pressure in the aorta is equal to the peak systolic pressure of the left ventricle (LV). The notch seen in diastole (i.e., the dicrotic notch) represents a brief increase in aortic pressure that occurs as the aortic valve closes. The ascending and descending aortic waveforms are similar in the absence of coarctation. The dicrotic notch is more prominent in the descending aorta. The leftward-most scale correlates with the waveform (40–80 mmHg).

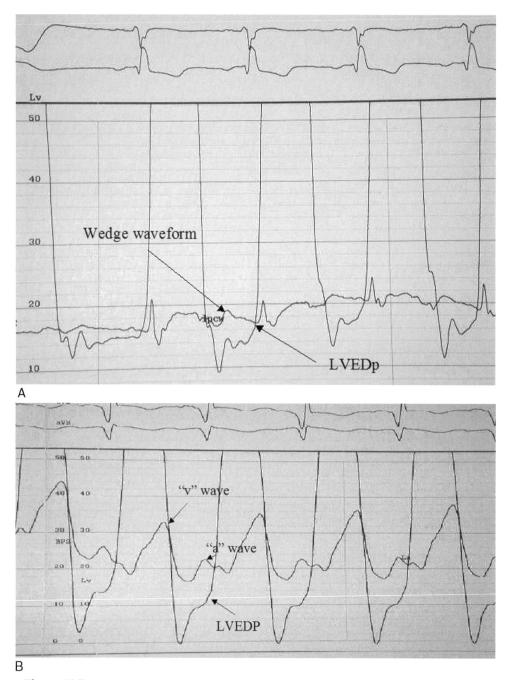

Figure 11-7   Simultaneous wedge and left ventricular end-diastolic pressure (LVEDP) measurement. **A,** The normal relationship between the pulmonary capillary wedge pressure and the LVEDP. In this example, simultaneous measurements reveal that the a wave, representing left atrial contraction, is equal to the LVEDP. The a wave is not clearly discernable. The wedge waveform approximates the LVEDP throughout the cardiac cycle. **B,** An example of mitral valve stenosis. There is a 10- to 12-mmHg gradient between the a wave and the LVEDP.

The left-sided pressure pullback begins with a pigtail catheter positioned in the left ventricular cavity. The catheter is withdrawn across the aortic valve, first into the ascending and then into the descending aorta. Figure 11-9 shows examples of both normal and abnormal left-sided pressure pullbacks.

Hemodynamic Calculations
Fick Principle
An important objective of a diagnostic cardiac catheterization is the collection of hemodynamic data. The measurements of pressure and oxygen saturation and calculations of

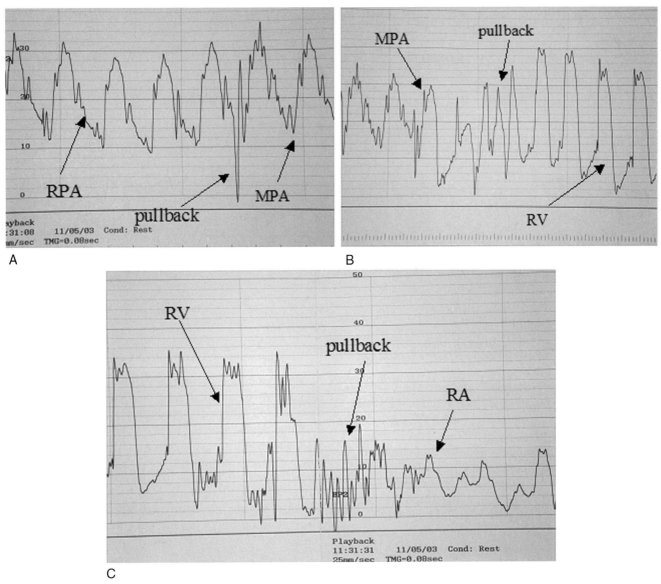

Figure 11-8   Right-sided pressure pullback. **A,** A normal right-sided pullback. Frame 1 shows the change in waveform as the catheter is withdrawn from the right pulmonary artery (RPA) to the main pulmonary artery (MPA). **B,** A high-frequency spike occurs in the waveform as the catheter is withdrawn proximally (marked as "pullback"). In a similar fashion, the catheter is withdrawn across the pulmonary valve into the right ventricle (RV). There is some respiratory variation in the systolic pressures; no gradient is seen. **C,** To complete the pullback, the catheter is withdrawn into the right atrium (RA). **D,** An abnormal right-sided pullback. As the catheter is withdrawn from the MPA into the RV, a mild gradient of 12 mmHg is revealed.

Continued

cardiac output, in conjunction with anatomic findings by angiography, are used to reach conclusions regarding the patient's condition and to make decisions regarding further management. Cardiac output (CO) is defined as the product of stroke volume (SV) and heart rate (HR); the units are L/m:

$$CO = SV \times HR$$

Because of the wide range in patient sizes encountered in pediatrics, the cardiac output is indexed (CI, cardiac index) to body surface area (BSA):

$$CI = CO / BSA$$

Normal values for the cardiac index are 3-5 L/min/m^2. Cardiac output is typically calculated in the catheterization laboratory using an indicator dilution technique. Historically, a known amount of indicator, green dye, was administered by bolus into a central vein. Blood was withdrawn from a systemic artery and the amount of green dye in the sample was determined. The cardiac output was then determined by measuring the area under the curve of dye concentration versus time. A commonly used variation on this method relies on using oxygen as

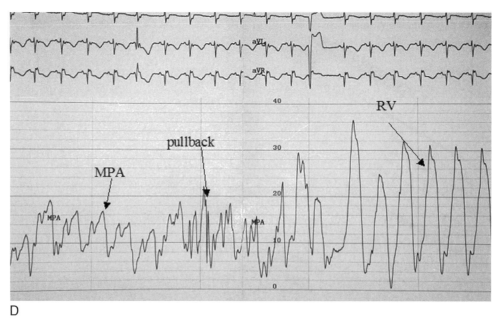

D

Figure 11-8, cont'd

the indicator. This method, based on the Fick principle, was originally described by Adolph Fick in 1870.[1,2]

The Fick principle is illustrated in Figure 11-10. In this example, a train moving along at given speed travels under a hopper. The hopper is delivering marbles into the cars of the train. The principle states that if one knows the number of marbles in each car before and after they cross under the hopper, and if one knows the rate at which the hopper delivers marbles, one can determine the train speed.

The train speed is cardiac output, the marbles are oxygen, the hopper is the lung delivering oxygen, and the rate of marble delivery is oxygen consumption (in a steady state the amount of oxygen the lungs deliver to the blood must equal the rate of oxygen consumption). Thus, the number of marbles per car before the hopper is the content of oxygen in mixed venous blood, and the number after the hopper is the oxygen content of arterial blood.[2] In other words, CO equals oxygen consumption (VO_2) divided by the arteriovenous oxygen difference (AVO_2):

$$CO \ (L/min) = VO_2 \ (mL/min) \ / \ AVDO_2 \ (mL/L)$$

Oxygen consumption can be measured or assumed based on published tables or nomograms. In order to complete the equation, the oxygen content of mixed venous and arterial blood must be determined. Oxygen content includes the oxygen bound to hemoglobin and that dissolved in plasma. The amount of oxygen hemoglobin carries when it is fully saturated is called the oxygen carrying capacity: O_2 cap (cc/L) = hemoglobin concentration (gm/L) $\times$ 1.36. The percentage of oxygen saturation (O_2 sat) of hemoglobin in a given sample of blood is determined by co-oximetry. The amount of oxygen dissolved in blood is the partial pressure of oxygen (pO_2, measured by standard blood gas analysis) times a constant (0.03). Thus,

$$O_2 \ content \ (cc/L) = pO_2 \times 0.03 + O_2 \ cap \times O_2 \ sat$$

If the patient is breathing ambient air, the amount of oxygen dissolved in blood is negligible and can be ignored. However, if supplemental oxygen is being administered, dissolved oxygen must be included in the calculation and, thus, pO_2 must be measured. Catheters are positioned in appropriate sites to sample blood for oxygen content analysis. The mixed venous sample is obtained from the most distal site in the systemic venous circulation, proximal to any left-to-right shunt. Thus, for hearts without shunt lesions, the pulmonary artery saturation is sampled. The arterial sample is typically obtained from the aorta.

An example of the application of the Fick equation to a normal child is as follows: A child with a body surface area of 1 m[2] has hemoglobin of 14.7 gm/dL. The oxygen consumption is measured at 130 cc/min, the oxygen saturation in the pulmonary artery is 77%, and that in the aorta 97%. Thus,

$$O_2 \ cap = 14.7 \times 1.36 = 20 \ cc/dL = 200 \ cc/L.$$

Systemic arterial O_2 content	$= O_2$ cap $\times O_2$ sat $= 200$ cc/L $\times 0.97$ $= 194$ cc/L.
Systemic venous O_2 content	$= 200$ cc/L $\times 0.77$ $= 154$ cc/L.

Finally, CO = VO_2 / $AVDO_2$ = 130 cc/min / (194 cc/L – 154 cc/L) = 130/40 L/min = 3.25 L/min/m[2].

Application of the Fick principle is very useful in the care of critically ill patients. For example, if oxygen consumption and hemoglobin are within the normal range,

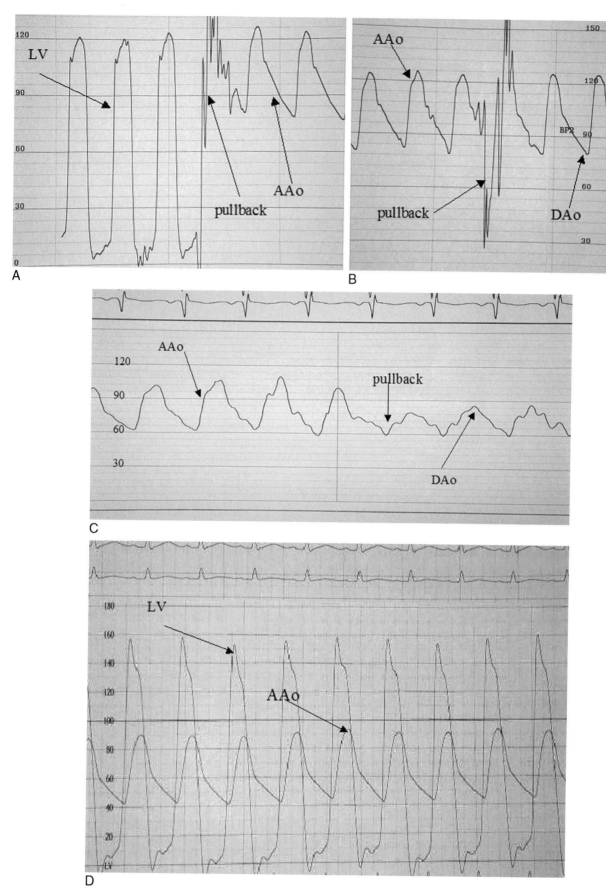

Figure 11-9   Left-sided pressure measurements.   **A-B,** A normal left-sided pullback. There are no gradients from the left ventricle (LV) to the descending aorta (DAo).   **C,** An example of mild coarctation of the aorta. Pullback from the ascending aorta (AAo) to the DAo reveals an 18- to 20-mmHg gradient.   **D,** Aortic valve stenosis with a 70- to 80-mmHg gradient from the LV to the AAo.

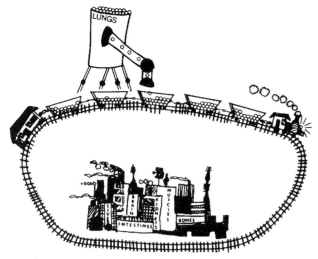

Figure 11-10 The Fick principle. The marbles represent molecules of oxygen. The difference between the number of marbles in each car before and after the hopper represents the arterio-venous oxygen difference (AVO_2). The rate at which the hopper delivers marbles represents the oxygen consumption (VO_2). The train's speed represents cardiac output ($CO = VO_2/[A - V]O_2$). (From Baim DS, Grossman W [eds]: Grossman's Cardiac Catheterization, Angiography, and Intervention, 6th ed. Philadelphia: Lippincott Williams & Wilkins, 2000.)

low mixed venous saturation is indicative of low cardiac output and may be used to monitor patients. By the same token, increased metabolic rate (e.g., fever or sepsis) or anemia will also lead to increased $AVDO_2$.

Thermodilution

Another frequently applied method to determine cardiac output is thermodilution. Thermodilution is another indicator dilution method in which the indicator is temperature.[1,2] A bolus of cold saline is administered in a central vein, and then temperature is measured from a thermistor positioned in the pulmonary artery. Because the indicator (i.e., cold) dissipates on recirculation, the thermodilution method has an enormous advantage over other indicator techniques in that it can be repeated multiple times without accumulation of the indicator. In certain conditions, such as intracardiac shunting, significant tricuspid regurgitation, or low cardiac output states, thermodilution is unreliable because there is loss of indicator (i.e., cold) prior to temperature measurement at the thermistor. The cold saline dissipates into the surrounding tissue, resulting in an overestimation of cardiac output.

Intracardiac Shunts

Intracardiac shunts can be identified by measurements of the oxygen saturation in the great vessels and the cardiac chambers. For example, a significant step-up in saturation between the right atrium and right ventricle is likely to

because the result of a ventricular septal defect. Oxygen saturations that are lower than normal (i.e., < 95%) on the left side of the heart may indicate a right-to-left shunt. In presence of intracardiac shunts or shunts of the great vessels, the concept of a single cardiac output is not applicable because systemic and pulmonary blood flow are not the same. The pulmonary blood flow (Qp) and systemic blood flow (Qs) can be calculated separately applying the Fick principle, first to the pulmonary and then to the systemic circulation. The denominator contains the difference of the oxygen content of the respective vascular bed.

$$Qp = \frac{VO_2}{CpvO_2 - CpaO_2}$$

and

$$Qs = \frac{VO_2}{CsaO_2 - CmvO_2}$$

($CpvO_2$, oxygen content of the pulmonary venous blood; $CpaO_2$, oxygen content of the pulmonary arterial blood; $CmvO_2$, oxygen content of the mixed venous blood; $CsaO_2$, oxygen content of the systemic arterial blood)

In certain cases of congenital heart disease, both a left-to-right and right-to-left shunt may exist at the same time. To adequately characterize this situation, an additional flow is calculated: the effective pulmonary blood (Qep). Qep is best conceptualized as the amount of mixed venous blood that is oxygenated in the lungs.

$$Qep = \frac{VO_2}{CpvO_2 - CmvO_2}$$

Once Qep has been determined, the wasted flow, termed "shunt flow," can be calculated. Left-to-right shunt flow is total Qp − Qep; similarly, right-to-left shunt flow is Qs − Qep.

The Qp/Qs ratio is often used as a convenient measure to describe the direction and magnitude of shunting. It can be quickly calculated because all values except for oxygen saturations (in patients breathing ambient air) are cancelled out of the equation:

$$\frac{Qp}{QS} = \frac{\text{Systemic artery} - \text{Systemic vein } O_2 \text{ saturation}}{\text{Pulmonary vein} - \text{Pulmonary artery } O_2 \text{ saturation}}$$

Vascular Resistance

The pulmonary and systemic vascular bed can be characterized by means of calculations of resistances from pressure measurements and flow calculation obtained during the cardiac catheterization. The relationship among pressure, flow, and resistance are described by Ohm's law ($R = \Delta P/Q$). Thus, the resistance of a vascular bed is the mean pressure difference across the particular vascular bed divided by the respective blood flow. The flows are indexed to body surface area. The equation for the systemic vascular resistance (Rs) is as follows:

$$Rs = \frac{AOp - RAp}{Qs}$$

Wood units per m2 = mmHg/L/min/m^2
(AOp, Aortic pressure; RAp, right atrial pressure;
Qs, systemic flow)

Normal values for the systemic vascular resistance in children range between 15 and 30 units/m^2. The resistance units may also be expressed as dynes $\times$ sec/cm^5, which equals Wood units $\times$ 80.

The pulmonary vascular (Rp) resistance is calculated as follows:

$$Rp = \frac{PA_p}{LA_pQp}$$

(PAp, pulmonary arterial pressure; LAp, left atrial pressure;
Qp, pulmonary flow)
The normal values for the pulmonary vascular resistance are
2–4 u/m^2.

Angiography

Angiography is used to define anatomy in the catheterization laboratory. Because blood and soft tissues have the same density on standard radiographic imaging, radiodense contrast media is used to opacify structures of interest. The catheter is positioned in the site of interest and a power injector delivers the contrast agent. Typically, biplane imaging is used for congenital heart lesions. The cameras can be moved to the desired angles to profile the anatomy of congenital heart defects. A variety of projections employing compound angles, so-called axial angiographic views, have been defined to profile various features of cardiac anatomy

Contrast agents are based on iodine, an organic preparation of triiodobenzoic acid derivatives. Recent improvements in these agents include nonionic agents with decreased osmolality. These advances have resulted in diminished toxicity. Nonetheless, all agents have potential toxic side effects, including nephrotoxicity, peripheral and coronary vasodilation, decreased myocardial contractility, arrhythmogenesis, pulmonary hypertensive crises, and pulmonary edema. Severe allergic reactions are very rare but well described. Anyone with a history of such allergies must be pretreated with corticosteroids and antihistamines. Patients known to be allergic to shellfish should also be considered at risk.[2]

Normal Angiographic Anatomy
The right ventricle has typical features by which it can be differentiated from the left ventricle. The right ventricle has coarse trabeculae and an outflow portion (conus or

infundibulum), which lies between the body of the chamber and the semilunar valve, resulting in discontinuity between the tricuspid and semilunar valves. The inflow and outflow form an angle of almost 90 degrees. The prominent muscle bundle of the right ventricle, the moderator band, can be visualized angiographically (Fig. 11-11). The left ventricle is finely trabeculated and bullet-shaped, and there is mitral valve to semilunar valve fibrous continuity (Fig. 11-12).

Angiography of Common Congenital Defects
Although echocardiography has become the mainstay of anatomic diagnosis, particularly for unoperated congenital defects, angiography remains important. This is particularly true in defining anatomy not well seen on echocardiography (i.e., distal pulmonary arteries), or as an additional modality to clarify or further define difficult anatomy (i.e., multiple ventricular septal defects). The ventricular septum has three portions: the inlet or atrioventricular canal portion, which is just under the tricuspid and mitral valves, posteriorly; the muscular septum, which makes up the major area; and the infundibular or outflow septum, anteriorly. Defects may occur in any of these regions (Fig. 11-13). Because the left ventricle is smooth-walled, ventricular septal defects are best profiled by left ventricular contrast injection. The ventricular septum has a complex three-dimensional topography; several different axial views are used to profile different portions of the

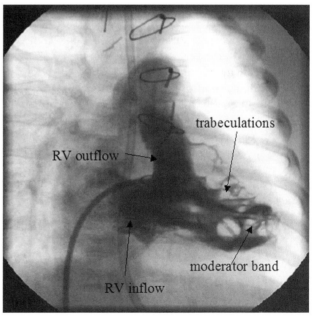

Figure 11-11   Right ventriculogram. The right ventricle (RV) is shown in an anteroposterior projection. The RV is coarsely trabeculated and can be divided into three portions: inflow, body, and outflow. The RV inflow and RV outflow are oriented at a 90-degree angle. The moderator band is prominently displayed within the body of the RV. A balloon-tipped catheter is shown, positioned in the apex of the RV. Wires are used to close the sternum after median sternotomy.

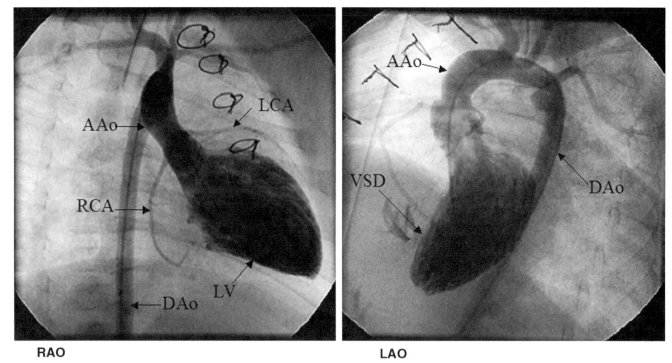

RAO   **LAO**

Figure 11-12 Left ventriculogram. The LV is shown in both the right anterior oblique (RAO) and left anterior oblique (LAO) projections. The LV cavity is smooth-walled, finely trabeculated, and bullet- or slipper-shaped. The right and left coronary arteries (RCA and LCA) originate from their respective coronary sinuses and branch in a normal distribution. Also labeled are the ascending and descending aortic portions (AAo and DAo). In the LAO projection, a small amount of contrast flows into the RV (anterior to the LV) through a small midmuscular ventricular septal defect (VSD). Sternal wires indicate a previous median sternotomy.

septum. Angiographic examples of several different ventricular septal defects are demonstrated in Figure 11-14.

Right ventricular angiography is used to delineate right ventricular outflow obstruction from sub- or valvar pulmonic stenosis. The former is typical in tetralogy of Fallot (Fig. 11-15).

Angiograms of the great arteries may be used to evaluate native or postoperative obstructions, for example, branch pulmonary artery stenosis and coarctation of the aorta (Fig. 11-16). Aortography is used to evaluate aortic insufficiency. Angiography of the aorta is particularly important in evaluating postoperative anatomy (Fig. 11-17).

Transcatheter Therapeutics or Interventional Cardiology

In 1966, William Rashkind reported the balloon atrial septostomy procedure for transposition of the great arteries,[3] heralding the beginning of the era of pediatric interventional cardiology. In the years since, the armamentarium of the interventional cardiologist has expanded to include balloons for dilating valves and stenotic vessels, stents for treatment of vascular and postoperative obstructions, coils and other materials for the embolization of vessels and surgical shunts, and devices for the

closure of intracardiac and extracardiac defects. It is fair to say that there are virtually no congenital heart lesions for which there is not a potential role for interventional treatment. Table 11-3 summarizes the spectrum of interventional procedures currently performed.

In this section, we will briefly describe transcatheter therapeutics to familiarize the reader with the range of procedures available, as well as their indications, expected results, and complications. The procedures can be divided into two main categories: (1) interventions designed to create or enlarge communications and (2) closure procedures.

Balloons and Stents

Stenoses of vessels and valves are common in congenital heart disease. In addition, some situations require creation of intracardiac communications (most commonly atrial septal defects) either to improve oxygen saturation (i.e., transposition) or to allow egress of blood from an atrium (i.e., mitral atresia or stenosis). Balloon dilations, balloon septostomy, and endovascular stent deployment are the procedures used to accomplish these ends. Balloon catheters are used to enlarge or to dilate stenotic cardiac

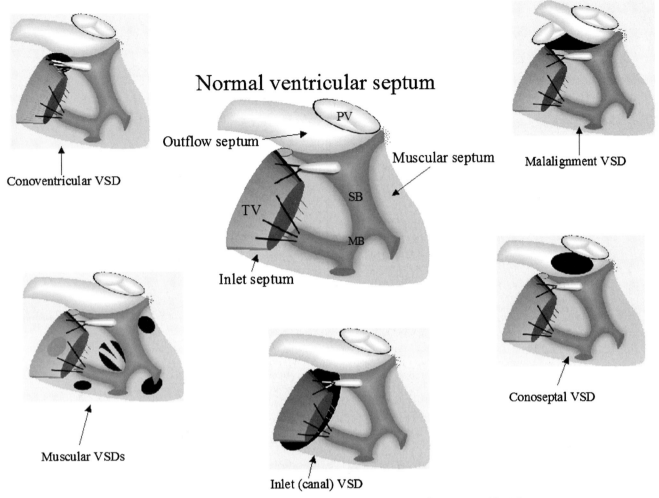

Normal ventricular septum

Conoventricular VSD

Outflow septum

PV

Muscular septum

Malalignment VSD

SB

TV

MB

Inlet septum

Muscular VSDs

Conoseptal VSD

Inlet (canal) VSD

Figure 11-13   Normal ventricular septum and ventricular septal defects (VSDs). The inlet, muscular, and outflow portions of the right ventricular septum are shown in the central illustration. VSDs may occur in any of these regions. Conoventricular, malalignment, muscular, conoseptal, and inlet (i.e., canal) VSDs are also shown. *MB,* Moderator band; *SB,* septal band; *PV,* pulmonary valve; *TV,* tricuspid valve. (From Kaiser LR, Kron IL, and Spray TL [eds]: Mastery of Cardiothoracic Surgery, 2nd ed. Philadelphia: Lippincott Williams and Wilkins, 1997.)

and vascular structures. Balloon dilation procedures were introduced to pediatric cardiology in the early 1980s for pulmonary valve stenosis[4] and are now the accepted treatment for many congenital heart and postoperative lesions. The balloon is made of a noncompliance or very-low-compliance synthetic polymer such as polyurethane, nylon, or polyethylene. Angioplasty balloons can be inflated to high pressures, allowing relief of stenosis. Catheters are designed for specialized purposes: small low-pressure balloons for dilation of stenotic valves in newborns can fit through 3F (i.e., 1 mm diameter) introducers, whereas large high-pressure balloons for lesions in older patients may require sheaths 12F or greater in diameter. Balloon dilation alone may be ineffective for treatment of pulmonary artery stenoses and coarctation because of vessel recoil or restenosis. In these situations,

balloon expandable stents have proven very effective.[2,5-7] Stents, made from tubular stainless steel lasers cut into a strutted framework, are usually used.

Balloon Atrial Septostomy
Since Rashkind and Miller first described the balloon septostomy, it has remained an essential part of the treatment of newborns with transposition of the great arteries who are cyanotic due to inadequate mixing of systemic and pulmonary blood. Less commonly, the procedure is used for other defects in which egress of blood from one of the two atria depends on an adequate-sized atrial communication (i.e., mitral atresia). Historically, the procedure was performed using fluoroscopic guidance, but now it is often done at the bedside using echocardiographic imaging.

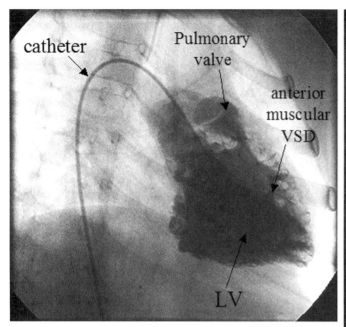

RAO

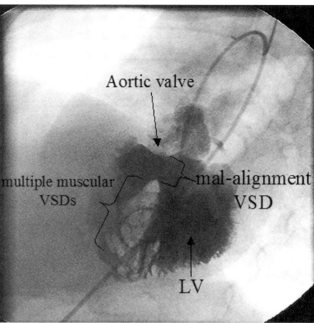

LAO

Figure 11-14   Angiographic examples of ventricular septal defects (VSDs). The figure above is a left ventriculogram shown in both the anterior and lateral projections (RAO and LAO). A pigtail catheter is placed retrograde into the LV cavity. Injection of contrast into the LV reveals multiple defects in the muscular portion of the ventricular septum, giving it a Swiss-cheese appearance. A large anterior malalignment VSD is profiled best in the LAO projection. The RAO projection best profiles the anterior portion of the muscular septum.

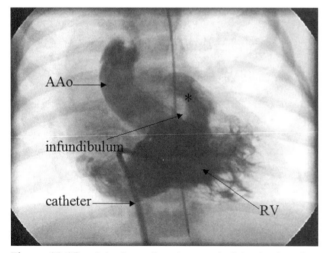

Figure 11-15   Subvalvar pulmonic stenosis. Injection into the right ventricle (RV) reveals subvalvar pulmonic stenosis (*) secondary to anterior malalignment of the infundibular septum. The opacification of the aorta (AAo) occurs secondary to right-to-left shunting across the malalignment VSD.

To perform a balloon atrial septostomy, the catheter is introduced through the umbilical or femoral vein and advanced from the right atrium, through the patent foramen ovale, and into the left atrium. The balloon at the catheter tip is filled with diluted contrast or saline and is

forcefully withdrawn to the right atrium to tear the thin portion of the atrial septum[5] (*see* Fig. 11-18). In severely cyanotic infants with D-transposition of the great arteries, the systemic saturations rise quickly and the pressure gradient between the atria nearly equalizes. After the newborn period or in patients with a thick or abnormal atrial septum, other techniques, such as blade atrial septostomy, balloon dilation of the atrial septum, or even stenting of the atrial septal defect, have been developed to create an adequate atrial communication.

Pulmonary Valve Stenosis

Transcatheter balloon dilation is the treatment of choice for pulmonary valve stenosis. Kan reported the first series of patients in 1982.[5] For several years, this technique had been used in neonates with severe and critical pulmonary valve stenosis. A child with a transvalvar gradient >40 mmHg is considered a candidate for valvuloplasty. Angiography of the right ventricle confirms the echocardiographic diagnosis and allows measurement of the dimensions of the pulmonary valve annulus. An oversized balloon, 1.2–1.4 times the size of the annulus, is used. During the inflation of the balloon, a waist, or indentation, that resolves with complete dilation can be observed on the balloon. Balloon valvuloplasty is very effective for typical valvar pulmonic

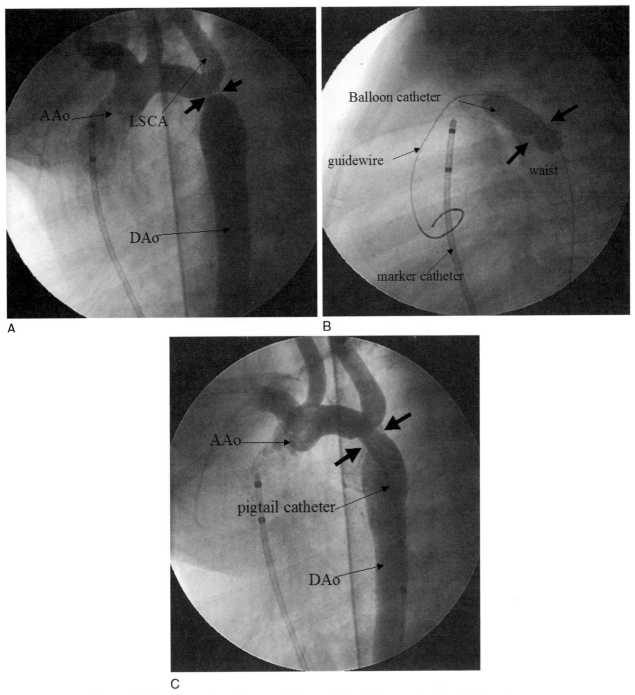

Figure 11-16   Coarctation of the aorta, before and after balloon angioplasty. **A,** A discrete coarctation of the aorta just distal to the origin of the left subclavian artery (LSCA). The *arrows* mark the narrowest diameter (~4 mm). **B,** A balloon angioplasty procedure. A balloon catheter is inflated across the point of narrowing and inflated until the balloon waist resolves. This image shows submaximal inflation of the balloon. The *arrows* mark the waist. **C,** An improvement in the diameter of the coarctation (*arrows*) after balloon dilation.

stenosis, and restenosis is uncommon.[4] In anatomic variants in which the pulmonary valve is dysplastic (common in Noonan syndrome), valvuloplasty is less effective. Balloon dilation is very effective in most newborns with critical pulmonic stenosis, although such patients may have cyanosis persisting after dilation because of a persistent right-to-left shunt at a patent foramen ovale as a result of the hypertrophied, noncompliant right ventricle. Usually this cyanosis improves as the right ventricle remodels.

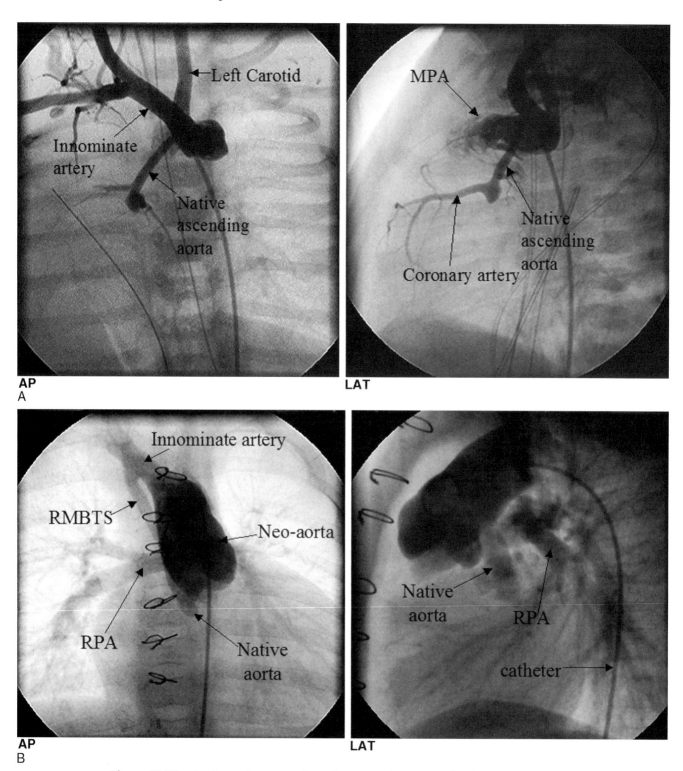

Figure 11-17   Aortic atresia, preoperative and postoperative angiography. **A,** An atretic ascending aorta associated with hypoplastic left heart syndrome (HLHS). Both the anteroposterior (AP) and lateral (LAT) projections are shown. A pigtail catheter is positioned in the innominate artery. Injection of contrast fills the native ascending aorta (AAo) in a retrograde fashion. The right and left coronary arteries originate from the atretic AAo, which measures approximately 2 mm in diameter. In the lateral view, the MPA opacifies through the patent ductus arteriosus. **B,** The postoperative anatomy following a Norwood reconstruction procedure. A pigtail catheter is positioned in the neoaorta. The native-to-neoaortic anastomosis is shown in both projections. The pulmonary arteries fill through a right modified Blalock–Taussig shunt (RMBTS).

Continued

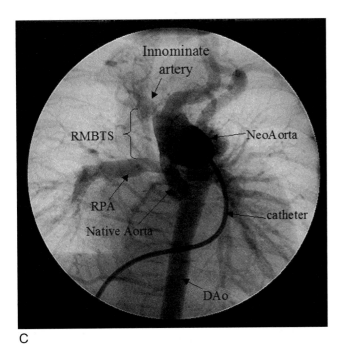

C

Figure 11-17, cont'd   C, Another example of the Norwood reconstruction for HLHS.

Some neonates with pulmonary atresia and intact ventricular septum are candidates for transcatheter treatment. In these patients, the atretic pulmonary valve plate is first perforated with a radiofrequency catheter and then is dilated in the standard manner[5,8] (Fig. 11-19).

Aortic Stenosis
In contrast to pulmonary valvotomy, interventions for aortic stenosis should be considered palliative procedures: restenosis and insufficiency usually will develop at some point after valvotomy (transcatheter or surgical). Most reports suggest that transcatheter intervention compares favorably with surgical valvotomy.[5,8] Given the fact that these patients will require multiple interventions, balloon valvuloplasty is generally felt to be the optimal first-line treatment for aortic stenosis in newborns, infants, and children. The success rate of percutaneous aortic valvotomy in children is reported to be about 90%, with a mortality of less than 1% beyond the newborn period. Patients with noninvasive evidence of moderate or severe aortic stenosis are referred for cardiac catheterization. Invasive diagnostics are performed, including pressure measurement to determine the severity of obstruction and angiography to demonstrate the location of narrowing. When the peak gradient at the aortic valve exceeds 50 mmHg and the obstruction is determined to be valvar, balloon dilation is performed. Balloon dilation usually results in a mild increase in aortic regurgitation. Restenosis, progressive aortic insufficiency, or both are common after balloon aortic valvuloplasty. Most patients will derive several years of benefit after a successful procedure. If restenosis develops, repeat dilation is appropriate, but surgical intervention is required when aortic insufficiency becomes significant. Subaortic stenosis is not effectively treated by balloon dilation and must be approached surgically.

Mitral Stenosis
Balloon dilatation of the mitral valve has proven very effective in rheumatic mitral stenosis.[1,2,5] The procedure has been applied to congenital mitral valve stenosis as well. In this relatively rare disorder, in which the mitral

Table 11-3   Spectrum of Interventional Procedures in Children

Balloon dilation and stents for stenotic or restrictive structures	Transcatheter occlusion of cardiac and vascular abnormalities	Emerging therapeutics
Atrial septostomy	Atrial septal defects (secundum ASD)	Percutaneous pulmonary valve replacement
Pulmonary valve stenosis/atresia	Patent foramen ovale	Percutaneous aortic valve replacement
Branch pulmonary artery stenosis	Patent ductus arteriosus	Atrioventricular valve repair (mitral, tricuspid)
Aortic valve stenosis	Ventricular septal defects	
Aortic coarctation	Collateral arteries (ToF, TGA)	
Mitral stenosis	Decompressing venous structures (e.g., LSVC to coronary sinus) after Fontan	
Postoperative stenoses:		
• Recoarctation of the aorta		
• Conduit obstruction		
• Branch pulmonary arteries		
• Fontan circuit (baffle, veins, pulmonary arteries)		
• Fontan fenestration		
• Mustard / Senning baffle		

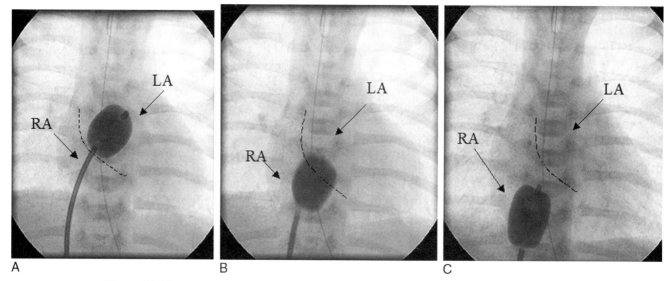

Figure 11-18   Balloon atrial septostomy. **A,** The tip of the septostomy balloon catheter is positioned in the left atrium (LA). The balloon is filled with dilute contrast. The atrial septum is represented by the dashed line. **B,** The septostomy balloon is forcefully "jerked" from the LA across the atrial septum and into the right atrium (RA). As a result, the atrial septum is torn. **C,** The balloon positioned in the RA after septostomy.

anatomy is quite disturbed, often with absence of true chordae tendinea (i.e., mitral arcade), dilation rarely seems to be of clinically significant benefit.

Branch Pulmonary Arteries

Stenosis and hypoplasia of branch pulmonary arteries are common problems in pediatric cardiology. These lesions occur congenitally in association with other congenital heart defects such as in tetralogy of Fallot. Isolated congenital narrowing of the pulmonary arteries occurs in Williams syndrome, congenital supravalvar aortic stenosis, and Alagille syndrome. Pulmonary artery stenosis is common after surgical interventions such as arterial-to-pulmonary shunts, arterial switch operations, and repairs of truncus arteriosus or tetralogy of Fallot. Balloon angioplasty for pulmonary artery stenoses was first described by Lock in the early 1980s.[5] The procedure is successful in 70–80% of lesions. Significant residual narrowing is common after successful dilation, as is restenosis, which occurs in approximately one third of lesions.

Suboptimal results after balloon angioplasty led to the application of balloon expandable stents for pulmonary artery stenosis. Stents can be very effective, often resulting in complete relief of vascular obstruction (Fig. 11-20). Stents can be redilated to accommodate for growth. Their use in small children guarantees the need for further procedures. They may be contraindicated if pulmonary artery stenoses involve more than one branching artery as the stent can bridge branch points and occlude or reduce flow into segments of lung. Standard indications for pulmonary artery intervention include stenosis severe enough to result in elevated right ventricular pressure, markedly decreased flow to the affected lung, or pulmonary hypertension in the contralateral lung. As successful dilation of pulmonary arteries results in tearing in the intima and often part of the media in most instances, it should not be surprising that vascular injury is an important potential complication, with vessel disruption or aneurysm formation occurring in roughly 1%.

Another important potential complication of pulmonary artery dilation or stenting is so-called reperfusion pulmonary edema. This problem is most likely to occur in patients who have multiple bilateral pulmonary artery stenoses and only some of the stenoses are effectively treated. This results in redirection of most of the cardiac output to the small portion of lung, perfused by the now unobstructed pulmonary artery, resulting in edema in that segment. Patients can become profoundly hypoxemic in this situation and mortality has been reported.

Coarctation of the Aorta

As with the other simple left-sided obstructive lesion, aortic stenosis, the clinical presentation of patients with coarctation varies depending on the lesion severity. Patients may present with shock as newborns at one extreme or with asymptomatic hypertension in adulthood at the other. Balloon dilation of aortic coarctation has been performed since the mid-1980s.[5,9] Restenosis is very common when the procedure is performed in young infants, leading most centers to refer such patients for surgical treatment. Although dilation in older infants and children is standard practice in many centers, others continue to refer the younger patients for surgical repair because of restenosis rates and concerns about the risk

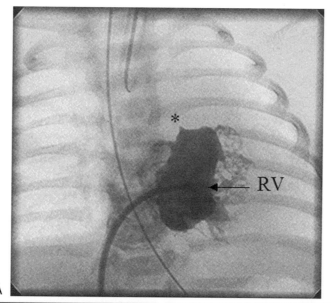

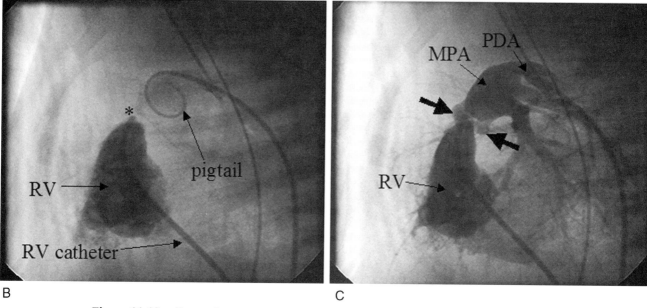

Figure 11-19   Transcatheter intervention for pulmonary atresia. **A,** A right ventriculogram in a patient with pulmonary atresia. The RV outflow tract ends blindly at the level of the atretic pulmonary valve (*). No contrast crosses the pulmonary valve plate, and therefore the pulmonary arteries do not opacify. **B,** The lateral view of an RV injection. The RV catheter is positioned just below the atretic pulmonary valve plate (*). As above, the RV ends blindly. There is a pigtail catheter positioned in the MPA retrograde through the patent ductus arteriosus (PDA). **C,** A simultaneous injection into the RV and the MPA. The bold arrows mark the atretic pulmonary valve.

Continued

of aneurysm formation. More recently, endovascular stenting of coarctation in older individuals has been applied. Acute (97% success) and intermediate results are encouraging, with very low rates of either aneurysm formation or restenosis. Although long-term results are not available for this therapy, it appears an appropriate strategy for management in these age groups.

When coarctation recurs after surgical repair of the aorta, balloon angioplasty is the treatment of choice in patients with simple coarctation as well as in those with complex disorders such as hypoplastic left heart syndrome (see Fig. 11-16).

Device Closure and Vascular Occlusions

An ever-increasing array of catheter-delivered devices allow for the closure of cardiac defects. In catheter embolizations, metal coils or other materials are delivered

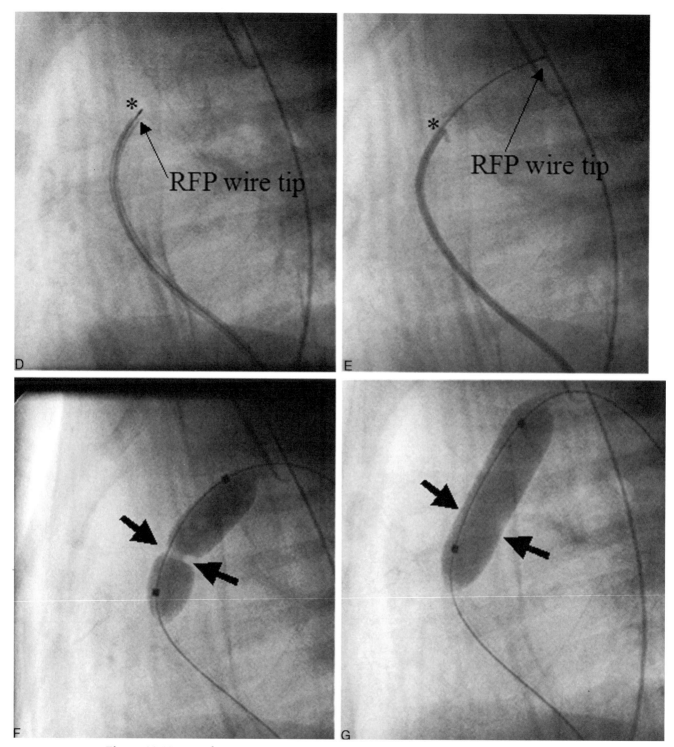

Figure 11-19, cont'd   **D,** The tip of the radio frequency perforation (RFP) wire positioned just below the atretic pulmonary valve plate (*). **E,** The tip of the wire is advanced across the atretic plate after perforation of the valve. **F,** A balloon catheter submaximally inflated across the atretic valve (*arrows*). **G,** The balloon is fully inflated and the waist resolves.

Continued

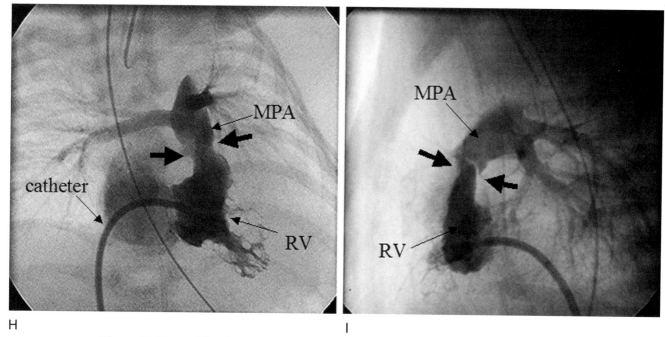

H   I

Figure 11-19, cont'd   H, I, Continuity has been established between the RV and the MPA. The *arrows* mark the pulmonary annulus.

by catheter in order to occlude vascular connections or to surgically created shunts. Gianturco et al. described embolization procedures using stainless steel coils nearly 30 years ago.[11] Since that time, a wide variety of devices and materials have been developed to occlude abnormal connections and to relieve or reduce the hemodynamic burden that they impose.

Patent Ductus Arteriosus

The incidence of an isolated patent ductus arteriosus (PDA) in term infants is estimated at 1 in 2000 live births, accounting for approximately 10% of all congenital heart disease.[1] PDA occurs much more frequently in premature infants (30–40% of premature births). Most commonly, the PDA originates from the proximal descending aorta, just beyond the left subclavian artery, coursing anteriorly and entering the main pulmonary artery superior to the origin of the left pulmonary artery. The hemodynamic sequelae of an isolated PDA are related to the magnitude of the left-to-right shunt across the ductus. The size of the shunt is a function of the diameter of the PDA and the ratio of systemic to pulmonary vascular resistance. As with most left-to-right shunt lesions, newborns have few symptoms because pulmonary vascular resistance remains high right after birth. Declining pulmonary resistance leads to an increased left-to-right shunt, and heart failure develops in the presence of a large PDA. With the exception of premature infants, most patients have a restrictive PDA and are asymptomatic at the time of presentation. The age of presenta-

tion varies from the newborn period through to adulthood. The initial diagnosis is often made when a murmur is noted as an incidental finding upon physical examination.

The rationale for closure of a PDA depends on the size of the ductus in question. Moderate to large PDAs result in significant left-to-right shunting. Over time, this can lead to congestive heart failure, pulmonary hypertension, or both. More commonly, the PDA is not hemodynamically significant. The small PDA carries an increased risk for infective endarteritis and, given the low risk of treatment, should be closed. This recommendation was based primarily on necropsy studies published in the preantibiotic era, although a recently published report suggests that the risk of endarteritis remains significant, particularly in patients not receiving antibiotic prophylaxis.[14] When the PDA is very small, the characteristic continuous murmur is absent. The natural history of these so-called silent PDAs is not well documented and the indications for closure are controversial. Recent studies suggest that the risk of infective endarteritis is not very different from the risk in the general population.

Porstmann and colleagues first described transcatheter occlusion of the PDA in 1971.[10] An Ivalon plug was positioned into the ductus through a large arterial catheter. Since that time, devices and techniques for ductal occlusion have evolved and PDA closure in the catheterization lab has become a well-established method of treatment. There are a variety of

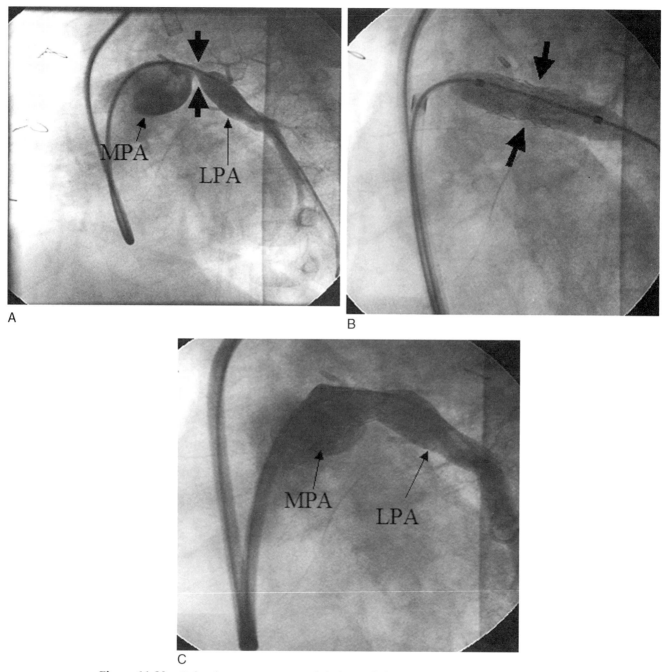

Figure 11-20   Left pulmonary artery stenosis, before and after stent placement. **A,** A lateral projection of a left pulmonary artery (LPA) injection. Severe stenosis of the proximal LPA is shown (diameter = 2 mm). **B,** The stent is deployed using a balloon catheter. **C,** Follow-up injection reveals a significant improvement in the diameter of the proximal LPA.

devices in use today. The most widely used are metallic coils (stainless steel or platinum) interwoven with Dacron fiber to encourage thrombus formation and the Amplatzer device, which is manufactured from nitinol wire and Dacron (an Amplatzer ASD device is shown in Fig. 11-22).[7] To close the PDA, it is usually crossed from the venous (pulmonary artery) side, and the occlusion device is positioned in the ductus.

Angiography is performed to confirm appropriate device placement and effective occlusion of the ductus (Fig. 11-21).

In current practice, occlusion rates should be greater than 96%. Serious complications, which are rare but have been reported, include device embolization, malposition, and persistent hemolysis in association with residual shunting across a partially occluded PDA.

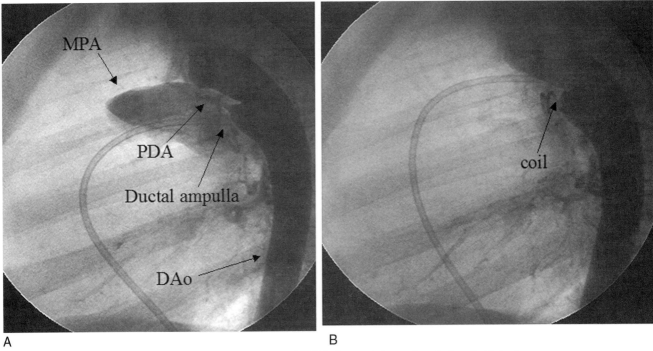

Figure 11-21   Patent ductus arteriosus (PDA) before and after coil occlusion. **A,** A lateral projection revealing a patent ductus arteriosus. Injection into the descending aorta (DAo) reveals left-to-right shunting across the PDA into the MPA. The ductal ampulla is prominent. **B,** Successful occlusion of the PDA with a single coil. No significant residual left-to-right shunting is observed.

Other Embolization Procedures

Coil embolization is also used in a host of other settings.[6,11] Systemic to pulmonary collateral arteries occur in tetralogy of Fallot with pulmonary atresia, transposition of the great arteries, and many cases of univentricular heart disease. These vessels may result in excess hemodynamic burden on the heart (i.e., left-to-right shunt), pulmonary hypertension, or hemoptysis. Most can be occluded with steel or platinum coils. Patients with hemoptysis are usually treated with particle embolization of bronchial arteries.

Atrial Septal Defects

Atrial septal defects (ASDs) are abnormalities characterized by a structural deficiency in the atrial septum. There are several types of ASD, each classified by its proposed embryogenesis and location. The most common ASD is the secundum type, which results from a deficiency or absence of the septum primum. Isolated secundum defects occur in 1 out of every 1500 live births and account for 10% of all congenital heart disease.[1,2] The hemodynamic sequelae are related to the magnitude of the shunt across the atrial septum. The size of the shunt is a function of the diameter of the defect and the relative compliances of the two ventricles. Outside of the newborn period, the right ventricle is more compliant than the left, resulting in a left-to-right shunt across the ASD.

The hemodynamic consequences of atrial defects change with age; in later adulthood, the left ventricle becomes less compliant, and this may result in a dramatic increase in the degree of shunting through a pre-existing ASD.

Although most ASDs are detected by 4 years of age, diagnosis may be delayed until late adulthood. Diagnosis of ASD is usually made in asymptomatic individuals after auscultation of a murmur. Large defects may lead to complaints of fatigue and exercise intolerance in older children, but this is rare. Adults with unrecognized ASD may present with atrial arrhythmias, exercise intolerance, pulmonary hypertension, or paradoxical embolism and stroke. To avoid these complications, it is recommended that all moderate to large ASDs be repaired in childhood regardless of symptoms. Whereas elective surgical repair has negligible mortality (< 1%), the risks associated with open-heart surgery and cardiopulmonary bypass are not trivial. Transcatheter ASD closure has evolved over the past 30 years and is now the method of choice for the closure of most secundum ASDs.[7]

Device occlusion of ASD was first described by King and Mills in 1974.[12] This first device consisted of left and right atrial disks that were opened and fastened together, thereby occluding the defect. Numerous devices have been developed since that time.[7,13-16] Currently, there are two Food and Drug Administration (FDA)–approved devices applicable to ASD (one approved specifically for

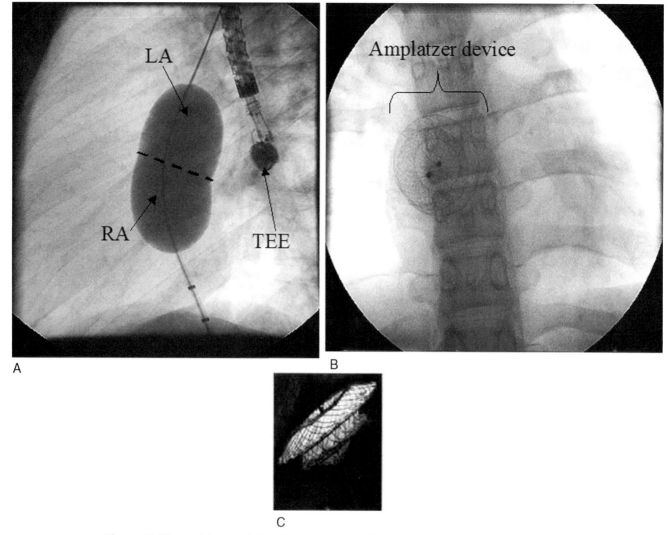

Figure 11-22   Atrial septal defect closure with an Amplatzer device. **A,** A sizing balloon inflated across the atrial septal defect (ASD). The left atrium (LA) is posterior to the right atrium (RA) in the lateral projection. The dashed line marks the stretched diameter of the ASD (approximately 26 mm). A transesophageal echocardiography probe (TEE) is often used to help visualize the ASD during device deployment. **B,** An Amplatzer atrial septal occluder device successfully deployed across the ASD (anterior projection). **C,** The Amplatzer ASD septal occluder itself.

ASD, the other for ventricular defects—see below). Several other devices are in various phases of clinical trials in the United States and have been approved in Europe.

The Amplatzer septal occluder (ASO) is the only device with FDA approval for the indication of ASD closure. The ASO is constructed from a fine mesh of the nickel titanium alloy nitinol.[7] Nitinol is a super-elastic metal with memory. Thus, the device can be collapsed into a catheter and, when extruded, will reassume its pre-formed shape. In the Amplatzer device, the nitinol is woven into a shape with two atrial disks and a central waist. There are woven Dacron disks inside the nitinol frame to promote occlusion of the defect (Fig. 11-22C).

ASD devices are delivered antegrade by femoral venous access. The left atrial disk is delivered first, followed by the right atrial disk. The ASO differs from other devices in that it occludes the ASD by filling the defect with the central waist of the device rather than by sandwiching the defect between two disks.

Studies have demonstrated that endothelialization of the device is complete 3–6 months after implantation.[7] Intermediate follow-up studies have shown complete closure rates of 93–98% at 1 year. Most residual leaks have been too small to be significant. Reported complication rates are on the order of 10%. Although most of these complications have been minor, major reported complications have included device displacement, complete heart block, atrial arrhythmias, deep venous thrombosis, air embolus, and stroke. Several studies comparing device closure to surgery have demonstrated that the techniques are of comparable efficacy with no difference in the frequency of major complications but with a higher rate of minor complications after surgery.[7] It should be emphasized that not all ASDs are amenable to device closure; defects that are too large or that lack an adequate rim of atrial septum may require surgery. Figure 11-22B shows an example of transcatheter ASD occlusion using the Amplatzer device.

Patent Foramen Ovale

Autopsy series have revealed that a patent foramen ovale (PFO) persists in 20–30% of adults.[1,2] In most cases, this is a normal anatomic variant without associated symptoms. Several studies have implicated paradoxical embolism across a PFO as a cause of unexplained strokes and transient ischemic attacks. Because the prevalence of PFO is so high in the normal population, the presence of a PFO in an individual who has sustained an unexplained embolic stroke is by no means proof that the PFO played a role in the event. An extensive evaluation must be undertaken in these cases, including thorough neurologic evaluation studies, to rule out prothrombotic conditions, and contrast echocardiography. Several trials comparing device closure of PFOs after a presumed paradoxical embolus with either antiplatelet or anticoagulant therapy are ongoing. There is general agreement that when neurologic events are recurrent despite antiplatelet or anticoagulation therapy, or when patients are not candidates for medical therapy, transcatheter PFO closure is appropriate. The techniques employed for PFO closure are similar to those for atrial septal defects; the devices are slightly different because a PFO is often more of a tunnel than a hole.

Ventricular Septal Defects

Ventricular septal defects (VSDs) represent approximately 30% of all congenital heart disease.[1,2] As is the case with atrial defects, there are several types of VSD.

In general, transcatheter VSD closure is a more complicated procedure than ASD closure. The right ventricular septum has deep trabeculations that make the VSD difficult to cross from a venous approach. Additionally, device encroachment on vital conduction and valve tissue could lead to severe complications (i.e., heart block, arrhythmia, or valvar regurgitation). For this reason, most of the early transcatheter VSD interventions focused on defects in the muscular portion of the ventricular septum, remote from valves and conduction system.

Lock and colleagues first described muscular VSD closure with the Rashkind double-umbrella PDA occluder in 1988.[13] Numerous studies with different devices have been published since that time. The reported rate of technical success varies, ranging from 72% to 95%. Complete defect occlusion ranges from 17% to 95%.[7,18,19] Several devices are in clinical trials in the USA and have been approved in Europe. The CardioSEAL (*see* Fig. 11-23) is the only device currently approved by the FDA.

Transcatheter closure of conoventricular (i.e., perimembranous) VSDs has recently been reported using the Amplatzer membranous VSD occluder (*see* Fig. 11-23). This unique device is designed to occlude defects in the membranous ventricular septum without interfering with the aortic valve. Early results have shown technical success in 95% of patients.[7] Currently, the device is under trial in the United States and is approved for use in Europe.

In summary, transcatheter closure of ventricular septal defects can be considered standard therapy for many muscular defects and is likely to become routine for many patients with membranous VSD in the near future.

MAJOR POINTS

- Cardiac catheterization remains the gold standard for assessment of intracardiac and intravascular anatomy and hemodynamics. Anatomic data are obtained by angiography and hemodynamics are determined by measuring pressures, oxygen saturations, and cardiac output.
- Pressure measurements are made with fluid-filled catheters attached to a transducer and are reported in millimeters of mercury (mmHg). Values from the intracardiac chambers and great vessels are evaluated in combination to assess function and to identify gradients. Table 11-2 shows the range of normal pressure values in children.
- Cardiac output is defined as the product of stroke volume and heart rate (CO = SV × HR). Because of the wide range in patient sizes encountered in pediatrics, the cardiac output is indexed to body surface area (BSA) and reported as the cardiac index (CI = CO / BSA). Normal values for cardiac index are 3–5 L/min/m^2.
- The cardiac index is typically calculated in the catheterization laboratory using one of the modified indicator dilution techniques. The Fick method uses oxygen as the indicator and the thermodilution method uses temperature.
- Pulmonary and systemic vascular resistances (R) are calculated using Ohm's law (R = ΔP / Q). Normal values for systemic vascular resistance (SVR) range from 15–30 Wood units. The normal values for pulmonary vascular resistance (PVR) are 2–4 Wood units.

Continued

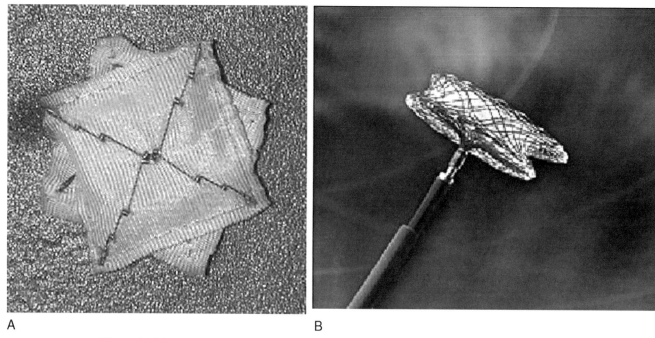

A   B

Figure 11-23   Ventricular septal defect (VSD) closure devices. **A,** An example of the CardioSEAL device used for the transcatheter closure of muscular VSDs. **B,** An artist's rendering of an Amplatzer membranous VSD occluder. This device is used to close defects in the conoventricular septum without interfering with the aortic valve.

MAJOR POINTS—CONT'D

- Angiography is used to define anatomy in the catheterization laboratory. Contrast agents based on iodine are used to opacify structures of interest. Potential side effects of the contrast agents include allergic reaction, nephrotoxicity, coronary vasodilation, decreased myocardial contractility, arrhythmia, pulmonary hypertension, and pulmonary edema.
- In 1966, William Rashkind reported the balloon atrial septostomy procedure for transposition of the great arteries, heralding the beginning of the era of pediatric interventional cardiology.
- Interventional procedures can be divided into two general categories: (1) interventions designed to create or enlarge communications and (2) closure procedures. Table 11-3 shows the spectrum of procedures in children.
- Balloon catheters are used to enlarge or to dilate stenotic cardiac and vascular structures. Expandable stents are used to prevent vessel recoil and restenosis after balloon dilation.
- Vascular occlusion procedures are performed in a host of different settings (e.g., patent ductus arteriosus, systemic to pulmonary collaterals, and surgically created shunts) to reduce the excess hemodynamic burden on the heart. Catheter embolization is usually accomplished with metal coils, microparticles, or both.

- The Amplatzer septal occluder is the only device with FDA approval for the indication of atrial septal defect closure. Several other devices are in various phases of clinical trial in the United States and have been approved for use in Europe.
- Transcatheter closure of muscular ventricular septal defect is well described. The Amplatzer membranous VSD occluder is currently under trial in the United States and has been approved for use in Europe. Early results are promising.

REFERENCES

1. Allen HD, Gutgesell HP, Clark EB, Driscoll DJ: Moss and Adam's Heart Disease in Infants, Children, and Adolescents: Including the Fetus and Young Adult, 6th ed. Philadelphia: Lippincott Williams & Wilkins, 2001.

2. Baim DS, Grossman W: Grossman's Cardiac Catheterization, Angiography, and Intervention, 6th ed. Philadelphia: Lippincott Williams & Wilkins, 2000.

3. Rashkind WJ, Miller WW: Transposition of the great arteries: Results of palliation by balloon atrioseptostomy in thirty-one infants. Circulation 38:453–457, 1968.

4. Mckrindle BW, Kan JS: Long-term results after balloon pulmonary valvuloplasty. Circulation 83:1915–1922, 1991.

5. Lock JE, Keane JF, Perry SB: Diagnostic and Interventional Cardiac Catheterization in Congenital Heart Disease, 2nd ed. Boston: Kluwer, 2000.

6. Mendelsohn AM, Shim D: Inroads in transcatheter therapy for congenital heart disease. J Pediatr 133(3):324-333, 1998.

7. Rao, PS: Summary and comparison of patent ductus arteriosus closure devices. Curr Interv Cardiol Rep 3:268-274, 2001.

8. Rao PS: Interventional cardiology: State of the art and future directions. Pediatr Cardiol 19:107-124, 1998.

9. Mendelsohn AM, Lloyd TR, Crowley DC, et al: Late follow-up of balloon angioplasty in children with native coarctation of the aorta. Am J Cardiol 74:696-700, 1994.

10. Rao, PS: Summary and comparison of patent ductus arteriosus closure devices. Curr Interv Cardiol Rep 3:268-274, 2001.

11. Rothman A: Pediatric cardiovascular embolization therapy. Pediatr Cardiol 19:74-84, 1998.

12. King TD, Mills NL: Nonoperative closure of atrial septal defects. Surgery 75:383-388, 1974.

13. Hijazi ZM, Cao QL, Patel HT, et al: Transcatheter closure of secundum atrial septal defects using the Amplatzer septal occluder: Results of Phase II US multicenter clinical trial. Circulation 100(Suppl I):804, 1999.

14. Latson LA: Per-catheter ASD closure. Pediatr Cardiol 19:86-93, 1998.

15. Rome JJ, Keane JF, Perry SB, et al: Double-umbrella closure of atrial septal defects: Initial clinical applications. Circulation 82:751-758, 1990.

16. Thanopoulos BD, Laskari CV, Tsaousis GS, et al: Closure of atrial septal defects with the Amplatzer occlusion device: Preliminary results. L Am Coll Cardiol 31:1110-1116, 1998.

17. Lock JE, Block PC, McKay RG, et al: Transcatheter closure of ventricular septal defects. Circulation 78:361-368, 1988.

18. Hijazi ZM, Hakim F, Haweleh AA, et al: Catheter closure of perimembranous ventricular septal defects using the new Amplatzer membranous VSD occluder: Initial clinical experience. Cathet Cardiovasc Interv 56(4):508-515, 2002.

19. Tofeig M, Patel RG, Walsh KP: Transcatheter closure of a mid-muscular ventricular septal defect with an Amplatzer VSD occlusion device. Heart 81:438-440, 1999.

20. Lock JE, Rome JJ, Davis R, et al: Transcatheter closure of atrial septal defects: Experimental studies. Circulation 79:1091-1099, 1989.

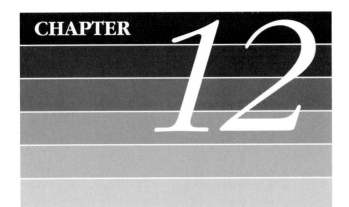
Fetal Cardiovascular Disease

JACK RYCHIK

Ultrasonic technologies have developed such that tiny structures only millimeters in size can be visualized and evaluated at relatively great distances from the ultrasound emitting source. This technology has been applied to the evaluation of the cardiovascular system of the developing human fetus and is called fetal echocardiography. Fetal echocardiography can provide detailed information about the cardiovascular system, and precise and reliable diagnosis of complex congenital heart disease can be made prior to birth. In addition, fetal echocardiography provides insight into the pathophysiology of complex disease processes that can affect the developing cardiovascular system.

The ability to peer into the womb and observe the growing fetus has furthered our understanding of human development and has significantly impacted on our management strategies for treatment of congenital heart disease. Although conventional diagnosis of congenital heart disease has taken place after birth in infancy and childhood, this arbitrary point in time is falling to the wayside as more and more patients are identified prior to birth in the third and second trimesters of gestation. In this chapter, we review the physiology of the developing fetal cardiovascular system and the basic tenets of the fetal echocardiographic evaluation, and we explore a variety of disease processes that affect the fetal cardiovascular system.

WHY PERFORM FETAL ECHOCARDIOGRAPHY?

The first ultrasonic images of the human fetal heart were generated over 25 years ago.[1] Ultrasound energy travels best in a fluid medium; hence, utilization of this technology for observation of the growing fetus in the naturally fluid-filled amniotic environment is logical. Approximately 80% of pregnant women in the United States currently undergo some form of fetal ultrasonic evaluation for gender discernment, gestational count (i.e., twins or triplets), or evaluation of a disease processes or congenital anomaly.

The most common type of congenital anomaly in the human species is congenital heart disease. It occurs in approximately 8 per 1000 live births and in approximately 10–12 per 1000 pregnancies. The incidence is somewhat lower in live births than it is in pregnancy because some fetuses undergo demise during gestation, oftentimes in relation to associated genetic or chromosomal abnormalities that limit viability. However, the majority of fetuses with congenital heart disease present without associated abnormalities (genetic, chromosomal, or extracardiac).

Is ultrasound scanning of the fetus helpful in diagnosing congenital heart disease? The answer depends upon the way in which the fetal echocardiographic evaluation is performed. In a landmark study by Ewigman et al.,[2] over 15,000 pregnant women underwent routine prenatal ultrasound evaluation. The investigators found very little impact on perinatal outcome and concluded that routine ultrasound scanning was not helpful. Of note, the cardiac examination consisted of only a "four-chamber view." In other words, if the operator could count the presence of four chambers of the heart, then the fetus was considered to have a normal cardiovascular system. Buskens et al.[3]

reported on the ultrasonic evaluation of nearly 7000 pregnant women, performing the four-chamber view alone and compared the fetal examination findings to the postnatal echocardiogram. They reported only 4.5% sensitivity for detection of congenital heart disease, a very low number. Using a different approach to imaging, Stumpflen et al.[4] reported on data from a single center in which over 3000 women were scanned. The operators were all trained to perform a more detailed fetal examination, consisting of the four-chamber view as well as identification of the right and left outflow tracts and the use of pulse-wave Doppler and color Doppler flow imaging. In their series, sensitivity and specificity for the detection of congenital heart disease was 86% and 100%, respectively, a marked improvement over the previous reports.

These studies highlight the fact that methodology and technique used in performing fetal echocardiography are essential in defining its utility. Proper technique, training, equipment, and fund of knowledge all contribute to the very effective diagnostic yield of fetal echocardiography as it currently exists today.

Let us assume that a skilled examination provides for a complete and accurate prenatal diagnosis. Does a correct fetal diagnosis of congenital heart disease impact upon outcome? This question is yet to be definitively answered. Intuitively, one would predict that identification of congenital heart disease prior to birth would provide some benefit to the newborn infant. However, in the current era of rapid neonatal diagnosis, efficient interhospital transport, and excellent surgical results, differences in early outcome between prenatally and postnatally diagnosed infants have not been uniformly seen.[5] However, some centers have begun to report differences in outcome, in particular for complex lesions. Tworetzky et al.[6] at the University of California, San Francisco, found improved survival for first stage palliation of hypoplastic left heart syndrome in prenatally diagnosed infants when compared to infants diagnosed after birth. An important contributing factor to overall improvement may be the better physiological state of prenatally diagnosed infants. Verheijen et al.[7] reported on a multicenter study in which comparison was made of the metabolic state of infants with and without prenatal diagnosis of congenital heart disease. They found that prenatal diagnosis improved infant blood pH and lactate levels to a significant degree.

There are many potential benefits to the prenatal diagnosis of congenital heart disease (Box 12-1). First is the importance of dissemination of knowledge and information. We live in an era in which information is a critical commodity. Parents are strongly desirous of any and all information concerning their unborn child, as witnessed by the current interest in "fetal photography" and the rendering of facial images of the fetus, both of which are now commercially available. Knowledge of the pres-

---

Box 12-1 Potential Benefits of Prenatal Diagnosis of Congenital Heart Disease

- Information and parental education
- Parental counseling with choice of termination
- Psychological and social preparation
- Choice of site for care
- Stable transition from pre- to postnatal life
- Reduction in acidosis
- Improved surgical survival
- Improved neurological outcome (?)
- Long-term benefits (?)
- Cost-effectiveness (?)

---

ence of a fetus with congenital heart disease allows the family to prepare psychologically for the rigors of care for an infant with a birth defect. Parents have the opportunity to spend time learning about the anomaly, its management, and its lifelong ramifications. Families can meet with physicians and nurses to discuss and develop a treatment strategy and can tour facilities such as the delivery suites and the intensive care unit. Prior knowledge of a congenital heart defect allows for a family to investigate and choose a site for delivery and care, one that is comfortable and experienced in the management of these patients. Alternatively, some families may choose to terminate a pregnancy after identification of congenital heart disease. Knowledgeable, compassionate, and nondirected counseling must accompany the revelation of the diagnosis. Emotional support should be available to families as they move through this decision process. Physicians and nurses offering such counseling must be fully aware of the latest strategies and outcomes for congenital heart disease so that families can make educated and informed decisions.

Of great promise is the possibility that prenatally diagnosed infants with congenital heart disease will do better in the long term than those diagnosed after birth. Much investigational focus is currently aimed at neurological outcome after repair of congenital heart disease. Studies have demonstrated impaired neurocognitive outcome and deficits in school performance in some children after surgical repair of congenital heart disease.[8] Perhaps prenatal diagnosis will have a positive impact on these long-term neurocognitive parameters since the occurrence of hypotension, hemodynamic instability, and acidosis in the early neonatal period should be minimized. Prenatal diagnosis may also prove to be cost-effective in both the short- and long-term if hospital outcome is improved and late complications are minimized.[9]

As a consequence of the increasing number of fetal echocardiograms performed, standards of practice are shifting. In a recent review of newborns with complex congenital heart disease admitted to the Cardiac Intensive Care Unit at The Children's Hospital of Philadelphia, more than half were diagnosed prenatally. The impact of this changing trend on overall outcome is of great interest and will be the subject of much study in the years to come.

UNIQUENESS OF THE FETAL CARDIOVASCULAR SYSTEM

The fetal cardiovascular system differs from the mature, adult system in many ways. First, the structural elements of the fetal myocardium are unique. Early fetal myocytes can undergo replication with development of hyperplasia, or an increase in cell number, whereas mature adult myocytes undergo hypertrophy, or increase in cell size. Second, the fetal heart is much stiffer than the adult heart, with impaired relaxation properties relative to the adult. The fetal myocardium is made up of approximately 60% noncontractile elements vs. 30% in the adult heart.[10] In addition, the uptake of calcium through the sarcoplasmic reticulum differs in the fetus from the adult.[11] In the fetus, the notion of ventricular "constraint" arising from a compressed chest wall, lungs, and pericardium limits ventricular preload, which is relieved with the first few breaths after birth.[12]

The fetal circulation is quite unique. Unlike after birth, in which the pulmonary and systemic circulations are in series (deoxygenated blood is pumped by the right side into the lungs, returns as oxygenated blood to the left side, and is pumped out to the body), the fetal right and left flows are in parallel, with oxygenation taking place at a site external to the fetus, the placenta (Fig. 12-1). A variety of structures such as the ductus venosus, the patent foramen ovale, and the ductus arteriosus provide for unique blood flow pathways specific to the fetus.

The fetal circulation is designed in a manner adaptive to the fetus' needs. The placenta is a richly vascularized organ and is of extremely low vascular resistance. The two fetal iliac arteries originating from the descending aorta give rise to the two umbilical arteries, which exit the fetus and travel toward the placenta. The umbilical arteries carry an admixture of deoxygenated arterial blood toward the oxygenating organ, the placenta. A single venous structure, the umbilical vein, carries richly oxygenated blood back to the fetus through the umbilical cord. The umbilical vein inserts into the ductus venosus, a structure that traverses the liver and connects into the inferior vena cava just as it enters the right atrium. The angle with which the ductus venosus inserts into the inferior vena cava/right atrial junction is such that the stream of flow is directed toward the foramen ovale and into the left atrium and left ventricle. In this manner, the most richly oxygenated blood returning from the placenta is directed toward the developing organs most in need of oxygen delivery—the myocardial and cerebral circulations—both of which are perfused by the left ventricle. Similarly, the most deoxygenated blood in the fetus drains from the superior vena cava and is directed toward the tricuspid valve. This column of blood is then ejected by the right ventricle into the main pulmonary artery. The pulmonary vasculature is of very high resistance during prenatal life; hence, little flow enters the pulmonary circulation and the majority of flow is directed toward the ductus arteriosus, the descending aorta, and the umbilical arteries. The fetal cardiovascular architecture is designed to maximize delivery of oxygenated blood to the organs in greatest need and to deliver the most deoxygenated blood in the most direct manner possible to the placenta.

FETAL ECHOCARDIOGRAPHY: IN WHOM, WHEN, AND HOW?

High-quality fetal cardiovascular imaging is being performed with increasing frequency. From 1998 to 2004, fetal echocardiograms performed at The Children's Hospital of Philadelphia have more than tripled in number, with over 1400 studies currently performed annually.

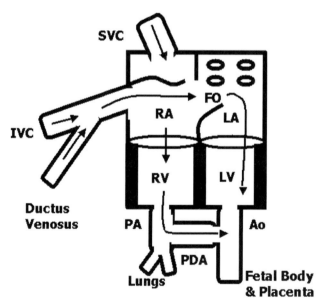

Figure 12-1   Schematic drawing of the fetal circulation. Ductus venosus flow (highly oxygenated) is channeled right to left across the foramen ovale (FO) and into the left atrium (LA) and left ventricle (LV). This blood is then delivered to the upper portion of the body. Superior vena caval (SVC) flow (highly deoxygenated) is directed toward the tricuspid valve and right ventricle (RV) and is ejected across the ductus arteriosus (PDA) to the lower part of the body. *IVC,* Inferior vena cava; *PA,* pulmonary artery.

Whereas many pediatric cardiologists have taken up an interest in developing the skills necessary to perform fetal echocardiography, maternal-fetal medicine specialists, perinatologists, and ultrasound radiologists have also mastered these skills and may perform high-quality scanning. Guidelines for performance of fetal echocardiography were recently established by the Pediatric Council of the American Society of Echocardiography.[13]

Indications for performing a fetal echocardiogram can be divided into maternal and fetal indications (Box 12-2). A family history of congenital heart disease is a common indication for referral for fetal echocardiography. Maternal diabetes mellitus is a risk factor for congenital heart disease and should prompt examination. In addition, diabetes can cause an increase in fetal ventricular wall thickness, which can deleteriously affect ventricular function after birth. Maternal exposure to a teratogen or maternal infection with rubella may increase the likelihood of fetal heart disease. Maternal autoimmune diseases such as lupus erythematosus or Sjögren's syndrome (SS) can lead to diseases of the fetal conduction system or the development of fetal cardiomyopathy.[14] Often, identification of fetal heart block may be the heralding sign of maternal autoimmune disease in an otherwise healthy, asymptomatic mother who may be positive for Sjögren's syndrome A (SS-A) or Sjögren's syndrome B (SS-B) antibodies. Recent data confirms an increased incidence of congenital anomalies in fetuses conceived by in vitro fertilization techniques[15,16]; hence, all such women should have careful fetal echocardiography performed.

Box 12-2 Indications for Performance of the Fetal Echocardiogram

MATERNAL INDICATIONS

- Family history of CHD
- Heritable disorders (e.g., Marfan syndrome)
- Metabolic disorders (e.g., diabetes or phenylketonuria)
- Teratogen exposure (e.g., lithium)
- Rubella infection
- Maternal autoimmune disease (e.g., lupus or Sjögren's)
- In vitro fertilization
- Advanced maternal age (> 40 yrs) (?)

FETAL INDICATIONS

- Aneuploidy
- Extracardiac abnormality
- Fetal heart beat irregularity
- Fetal hydrops
- Increased nuchal translucency (first trimester)
- Abnormal obstetrical ultrasound screen

Fetal indications include the presence of aneuploidy (e.g., trisomies 13, 18, or 21) or extracardiac anomalies (e.g., diaphragmatic hernia or teratoma). The presence of fetal hydrops should precipitate an investigation of possible cardiac causes through fetal echocardiography. Fetal heartbeat irregularity or suspicion of a structural abnormality on routine obstetrical screening should lead to a more detailed and comprehensive fetal echocardiogram. Recently, great interest has been generated in the use of first-trimester (at 10–13 weeks' gestation) imaging of the posterior aspect of the fetal neck, looking at nuchal translucency. Normally, a small clear space can be seen in this region, with standard normative measures established. However, fetuses with increased nuchal translucency have a significantly increased incidence of aneuploidy or of congenital heart disease alone, even in the absence of aneuploidy.[17] Some investigators have predicted that increased nuchal translucency may yet become the most reliable predictor of the presence of congenital heart disease. There is no question that current practice should include referral for fetal echocardiography at the second trimester if first trimester nuchal translucency examination is performed and is noted to be increased.

The optimal timing for performance of a fetal echocardiogram is at approximately 18–20 weeks' gestation. The earliest four-chamber view can be obtained at approximately 14 weeks; however, visualizing the outflow tracts at this age can be difficult. Often, image resolution and acoustic window diminishes after 34 weeks when the amniotic fluid-to-infant mass ratio decreases. Transvaginal fetal echocardiography using specially designed equipment can be performed at 10–12 weeks with good visualization of cardiac chambers; however, views are limited due to restrictions in mobility of the transducer and an inability to optimize scanning angles.[18]

As lesions and disease processes are dynamic in the growing fetus, identification of congenital heart disease or other disorders of the cardiovascular system requires repeat, serial fetal echocardiographic evaluation. It is our current practice to monitor fetuses with congenital heart disease with echocardiographic scans every 4–6 weeks to observe for any developmental progression (e.g., worsening of valvar stenosis) or physiological changes (e.g., ventricular dysfunction or atrioventricular valve insufficiency) that may occur. Many fetuses with arrhythmia, hydrops, or progressive disease processes or those undergoing treatment require more frequent surveillance, as necessary.

Specific instrumentation (beyond general obstetrical ultrasound) is necessary in order to perform fetal echocardiography. Fetal imaging is carried out using ultrasound frequencies of 3–7 MHz. Echocardiographic modalities of two-dimensional Doppler, pulsed Doppler, continuous wave Doppler, and color Doppler flow imaging should all be available. Unlike for general obstetrical ultrasound, still-frame storage of images is inadequate for analysis of the fetal cardiovascular system. Because the heart is a dynamic structure undergoing continuous change in a spacial-temporal manner, images must be stored and reviewed in motion. Videotape storage or digital media are currently available and provide excellent quality for review and analysis.

Standardized imaging views have been suggested and are illustrated in Figure 12-2. These views provide for a comprehensive assessment of the fetal cardiovascular system.

EVALUATING THE HEALTH OF THE FETAL CARDIOVASCULAR SYSTEM: ANALYSIS OF DOPPLER FLOW PATTERNS

Fetal echocardiography allows for evaluation of structural and functional abnormalities of the heart. One simple measure of cardiac status is determining the heart size. Fetal cardiomegaly is assessed by comparing the measured cross-sectional area of the heart relative to the cross-sectional area of the chest wall (Fig. 12-3). The cardiothoracic area ratio should be <0.33, or, upon visual inspection, one should normally be able to fit three hearts in the chest.

Application of Doppler techniques to various sites with the cardiovascular system allows for an understanding of physiological processes. Normal patterns of blood flow at these sites have been established; deviations from these normal patterns suggest pathology. Derangements of the fetal cardiovascular system commonly result in an alteration of ventricular compliance and stiffness of the ventricles with elevation in atrial filling pressures, reflected as impediment to forward flow or reversal of direction of flow in the venous system. Analyses of these patterns of flow offer a deeper understanding of the derangement at hand.

The following are common cardiovascular sites interrogated and analyzed with Doppler echocardiography in the fetus:

- Atrioventricular valves: There are normally two peaks of flow across the tricuspid or mitral valve, representing (1) early passive diastolic filling with opening of the valve and (2) active diastolic filling in relation to atrial contraction. In the fetus, the second wave (i.e., the atrial contraction) is normally of higher velocity (Fig. 12-4). When ventricular compliance is altered, fusion of the two beats can occur.
- Inferior vena cava: Flow is normally phasic, with a small amount of reversal (Fig. 12-5). Altered right ventricular compliance, restriction to flow, or ventricular dysfunction results in increased reversal.
- Ductus venosus: Flow is normally phasic and all forward with no reversal (Fig. 12-6). The presence of reversal suggests elevated right atrial pressure.

- Umbilical artery: Pulsatile flow with a systolic and diastolic phase is noted in each of the two umbilical arteries. Assessment of umbilical arterial flow provides important information on the health of the placenta. The placenta is an organ of very low vascular resistance, so there should be a large amount of diastolic flow present in the umbilical artery. Diminished diastolic flow reflects elevated placental resistance and is seen in a variety of diseases including infection, fetal intrauterine growth retardation, maternal preeclampsia, or the twin–twin transfusion syndrome. Placental vascular resistance can be measured by analyzing umbilical arterial flow and calculating the pulsatility index, which equals (systolic velocity – diastolic velocity) / time-velocity integral, or area under the Doppler spectral curve (Fig. 12-7).
- Umbilical vein: Continuous low-velocity, non-pulsatile flow is expected in the normal umbilical vein (see Fig. 12-7).

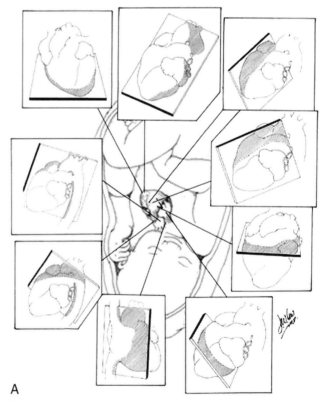

A

Figure 12-2 Tomographic views used for imaging of the fetal heart. Nine standardized views have been established. *Ao,* Aorta; *IVC,* inferior vena cava; *LA,* left atrium; *LV,* left ventricle; *MV,* mitral valve; *PA,* pulmonary artery; *RA,* right atrium; *RV,* right ventricle; *SVC,* superior vena cava. (Reprinted from J Am Soc Echocardiogr 17: Rychik, Ayres, Cuneo, et al, American Society of Echocardiography guidelines and standards for performance of the fetal echocardiogram, pp. 803–810. © 2004, with permission from the American Society of Echocardiography.)

Continued

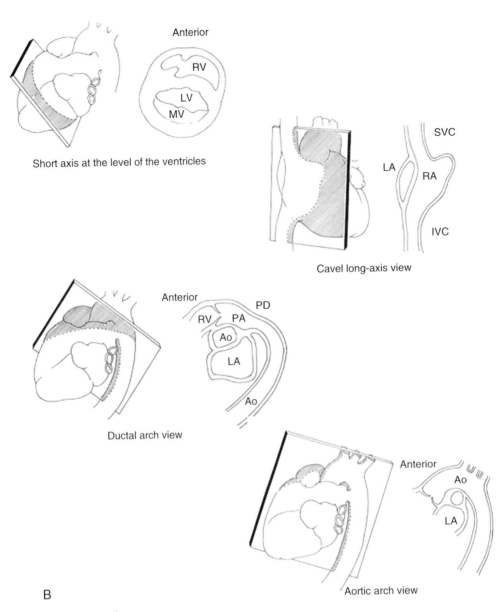

B

Figure 12-2, cont'd

FETAL CARDIOVASCULAR DISEASE: CONGENITAL HEART ANOMALIES

Simple and complex forms of congenital heart disease can be discerned by fetal echocardiography. Examples are shown in Figures 12-8 through 12-16.

Structural abnormalities of the heart rarely result in any disturbance of fetal well-being; hence, nearly all will make it to term without hydrops or heart failure. Marked hypoplasia of the right or left ventricle, or even severe outflow tract obstructions, are of little hemodynamic consequence since (1) the placenta, not the fetal lungs, provide for oxygenation, and (2) fetal structures such as

the ductus arteriosus and the foramen ovale allow for bypass of maldeveloped structures and maintenance of flow. In cases of right heart maldevelopment, flow crosses the foramen from right to left and the left ventricle can provide for fetal perfusion. Similarly, if the left ventricle is maldeveloped, flow crosses the foramen from left to right and enters the right ventricle, which can then perfuse the fetal body through the patent ductus arteriosus. Exceptions to this principle include fetuses with (1) genetic or chromosomal abnormalities, (2) hemodynamically significant atrioventricular valve regurgitation, or (3) ventricular dysfunction or myocardial (pump) failure.

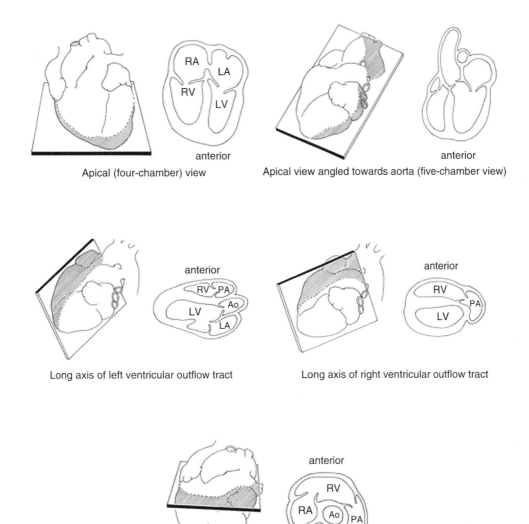

anterior
Apical (four-chamber) view

anterior
Apical view angled towards aorta (five-chamber view)

anterior

Long axis of left ventricular outflow tract

anterior

Long axis of right ventricular outflow tract

anterior

C

Short axis at the level of the great vessels

Figure 12-2, cont'd

Progression of congenital heart disease has been identified in the fetus. For example, pulmonary stenosis with a patent pulmonary valve identified at 18 weeks gestation can progress to pulmonary atresia with subsequent right ventricular hypoplasia in some cases.[19] Dramatic changes with progression in left sided anomalies have also been reported. For example, aortic stenosis with a dilated, poorly functional left ventricle at 16 weeks may undergo arrest of left ventricular development with manifestation of hypoplastic left heart at birth. Identifying precisely who will progress from simple lesion A to more complex lesion B cannot yet reliably be done. Nonetheless, techniques are being developed to allow for prenatal intervention in order to improve flow characteristics in the fetal heart and to potentially prevent progression of disease. Recently, investigators reported on the experience with performance of balloon valvuloplasty in the

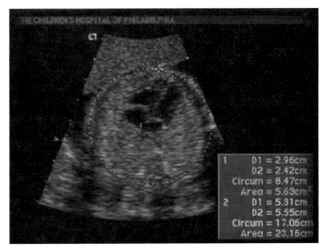

Figure 12-3   Cardiac area and thoracic area ratio measurement. This ratio should normally be <0.33.

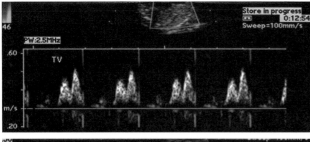

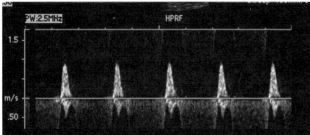

Figure 12-4   Doppler spectral display of the tricuspid inflow pattern. Top panel is the normal flow pattern expected, with a double peak. The bottom panel is from a fetus with an abnormally hypertrophied heart and displays a Doppler tricuspid inflow pattern with a single peak.

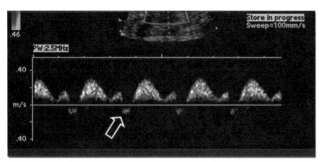

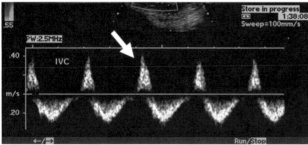

Figure 12-5   Inferior vena cava flow. Top panel is a Doppler spectral display from a normal fetus with a small amount of flow reversal *(open arrow)*. Bottom panel is from a fetus with poor right ventricle compliance and demonstrates an increased degree of flow reversal *(closed arrow)*.

fetus with aortic stenosis in the hopes of preventing development of left ventricular hypoplasia.[20] Although the technique itself appeared to be a success in some, a number of fetuses continued toward the pathway of developing left ventricular hypoplasia. This exciting avenue of investigation is still in its infancy but promises to open a whole new arena for the potential preemptive treatment of congenital heart disease.

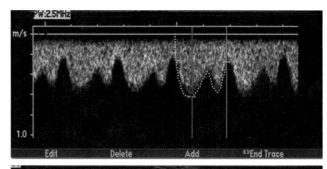

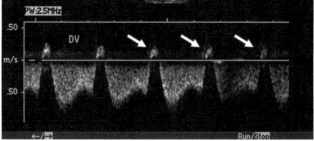

Figure 12-6   Ductus venosus flow. Top panel is the normal flow pattern with continuous forward flow. The bottom panel demonstrates some reversal of flow *(arrows)*, suggesting a stiff abnormal heart.

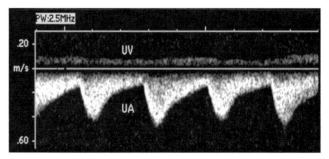

Figure 12-7   Doppler sample obtained from the umbilical cord. Both the umbilical artery (UA) and the umbilical vein (UV) flow patterns are displayed. Note the pulsatile systolic and diastolic components to the UA flow *(arrow)*, while UV flow is continuous, nonpulsatile, and of low velocity.

RHYTHM DISTURBANCES IN THE FETUS

Electrocardiography (ECG) is difficult, but not impossible, to perform in the fetus. Fetal ECG signals are weak due to the distance to the maternal abdominal surface as well as interference from maternal signal. Computer processing algorithms can provide for impressions of fetal electrical activity; however, reliable fetal ECG monitoring is still clinically unavailable. Alternatively, fetal arrhythmia can be diagnosed by observation of the mechanical sequelae of electrical activity, namely motion of the cardiac structures and blood flow patterns studied through fetal echocardiography.

Fetal heart rates normally range from 120 to 180 beats per minute (bpm) with synchronous atrial and ventricular contraction. Transient increase in heart rate can

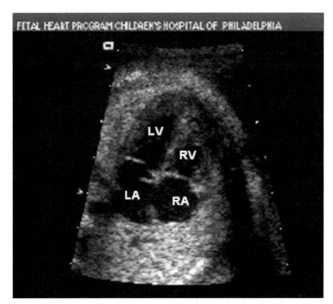

Figure 12-8   Normal four-chamber view of the fetal heart. *LA,* Left atrium; *LV,* left ventricle; *RA,* right atrium; *RV,* right ventricle.

be seen during fetal activity, whereas transient fetal bradycardia can be noted during maternal abdominal compression with temporary cord compression.

Premature atrial contractions are the most common arrhythmia seen in the fetus. As seen on fetal echocardiography, these are typically due to a floppy atrial septum touching the back of the atrium during the various phases of the cardiac cycle. Maternal nicotine use and placental insufficiency may also be the cause. These are benign and typically resolve after birth.

Maternal autoimmune disease resulting in SS-A or SS-B antibodies can result in fetal conduction system abnormalities, namely development of compete heart block.[14] Early signs of heart block such as first or second degree can be discerned on fetal echocardiography by measuring the time intervals between onset of flow across the mitral valve in conjunction with atrial contraction (i.e., a wave) and onset of flow across the aortic valve. This interval is called the mechanical PR interval and can provide information about the delay in conduction at the atrioventricular node.[21] This time interval should be less than 130 milliseconds in the fetus. Treatment regimens with steroids have improved the outcome for the fetus with maternal autoimmune-derived complete heart block.

In the fetus, rapid heart rates seem to be well tolerated for relatively long periods of time, even days. These rapid heart arrhythmias may include supraventricular tachycardia (SVT) (rates of 220–280 bpm) or atrial flutter, with rapid conduction (may be >300 bpm). SVT is distinguished from atrial flutter in the fetus by identifying a 1:1 ratio of motion of the atria and ventricles on fetal echocardiography. Ultimately, elevated heart rates may impair ventricular filling, resulting in diminished cardiac output. Alternatively, myocardial dysfunction can occur after prolonged periods of tachyarrhythmia, resulting in impaired perfusion and hydrops. Treatment with transplacental therapy such as maternal administration of digoxin, amiodarone, or sotalol can be effective in most cases.[22] Often, direct administration to the fetus is necessary through umbilical vein puncture or intramuscular injection into the

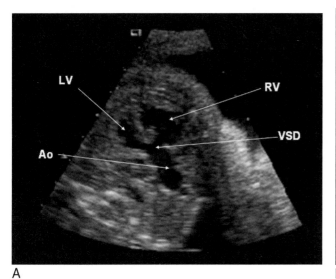

A

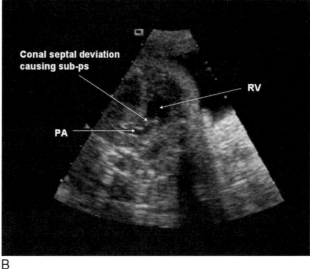

B

Figure 12-9   Fetal heart with tetralogy of Fallot. **A,** Fetal heart with a large ventricular septal defect (VSD) and large overriding aorta (Ao). The pulmonary artery (PA) is not seen in this panel. **B,** With anterior angulation, the small PA can be seen. The portion of the ventricular septum just beneath the great vessels called the conal septum can be seen deviated into the right ventricular outflow tract, causing subpulmonic obstruction. This is one of the hallmark findings in tetralogy of Fallot. *Ao,* Aorta; *LV,* left ventricle; *PA,* pulmonary artery; *RV,* right ventricle; *VSD,* ventricular septal defect.

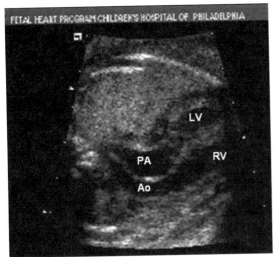

Figure 12-10   Example of transposition of the great arteries in the fetus. Both great vessels arise from the heart in parallel, suggesting a conotruncal anomaly. The aorta *(Ao)* is seen arising from the right ventricle *(RV)*, and the pulmonary artery *(PA)* is seen arising from the left ventricle *(LV)*.

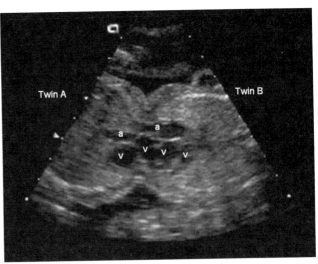

Figure 12-12   Example of fetal thoracopagus (i.e., conjoined twins, joined at the chest). The twins share a single heart with two atria *(a)* and four identifiable ventricles *(v)*, all combined into one amalgam of cardiac mass.

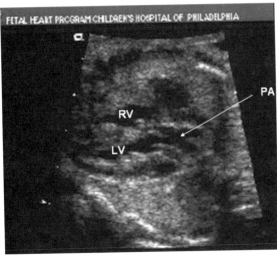

Figure 12-11   Example of transposition of the great arteries. The great vessel arising from the left ventricle bifurcates early and is the pulmonary artery. *RV,* Right ventricle; *LV,* left ventricle; *PA,* pulmonary artery.

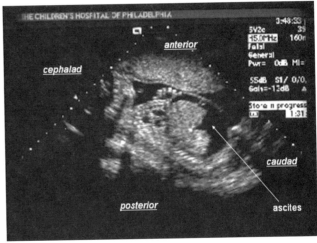

Figure 12-13   Example of a fetus with complete heart block who has developed hydrops, manifested primarily as ascites.

fetus. Failure of therapeutic measures in treating either brady- or tachyarrhythmias in the viable fetus should prompt consideration of delivery and direct administration of treatment to the premature infant if impending fetal demise seems imminent.

FETAL CARDIOVASCULAR DISEASE: NONCONGENITAL HEART DISEASE

A variety of anomalies and disorders affecting the fetus may secondarily impact the fetal cardiovascular system. Some examples and ways in which fetal echocardiography play an important role include the following:

1. Congenital diaphragmatic hernia is associated with congenital heart disease in approximately 10% of cases.[23] Abdominal contents in the thoracic cavity may limit pulmonary vascular development, which can impact upon neonatal physiology. A number of findings are seen on fetal echocardiography. Branch pulmonary artery measurements may reveal smallness on the side of the hernia, commensurate with the degree of pulmonary hypoplasia present.[24] In addition, mild left ventricular hypoplasia can be seen in accordance with limited right-to-left flow across the foramen and decreased fetal pulmonary venous return as a consequence of pulmonary hypoplasia.

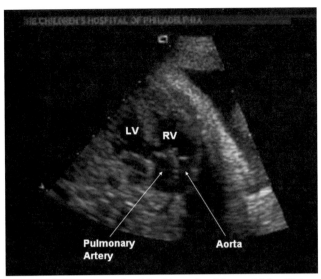

Figure 12-14   Example of double-outlet right ventricle. Note the large ventricular septal defect beneath the great vessels, both of which arise from the right ventricle.

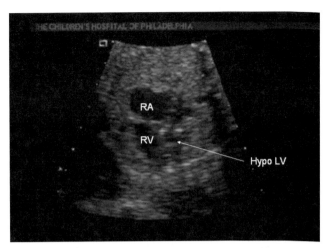

Figure 12-16   Example of hypoplastic left heart syndrome. This is one of the most commonly diagnosed forms of heart disease in the fetus due to its ease of recognition. *Hypo LV,* Hypoplastic left ventricle; *RA,* right atrium; *RV,* right ventricle.

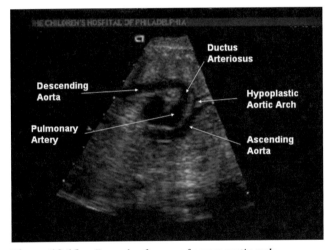

Figure 12-15   Example of a case of severe aortic arch hypoplasia. Both vascular arches of the fetal circulation are seen, with the hypoplastic aortic arch and the ductal arch arising from the pulmonary artery and connecting to the descending aorta. This fetus will likely require patency of the ductus arteriosus at birth in order to maintain the fetal circulatory pathways and to provide for systemic perfusion. Prostaglandin infusion should be offered to the neonate after delivery.

2. Chest masses such as congenital cystic adenomatoid malformation (CCAM) can grow to giant size, resulting in compression of the thoracic contents and a cardiac tamponade–type physiology.[25] Hydrops can be seen when cardiac compression is significant, with a high likelihood of fetal demise. Changes in the echocardiography-derived Doppler filling patterns across the tricuspid and mitral valves may herald the findings of impending tamponade and fetal hydrops.

3. Arteriovenous malformations such as sacrococcygeal teratoma (SCT) or vein of Galen malformations can result in massive degrees of increased venous return and volume overload on the fetal heart.[26] Because the fetal heart tolerates volume loads poorly, fetal hydrops and demise possible if these vascular lesions are large with high-volume loads. One measure of the consequence of these lesions is the fetal combined cardiac output. This can be calculated by echocardiography and is the sum of ejection volumes across both the pulmonary (i.e., right ventricle) and aortic (i.e., left ventricle) tracts. Normal fetal combined cardiac outputs are in the 400- to 500-mL/min/kg range, and the fetus with SCT may manifest values as high as >1000 mL/min/kg.[27] At these elevated levels, one can also commonly see cardiomegaly, ventricular dilation, and atrioventricular valve regurgitation.

4. Maternal diabetes can increase the risk of development of congenital heart disease. However, in addition, elevated levels of maternal glucose can trigger hyperinsulinism in the fetus, which promotes cardiac hypertrophy. Asymmetric septal hypertrophy of the fetal heart may occur, with development of left ventricular outflow tract obstruction as well as ventricular stiffness and diastolic dysfunction.

SUMMARY

Through advances in imaging, we are currently able to visualize and understand many aspects of the developing fetal cardiovascular system, previously hidden and unknown. Fetal echocardiography provides a window to the womb that is changing the way congenital heart anomalies are detected. Fetal echocardiography will provide a way for prenatal interventional treatment to take place safely, effectively, and reliably, which will dramatically alter the way we treat congenital heart disease.

MAJOR POINTS

- Fetal echocardiography provides for high-resolution images of the fetal cardiovascular system and is an accurate and reliable way to diagnose congenital heart disease prior to birth.
- The increasing application of fetal echocardiography is resulting in a shift in demographics, with a greater percentage of patients with congenital heart disease being diagnosed prior to birth.
- Fetal echocardiography provides for a number of benefits, including improved hemodynamic state prior to intervention and improved surgical outcome.
- The fetal cardiovascular system is uniquely different from the mature postnatal system in the presence of a number of unique shunting pathways (i.e., the foramen ovale, the ductus venosus, and the ductus arteriosus) and a different myocardial compliance.
- Indications for performing a fetal echocardiogram have been established and recategorized as either maternal or fetal indications.
- Evaluation of Doppler flow patterns in the venous and arterial systems can provide important information about the physiological state of the developing fetus.
- Some forms of congenital heart disease undergo marked progressive changes from the early second to the third trimester of gestation, which may alter the postnatal management strategies. Serial evaluation using fetal echocardiography during gestation is warranted in the fetus with congenital heart disease.
- A variety of rhythm disturbances can be diagnosed when applying fetal echocardiography by looking for mechanical correlates of conduction disturbances. Appropriate treatment regimens can then be applied to the mother and the fetus.
- A variety of disease processes other than primary congenital heart disease can seriously affect the fetal cardiovascular system and can be diagnosed and monitored using fetal echocardiography.
- With clearer delineation of the prenatal natural history of congenital heart disease, strategies for fetal intervention using catheter techniques or fetal surgery can be applied toward treating congenital heart disease prior to birth.

REFERENCES

1. Kleinman CS, Hobbins JC, Jaffe CC, et al: Echocardiographic studies of the human fetus: Prenatal diagnosis of congenital heart disease and cardiac dysrhythmias. Pediatrics 65: 1059-1067, 1980.

2. Ewigman BG, Crane JP, Frigoletto FD, et al: Effect of prenatal ultrasound screening on perinatal outcome. RADIUS Study Group. N Engl J Med 329:821-827, 1993.

3. Buskens E, Grobbee DE, Frohn-Mulder IM, et al: Efficacy of routine fetal ultrasound screening for congenital heart disease in normal pregnancy. Circulation 94:67-72, 1996.

4. Stumpflen I, Stumpflen A, Wimmer M, Bernaschek G: Effect of detailed fetal echocardiography as part of routine prenatal ultrasonographic screening on detection of congenital heart disease. Lancet 348:854-857, 1996.

5. Mahle WT, Clancy RR, McGaurn SP, et al: Impact of prenatal diagnosis on survival and early neurologic morbidity in neonates with the hypoplastic left heart syndrome. Pediatrics 107:1277-1282, 2001.

6. Tworetzky W, McElhinney DB, Reddy VM, et al: Improved surgical outcome after fetal diagnosis of hypoplastic left heart syndrome. Circulation 103:1269-1273, 2001.

7. Verheijen PM, Lisowski LA, Stoutenbeek P, et al: Lactacidosis in the neonate is minimized by prenatal detection of congenital heart disease. Ultrasound Obstet Gynecol 19:552-555, 2002.

8. Mahle WT: Neurologic and cognitive outcomes in children with congenital heart disease. Curr Opin Pediatr 13:482-486, 2001.

9. DeVore GR: Influence of prenatal diagnosis on congenital heart defects. Ann N Y Acad Sci 847:46-52, 1998.

10. Friedman, WF: The intrinsic physiologic properties of the developing heart. Prog Cardiovasc Dis 15:87-111, 1972.

11. Mahoney L: Calcium homeostasis and control of contractility in the developing heart. Sem Perinatol 20:510-519, 1996.

12. Grant DA: Ventricular constraint in the fetus and newborn. Can J Cardiol 15:95-104, 1999.

13. Rychik J, Ayres N, Cuneo B, et al: American Society of Echocardiography guidelines and standards for performance of the fetal echocardiogram. J Am Soc Echocardiogr 17:803-810, 2004.

14. Jaeggi ET, Fouron JC, Silverman ED, et al: Transplacental fetal treatment improves the outcome of prenatally diagnosed complete atrioventricular block without structural heart disease. Circulation 110:1542-1548, 2004.

15. Koivurova S, Hartikainen AL, Gissler M, et al: Neonatal outcome and congenital malformations in children born after in vitro fertilization. Hum Reprod 17:1391-1398, 2002.

16. Hansen M, Kurinczuk JJ, Bower C, Webb S: The risk of major birth defects after intracytoplasmic sperm injection and in vitro fertilization. N Engl J Med 346:725-730, 2002.

17. Ghi T, Huggon IC, Zosmer N, Nicolaides KH: Incidence of major structural cardiac defects associated with increased nuchal translucency but normal karyotype. Ultrasound Obstet Gynecol 18:610-614, 2001.

18. Gembruch U, Knopfle G, Bald R, Hansmann M: Early diagnosis of fetal congenital heart disease by transvaginal echocardiography. Ultrasound Obstet Gynecol 3:310-317, 1993.

19. Tulzer G, Arzt W, Franklin RC, et al: Fetal pulmonary valvuloplasty for critical pulmonary stenosis or atresia with intact septum. Lancet 360:1567-1568, 2002.

20. Tworetzky W, Wilkins-Haug L, Jennings RW, et al: Balloon dilation of severe aortic stenosis in the fetus: Potential for prevention of hypoplastic left heart syndrome: Candidate selection, technique, and results of successful intervention. Circulation 110:2125-2131, 2004.

21. Van Bergen AH, Cuneo BF, Davis N: Prospective echocardiographic evaluation of atrioventricular conduction in fetuses with maternal Sjögren's antibodies. Am J Obstet Gynecol 191:1014-1018, 2004.

22. Oudijk MA, Michon MM, Kleinman CS, et al: Sotalol in the treatment of fetal dysrhythmias. Circulation 101: 2721-2726, 2000.

23. Cohen MS, Rychik J, Bush DM, et al: Influence of congenital heart disease on survival in children with congenital diaphragmatic hernia. J Pediatr 141:25-30, 2002.

24. Sokol J, Bohn D, Lacro RV, et al: Fetal pulmonary artery diameters and their association with lung hypoplasia and postnatal outcome in congenital diaphragmatic hernia. Am J Obstet Gynecol 186:1085-1090, 2002.

25. Mahle WT, Rychik J, Tian ZY, et al: Echocardiographic evaluation of the fetus with congenital cystic adenomatoid malformation. Ultrasound Obstet Gynecol 16:620-624, 2000.

26. Silverman NH, Schmidt KG: Ventricular volume overload in the human fetus: Observations from fetal echocardiography. J Am Soc Echocardiogr 3:20-29, 1990.

27. Rychik J, Tian Z, Cohen MS, et al: Acute cardiovascular effects of fetal surgery in the human. Circulation 110:1549-1556, 2004.

CHAPTER 13

Pharmacologic Treatment of Heart Disease

RONN E. TANEL

MARK D. LEVIN

Adrenergic Agonists (Inotropic Agents)
  Dopamine
  Dobutamine
  Epinephrine
  Norepinephrine
  Isoproterenol
  Calcium
Phosphodiesterase Inhibitors
  Amrinone
  Milrinone
Vasodilators
  Nitroprusside
  Nitroglycerin
  Hydralazine
  Enalaprilat
Pharmacologic Agents That Affect Pulmonary Hypertension
  Nitric Oxide
  Prostacyclin
  Iloprost
  Bosentan
  Sildenafil
Vasoconstrictors
  Phenylephrine
Congestive Heart Failure
Diuretics
  Furosemide
  Ethacrynic Acid
  Bumetanide
  Chlorothiazide and Hydrochlorothiazide
  Metolazone
  Spironolactone
Angiotensin-Converting Enzyme Inhibitors
  Captopril
  Enalapril
Angiotensin II Receptor Blockers
  Losartan
  Candesartan

Antiarrhythmic Medications
Class IA Agents
  Procainamide
  Disopyramide
Class IB Agents
  Lidocaine
  Mexiletine
Class IC Agents
  Flecainide
Class II Agents
  Esmolol
  Propranolol
Class III Agents
  Amiodarone
  Sotalol
Class IV Agents
  Verapamil
Non-Classified Antiarrhythmics
  Digoxin
  Adenosine
Ductal Manipulators
  Prostaglandin E1
  Indomethacin

The pharmacologic management of pediatric cardiac patients is complex and includes many therapeutic options that are growing at a rapid pace. Many of the drugs are relatively new with little scientific experience upon which to base clinical decision making. Nonetheless, information and recommendations exist and are determined by anecdotal experience, case reports, in vitro experiments, animal models, and extrapolation from large adult clinical trials. This chapter is an effort to clinically categorize, describe, and apply the knowledge available regarding cardiovascular drugs prescribed in pediatric practice.

Historically, children have been underrepresented as subjects of cardiovascular clinical trials, resulting in a small proportion of drugs that have been studied and labeled for pediatric use. In order to encourage pediatric studies and to identify potential therapeutic benefits in this population, Congress passed the Food and Drug Administration Modernization Act, also known as the Pediatric Exclusivity Provision, in 1997, which provided a 6-month patent extension to manufacturers who sponsored studies in children. This legislation has been the most successful stimulus for pediatric drug studies and prescribing information. The agreement was extended by 6 years when Congress passed the Best Pharmaceuticals for Children Act in January 2002. In addition to these incentives, The Pediatric Rule, enacted in 1999, now requires manufacturers of new drugs to conduct studies that allow for labeling for pediatric patients if the drug is thought to have a significant clinical impact in children.

The drugs that have significant effects on the cardiovascular system and are routinely used in the pediatric population are described here. In order to understand effects on the heart and vasculature, there must be an appreciation of the dynamic regulation of the cardiovascular system. Central nervous system control of the cardiovascular system, including the heart and arterial and venous circulations, is a complex and highly differentiated feedback process that occurs primarily through the sympathetic and parasympathetic components of the autonomic nervous system. In general, the cardiovascular reflex arc includes the sensory neurons from the heart and vasculature, the autonomic efferent neurons in the brainstem, the central nervous system processing centers, and the sympathetic and parasympathetic preganglionic efferent neurons that synapse with postganglionic neurons. It is these autonomic neurons that allow control of the target organs by the brain and spinal cord. In addition, autonomic responses are modified by factors outside the reflex arc, including local tissue pH and adrenergic receptor status. In pediatrics, autonomic dysfunction generally occurs as a congenital or developmental problem caused by a primary nervous system or cardiovascular disease. Maturational differences, as well as the existing developmental stage of end-organs, neurons, neurotransmitters, and receptors, will influence the autonomic response.

Neurohormonal regulation occurs through the adrenergic receptors that are present on the surface of vascular tissues and sympathetic nerves. The extracellular catecholamines regulate intracellular processes through these receptors. The α-adrenergic receptors occur primarily in the peripheral vasculature and have a greater affinity for norepinephrine. The vascular postsynaptic α_1-receptor mediates vasoconstriction, whereas activation of the α_2-receptor, located on the sympathetic nerve terminus, inhibits release of norepinephrine from the sympathetic nerve. The β-receptors occur primarily within the myocardium and are more responsive to epinephrine. The β_1-receptor activation results in cardiac inotropic and chronotropic responses, as well as intestinal relaxation and renal renin release. Activation of the β_2-receptor results in vascular and bronchial smooth muscle dilation, whereas β_2–receptors on the sympathetic nerve terminus enhance sympathetic nerve release of norepinephrine.

ADRENERGIC AGONISTS (INOTROPIC AGENTS)

The adrenergic agonists have their cardiac effects through cardiac and vascular adrenergic receptors (Table 13-1). All of these inotropic agents have some effect on the myocardial β_1-receptor. The adrenergic receptor activation increases adenyl cyclase activity, which increases cyclic adenosine monophosphate levels and cyclic adenosine monophosphate-dependent protein kinase activity. Phosphorylation by protein kinase results in increased activity of many intracellular cardiac proteins. This results in an increased speed and force of contraction of the myocardium and an increased heart rate.

Dopamine

Indications
At low to moderate doses, dopamine enhances myocardial contractility and results in renal, mesenteric, cerebral, and coronary vasodilation. However, there is little effect on the pulmonary vascular bed. Dopamine can have effects on α_1-receptors at high doses, resulting in vasoconstriction. Dopamine is used clinically for its inotropic effects in situations of shock, hypotension, and low cardiac output syndrome after cardiac surgery, as well as for other conditions resulting in myocardial failure. In lower doses, the medication can enhance or

Table 13-1	Adrenergic Receptors Effects of Inotropic Agents			
Drug	DA	α	β_1	β_2
Dopamine	+	0/+ (high dose)	+	+
Dobutamine	0	0	+	0
Epinephrine	0	+	+	+
Norepinephrine	0	+	+	0
Isoproterenol	0	0	+	+

+, Positive effect; 0, no significant effect; α, α-adrenergic receptor; β_1, β_1 adrenergic receptor; β_2, β_2-adrenergic receptor; DA, dopaminergic receptor.

maintain urine output. Dopamine has less potent chronotropic effects at standard doses.

Mechanism of Action

Dopamine is an endogenous catecholamine that is the immediate precursor of norepinephrine. It has potent direct cardiac β_1-receptor activity as well as indirect effects on the β_1-receptor by release of norepinephrine from the cardiac sympathetic nerve terminal. Dopamine also has an effect on specific dopamine receptors, but it has less of an effect on β_2-receptors. Higher doses stimulate α-adrenergic receptors.

Dosage

Dopamine is only available in the intravenous form and should be administered through a central venous catheter. The standard dose range for a continuous infusion is 1–20 mcg/kg/min, but higher dosing may be used, titrated to effect. The hemodynamic effects are dose dependent: a low dose of 1–3 mcg/kg/min increases renal blood flow and urine output; an intermediate dose of 3–10 mcg/kg/min increases renal blood flow, heart rate, cardiac contractility, and cardiac output; a high dose of > 10 mcg/kg/min elicits α-adrenergic effects, such as vasoconstriction, leading to increased blood pressure.

Metabolism and Half-Life

Dopamine is metabolized by both hepatic and renal mechanisms. The half-life is 2 minutes. It must be mixed only with nonalkaline solutions because alkaline preparations inactivate the drug.

Adverse Effects

Side effects are most commonly encountered with high-dose infusions and include those related to vasoconstriction and tachycardia. Arrhythmias may be provoked with high doses. Other side effects include headache, nausea, vomiting, and dyspnea.

Monitoring

Due to its potent cardiovascular effects, intensive hemodynamic monitoring is necessary during the administration of dopamine to ensure accurate titration to effect.

Pearls

Peripheral extravasation may cause local ischemia, requiring careful observation leading to early recognition and appropriate therapy.

Dobutamine

Indications

Dobutamine acts to improve contractility without a significant effect on heart rate. Peripheral vascular effects favor the coronary and skeletal muscle beds over the mesenteric, pulmonary, and renal vasculature. In fact, there are significant beneficial vasodilating effects on the systemic vasculature, but there is little effect on the pulmonary vascular bed. Therefore, dobutamine may decrease the central venous pressure and capillary wedge pressure, but it does not significantly change the pulmonary vascular resistance. Dobutamine increases cardiac output by increasing stroke volume, which allows for a decrease in systemic vascular resistance and an overall increase in blood pressure. Dobutamine causes less peripheral vasoconstriction than dopamine. These effects of dobutamine have been studied in pediatric patients with cardiogenic shock, with a much lower effectiveness in patients with septic shock and in infants younger than 12 months of age.[1,2] Dobutamine may be used as a short-term infusion to improve symptoms of congestive heart failure and may continue to have benefit beyond the duration of the infusion. It is not known whether short-term dobutamine use in end-stage congestive heart failure improves outcome.

Mechanism of Action

Dobutamine is a synthetic catecholamine that has a primary effect on the β_1-adrenergic receptor without significant effects on the β_2- or α-receptors.

Dosage

Dobutamine is only available in the intravenous form and should be administered through a central venous catheter. Standard doses are 1–20 mcg/kg/min. Higher doses are used in selected circumstances. A combination of dobutamine and dopamine can be used with lower doses of each, resulting in improved cardiac performance. This may preserve the renal effects of dopamine while minimizing potential toxicity. Dobutamine should not be mixed with sodium bicarbonate.

Metabolism and Half-Life

Dobutamine is metabolized in tissues and in the liver to inactive metabolites. The half-life is 2 minutes.

Adverse Effects

Side effects include arrhythmias, nausea, headache, palpitations, angina, and increases or decreases in heart rate or blood pressure. High-dose dobutamine may adversely affect myocardial oxygen demand. Peripheral infusion may be associated with phlebitis and pain, and extravasation may cause localized ischemia.

Monitoring

Intensive hemodynamic monitoring is necessary during dobutamine infusion for accurate titration to effect. The serum potassium level should be followed.

Pearls

Dobutamine is ineffective in the presence of mechanical obstruction, such as valvar aortic stenosis, and is contraindicated for use in patients with hypertrophic cardiomyopathy.

Epinephrine

Indications

Epinephrine is reserved for situations of low cardiac output resulting in cardiovascular collapse when acute inotropic and chronotropic effects are desired. Specific clinical indications include septic shock, low cardiac output syndrome after cardiac surgery, and dilated cardiomyopathy, especially after trials of other drugs have failed.

Mechanism of Action

Epinephrine is an endogenous catecholamine that has potent α-, β_1-, and β_2-adrenergic effects. At low concentrations, cardiovascular effects include increased heart rate, increased contractility, and increased systolic blood pressure caused by stimulation of β_1-receptors. Thus, it serves as both an inotrope and a chronotrope. With increasing dosage, the diastolic blood pressure decreases because of stimulation of the peripheral vascular β_2-receptors. At high doses, vasoconstriction occurs as the α-receptors become stimulated. At excessive infusion rates, the cardiac index will decrease in association with greatly increased systemic vascular resistance. Epinephrine has variable effects on the pulmonary vasculature, which contains both α- and β_2-receptors. The result of vasodilation vs. vasoconstriction depends on the epinephrine infusion rate, the duration of drug exposure, the presence of hypoxia, and the underlying pulmonary vascular tone.[3-6]

Dosage

The acute dose for adult patients is 0.5–1.0 mg, intravenously. Pediatric guidelines recommend 10 mcg/kg/dose for cardiac arrest. High-dose epinephrine is controversial but may be considered at 100 mcg/kg in cases in which lower doses are ineffective.[7,8] Infusion rates of 0.03–0.2 mcg/kg/min are used to enhance myocardial contractility. The infusion rate is generally started at the low end of the dosage range and is titrated upward to effect. The medication should be infused through a central catheter due to the risk of tissue necrosis with subcutaneous infiltration. Epinephrine may be administered through the endotracheal tube at 100 mcg/kg or intracardiac at 0.1–0.2 mg. Epinephrine may also be administered through an intraosseous needle.

Metabolism and Half-life

Epinephrine is metabolized in the adrenergic neuron by monoamine oxidase and catechol-O-methyltransferase. In addition, the circulating drug is metabolized in the liver and metabolites are excreted in the urine along with small amounts of unchanged drug. The half-life is 2 minutes.

Adverse Effects

Arrhythmia induction is an important potential side effect. Epinephrine may cause myocardial ischemia by increasing myocardial oxygen demand and tissue ischemia, caused by vasoconstriction at high doses. Extravasation of the drug into the subcutaneous tissues may cause necrosis. Other side effects include tachycardia, hyperglycemia, hypokalemia, anxiety, headache, cold extremities, cerebral hemorrhage, and pulmonary edema. Newborn infants appear to be more susceptible to myocardial injury during epinephrine infusions, and this has been associated with sarcolemmal rupture and mitochondrial calcium granule deposition.[9]

Monitoring

Cardiac monitoring is necessary for evaluation of heart rate and blood pressure. The possibility of arrhythmias must be monitored, especially in patients with underlying myocardial disease and diagnoses with greater arrhythmia potential. The site of the infusion must be assessed for blanching or extravasation.

Pearls

If possible, epinephrine should be avoided in patients at high risk for ventricular arrhythmias, such as those with myocarditis, hypokalemia, and hypercapnia, particularly during inhaled anesthesia.

Norepinephrine

Indications

Norepinephrine is a potent inotropic agent, but it has limited applications because it causes profound vasoconstriction. It is often avoided because of the associated increased myocardial oxygen demand, reduced renal blood flow, and potential for the induction of arrhythmias. In situations of severe low cardiac output, it is used for temporary support of the central blood pressure. Specifically, norepinephrine may be useful in vasodilatory shock that is not responsive to dopamine or epinephrine. Norepinephrine may enhance coronary blood flow by increasing systemic diastolic pressure.

Mechanism of Action

Norepinephrine, the postganglionic sympathetic neurotransmitter, is an endogenous catecholamine with β_1-, but not β_2-, and α-adrenergic receptor effects. Stimulation of these receptors results in an increase in the systolic and diastolic blood pressure, an increase in the systemic vascular resistance, and enhanced contractility. Although there are β_1-adrenergic effects, the heart rate may not increase and may actually decrease due to the stimulation of baroreceptors. The systemic vasoconstriction due to α-receptor stimulation may result in end-organ hypoperfusion.

Dosage

Norepinephrine should be infused through a central venous catheter. The dose is 0.05–0.1 mcg/kg/min and may be titrated to effect. The maximum dose is 1–2 mcg/kg/min. The drug should not be mixed with sodium bicarbonate.

Metabolism and Half-Life

Norepinephrine is metabolized by the monoamine oxidase and catechol-O-methyltransferase enzyme systems in the adrenergic neuron. Metabolites are excreted in the urine. The half-life of the drug is 3 minutes. The drug should be protected from light since it is readily oxidized.

Adverse Effects

The potency of norepinephrine makes arrhythmias and tissue ischemia caused by marked vasoconstriction important risks. Extravasation into the cutaneous tissues may result in tissue necrosis. Extravasation of the drug should be treated with the subcutaneous administration of phentolamine into the extravasation area.

Monitoring

Monitoring for ventricular arrhythmias is important during the use of norepinephrine. In addition, there must be ongoing assessment for reduced end-organ perfusion.

Pearls

The drug should not be used for patients with hypotension because of hypovolemia. An adequate circulatory volume should be established before giving the drug.

Isoproterenol

Indications

Isoproterenol may be used in patients with low cardiac output caused by impaired contractility, especially if this is associated with elevated systemic resistance. Because of its positive chronotropic effect, isoproterenol may be helpful in augmenting the heart rate in patients with bradycardia caused by sinus node dysfunction or atrioventricular block. It may directly increase the sinus rate, enhance atrioventricular conduction, or improve the junctional or ventricular escape rate. This is generally a temporizing measure until more definitive therapy for bradycardia can be arranged. Isoproterenol must be used cautiously in the treatment of bradycardia because a decrease in systemic vascular resistance, in combination with a low heart rate, could aggravate hypotension, especially in the hypovolemic patient. Isoproterenol has utility for the cardiac transplant patient as it can maintain the heart rate and decrease afterload in the immediate postoperative period. Isoproterenol is also known as a potent bronchodilator, resulting in additional benefit for patients with reactive airway disease. However, other more selective β_2-receptor agonists are usually chosen for management of status asthmaticus because of the potential for myocardial ischemia with isoproterenol.

Mechanism of Action

Isoproterenol is a synthetic catecholamine with nearly exclusive nonselective β-receptor agonistic activity. The combination effect on the myocardial β_1- and peripheral β_2-receptors ($\beta_1 > \beta_2$) results in enhanced myocardial contractility, a positive chronotropic response, and decreased systemic vascular resistance. As a result, the systolic blood pressure is elevated and the diastolic blood pressure is reduced. Although isoproterenol increases myocardial and systemic oxygen consumption, the increase in oxygen delivery allows improvement of the mixed venous saturation.[10] Isoproterenol has potent effects on reducing pulmonary vascular resistance and may be particularly helpful in the management of patients with pulmonary hypertension of any cause. The peripheral effects of isoproterenol are most potent in the skeletal muscle and the renal and splanchnic vascular beds.

Dosage

Isoproterenol is only available in the intravenous form and may be administered peripherally, but central administration is preferred. The dosage range for isoproterenol is 0.05–1.0 mcg/kg/min. Postoperative cardiac patients require lower infusion rates than patients receiving isoproterenol for reactive airway disease. This may be due to decreased clearance in the more critically ill cardiac patients.

Metabolism and Half-Life

Isoproterenol is metabolized in the liver, the lungs, and many other tissues by catechol-O-methyltransferase. It is then excreted in the urine, primarily as sulfate conjugates. It is metabolized relatively less by monoamine oxidase. The half-life is 2 minutes.

Adverse Effects

Side effects of isoproterenol include tachycardia, arrhythmias, and nausea. Other side effects include headache, tremor, and sweating. Beneficial effects of the medication may be limited by increased myocardial oxygen consumption as a result of increased contractility and heart rate. For example, patients with compromised coronary perfusion may respond poorly to isoproterenol since the myocardial oxygen consumption may increase, whereas there is decreased perfusion pressure (i.e., diastolic blood pressure) caused by vasodilation. The β_2-receptor activity exerts its effects on vasodilation in the skeletal muscle more than in the renal or mesenteric vasculature, potentially resulting in hypotension. Patients with fixed ventricular outflow tract obstruction should not be administered isoproterenol because of the risk for an increased flow gradient when there is systemic afterload reduction from isoproterenol.

Monitoring

Hemodynamic and electrocardiographic monitoring is necessary during isoproterenol infusion.

Pearls

Isoproterenol should be avoided in patients with compromised coronary blood flow because of potential intolerance of the increased myocardial oxygen consumption. Patients with hypertrophic cardiomyopathy are particularly susceptible because the ventricular outflow tract gradient may increase along with an increase in myocardial oxygen consumption. Isoproterenol should be avoided in patients with arrhythmias.

Calcium

Indications

Calcium is administered for clinical improvement in myocardial contractility and for support of the systemic blood pressure. The hemodynamic effects of calcium appear to be more significant in the newborn, possibly because of intrinsically lower intracellular calcium concentrations in the immature myocardium.[11] Calcium metabolism is of particular interest in the newborn with hypoparathyroidism because of a 22q11 microdeletion that is relatively common in patients with conotruncal cardiac lesions. Although controversy exists regarding the administration of calcium without documented hypocalcemia, its use has been beneficial in patients with electromechanical dissociation.[12] Other current indications for treatment with calcium include hyperkalemia, hypermagnesemia, and calcium-channel blocker toxicity.

Mechanism of Action

Ionized calcium appears to be important for the maintenance of blood pressure and cardiac output, probably because of diminished intracellular calcium stores in young patients. Calcium supplementation seems appropriate for critically ill children, especially when hypocalcemia is documented.[13] Hypocalcemia in this group of patients is sometimes associated with transient hypoparathyroidism. Finally, in infants and children who have had surgery to repair congenital heart disease, supplemental calcium may be important because of the use of citrated blood products.

Dosage

Calcium chloride and calcium gluconate are administered intravenously. The dose of calcium chloride is 0.1–0.3 mg/kg, and the dose of calcium gluconate is 50–100 mg/kg. Doses may be repeated every 30–60 minutes, as necessary. Calcium chloride seems to result in a more significant increase in ionized calcium levels and in an improvement in blood pressure, compared with calcium gluconate.[14]

Metabolism

Calcium chloride and calcium gluconate are excreted primarily in the feces as unabsorbed calcium. There is a small amount of calcium excreted in the urine.

Adverse Effects

The most significant side effects of calcium administration are bradycardia and asystole. This is of particular importance when calcium is being infused directly into the heart through an intracardiac catheter.

Monitoring

Hypocalcemia is detected more accurately by measurement of the serum-ionized calcium rather than total serum calcium. Heart rate and blood pressure monitoring must occur while calcium is being administered.

Pearls

Calcium must be used with caution in the presence of digoxin because it potentiates digoxin and can result in digoxin toxicity, causing ventricular arrhythmias.

PHOSPHODIESTERASE INHIBITORS

The most commonly used phosphodiesterase inhibitors block cyclic nucleotide phosphodiesterase III and increase intracellular myocardial and vascular cyclic adenosine monophosphate. This results in a positive inotropic effect caused by an increased intracellular myocardial calcium concentration. Increased vascular intracellular cyclic adenosine monophosphate concentrations result in vascular relaxation and decreased afterload. Amrinone and milrinone are bipyridine derivatives and may have an additional role as anti-inflammatory agents in septic shock.[15] Milrinone has been shown to increase cardiac index, stroke volume, and oxygen delivery and to decrease systemic and pulmonary vascular resistance while not significantly affecting heart rate in children with septic shock.[16]

Amrinone

Indications

Amrinone has been used most frequently in pediatric patients in the setting of postoperative low cardiac output syndrome, but other indications have been evaluated in which there is depressed cardiac function.[17,18]

Mechanism of Action

Amrinone was one of the first phosphodiesterase inhibitors to be developed and is relatively weak and nonspecific. Amrinone increases cardiac output and reduces filling pressures and systemic vascular resistance without having much effect on heart rate. It has been shown to decrease pulmonary artery pressure without causing systemic hypotension in children.[19]

Dosage

Amrinone is administered as an intravenous bolus loading dose over 10–20 minutes, followed by an infusion. The loading dose is 1–3 mg/kg, and the infusion rate is 5–15 mcg/kg/min.

Metabolism and Half-Life

Amrinone is excreted in the kidney with some metabolism occurring through glucuronidation and acetylation. Amrinone is sensitive to light and cannot be mixed with glucose. Amrinone binds to cardiopulmonary bypass circuitry. Elimination occurs in 5–6 hours in children, is faster in adults, and takes as long as 12–44 hours in neonates.

Adverse Effects

Long-term oral use of amrinone is associated with thrombocytopenia, fever, gastrointestinal complaints, hepatic dysfunction, arrhythmias, and central nervous system abnormalities. Short-term intravenous use usually is well tolerated, but hypotension and ventricular arrhythmias are possible. Hypotension can be prevented by administering the loading dose slowly or by maintaining preload with volume expansion.

Monitoring

Patients receiving amrinone should be monitored for the development of new arrhythmias and hypotension. The complete blood count should be followed, especially with attention to the platelet count.

Pearls

The phosphodiesterase inhibitors usually are used in combination with other inotropic agents, such as the β-adrenergic agonists, for potentially greater effect.

However, this clinical approach has not been studied in detail. Amrinone should be avoided in patients with severe ventricular outflow tract obstruction.

Milrinone

Indications

Currently, milrinone is the most commonly used phosphodiesterase inhibitor in pediatric patients, usually used in the postoperative patient with low cardiac output syndrome or in patients with a variety of causes of congestive heart failure.[20,21]

Mechanism of Action

Milrinone is approximately 15–20 times more potent than amrinone and is a more selective phosphodiesterase inhibitor than amrinone. As a phosphodiesterase inhibitor, milrinone causes vasodilation, which decreases systemic vascular resistance, reduces filling pressures, and augments cardiac output.

Dosage

Milrinone is restricted to intravenous use. It is prescribed as a loading dose, followed by an infusion. The loading dose is 50 mcg/kg, followed by an infusion of 0.5–1.0 mcg/kg/min.

Metabolism and Half-Life

Milrinone is primarily excreted by the kidney. Milrinone does not bind to cardiopulmonary bypass circuitry. The half-life is 136 minutes in patients with congestive heart failure and is longer in cases of more severe congestive heart failure. Elimination of milrinone is much more rapid in children than in adults.

Adverse Effects

Milrinone has some of the same side effects as amrinone, but it seems to have less potential for arrhythmia development and has much less of an effect on platelet count and function.

Monitoring

Cardiac monitoring of the heart rate and blood pressure is important while assessing for improvement in signs and symptoms of congestive heart failure. Continuous telemetry should assess for the development of ventricular ectopy, although life-threatening arrhythmias are rare. Adults should be evaluated for any exacerbation of angina. The serum potassium should be checked and followed during the infusion of milrinone.

Pearls

Milrinone should be avoided in patients with severe ventricular outflow tract obstruction since vasodilation may result in profound hypotension.

VASODILATORS

Changes in the peripheral vascular resistance and capacitance, as well as changes in preload, affect cardiac performance. Arterial vasodilation results in decreased afterload by decreasing the systemic and pulmonary vascular resistance. This decrease in afterload and resistance against which the heart must pump effectively decreases the work of the heart. Vasodilators may have a preferential effect on either the pulmonary vasculature or the systemic vasculature, or they may have no significant differential effect on the two. Although adequate preload is necessary for maintaining cardiac output, an elevated preload has the potential to result in pulmonary or systemic venous congestion. Venous vasodilators increase venous capacitance, decrease venous return, and result in decreased preload, which can reduce venous pressure and symptoms without compromising cardiac output. The vasodilators may have a preferential effect on either the venous or the arterial side of the circulation, but many affect both. Because most drugs affect both afterload and preload, they are frequently used in patients with congestive heart failure who have both increased systemic vascular resistance and increased filling pressures.

Nitroprusside

Indications

As a mixed vasodilator, nitroprusside results in arterial and venous vasodilation without any significant direct cardiac effects. The clinical effect is a reduction in both afterload and preload. A reduction in systemic afterload is beneficial for patients with left ventricular failure caused by dilated cardiomyopathy and for patients with mitral regurgitation in whom the decreased afterload may improve cardiac output.[22-24] Postoperative cardiac patients with low cardiac output syndrome may benefit from nitroprusside, especially when it is used in combination with an inotropic agent and volume expansion.[25-27] Nitroprusside is an excellent therapy for hypertensive emergencies because of the controlled manner in which the medication can be titrated to effect. This has been established in hypertensive pediatric patients. In addition, cardiac patients who are hypertensive following repair of coarctation of the aorta have also been shown to benefit from the rapid onset of the drug.[28-30] Finally, nitroprusside has been used for controlled hypotension during surgery when there is significant blood loss.[31] The goal in this situation is to maintain perfusion of the end-organs despite a lower mean arterial pressure. The nitrates are contraindicated in patients with obstructive valvar heart disease.

Mechanism of Action

Nitroprusside interacts with oxyhemoglobin to release cyanide and nitric oxide. Nitric oxide results in vasodilation, either directly or through a related nitrosothiol. Nitric oxide is a potent activator of guanylate cyclase, which is found in vascular smooth muscle and results in increased intracellular cyclic guanosine monophosphate concentrations. Cyclic guanosine monophosphate interferes with calcium entry into vascular smooth muscle cells and may increase calcium uptake by the smooth muscle endoplasmic reticulum. All of these cellular activities result in vasodilation. Nitric oxide is also thought to have a possible direct effect on the myocardium.[32]

Dosage

Nitroprusside is administered intravenously at 0.5–8.0 mcg/kg/min. It may be administered through a peripheral or central intravenous catheter. Doses of 0.2–6.0 mcg/kg/min have been safe and effective in neonates. Due to its rapid onset and elimination, it is readily titrated to clinical effect as long as hypotension does not occur.

Metabolism and Half-Life

Nitroprusside metabolism occurs in the liver and kidney by rhodanase, a mitochondrial enzyme, and the coenzyme vitamin B_{12}. One of the five nitroprusside cyanide ions is inactivated by the formation of methemoglobin, and the remaining four cyanide ions combine with thiosulfate to form thiocyanate. The half-life of nitroprusside is less than 5 minutes. The thiocyanate metabolite is excreted in the urine, with a half-life of 4–7 days.

Adverse Effects

Hypotension is the most direct side effect during nitroprusside administration. Cyanide toxicity may occur if the nitroprusside infusion rate exceeds the rate at which nitroprusside and hydrocyanic acid are metabolized by rhodanase and thiosulfate to thiocyanate. Free cyanide interferes with oxidative phosphorylation by binding to cytochrome oxidase. Despite adequate oxygen delivery, there is metabolic acidosis caused by tissue hypoxia. The mixed venous saturation is elevated due to decreased oxygen consumption. If the thiocyanate metabolite accumulates because of either renal insufficiency or a prolonged high nitroprusside rate of infusion, psychosis, seizures, and abdominal pain may occur. Other side effects include nausea, vomiting, muscle twitching, and apprehension. If nitroprusside causes significant vasodilation, a ventilation-to-perfusion mismatch may occur, resulting in hypoxia.

Monitoring

Invasive arterial monitoring and measurement of serum lactate and thiocyanate levels are recommended during infusion of nitroprusside. Therapeutic thiocyanate levels are between 50 and 100 mg/L.

Pearls

Nitroprusside is light-sensitive, so it must be administered through intravenous tubing that is protected from light. Patients who are especially preload-dependent may require significant volume expansion during infusion of nitroprusside because of the venous vasodilation that occurs with its use. As such, patients should have a large bore intravenous catheter for fluid administration. Development of a metabolic acidosis, especially in the setting of an elevated mixed venous saturation, should alert the clinician to cyanide toxicity. Nitroprusside infusions are prepared with thiosulfate to help prevent cyanide toxicity. When nitroprusside is discontinued, there may be rebound hypertension.

Nitroglycerin

Indications

Nitroglycerin is indicated for the treatment of congestive heart failure. Children with postoperative low cardiac output syndrome after cardiac surgery benefit from nitroglycerin therapy. This is thought to be related to either improved myocardial oxygen supply or decreased myocardial oxygen demand. Nitroglycerin has been used as a pulmonary vasodilator for some children with reactive pulmonary hypertension.[33,34] Nitroglycerin is a coronary vasodilator, which is the basis for its most widely used application for myocardial ischemia in adult medicine. Patients with fixed pulmonary vascular disease, sepsis, and chronic lung disease do not seem to have a favorable response to nitroglycerin. In fact, nitroglycerin has been replaced by nitric oxide therapy in patients with isolated pulmonary hypertension. Finally, nitroglycerin may be used to treat severe systemic hypertension, especially that occurring after cardiac surgery.

Mechanism of Action

The mechanism of action of nitroglycerin is the same as for nitroprusside. The primary clinical effect of nitroglycerin is venous vasodilation, with a lesser effect on the arterioles. As a result, there is decreased preload with low atrial pressures but less of an effect on the blood pressure. Nitroglycerin reduces myocardial oxygen demand by decreasing the left ventricular pressure and the systemic vascular resistance.

Dosage

The continuous infusion of nitroglycerin is started at 0.25-0.5 mcg/kg/min and is titrated to effect by 1-mcg/kg/min increments at 20- to 60-minute time intervals. The standard dose of nitroglycerin is

2-5 mcg/kg/min, but higher doses may be needed for the treatment of pulmonary hypertension. Tolerance to nitrates occurs, often within 24-48 hours of continuous administration, and may be minimized by drug-free periods of 10-12 hours per day.

Metabolism and Half-Life

Nitroglycerin is metabolized by an extensive first-pass effect and has a half-life of 1-4 minutes.

Adverse Effects

As a result of the decreased preload, nitroglycerin may result in lower systemic and pulmonary arterial pressures and reflex tachycardia. Nitroglycerin has less potential for a ventilation-to-perfusion mismatch than nitroprusside. Nitroglycerin is contraindicated in patients using phosphodiesterase-5 inhibitors.

Monitoring

During nitroglycerin infusion, the patient should be monitored for hypotension and tachycardia.

Pearls

Nitroglycerin should not be used in patients with increased intracranial pressure. Nitroglycerin can be absorbed by plastic, so the drug is prepared in glass bottles and is administered through special infusion sets.

Hydralazine

Indications

Hydralazine is approved for children for the treatment of severe hypertension, congestive heart failure, and pulmonary hypertension. Hydralazine has potential clinical benefit in pediatric patients with a large left-to-right shunt, cardiomyopathy, or postoperative hypertension.

Mechanism of Action

Hydralazine is a smooth muscle vasodilator specific to the arterioles. As a result, there is decreased systemic resistance. There is little effect on the venous capacitance.

Dosage

Hydralazine is administered orally at a dose of 0.75-3 mg/kg/day in 2-4 divided doses or intravenously at 0.1-0.5 mg/kg/dose, injected over 1 minute, every 4-6 hours. The dose may be titrated to effect, but the response may be delayed or unpredictable in some patients.

Metabolism and Half-Life

Hydralazine is metabolized primarily in the liver with a small amount of the drug being excreted unchanged by the kidney. The half-life of the drug is 2-8 hours.

Adverse Effects

Side effects of hydralazine include hypotension, headache, nausea, vomiting, tachycardia, drug-induced fever, rash, and a lupus-like syndrome. The drug-induced lupus-like syndrome is more likely to occur with larger doses over a longer period of time. The syndrome may resolve after discontinuation of the drug. Hydralazine may cause sodium and fluid retention.

Monitoring

Particular care should be used when administering hydralazine to patients with pulmonary hypertension because of the possibility of systemic hypotension, and to patients with a cardiomyopathy who might be sensitive to the increased myocardial oxygen demand that accompanies a reflex tachycardia. The blood pressure and heart rate should be followed closely, especially with intravenous use. The antinuclear antibody may be followed during chronic use to assess for the potential of a drug-induced lupus-like syndrome.

Pearls

The combination of hydralazine and isosorbide dinitrate has been associated with decreased morbidity and mortality in patients with congestive heart failure.[35]

Enalaprilat

Indications

Enalaprilat is an intravenous angiotensin-converting enzyme inhibitor that has not been studied in children except for the treatment of hypertensive emergencies. The use of enalaprilat in children for other indications can only be extrapolated from studies of the oral angiotensin-converting enzyme inhibitors.

Mechanism of Action

The angiotensin-converting enzyme inhibitors may be particularly helpful in patients with congestive heart failure who have activation of the renin-angiotensin system. These patients are subject to vasoconstriction and increased afterload. The angiotensin-converting enzyme inhibitors decrease systemic vascular resistance and increase venous capacitance. If the cardiac output can increase to compensate for the lower systemic vascular resistance and decreased filling pressures, then the blood pressure will be maintained.

Dosage

The dose of enalaprilat should be started low and gradually increased. The usual adult dose is 1.25 mg every 6 hours, given over 5 minutes. Infants have been given 5–10 mcg/kg/dose every 8–24 hours for hypertension. The dose is halved for patients with renal insufficiency, existing diuretic therapy, or other reasons to suspect a hypotensive response.

Metabolism and Half-Life

There is a 15-minute onset of action. The drug is almost entirely excreted by the kidney. The half-life is 6–10 hours in young infants and 35–38 hours in adults.

Adverse Effects

Hypotension is the most significant potential adverse effect, especially at high doses or in young infants. Renal insufficiency may occur as a result of inadequate glomerular filtration. Therefore, the angiotensin-converting enzyme inhibitors should be used carefully in patients receiving potassium supplements or potassium-sparing diuretics.

Monitoring

The blood pressure should be monitored carefully while starting therapy with any of the angiotensin-converting enzyme inhibitors.

Pearls

Patients with restrictive cardiac physiology, such as those with constrictive pericarditis, respond poorly to angiotensin-converting enzyme inhibitors because they cannot increase their cardiac output. As a result, the decrease in systemic vascular resistance results in hypotension.

PHARMACOLOGIC AGENTS THAT AFFECT PULMONARY HYPERTENSION

Pulmonary hypertension may occur as a primary condition that is defined as a sustained elevation of the mean pulmonary artery pressure to greater than 25 mmHg at rest without a demonstrable cause. Alternatively, pulmonary hypertension may be associated with left-sided cardiac valvar disease, myocardial disease, congenital heart disease, respiratory disease, connective tissue disease, chronic thromboembolic disease, or pulmonary vascular disease in patients with portal hypertension, human immunodeficiency virus infection, or history of appetite-suppressant drug use.[36-38] Regardless of the cause, pulmonary hypertension is due to increased vascular resistance produced by vasoconstriction, vascular wall remodeling, or thrombosis in situ, or a combination thereof. Because pulmonary hypertension is a progressive disease without a known cure, medical therapy is generally directed at alleviating symptoms with strategies for pulmonary vasodilation. Many of the drugs used for treatment of pulmonary hypertension are administered as an inhaled preparation in an attempt to provide selectivity of the hemodynamic effects to the pulmonary vasculature and to avoid systemic side effects.

Nitric Oxide

Indications

Nitric oxide is a specific pulmonary vasodilator with rapid metabolism of the inhaled preparation. Clinical indications for inhaled nitric oxide therapy in pediatric patients include persistent pulmonary hypertension of the newborn, congenital heart disease complicated by pulmonary hypertension, and postoperative pulmonary hypertension. Due to its rapid onset, patients with pulmonary hypertension who are potential surgical candidates, such as patients with atrioventricular septal defects or total anomalous pulmonary venous connection, can be evaluated acutely for pulmonary vascular reactivity preoperatively with nitric oxide.[39,40] The same evaluation can be performed in patients with pulmonary hypertension (with or without congenital heart disease) to assess for candidacy for heart transplantation alone versus combined heart–lung transplantation.[41] Postoperative pulmonary hypertension is regarded as an effect of inflammatory mediators that are activated by cardiopulmonary bypass, which is utilized in the majority of patients who have surgery for congenital heart disease. Nitric oxide has been shown to be very effective in improving hemodynamics and stabilizing these postoperative cardiac patients.[39,42]

Mechanism of Action

Nitric oxide, an important endothelium-derived relaxation factor, is an endogenously produced vascular smooth muscle relaxant. This vasodilatory effect is strong and can override simultaneous competing sources of pulmonary vasoconstriction.[43] Nitric oxide synthase is responsible for the production of nitric oxide in vascular endothelial cells, as well as at other sites. Nitric oxide activates guanylate cyclase, which increases cyclic guanosine monophosphate and results in the relaxation of vascular smooth muscle through the activity of protein kinases. Nitric oxide is also a bronchodilator.

Dosage

Inhaled nitric oxide therapy is delivered at concentrations of 5–80 ppm through a face mask, a nasal cannula, a conventional ventilator, or a high-frequency oscillator.

Metabolism and Half-Life

Nitric oxide is rapidly inactivated upon binding to hemoglobin and has an affinity to hemoglobin much greater than that for other compounds. The metabolites include methemoglobin, which is reduced to ferrous hemoglobin by methemoglobin reductase. The rapid inactivation prevents inhaled nitric oxide from ever reaching the systemic circulation. As a result, there is no significant systemic vasodilation from inhaled nitric oxide. The half-life is 15–30 seconds.

Adverse Effects

Toxic byproducts of nitric oxide use are methemoglobin and nitric dioxide. Elevated methemoglobin reduces oxygen delivery capacity, and elevated nitric dioxide may result in acute lung injury. Fortunately, studies have demonstrated serum methemoglobin levels that are usually not elevated when drug concentrations are within the typical dosing range, even for moderately prolonged periods of time.[39,41,44] In addition, the currently used doses of nitric oxide have not resulted in the detection of nitric dioxide by current airway monitoring techniques.[45] Other side effects include hypotension, hyperglycemia, and sepsis.

Monitoring

Because methemoglobin and nitric dioxide are metabolites, nitric oxide therapy must be monitored to avoid methemoglobinemia and the formation of nitric dioxide. In addition, respiratory status, including arterial blood gases, blood pressure, blood sugar, and signs and symptoms of infection, should be assessed.

Pearls

Nitric oxide must be administered with special care to patients with left ventricular failure, because the increased preload that occurs with a decrease in pulmonary vascular resistance may not be tolerated by the failing left ventricle.

Prostacyclin

Indications

Because of the rapid onset of action and short half-life, prostacyclin is used to test pulmonary vascular reactivity, particularly during cardiac catheterization. Responders to prostacyclin infusion have a decrease in pulmonary vascular resistance and an increase in cardiac output. Prostacyclin improves hemodynamic characteristics, exercise tolerance, and quality of life, and it was the first therapy to reduce long-term mortality in patients with severe pulmonary hypertension.[46] In addition, these positive effects have been shown to provide long-term benefit in pediatric patients.[47]

Mechanism of Action

Prostacyclin, also referred to as prostaglandin I_2 or epoprostenol, is a potent systemic and pulmonary artery vasodilator. Other properties of prostacyclin that may contribute to its long-term benefit include effects on vascular remodeling and inhibition of platelet aggregation.

Dosage

Therapy is usually started with a low dose of 1–2 ng/kg/min, and the rate of infusion is increased by 1–2 ng/kg/min daily until a positive effect is seen or until hypotension occurs. The dosage range is generally between 2 and 20 ng/kg/min, with studies reporting an effective dose of 5 ng/kg/min.[48,49] Most patients reach a plateau dose above which little additional benefit is achieved, but the ultimate effective dose is highly individual.

Metabolism and Half-Life
The half-life is 3–5 minutes. As a result, the medication can be titrated to clinical effect. The short half-life necessitates administration by a continuous infusion. This is achieved by using a portable infusion pump and a permanent indwelling central venous catheter. Prostacyclin cannot be administered orally because it is inactivated by the acidic stomach environment.

Adverse Effects
As a result of its nonselective arterial effects on the systemic and pulmonary vasculature, prostacyclin can result in profound hypotension. Over the long term, prostacyclin can result in edema, hypoxia, diarrhea, flushing, headache, nausea, vomiting, rash, and jaw pain. The long-term use of prostacyclin requires an indwelling central venous catheter, which increases the risk of infection and thrombosis. Interruption of the infusion may result in the immediate return of life-threatening symptoms.

Monitoring
Because of the nonselective arterial vasodilation properties, invasive blood pressure monitoring is essential during the initiation of infusion of prostacyclin.

Pearls
Because of tachyphylaxis, the prostacyclin infusion usually requires escalating doses. Once an effective dose is achieved, the rate is empirically increased by 1- to 2-ng/kg/min increments weekly over the long term.

Iloprost

Indications
Iloprost is indicated for the treatment of moderate to severe primary and secondary pulmonary hypertension. Open-label uncontrolled studies of patients with severe pulmonary hypertension and congestive heart failure show that long-term use of aerosolized iloprost results in clinical improvement.[50,51] Both hemodynamic values and exercise capacity are improved. Information regarding the use of iloprost in pediatric patients is limited. Iloprost is currently not approved and not available in the United States.

Mechanism of Action
Iloprost is a stable analogue of prostacyclin that, when delivered in the aerosolized form, is as potent as prostacyclin but has effects that last two to six times longer. Iloprost differs from prostacyclin in that iloprost is a selective pulmonary vasodilator.

Dosage
Iloprost is aerosolized by a nebulizer in doses of 2.5–5.0 mcg at a frequency of six to nine times per day over 10–15 minutes. It is also available as an intravenous infusion in a dose of 0.5–2.0 ng/kg/min, to run over 6 hours per day.

Metabolism and Half-Life
Iloprost has better chemical stability than other prostacyclin analogues. The half-life is 20–25 minutes.

Adverse Effects
Systemic side effects from inhaled iloprost are uncommon and include cough, headache, flushing, and hypotension.

Monitoring
Patients receiving iloprost should be monitored for systemic hemodynamic effects, especially hypotension. This is most relevant for acute therapy.

Pearls
The inhaled administration of iloprost decreases the incidence of systemic side effects and intravenous catheter complications. In addition, this route also allows adequate delivery of the drug with clinical effect in patients with intrapulmonary right-to-left shunts. However, the frequency of inhaled therapy is a potential limitation for clinical application.

Bosentan

Indications
Bosentan is a new, potentially effective treatment for pulmonary hypertension. It is administered orally, thus avoiding many of the problems and risks of therapies that are delivered by continuous intravenous infusion. It appears to be well tolerated, but pediatric experience is very limited. The drug is not yet approved for pediatric use.

Mechanism of Action
Bosentan is an oral antagonist of the vascular endothelial and smooth muscle endothelin (ET_A and ET_B) receptors. This is important as endothelin-1 is a potent vasoconstrictor and a smooth-muscle mitogen. Bosentan has been shown to improve exercise capacity and cardiopulmonary hemodynamics and to decrease the rate of clinical deterioration in patients with pulmonary arterial hypertension.[52,53]

Dosage

The recommended oral dose of bosentan is 62.5–250 mg twice daily, with the lower end of the dose range used initially followed by upward titration as tolerated. There is limited pediatric data, but one recent pediatric pharmacokinetic study demonstrated that doses of 31.25–125 mg appear to be safe and effective.[54] The use and possible dose adjustment of bosentan should be carefully considered in patients with hepatic impairment. In patients with baseline moderate to severe hepatic insufficiency, bosentan should be avoided. When discontinuing the drug, the dose should be weaned to avoid clinical deterioration.

Metabolism and Half-Life

Bosentan is metabolized almost exclusively in the liver through the cytochrome P450 enzyme pathway. The half-life of the drug is 5 hours. One of the three metabolites remains active. Bosentan may decrease cyclosporine levels by 50% through enhanced drug metabolism, whereas cyclosporine use increases serum bosentan levels. Therefore, simultaneous cyclosporine use is contraindicated. Many drugs that affect the hepatic cytochrome P450 enzyme pathway alter bosentan levels. Some of these drugs include phenobarbital, phenytoin, sulfonamides, nonsteroidal anti-inflammatory agents, azole antifungals, erythromycin, propofol, and verapamil. Bosentan may increase the metabolism of warfarin.

Adverse Effects

Side effects of bosentan include anemia, fluid retention and edema, transaminase elevation, headache, flushing, hypotension, palpitations, and pruritus. Fluid retention may exacerbate symptoms of congestive heart failure. As bosentan has produced major birth defects in animal studies, bosentan administration is contraindicated during pregnancy. In addition, the efficacy of hormonal contraception may be decreased, necessitating the use of an alternative form of birth control.

Monitoring

Hepatic function should be monitored closely and the medication should be discontinued if there is a rise in transaminases, an elevation of serum bilirubin, or symptoms of jaundice, nausea, vomiting, abdominal pain, or fever. The hemoglobin should be monitored, and the international normalized ratio (INR) should be followed in patients taking warfarin. A negative pregnancy test must be documented before starting treatment in women.

Pearls

Bosentan is currently available only through limited distribution directly from the manufacturer.

Sildenafil

Indications

Sildenafil is used for treatment of pulmonary hypertension on an investigational basis. It appears to have a beneficial effect on the pulmonary vascular smooth muscle, resulting in a decrease in pulmonary vascular resistance. Hemodynamic effects usually include a mild drop in blood pressure without a significant change in heart rate.

Mechanism of Action

Sildenafil is a phosphodiesterase type 5 enzyme inhibitor. Since the enzyme is responsible for the degradation of cyclic guanosine monophosphate, decreased enzyme activity results in increased cyclic guanosine monophosphate levels and vascular smooth muscle relaxation. Cyclic guanosine monophosphate levels are mediated by nitric oxide.

Dosage

Sildenafil is available in the oral form only. The adult dose for pulmonary hypertension is 25 mg twice daily, but dosages up to 100 mg five times per day have been used. The usual starting pediatric dosage is 0.5–1.0 mg/kg/day, divided into three to four doses. The dose is then increased to effect. Dosage may need to be adjusted in cases of hepatic failure, renal insufficiency, or when other drugs that interfere with metabolism are being used.

Metabolism and Half-Life

Sildenafil has an onset of action within 60 minutes and has a half-life of 4 hours. It is metabolized through the cytochrome P450 enzyme pathway in the liver. There is a small amount of drug that is eliminated by the kidneys. Important drug interactions include medications that can potentiate the effects of hypotension, such as nitrates, α-receptor blockers, and other vasodilators. Other medications that can increase sildenafil effects by interfering with metabolism and by raising serum levels include the macrolide antibiotics, azole antifungals, protease inhibitors, propofol, verapamil, and quinidine.

Adverse Effects

Because side effects of sildenafil include hypotension, the simultaneous use with other vasodilators should be avoided. Other side effects include headache, dyspepsia, vision changes, flushing, dizziness, and rash.

Monitoring

The most important parameter to be monitored during the administration of sildenafil is blood pressure, especially in cases of hypovolemia, congestive heart failure, or simultaneous use of other drugs that can cause hypotension.

Pearls

Because of the potential vasodilator effects, sildenafil may not be tolerated in patients with primary pulmonary hypertension who have congestive heart failure since the drug may provoke hypotension, especially when hypovolemia is present.

VASOCONSTRICTORS

There are few pure vasoconstrictors in clinical use. Most medications that have a vasoconstrictor effect also have other simultaneous effects. The nearly pure α-adrenergic receptor effect of phenylephrine places it in a category of its own. It is a particularly helpful clinical tool in specific clinical situations that include hypotension, vascular collapse in shock, and hypercyanotic episodes in tetralogy of Fallot.

Another vasoconstrictor with poorly defined utility in pediatrics is vasopressin. Vasopressin, or antidiuretic hormone, is a neuropeptide secreted during serum hyperosmolality or hypovolemia. At low concentrations, vasopressin causes water retention, but at high concentrations it causes vasoconstriction. Postoperative pediatric cardiac surgery patients with adequate cardiac function and vasodilatory shock that is refractory to the usual inotropes have a significantly increased systemic blood pressure during vasopressin infusion.[55]

Phenylephrine

Indications

The most common use of phenylephrine in pediatric cardiology is to reverse and to treat hypercyanotic episodes in patients with tetralogy of Fallot. The increase in systemic vascular resistance, in excess of the pulmonary vascular resistance, decreases the right-to-left shunt at the ventricular septal defect, which increases pulmonary blood flow, and improves arterial oxygenation. Historically, phenylephrine was used to treat atrioventricular reciprocating supraventricular tachycardia by blocking the atrioventricular node and terminating the arrhythmia. This occurs through parasympathetic input to the heart, which is increased when the vasoconstrictor causes systemic hypertension. In a more general sense, phenylephrine is used to treat hypotension and shock caused by peripheral vasodilation.

Mechanism of Action

Phenylephrine is a potent systemic vasoconstrictor because of its α-1–receptor agonist activity. It has essentially no β-receptor effect. As a result of its greater systemic effect, phenylephrine increases systemic vascular resistance and systemic arterial pressure more than pulmonary vascular resistance and pulmonary arterial pressure. There may be a reflex bradycardia during the administration of phenylephrine.

Dosage

Phenylephrine is administered intravenously in a bolus dose of 5–20 mcg/kg every 15 minutes as needed, followed by a continuous infusion at 0.1–0.5 mcg/kg/min. Phenylephrine can also be given through the intramuscular or subcutaneous route at a dose of 0.1 mg/kg/dose every 1–2 hours, as needed.

Metabolism and Half-Life

Phenylephrine is metabolized in the liver and is excreted in the urine. The half-life of the drug is 2.5 hours, but it is longer after a long-term infusion.

Adverse Effects

The most significant side effect seen with phenylephrine is the reflex bradycardia. Other side effects include hypertension, ventricular ectopy, chest pain, headache, tremors, metabolic acidosis, and decreased renal output.

Monitoring

Monitoring of the blood pressure and heart rate are obviously most important. The intravenous catheter site should be watched carefully during a phenylephrine infusion as extravasation of the drug may lead to necrosis.

Pearls

Phenylephrine should not be the primary therapy in patients with hypotension caused by aortic valve dysfunction. The increased afterload in this situation could exacerbate the aortic valve disease. Hypovolemia should be treated with volume expansion before the consideration of phenylephrine.

CONGESTIVE HEART FAILURE

Congestive heart failure may be the result of a variety of underlying conditions, and each condition may have a very specific therapy that is inappropriate in another situation. There are several fundamental principles to consider across the spectrum of causes of heart failure. Therapy is generally directed at improving pump function, decreasing the workload, and limiting salt and water retention. Current strategies include improvement of cardiac performance with digitalis and other inotropic agents, decreasing preload with diuretics, and decreasing afterload with vasodilators or angiotensin-converting enzyme inhibitors. The diuretics, angiotensin-converting enzyme inhibitors, and angiotensin

II receptor blockers are discussed below. Finally, certain β-blockers have been shown to improve morbidity and mortality in patients with mild to moderate heart failure. Guidelines now recommend β-blocker therapy for all patients with New York Heart Association Class II–III heart failure who are clinically stable with standard therapy.[56]

DIURETICS

Diuretics have been a mainstay of anticongestive therapy for many years as they improve signs and symptoms of congestion and pulmonary edema by decreasing preload. Their role in patients with congestive heart failure is based on the fact that sodium retention results in volume expansion. Diuretic efficacy depends on the delivery of salt and water to the renal tubule. There are three general classes of diuretics: loop diuretics, thiazide diuretics, and potassium-sparing diuretics (Table 13-2). The loop diuretics are the ones most commonly used in pediatric patients and act in the loop of Henle. Loop diuretics inhibit the chloride–sodium–potassium cotransporter in the ascending loop of Henle. Water is excreted as a result of the decreased reabsorption of electrolytes. Increasing doses of the loop diuretics result in an increased diuresis until a maximum effect is achieved. This concept is true of the individual loop diuretics as well as combination loop diuretic therapy. Therefore, the simultaneous use of multiple loop diuretics is usually not helpful and is not recommended. The thiazide diuretics act by inhibiting sodium and chloride transport

in the distal convoluted tubule. Spironolactone is the most commonly used potassium-sparing diuretic in pediatric patients and acts by competitively inhibiting aldosterone. In general, all diuretics should be used with caution with respect to intravascular volume status and electrolyte balance. The use of diuretics in combination with other antihypertensive agents or angiotensin-converting enzyme inhibitors may result in hypotension, volume depletion, and renal insufficiency.

Furosemide

Indications
Furosemide is an established first-line diuretic used most commonly for treatment of acute and chronic congestive heart failure, pulmonary edema, and diuresis in the patient who has recently had cardiac surgery.

Mechanism of Action
As a loop diuretic, furosemide prevents reabsorption of approximately 25% of the filtered sodium. Water is then excreted along with the sodium. Furosemide also increases renal blood flow, increases renin release, and reduces renal vascular resistance, primarily through the stimulation of renal prostaglandins. Furosemide also has direct pulmonary effects and reduces pulmonary transvascular fluid filtration. Finally, furosemide promotes venodilation and preload reduction.

Dosage
Furosemide may be administered either intravenously or orally. Intravenous use is usually as a bolus, but infusions may be particularly useful for increasing net drug effect and for allowing diuresis in patients who are hypotensive. Intravenous furosemide is usually given as a 1-mg/kg/dose bolus. Larger doses may be used in refractory cases, and patients with poor cardiac output generally need higher doses. The oral maintenance dose is 2–6 mg/kg/day in two to three divided doses. The drug dosage must be adjusted in patients with renal or hepatic disease. Due to decreased luminal excretion in patients with renal insufficiency, doses as high as 250–2000 mg may be needed to achieve the desired effect. In young and premature infants who have immature renal function, it is recommended that lower doses be used to avoid toxicity. The drug should be avoided in oliguric or anuric patients. Furosemide is not dialyzed, so additional doses should not be given in those patients.

Metabolism and Half-Life
Furosemide is excreted in the kidneys. The drug half-life is 8 hours in infants, 1 hour in adults, and up to 20 hours in premature infants.

Table 13-2 Diuretics		
Drug	**Site of Action**	**Effects**
Furosemide	Loop of Henle	Inhibits sodium absorption, increases potassium excretion
Ethacrynic acid	Loop of Henle	Inhibits sodium absorption, increases potassium excretion
Bumetanide	Loop of Henle	Inhibits sodium absorption, Increases potassium excretion
Thiazides	Early distal tubule	Inhibits sodium absorption, Increases potassium excretion
Metolazone	Proximal tubule, early distal tubule	Inhibits sodium absorption, Increases potassium excretion
Spironolactone	Late distal tubule	Inhibits sodium absorption, Decreased potassium excretion

Adverse Effects

Side effects of furosemide include hypovolemia, electrolyte abnormalities, and ototoxicity. Hypovolemia can aggravate an already low cardiac output. Hypokalemia is usually not a significant problem during chronic outpatient use, but higher oral doses and aggressive intravenous dosing should be accompanied by monitoring of serum electrolytes, possible potassium chloride supplementation, or the addition of a potassium-sparing diuretic. Hyponatremia in patients with congestive heart failure is usually dilutional, but chronic furosemide use may result in decreased total body sodium levels. In this situation, water restriction may be necessary. Chronic furosemide use frequently results in a hypochloremic metabolic alkalosis. In that situation, carbonic anhydrase inhibitors, such as acetazolamide, can be helpful by interfering with bicarbonate reabsorption and acting as a weak diuretic. Potassium chloride and ammonium chloride supplementation should be considered. Hyperuricemia can occur and pediatric patients can develop nephrocalcinosis. Other side effects include dermatitis, nausea, vomiting, hyperglycemia, and anemia.

Monitoring

Patients receiving furosemide should have serum electrolyte concentrations followed and renal function assessed, especially during aggressive intravenous diuresis. Premature babies and young infants with immature renal function and those who receive large doses of furosemide should have their hearing screened in follow-up.

Pearls

Furosemide should be used sparingly in patients with renal dysfunction, particularly in premature infants with immature kidney function. Patients who are receiving other ototoxic medications, such as aminoglycosides, should be prescribed furosemide with particular attention to additive effects. Furosemide may precipitate digitalis toxicity both by decreasing renal excretion in cases of hypovolemia and by causing hypokalemia.

Ethacrynic Acid

Indications

Ethacrynic acid is used less commonly than furosemide and is generally used after a failed response to other diuretics in patients with edema caused by congestive heart failure or renal disease. It can also be used to treat ascites and pulmonary edema from other causes. It is sometimes used in conjunction with other loop diuretics.

Mechanism of Action

As a loop diuretic, ethacrynic acid interferes with sodium and chloride reabsorption in the ascending loop of Henle. This occurs through interference with the chloride-binding cotransport system. As a result, there is increased urinary excretion of water, sodium, and chloride.

Dosage

Ethacrynic acid may be administered orally or intravenously. The adult oral dose is 25–100 mg/dose and may be given once or twice per day. Increasing incremental doses, up to 200 mg twice daily, may be needed in the most severe cases. The dose for children is 1 mg/kg/dose once daily and may be increased to 3 mg/kg/day. The intravenous dose is 0.5–1.0 mg/kg/dose, to a maximum of 100 mg/dose, and may be repeated every 8–12 hours. The intravenous form should be infused over several minutes.

Metabolism and Half-Life

Ethacrynic acid is metabolized in the liver to an active metabolite and is excreted in the urine and stool. The half-life of the drug is 2–4 hours. Ethacrynic acid is not removed by hemodialysis or peritoneal dialysis.

Adverse Effects

Side effects of ethacrynic acid include headache, dizziness, fatigue, rash, electrolyte abnormalities, hypovolemia, anorexia, abdominal pain, renal insufficiency, hematuria, agranulocytosis, and jaundice. Ethacrynic acid is associated with a higher incidence of ototoxicity than the other loop diuretics. It may be necessary to administer supplemental potassium while treating with ethacrynic acid.

Monitoring

Electrolytes, renal function, blood pressure, and intravascular volume status should all be monitored during the use of ethacrynic acid.

Pearls

Ethacrynic acid, unlike the other loop diuretics, has no cross-reactivity to sulfonamides. Therefore, the drug may be used in patients who are sulfa allergic. Ethacrynic acid may have a synergistic effect with the thiazide diuretics. Intravenous ethacrynic acid has the potential to be irritating and may cause thrombophlebitis.

Bumetanide

Indications

Bumetanide is a relatively new and more potent loop diuretic that has had increased use in pediatric patients, especially in those with refractory heart failure. It is used to manage hypertension and fluid retention caused by heart failure, renal insufficiency, or hepatic dysfunction.

Mechanism of Action

The mechanism of action and effects of bumetanide are similar to those of furosemide. The drug increases urinary excretion of water, sodium, and chloride by inhibiting reabsorption of sodium and chloride through interference with the chloride-binding cotransport system in the ascending loop of Henle.

Dosage

Bumetanide can be administered orally or intravenously. Bumetanide is thought to be approximately 40-70 times more potent than furosemide. The usual adult oral dose is 0.5-2.0 mg and may be given once or twice per day. The intravenous dose of 0.5-3 mg is given over 1-2 minutes and can be repeated every 2-3 hours, with a maximum total daily dose of 10 mg. For infants and children, an oral dose of 0.015-0.1 mg/kg/dose may be given every 6-24 hours, with a maximum total daily dose of 10 mg. Patients with hepatic disease may require a reduced dose, whereas patients with renal insufficiency may need a larger dose to achieve the same therapeutic effect.

Metabolism and Half-Life

Bumetanide is partially metabolized by the liver and is excreted in the urine as drug and metabolite. The half-life of bumetanide is variable, depending on patient age: neonates, approximately 6 hours; infants, approximately 2.4 hours; and adults, 1.0-1.5 hours.

Adverse Effects

The side effects of bumetanide are similar to those of furosemide.

Renal toxicity from bumetanide may be more than is seen with furosemide. The simultaneous use of antihypertensive agents may result in hypotension. Bumetanide can increase the serum bilirubin concentration, so neonates at risk for kernicterus should not receive the drug. Patients with a sulfonamide allergy may be more sensitive to bumetanide, but an allergy to furosemide does not preclude the use of bumetanide.

Monitoring

Because bumetanide is such a potent diuretic, patients should be monitored for electrolyte abnormalities, volume depletion, and associated clinical signs and symptoms. Specifically, the blood pressure, serum electrolytes, and renal function should be assessed. Patients with hepatic dysfunction should be monitored with particular caution.

Pearls

The use of other potentially nephrotoxic or ototoxic drugs should be avoided when bumetanide is being administered. Currently, bumetanide is used as a second-line loop diuretic unless there is specific reason to avoid furosemide, such as allergy or ototoxicity.

Chlorothiazide and Hydrochlorothiazide

Indications

The thiazide diuretics have been available for many years. The two thiazide diuretics most commonly used in pediatric patients are chlorothiazide and hydrochlorothiazide. They are similar in structure, mechanism of action, and side effects. They differ in dosage, absorption, and excretion. They are both used for the management of hypertension and edema secondary to congestive heart failure or nephrotic syndrome. There may be a synergistic effect with angiotensin-converting enzyme inhibitors or β-blockers when they are used to treat hypertension.

Mechanism of Action

The thiazide diuretics inhibit sodium reabsorption in the distal convoluted tubule, resulting in increased sodium, potassium, and water excretion. Hydrochlorothiazide is the more potent of the two thiazides.

Dosage

Intravenous and oral doses of chlorothiazide are equivalent according to the manufacturer, but intravenous dosing has not been well established in children. The recommended oral dose of chlorothiazide is 250-1000 mg or 10-50 mg/kg/day in two divided doses. The intravenous dose of chlorothiazide is 2-8 mg/kg/day in two divided doses. Hydrochlorothiazide is available only in an oral preparation at a dose of 25-100 mg/day in one to two doses for congestive heart failure and 12.5-50 mg/day for hypertension. For children, the dose is 2-3 mg/kg/day in two divided doses. Chlorothiazide may be preferred in young pediatric patients since there is a suspension formula available.

Metabolism and Half-Life

Chlorothiazide is excreted unchanged in the urine and has a half-life of 1-2 hours. Hydrochlorothiazide is also excreted unchanged in the urine but has a longer half-life of 5.6-14.8 hours.

Adverse Effects

Side effects of the thiazide diuretics include hypotension, hypokalemia, hyponatremia, hypochloremic alkalosis, and hyperuricemia. Adult patients may have elevation of cholesterol and triglyceride levels. A risk of cross-reaction exists in patients with sulfonamide allergy. The thiazides may activate or exacerbate systemic lupus erythematosus. Other rare side effects of thiazide diuretics include intrahepatic jaundice, photosensitivity, pancreatitis, blood dyscrasias, pneumonitis, and interstitial nephritis.

Monitoring

Serum electrolytes, renal function, blood pressure, and intravascular volume status should all be monitored during the administration of thiazide diuretics.

Pearls

The use of thiazide diuretics may result in more severe hypotension if they are administered in combination with angiotensin-converting enzyme inhibitors or in patients who are hypovolemic for any reason. The serum potassium and intravascular volume status should be assessed before the administration of a thiazide diuretic.

Metolazone

Indications

Metolazone is used to treat hypertension and symptoms related to fluid retention in patients with congestive heart failure and nephrotic syndrome. Metolazone appears to be particularly effective in patients with impaired renal function. Metolazone is used for refractory cases and may be synergistic with furosemide, resulting in marked diuresis, hypovolemia, and electrolyte abnormalities.

Mechanism of Action

Although metolazone does not have the same structure as the other thiazide diuretics, it increases the excretion of sodium, potassium, and water by inhibiting sodium reabsorption in the distal and proximal convoluted tubule.

Dosage

In adults, metolazone is administered orally in a dose of 2.5–5 mg every 24 hours. For children, the dose is generally 1 mg daily for toddlers and preschool-age children, 2.5 mg for school-age children, and 5 mg for adolescents and young adults.

Metabolism and Half-Life

Metolazone undergoes enterohepatic recirculation and is excreted primarily in the urine. The dose may need to be adjusted for patients with severe hepatic dysfunction or renal impairment. The drug should be used with caution in patients with elevated serum cholesterol levels. Loop diuretics may increase the effect of metolazone, whereas nonsteroidal anti-inflammatory drugs can decrease the efficacy of thiazide diuretics. The half-life of metolazone is dependent on renal function and varies between 6 and 20 hours. The drug is not dialyzable.

Adverse Effects

Side effects of metolazone include electrolyte disturbances, dizziness and orthostatic hypotension, palpitations, headache, fatigue, rash, nausea, vomiting, cough, photosensitivity, and exacerbation or activation of systemic lupus erythematosus. A risk of cross-reaction exists in patients with sulfonamide allergy because of the chemical similarities of the compounds.

Monitoring

Serum electrolytes, including potassium, sodium, chloride, and bicarbonate, should be monitored. In addition, renal function and orthostatic vital signs should be measured on a regular basis.

Pearls

Because loop diuretics may enhance the effects of metolazone, the two drugs are sometimes used together for better diuresis, especially in patients who are refractory to single-diuretic therapy. However, profound hypovolemia may occur.

Spironolactone

Indications

Spironolactone is the most commonly used potassium-sparing drug in pediatric patients. It is used to treat edema and hypertension, especially in combination with other diuretics that result in hypokalemia. Its utility as an adjunct to therapy for congestive heart failure was appreciated when the Randomized Aldactone Evaluation Study (RALES) showed that spironolactone, an aldosterone receptor antagonist, reduced the risk of morbidity and death among patients with severe heart failure who were treated with maximal standard therapy. The 30% mortality reduction was due to a lower risk of death from progressive heart failure and sudden death from cardiac causes. This finding was attributed to speculation that aldosterone receptor antagonism prevented sodium retention and myocardial fibrosis.[57]

Mechanism of Action

Spironolactone acts by inhibiting aldosterone. The blocked aldosterone receptor in the distal renal tubule prevents aldosterone effects and results in decreased sodium absorption and decreased potassium secretion in the distal tubule. Because it is the weakest of the diuretics, spironolactone is usually used in combination with a loop diuretic or a thiazide diuretic.

Dosage

Spironolactone is an oral medication and should be administered once a day in a dose of 1–2 mg/kg/day. Patients in the RALES trial received a dose of 25 mg/day along with standard maximal therapy for heart failure, including an angiotensin-converting enzyme inhibitor, diuretic, and sometimes digoxin.

Metabolism and Half-Life

Spironolactone is metabolized both in the liver and kidney. The half-life of spironolactone is 78–84 minutes.

Adverse Effects

The most significant side effect is hyperkalemia, which does not usually become a problem except in cases of renal dysfunction, liver dysfunction, or potassium supplementation. Due to the risk of hyperkalemia, spironolactone should be used carefully in combination with angiotensin-converting enzyme inhibitors. Spironolactone may cause gynecomastia, which is related to dose and duration of therapy. Other side effects include lethargy, headache, rash, hyponatremia, impotence, anorexia, gastritis, and agranulocytosis.

Monitoring

Blood volume status and electrolyte monitoring, especially of the serum potassium, is important during the administration of spironolactone.

Pearls

Patients who are prescribed spironolactone should not receive potassium supplements, potassium-containing salt substitutes, a potassium-rich diet, or other drugs that can cause hyperkalemia.

ANGIOTENSIN-CONVERTING ENZYME INHIBITORS

The angiotensin-converting enzyme (ACE) inhibitors have become more widely used for the treatment of hypertension and congestive heart failure. Adult studies have confirmed their utility, especially in comparison to other, more conventional, vasodilators.[58,59] Use in the pediatric population has increased over the last decade. The group of drugs acts by inhibiting the conversion of angiotensin I to angiotensin II by interfering with the converting enzyme. The angiotensin-converting enzyme inhibitors also reduce the inactivation of bradykinins and decrease aldosterone production, both of which ultimately enhance vasodilation. As a result, this class of medications results in decreased systemic vascular resistance, lower systemic blood pressure, and increased venous capacitance. Captopril and enalapril are the most commonly used angiotensin-converting enzyme inhibitors in children, but others are also available with less pediatric clinical experience.

Captopril

Indications

Captopril was the first widely available angiotensin-converting enzyme inhibitor and is used for hypertension and afterload reduction. Patients with congestive heart failure due to a left-to-right shunt, dilated cardiomyopathy, or diastolic dysfunction may benefit.[60–62] Some investigators have proposed that single ventricle patients may also benefit, but no corroborative data currently exist.

Mechanism of Action

As a competitive inhibitor of the angiotensin-converting enzyme, captopril prevents conversion of angiotensin I to angiotensin II. Because angiotensin II is a potent vasoconstrictor, captopril reduces systemic vascular resistance and increases venous capacitance, resulting in increased cardiac output and decreased filling pressures. Captopril decreases the pulmonary vascular resistance, increases renal blood flow, reduces aldosterone production, and minimally affects heart rate.

Dosage

Captopril is available for oral administration with a recommended dose of 0.5–3.0 mg/kg/day, divided into three doses. The dose is titrated to effect with a maximum dose of 6 mg/kg/day. Initially, a smaller test dose is usually given in order to determine whether the effect on the blood pressure will allow the patient to tolerate the medication.

Metabolism and Half-Life

Captopril is primarily excreted by the kidney, with a half-life of 2 hours. The half-life is longer in patients with congestive heart failure.

Adverse Effects

The most important side effect of captopril is hypotension, especially in patients with congestive heart failure and in those taking diuretics. One of the most common and troublesome side effects is cough, which is due to an increased sensitivity of the cough reflex, resulting in a dry, irritating, nonproductive cough. The cough may be mediated by bradykinins and prostaglandins. The cough can be relieved by the calcium antagonist nifedipine, nonsteroidal anti-inflammatory agents, or time.[63,64] Renal failure can occur and is precipitated by hypotension, congestive heart failure, and renal artery disease. This is usually a reversible process, but captopril is contraindicated in patients with bilateral renal artery stenosis. Hyperkalemia may occur as a result of potassium retention, especially when potassium-sparing diuretics are being used or in patients with renal insufficiency. Neutropenia seems to be most frequently associated with high-dose captopril use in patients with renal failure or collagen vascular disease. Captopril can cause potentially life-threatening angioedema and is contraindicated in pregnancy.

Monitoring

Blood pressure monitoring is mandatory for 2–4 hours after a dose, especially around the time of the test dose.

In addition, the neutrophil count, renal function, serum potassium, and baseline pregnancy test should be documented and followed.

Pearls
Because the duration of action of captopril is shorter than that of other angiotensin-converting enzyme inhibitors, the drug must be administered three times per day.

Enalapril

Indications
Enalapril is similar to captopril and has been extensively studied in heart failure trials. Enalapril was originally shown to decrease mortality in patients with severe heart failure when added to a prior treatment regimen of digoxin and diuretics.[65] Subsequently, enalapril has been shown to decrease morbidity and mortality in patients with symptomatic and asymptomatic ventricular dysfunction by decreasing the number of hospitalizations and slowing progression to congestive heart failure.[66,67] The most significant differences from captopril include a longer half-life and a slower onset of action, caused by the necessary hydrolysis in the liver of the prodrug to the active form, enalaprilat. The most significant structural difference, compared with captopril, is the absence of the SH group. Enalapril is effective for the treatment of hypertension and congestive heart failure in pediatric patients and is being studied for these indications in neonates and young infants.[68-70]

Mechanism of Action
As a competitive inhibitor of the angiotensin-converting enzyme, enalapril prevents conversion of angiotensin I to angiotensin II. Because angiotensin II is a potent vasoconstrictor, enalapril reduces systemic vascular resistance and increases venous capacitance, resulting in increased cardiac output and decreased filling pressures. Due to the lower angiotensin II levels, there is an increase in plasma renin activity and a reduction of aldosterone secretion.

Dosage
As with captopril, a test dose is recommended. For hypertension, the recommended starting dose is 0.08 mg/kg, with a maximum dose of 5 mg daily. This dose may be titrated to effect, as tolerated. For congestive heart failure, the dosage is 0.1 mg/kg/day, with an increase, as needed, to 0.5 mg/kg/day over 2 weeks. Dosing for the treatment of heart failure should be twice daily. The dose should be lower in patients with renal insufficiency. In addition, these patients should begin therapy with a single daily dose, which may be increased as needed and as tolerated.

Metabolism and Half-Life
The therapeutic effect of enalapril depends on hepatic function since the prodrug must be hydrolyzed to the active form, enalaprilat. Therefore, in patients with hepatic failure, the dose may need to be increased. The peak serum concentration is 2 hours after administration and nearly all of the drug and active metabolite is excreted by the kidney. The half-life is 2 hours and is longer in patients with congestive heart failure.

Adverse Effects
Many of the side effects of enalapril are similar to those encountered with captopril. Cough, hypotension, renal insufficiency, neutropenia, and angioedema have been reported. Enalapril may be safer with respect to skin rash. In addition, the immune-based adverse effects may be less common due to the absence of the SH group. As with captopril, enalapril is contraindicated in patients with bilateral renal artery stenosis and in pregnancy.

Monitoring
Blood pressure monitoring is mandatory, especially around the time of the test dose. In addition, the neutrophil count, renal function, serum potassium, and baseline pregnancy test should be documented and followed.

Pearls
Enalapril may induce severe hypotension in patients who are sodium or volume depleted. Enalapril may cause a significant rise in serum potassium and creatinine, especially in those with bilateral renal artery stenosis.

ANGIOTENSIN II RECEPTOR BLOCKERS

The angiotensin II receptor blockers are selective antagonists of the angiotensin II type 1 (AT1) receptor. This interferes with the action of angiotensin II on vascular smooth muscle and its adverse effects on cardiovascular remodeling. Because the angiotensin II receptor blockers act primarily at the AT1 receptor and are independent of the pathway by which angiotensin II is generated, they have a distinctly different mechanism from the angiotensin-converting enzyme inhibitors (Fig. 13-1). In the presence of an angiotensin II receptor blocker, the angiotensin II that this inhibited from binding to the AT1 receptor is then available to bind to the AT2 receptor. The AT2 receptor has its own beneficial cardiovascular effects, such as vasodilation, improved endothelial function, and decreased renal tubular sodium reabsorption. Candesartan is the drug in this group with the greatest binding affinity to the AT1 receptor.

The angiotensin II receptor blockers are thought to be an appropriate therapy for hypertension in patients with diabetes, chronic kidney disease, left ventricular

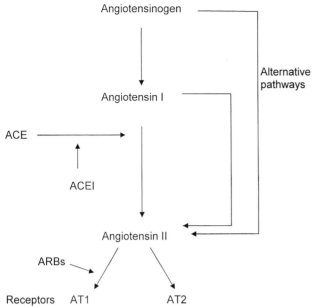

Figure 13-1   Angiotensin II generation pathways. *ACE,* Angiotensin converting enzyme; *ACEI,* angiotensin-converting enzyme inhibitor; *ARB,* angiotensin receptor blocker; *AT1,* angiotensin II type 1 receptors; *AT2,* angiotensin II type 2 receptors.

hypertrophy, and heart failure. In addition, recent multi-center studies in adult patients with heart failure have demonstrated reduced cardiovascular morbidity and mortality with losartan, candesartan, and valsartan. As a group, the drugs appear to be as effective as the angiotensin-converting enzyme inhibitors in patients with heart failure and myocardial infarction.[71-74] Valsartan has been shown to be beneficial in cardiac remodeling by improving left ventricular structure and function.[75]

Despite their promising clinical applications, the angiotensin II receptor blockers should not replace the angiotensin-converting enzyme inhibitors in the treatment of heart failure, but they may be used in patients who are intolerant to the angiotensin-converting enzyme inhibitors. The angiotensin II receptor antagonists seem not to result in as much cough and angioedema as the angiotensin-converting enzyme inhibitors. This may be because they cause more complete inhibition of the renin-angiotensin system, resulting in less of an effect on the response to bradykinin. Therefore, the cough and angioedema associated with the use of angiotensin-converting enzyme inhibitors, which are thought to be related to bradykinin, are less likely to occur with angiotensin II receptor blockers. However, there are reports of patients who have had angioedema related to both angiotensin-converting enzyme inhibitors and angiotensin II receptor blockers. The current strategy is to treat heart failure patients with angiotensin-converting enzyme inhibitors as first-line agents. Angiotensin II receptor blockers remain avail-

able as good alternatives for patients who are intolerant of angiotensin-converting enzyme inhibitors and may be helpful in some patients as a second-line therapy that can be used in combination with diuretics, β-blockers, and digoxin.

Losartan

Indications
Losartan is used for the treatment of hypertension and diabetic nephropathy with hypertension. It was recently approved by the Federal Drug Administration to reduce the risk of stroke in patients with hypertension and left ventricular hypertrophy.

Mechanism of Action
Losartan is a selective, competitive angiotensin II receptor antagonist. Losartan blocks the effects of angiotensin II, which include vasoconstriction and aldosterone secretion. It is a selective angiotensin II receptor blocker with a greater affinity for the AT1, versus AT2, receptor. As a result, losartan results in vasodilation and decreased aldosterone secretion. Losartan increases urinary output.

Dosage
Dosing for losartan has been established for pediatric patients between 6 and 16 years of age. The standard dose is 0.7 mg/kg once daily to a maximum of 50 mg/day, but adjustments may be necessary and depend on the clinical response. Dosing may need to be decreased in patients with volume depletion, renal insufficiency, or hepatic dysfunction. In addition, the dose should be divided into two daily doses in cases of hepatic dysfunction. The drug may be continued in a patient whose serum creatinine is less than 35% above baseline unless there is associated hyperkalemia.

Metabolism and Half-Life
Losartan is metabolized by the cytochrome P450 enzyme system in the liver to an active metabolite, E-3174, which is much more potent. The half-life is 1.5–2 hours for losartan and 6–9 hours for the metabolite. Concomitant use of non-steroidal anti-inflammatory drugs may decrease the efficacy of losartan. The drug is not removed with hemodialysis.

Adverse Effects
The most common side effects include dizziness, chest pain, fatigue, headache, hypoglycemia, hyperuricemia, diarrhea, urinary tract infection, anemia, and cough, with most occurring more frequently in patients taking the drug for treatment of diabetic nephropathy. Toxic doses may result in hypotension and tachycardia. Losartan should be avoided during pregnancy because drugs that affect renin-angiotensin regulation can be associated with fetal and neonatal morbidity and death. It should also be avoided in

patients with bilateral renal artery stenosis. The drug should be used in lower doses or should be avoided in patients who are volume depleted or have pre-existing renal insufficiency. Patients with a creatinine clearance of less than 30 mL/minute should not receive the drug.

Monitoring
Blood pressure, electrolytes, serum creatinine, blood urea nitrogen, urinalysis, and blood counts should be monitored during the use of losartan.

Pearls
As an angiotensin II receptor blocker, losartan does not result in increased levels of bradykinin and is less likely to be associated with nonrenin-angiotensin effects such as cough and angioedema. The different sites of action of the angiotensin II receptor blockers and angiotensin-converting enzyme inhibitors have led to the speculation that these two classes of medications may be used in combination for greater effect in heart failure patients. Caution should be used when administering an angiotensin II receptor blocker to a patient already receiving a β-blocker since patients fared worse in the Val–HeFT study with this therapy regimen.[76]

Candesartan

Indications
Candesartan is used alone or in combination with other antihypertensive drugs to treat high blood pressure. Although candesartan is used for the treatment of congestive heart failure, it is not labeled for this use. Heart failure efficacy studies are currently being evaluated. Candesartan may be preferred over losartan due to its minimal metabolism requirements and its potential for use in patients with mild hepatic dysfunction.

Mechanism of Action
Candesartan is an angiotensin II receptor antagonist. Candesartan binds to the AT1 angiotensin II receptor, which prevents angiotensin II from binding to the receptor and interferes with its vasoconstriction and aldosterone-secreting effects.

Dosage
The dose of candesartan should be individualized and ranges from 4 to 32 mg daily in one or two doses. The blood pressure response is dose dependent. The usual adult starting dose is 16 mg daily when it is administered alone in a well-hydrated patient. For congestive heart failure, the target adult dose is 32 mg daily. It is preferable to take the medication on an empty stomach. It is important to consider a lower starting dose in patients with moderate hepatic dysfunction.

Metabolism and Half-Life
The drug is metabolized by the intestinal wall cells and is excreted in the urine. The half-life of candesartan is dose dependent and ranges from 5 to 9 hours. Nonsteroidal anti-inflammatory drugs may decrease the efficacy of candesartan, including the treatment of congestive heart failure.

Adverse Effects
The most common side effects include palpitations, flushing, dizziness, headache, fatigue, rash, angioedema, hyperglycemia, hematuria, and worsening renal function in patients dependent on the renin–angiotensin–aldosterone system. Overdose may result in hypotension and tachycardia. Candesartan should be avoided during pregnancy since drugs that affect renin–angiotensin regulation can be associated with fetal and neonatal morbidity and death. It should also be avoided in patients with bilateral renal artery stenosis. The drug should be used in lower doses or avoided in patients who are volume depleted or have preexisting renal insufficiency.

Monitoring
During the administration of candesartan, electrolytes, serum creatinine, blood urea nitrogen, urinalysis, and orthostatic vital signs should be monitored

Pearls
As an angiotensin II receptor blocker, candesartan does not result in increased levels of bradykinin and is less likely to be associated with nonrenin-angiotensin effects such as cough and angioedema. The different sites of action of the angiotensin II receptor blockers and angiotensin-converting enzyme inhibitors have led to the speculation that these two classes of medications may be used in combination for greater effect in heart failure patients.

ANTIARRHYTHMIC MEDICATIONS

The antiarrhythmic drugs are distinguished by their various effects on the two types of action potentials found in the cardiac tissues and their effects on the autonomic nervous system. The fast response action potential is rich with sodium channels and is found in atrial and ventricular myocytes, as well as in Purkinje fibers. The slow response action potential is primarily mediated by the slow calcium channels and is present predominantly in the pacemaker regions of the heart, the sinoatrial node and the atrioventricular node.

The initial phase 0 of the fast response action potential represents the rapid depolarization and results from the influx of sodium ions. The slope of the phase 0 depolarization influences the conduction velocity of cardiac tissue. Repolarization is the return of the action potential to the resting membrane potential and corresponds to phases 1–3, the width of the action potential. Repolarization results from inactivation of the inward sodium current as well as activation of the specialized potassium and calcium channels that direct current out of the cell. The period of repolarization determines the refractory period of the cardiac tissue (Fig. 13-2).

The Vaughn Williams classification of antiarrhythmic drugs, described in 1970, is based on pharmacologic effects on the types and phases of the cardiac cell action potential. The drugs are categorized into four major groups (Table 13-3).

Class I Antiarrhythmic Medications

The Class I antiarrhythmic agents include a diverse group of medications that block the rapid sodium channel and delay the upstroke of the action potential. In addition, there are effects on depolarization and repolarization. There is primarily a prolongation of conduction time in the fast response cells of the atrium, the ventricle, the Purkinje fibers, and accessory pathways, with a lengthening of the QRS duration and QT interval. Because of the varying degrees of sodium channel blockade and varying effects on the action potential duration, the medications are further subclassified into subgroups IA, IB, and IC.

Class IA Antiarrhythmic Medications

Procainamide, disopyramide, and quinidine are Class IA agents. In addition to delaying the rapid upstroke of

Table 13-3	Vaughn-Williams Classification of Antiarrhythmic Drugs	
Class	**Effect**	**Drugs**
I	Sodium channel blockade	
Subclass IA		Procainamide, disopyramide, quinidine
Subclass IB		Lidocaine, mexiletine, phenytoin
Subclass IC		Flecainide, propafenone, encainide
II	β-adrenergic receptor blockade	Propranolol, esmolol, atenolol, nadolol, carvedilol
III	Potassium-channel blockade	Amiodarone, sotalol, bretylium
IV	Slow inward calcium-channel blockade	Verapamil, diltiazem, nifedipine
Other		Digoxin, adenosine

the action potential, medications in this group delay repolarization resulting in slower conduction times and longer refractory periods. The Class IA drugs are unique in their significant effects on the autonomic nervous system. Anticholinergic effects result in increased sinoatrial node activity and in more rapid atrioventricular node conduction. Electrocardiographic changes that occur with this class of medications include widening of the QRS complex and prolongation of the QT interval. These medications are useful in treating atrial, ventricular, and atrioventricular reciprocating reentrant tachycardias. Quinidine is the member of the group with the longest history, but procainamide and disopyramide are currently used more frequently in practice, with procainamide being predominant. The Class IA agents all carry a risk of proarrhythmia with the aggravation of existing arrhythmias or the development of new atrial and ventricular arrhythmias, including torsades de pointes. The Cardiac Arrhythmia Suppression Trial showed higher mortality with some of the Class I drugs during the treatment of asymptomatic arrhythmias after myocardial infarction and increased proarrhythmia in patients with congestive heart failure. As a result, there has been a hesitance to use these drugs to treat arrhythmias in patients with structural heart disease or congestive heart failure. This has raised concern with the management of pediatric arrhythmias, but most reports of Class I agent use in children have been reassuring.

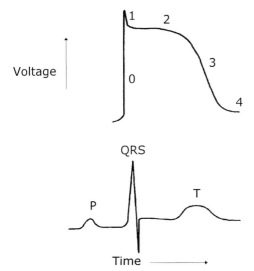

Figure 13-2   Fast response cardiac action potential and simultaneous correlation with surface electrocardiographic events.

CLASS IA AGENTS

Procainamide

Indications
Procainamide is used for the treatment or prevention of atrial, ventricular, and atrioventricular reciprocating reentrant tachycardias. Specific diagnoses that may be amenable to procainamide therapy include atrial fibrillation, atrial flutter, focal primary atrial tachycardias, Wolff–Parkinson–White syndrome, and other atrioventricular reentrant supraventricular tachycardias.

Mechanism of Action
Procainamide acts by blocking sodium channels, resulting in decreased myocardial excitability and slower conduction velocity. There is a greater prolonging on the effective refractory period than on the action potential duration. The electrophysiologic effects of procainamide, including sodium channel blockade, occur in a rate-dependent manner. There is some drug effect on potassium channels, primarily from the active N-acetyl procainamide metabolite. As a result of these cellular effects, procainamide does not affect the PR interval, prolongs the QRS duration, and prolongs the QT interval. Procainamide has the least anticholinergic effect of the Class I drugs. Finally, there may be a mild negative inotropic effect which appears to be less than for other Class IA agents. The hemodynamic effects are complex and not fully understood but seem to be dependent on the baseline level of myocardial function, the adrenergic state of the patient, the method of drug delivery, and concomitant therapy.

Dosage
Procainamide can be delivered by oral or intravenous routes. The intravenous loading dose is 5–15 mg/kg administered over 30 minutes. Continuous maintenance infusion rates range from 20 to 80 mcg/kg/min, with a maximum dose of 2 g/day. Infants and younger children may need higher doses of up to 100 mcg/kg/min. The recommended oral dose range is 15–50 mg/kg/day, divided into doses every 4 hours. The slow release preparation may be divided into four daily doses. Fortunately, there is now a preparation that allows twice-daily dosing. A much higher oral dosage may be necessary, depending on serum drug levels, since poor absorption and rapid elimination seem to be more significant problems in infants.

Metabolism and Half-Life
Procainamide is metabolized in the liver by acetylation to produce N-acetyl procainamide, which has active Class III antiarrhythmic effects. The rate of acetylation is bimodal with 55% of Caucasian and African-American patients having rapid acetylation. The kidneys excrete unacetylated procainamide and N-acetyl procainamide. The half-life of procainamide is 1.7 hours, and the half-life of N-acetyl procainamide is 6 hours.

Adverse Effects
Hypotension is the most significant side effect during the administration of intravenous procainamide. This is generally due to vasodilation and is most appropriately treated with volume expansion. Additional important cardiovascular side effects include ventricular arrhythmias, proarrhythmia, widening of the QRS complex, prolongation of the QT interval, and depressed ventricular function. Most other adverse effects are dependent on the plasma concentration and include nausea, vomiting, diarrhea, anorexia, headaches, rash, fever, blood dyscrasias, and a lupus-like syndrome. The syndrome occurs more commonly in patients who slowly acetylate procainamide. Acetylation of the procainamide amino group to form N-acetyl procainamide appears to block the lupus-inducing effect. Thus, the "slow acetylators" who have lower N-acetyl procainamide levels are more prone to a positive antinuclear antibody and a lupus-like syndrome. Symptoms of the drug-induced lupus-like syndrome occur in 20–30% of adult patients and include arthralgia, arthritis, fever, rash, and pericardial effusion. In children, this is less common. The drug does not necessarily need to be discontinued in situations of potentially life-threatening arrhythmias. The syndrome usually resolves upon discontinuation of the medication.

Monitoring
Procainamide and N-acetyl procainamide levels can be monitored and have therapeutic ranges of 4–10 mcg/mL and 1–10 mcg/mL, respectively. Combined levels >15–20 mcg/mL are considered toxic. Blood pressure and electrocardiographic monitoring are indicated, especially during intravenous drug administration. The complete blood count and liver function studies should be followed. The antinuclear antibody may be checked if there are clinical concerns for the development of signs and symptoms of systemic lupus erythematosus. However, a positive antinuclear antibody does not necessarily indicate a clinical diagnosis of systemic lupus erythematosus. The drug is usually started during an inpatient hospitalization due to the risk of proarrhythmia.

Pearls
When procainamide is used for the treatment of atrial fibrillation, there may be an increase in the ventricular response rate before conversion to sinus rhythm. This occurs as a result of the vagolytic effects of procainamide or effective slowing of the atrial tachycardia with an increased opportunity for atrioventricular node conduction. Therefore, before administering procainamide in

this situation, control of atrioventricular node conduction should be achieved with digoxin, a β-blocker, or a calcium-channel blocker.

Disopyramide

Indications
Disopyramide is an alternative Class IA agent that is available for oral administration for the treatment of atrial and ventricular arrhythmias. There is a role for the use of disopyramide in the treatment of patients with vasodepressor syncope, probably related to its potent effects on the autonomic nervous system.

Mechanism of Action
As a Class IA drug, disopyramide decreases myocardial excitability and slows cardiac tissue conduction velocity. It also diminishes differences in refractoriness between healthy and abnormal myocardium, results in peripheral vasoconstriction, has negative inotropic effects, and imparts anticholinergic effects.

Dosage
The oral dose is 20–30 mg/kg/day in infants, 10–20 mg/kg/day in children, and 5–15 mg/kg/day in adolescents, divided into four doses. The slow-release preparation allows for dosing twice daily.

Metabolism and Half-Life
The drug is metabolized equally in the liver and kidney and has a half-life of 4–10 hours.

Adverse Effects
The most limiting side effect of disopyramide is its negative inotropic effect. The drug should not be used in patients with congestive heart failure or significantly decreased ventricular function. Electrocardiographic findings include widening of the QRS complex, prolongation of the QT interval, and development of ventricular arrhythmias. Anticholinergic effects result in symptoms such as a dry mouth, constipation, urinary retention, and delirium.

Monitoring
The drug is usually started during an inpatient hospitalization because of the risk of proarrhythmia and depressed ventricular function. The patients must also be monitored for myocardial depression, hypotension, and signs and symptoms of congestive heart failure. The therapeutic serum drug level is 2.0–5.0 mcg/mL. The toxic range is considered >8 mcg/mL.

Pearls
There may be a synergistic effect on myocardial depression if disopyramide is administered in conjunction with β-blockers or calcium-channel blockers.

CLASS IB AGENTS

Medications in this group include lidocaine, mexiletine, and phenytoin. These medications act by shortening the duration of the action potential. They are primarily used for treatment of ventricular arrhythmias.

Lidocaine

Indications
Lidocaine is indicated for the treatment of complex ventricular ectopy, ventricular tachycardia, and ventricular fibrillation. It is effective for treating both reentrant and automatic arrhythmias by promoting uniformity in myocardial tissue refractoriness. It may also be useful for the emergent treatment of arrhythmias that occur in association with a prolonged QT interval. Lidocaine does not appear to be as effective in the treatment of atrial arrhythmias.

Mechanism of Action
Lidocaine blocks sodium channels, resulting in shortening of the action potential duration. This occurs preferentially in a diseased myocardium that generally has a prolonged refractory period. There is little effect on the phase 0 upstroke of the action potential. A decrease in the phase 0 slope and tissue conduction time becomes more noticeable in situations of acidosis, cell damage, and hyperkalemia. There is a minimal effect on impulse conduction but a significant decrease in refractoriness, especially in ventricular and Purkinje cells. Lidocaine has little effect on the slow response cells of the sinoatrial node and the atrioventricular node and has no significant effect on the autonomic nervous system.

Dosing
For acute treatment, a 1 mg/kg intravenous loading dose is administered, followed by a continuous infusion. The bolus may be repeated after 10 minutes to a maximum total dose of 250 mg. The usual starting infusion rate is 20 mcg/kg/minute, but this can be titrated to a maximum of 50 mcg/kg/min, depending on the clinical effect and serum levels.

Metabolism and Half-Life
Lidocaine is metabolized rapidly by the liver and is excreted by the kidney, and therefore must be administered intravenously or intraosseously. The half-life of the drug is 30 minutes. Drug interactions include those with β-blockers and cimetidine, which increase the serum lidocaine level; isoproterenol, phenobarbital, and phenytoin, which decrease the serum lidocaine level; and disopyramide, which increases the risk of adverse effects. Several different circumstances require adjustment in lidocaine

dosing.[77] Prolonged lidocaine infusions result in reduced drug clearance, requiring a lower infusion rate. In patients with congestive heart failure, shock, or low cardiac output, the drug volume of distribution is decreased so that the loading dose will need to be lower.

Adverse Effects
Major side effects involve the central nervous system and include nausea, tremors, headaches, seizures, vertigo, and altered mental status.

Monitoring
Serum levels and clinical signs and symptoms should be monitored for evidence of toxicity. The therapeutic serum level range for lidocaine is between 1.5 and 5 mcg/mL. The electrocardiogram usually shows no detectable change but may exhibit a slightly shorter QT interval.

Pearls
A negative inotropic effect is not usually seen with standard lidocaine dosing and drug levels that are <7 mcg/mL. Proarrhythmia is a rare adverse effect of lidocaine. There is no oral form of lidocaine, so mexiletine is used chronically in patients who respond to Class IB agents.

Mexiletine

Indications
As with lidocaine, mexiletine is used primarily to treat ventricular arrhythmias and is a natural choice for the patient who requires chronic outpatient therapy for an arrhythmia that is responsive to intravenous lidocaine.

Mechanism of Action
Mexiletine is structurally similar to lidocaine but has a longer half-life, allowing for oral administration. The half-life in adult patients is 10–14 hours and seems to be shorter in younger patients. At a cellular level, mexiletine has effects similar to those of lidocaine and results in decreased tissue refractoriness.

Dosage
Mexiletine is only available orally. Recommended mexiletine doses for children are in the range of 5–15 mg/kg/day and are higher for infants, at 8–25 mg/kg/day.[78] Adult doses range from 450 to 1200 mg/day. Administration is usually divided into two to three daily doses. The dose may need to be adjusted in cases of hepatic insufficiency.

Metabolism and Half-Life
The drug is metabolized primarily in the liver, with a half-life of 10–14 hours. Antacids, cimetidine, and narcotics slow drug absorption, rifampin and phenobarbital result in decreased serum levels, and theophylline and amiodarone result in increased serum levels.

Adverse Effects
The most common side effects seen during mexiletine administration are abdominal pain and discomfort, nausea, headache, rash, tremors, vision changes, and, rarely, hepatitis. Proarrhythmia occurs less commonly than with some other antiarrhythmic agents but appears to be more of a concern than with lidocaine.

Monitoring
Mexiletine serum levels can be measured but are usually not immediately available. The therapeutic serum level range is 0.5–2.0 mcg/mL.

Pearls
Mexiletine is not available for intravenous use.

CLASS IC AGENTS

Class IC agents include flecainide, propafenone, and encainide. As with the Class IA and Class IB agents, these medications inhibit sodium channels in fast-response cells and have a profound depressant effect on conduction velocity. There is relatively little effect in slow response cells. These agents also have relatively little effect on refractory periods or on the autonomic nervous system. As a whole, the group is used clinically to depress abnormal automaticity and to prevent the induction of atrial muscle, ventricular muscle, and accessory pathway reentry circuits. The Class IC agents have a relatively high potential for proarrhythmia, as suggested by the Cardiac Arrhythmia Suppression Trial (CAST) of the late 1980s, which demonstrated that patients with a history of myocardial infarction and asymptomatic ventricular ectopy actually had a significantly higher mortality rate when randomized to long-term therapy with flecainide or encainide.[79] A subsequent pediatric multicenter study confirmed a relatively high incidence of adverse events, including proarrhythmia, cardiac arrest, and death, with these drugs, but the events occurred predominantly among patients with underlying heart disease.[80]

Flecainide

Indications
Flecainide is used for the prevention and suppression of life-threatening and refractory arrhythmias caused by abnormal automaticity or atrial, ventricular, or atrioventricular reciprocating reentry tachycardias. In pediatrics, flecainide is most commonly used for the prevention of symptomatic disabling supraventricular arrhythmias in patients without structural heart disease.

Mechanism of Action

Flecainide depresses the phase 0 upstroke of the action potential by blocking sodium channels. This results in slowing of conduction in the fast-response cells. There is minimal effect on the action potential duration, repolarization, and refractory period.

Dosage

Flecainide is only available orally. The usual therapeutic dosing range is 3–6 mg/kg/day or 100–200 mg/m²/day in three divided doses in younger children and two divided doses in pediatric patients of school age and older. The maximum daily dose is 400 mg/day.

Metabolism and Half-Life

Flecainide is metabolized primarily by the liver. The half-life varies between 8 and 12 hours, depending on age. Flecainide use can increase digoxin and amiodarone serum levels, whereas cimetidine can increase the flecainide serum level.

Adverse Effects

Side effects include nausea, vomiting, headache, rash, and tremor. Flecainide has the potential to be a potent negative inotropic agent, especially when administered concurrently with other negative inotropic agents such as the β-blockers. Flecainide, like the other Class IC agents, is thought to have a higher incidence of proarrhythmia (4–17%).

Monitoring

Serum levels can be monitored but are not usually immediately available. Therapeutic serum levels range from 0.2 to 1.0 mcg/mL. The electrocardiogram shows a longer QRS duration because of intraventricular conduction delay. PR interval prolongation may be seen. The T wave itself is not significantly changed, but there may be prolongation of the QT interval due to QRS widening.

Pearls

Whereas the CAST study has shown an increase in mortality in a select group of patients not encountered in pediatric practice, studies of the medication in young patients without structural heart disease have demonstrated efficacy with an acceptable side effect profile.[80,81]

CLASS II AGENTS

Class II is designated for the β-blockers, which include propranolol, esmolol, atenolol, nadolol, and carvedilol. These medications work by several mechanisms, but primarily through competitive inhibition of the cardiac β-adrenergic receptor. By blocking endogenous catecholamines and decreasing sympathetic tone through an effect on the autonomic nervous system, the β-blockers slow spontaneous discharge from the sinus node as well as abnormal automaticity from other cardiac tissues. In addition, atrioventricular nodal conduction is slowed. Direct cellular and membrane effects of the β-blockers, seen particularly with high chronic doses, include prolongation of the action potential duration and an increase of the threshold for ventricular fibrillation. The medications are used to treat all arrhythmias of abnormal automaticity, especially those that are catecholamine driven. In addition, they may be used to treat reentry tachycardias by preventing the premature beats that act as initiating events or by affecting atrioventricular nodal conduction when that structure is part of the arrhythmia circuit. β-blockers are an important part of the management of long QT syndrome.

There are many β-blockers available, with those mentioned above representing a small subset. Esmolol and propranolol are discussed in more detail. Others that are used commonly or with increased frequency in pediatrics include atenolol, nadolol, and carvedilol. Atenolol has the advantages of more cardiac β-receptor selectivity, less central nervous system penetration, and a longer half-life, resulting in less frequent dosing. Nadolol requires less frequent dosing and has less penetration to the brain than other β-blockers, making the incidence of central nervous system side effects low. Carvedilol and metoprolol have been approved in the United States for the management of congestive heart failure in the adult population, but the experience in pediatrics is limited, with a randomized clinical trial in progress.[82,83] Patients with chronic congestive heart failure have increased sympathetic nervous system activity that is thought to be related to their clinical deterioration, and β-blocker therapy is thought to interfere with this debilitating neurohormonal pathway. Despite the different preparations having variable cardiac selectivity, most β-blockers affect the β-2 receptor at high doses. Thus, the choice of a specific β-blocker usually depends on factors such as route of administration, dosing interval, rate of metabolism, indications for therapy, cardiac selectivity, and interactions with other medications.

Esmolol

Indications

Esmolol has several roles in pediatric heart disease. It is indicated for treatment of supraventricular and ventricular arrhythmias, especially in emergent situations. It is well suited for therapeutic trials during intracardiac electrophysiologic studies. Aside from its use as an antiarrhythmic drug, esmolol is of particular benefit for the treatment of acute hypertensive events, especially in postoperative cardiac patients. Esmolol is frequently used to control hypertension, especially after surgical repair of coarctation of the aorta.[84,85] Patients with ventricular outflow tract obstruction may benefit from β blockade. Esmolol can relieve hypercyanotic episodes in patients with tetralogy of Fallot by decreasing the heart rate and the dynamic subpulmonic narrowing in the right ventricular outflow tract.[86] Although esmolol does not provide the benefits of long-term β-blocker therapy, it can help predict success and tolerance of the drug class for future transition to an oral preparation.

Mechanism of Action
Esmolol selectively and competitively inhibits β_1-adrenergic receptors, with little or no effect on β_2-receptors. It is particularly noted for its rapid onset and its short duration of action.

Dosage
Esmolol is available only for intravenous administration and is given as a loading dose of 500 mcg/kg over 1–2 minutes, followed by a continuous infusion usually at 50–200 mcg/kg/min. Esmolol infusions are sometimes titrated to much higher rates, with the specific dose ultimately being determined by a clinical effect or intolerance.[87,88]

Metabolism and Half-Life
Esmolol has particular advantages with regard to its rapid onset and elimination. It is rapidly hydrolyzed by red blood cell esterases and has an elimination half-life of 9 minutes in adults. The half-life of the drug has been reported to be as rapid as 4.5 minutes in children.[89,90]

Adverse Effects
Side effects include hypotension, bradycardia, nausea, hypoglycemia in the very young, and negative inotropy. Central nervous system symptoms and bronchospasm are rare. As with the other β-blockers, esmolol should be used very carefully with calcium-channel blockers. The administration of β-blockers simultaneously with calcium-channel blockers can result in hypotension and cardiovascular collapse, especially in young infants and in patients with ventricular dysfunction.

Monitoring
Serum drug levels are not routinely measured. Continuous hemodynamic and cardiac rhythm monitoring should occur, with particular attention to the blood pressure. Electrocardiographic findings include bradycardia and a prolonged P-R interval.

Pearls
The rapid volume distribution and metabolism of esmolol facilitate rapid adjustments in dosing to balance blood pressure and heart rate with desired drug effect.

Propranolol

Indications
Propranolol is indicated to treat supraventricular arrhythmias, selected ventricular arrhythmias, and long QT syndrome. It may be particularly useful for arrhythmias that are catecholamine sensitive. Like the other β-blockers, propranolol may be useful for the treatment of hypertension. β-blockers improve the long-term survival of pediatric patients with symptomatic hypertrophic cardiomyopathy and long QT syndrome.[91]

Mechanism of Action
Propranolol competitively blocks β_1- and β_2-adrenergic receptors in a nonselective manner.

Dosage
For treatment of arrhythmias, oral dosing begins at 0.5–1.0 mg/kg/day, divided into three or four doses. The dosage can be titrated upwards to 2–4 mg/kg/day until clinical effects are reached. The intravenous bolus dose range is from 0.01 to 0.1 mg/kg/dose and is given slowly over 10 minutes. This dose can be repeated every 6 hours, as needed.

Metabolism and Half-Life
Propranolol is metabolized by the liver. The half-life is 4–6 hours in children.

Adverse Effects
Side effects are similar to those for esmolol and include hypotension, bradycardia, nausea, hypoglycemia (especially in younger patients), atrioventricular block, and negative inotropy. Central nervous system symptoms and bronchospasm are more common than with the cardioselective β-blockers. Neonates are particularly susceptible to respiratory depression. As with the other β-blockers, propranolol should be used very carefully with calcium-channel blockers because of the possibility of a synergistic effect on myocardial depression.

Monitoring
Although serum drug levels are not routinely measured, blood glucose levels should be assessed while initiating propranolol, especially with neonates and infants. Electrocardiographic findings include bradycardia and a prolonged PR interval.

Pearls
There is a limited role for intravenous propranolol. Esmolol, with its shorter half-life, is a better choice in most clinical situations. In cases of β-blocker overdose, glucagon has been used with some success as a cardiac stimulant.

CLASS III AGENTS

The Class III agents include amiodarone, sotalol, and bretylium. By definition, Class III antiarrhythmic agents prolong the action potential duration through their actions, primarily on potassium channels. There is less of an effect on the phase 0 upstroke. These medications work primarily by prolonging the refractory period of myocardial tissue. Amiodarone and sotalol have additional effects on action potential propagation and variable effects on the autonomic nervous system. Amiodarone and sotalol are being used more commonly in pediatric practice and are described below, whereas bretylium has been removed from Advanced Cardiac Life Support (ACLS) algorithms. Despite its less frequent use, bretylium has a unique combination of antiarrhythmic and autonomic effects. Bretylium results in a biphasic norepinephrine response that is characterized by an initial increase and a subsequent decrease in circulating endogenous catecholamine levels. This correlates with a clinical tachycardia, an increase in blood pressure, and a potential worsening of arrhythmias, followed by hypotension and delayed Class III effects. Bretylium is traditionally used to treat refractory ventricular fibrillation and ventricular tachycardia and can be useful if its complex properties are understood and expected. Bretylium has been removed from ACLS treatment algorithms because of a high incidence of adverse events, the availability of safer agents, and its limited supply.

Amiodarone

Indications

Amiodarone is a potent antiarrhythmic agent that is usually reserved for the treatment of potentially life-threatening arrhythmias or arrhythmias that are refractory to other therapies. Amiodarone has also become the preferred treatment for other specific troublesome arrhythmias such as acute conversion of atrial fibrillation or atrial flutter in patients with repaired congenital heart disease, suppression of postoperative junctional ectopic tachycardia, and management of incessant atrioventricular reciprocating reentrant tachycardias that are refractory to less potent medical therapy.[92] Finally, amiodarone has been incorporated in ACLS treatment algorithms after defibrillation and epinephrine for unstable ventricular tachycardia or ventricular fibrillation.[93,94]

Mechanism of Action

Amiodarone is a unique antiarrhythmic drug in that it has a broad mechanism by which it affects cardiac tissue. The predominant effect is prolongation of the action potential by blocking the outward potassium current. This results in longer refractory periods in the fast response action potential of the atrium, the ventricle, the Purkinje fibers, and accessory pathways. Amiodarone affects the slow response cells of the sinoatrial node and the atrioventricular node, depressing discharge and conduction velocity in those structures. Finally, amiodarone has the ability to block both α-adrenergic and β-adrenergic receptors. As a result, there is reduced membrane excitability, decreased automaticity, and an increased fibrillation threshold. The corresponding electrocardiographic findings include sinus bradycardia, PR interval prolongation, widening of the QRS complex, and QT interval prolongation.

Dosage

Amiodarone can be administered by the oral or intravenous route. Loading is commonly performed with 2.5-mg/kg bolus infusions over 10–15 minutes. Doses can be repeated every 6 hours for a total intravenous dose of 10 mg/kg/day. The intravenous maintenance dose is 2–20 mg/kg/day and is administered as bolus dosing in young children but as a continuous infusion in older children and adolescents. Infants may require higher doses to achieve an effect. Loading can also be performed with oral drug administration, which usually requires a higher dose. The recommended oral loading dose is 10–20 mg/kg/day in one or two doses for up to 14 days or until there is adequate rhythm control. The loading phase is considered to occur over the first few weeks of therapy. Dosing for chronic oral therapy is generally 2.5–5 mg/kg once daily but may need to be as high as 10 mg/kg/day. Pediatric Advanced Life Support (PALS) dosing for pulseless ventricular tachycardia or ventricular fibrillation is 5 mg/kg of intravenous amiodarone.

Metabolism and Half-Life

Amiodarone is metabolized by the liver. Its peak concentration occurs 3–7 hours after a load. Both treatment response and elimination are delayed. The half-life is longer than 1 month. Because of its high lipid solubility, drug levels can persist months after discontinuation of the medication. This can be of particular importance in cases of toxicity.

Adverse Effects

Amiodarone has a number of serious side effects that limit its long-term utility. Many of these adverse effects are dose related and may occur with greater frequency when there has been a higher total cumulative dose or a longer duration of therapy. Children may tolerate this medication better than adults.[95] Cardiac side effects include proarrhythmia of new or worse arrhythmias, including torsades de pointes, congestive heart failure, intraventricular conduction delay, atrioventricular block, and sinus pauses. The more common noncardiac side effects include corneal microdeposits, hyper- or hypothyroidism, chemical hepatitis, pulmonary interstitial fibrosis, a blue-gray discoloration of the skin, peripheral neuropathy, and photosensitivity. Most of the adverse effects are reversible, but pulmonary toxicity and skin discoloration are chronic effects that are more likely to persist.

Monitoring

Serum drug levels are not usually followed, but the therapeutic range is 1–2 mcg/mL. The reverse T3 is a sensitive parameter to follow and correlates with drug tissue penetration and toxicity. Other laboratory tests to be monitored include the electrocardiogram, the complete blood count, thyroid function tests, liver function studies, the ophthalmologic exam, the chest radiograph, and pulmonary function tests. Electrocardiographic changes include prolongation of the PR interval, QRS complex, and corrected QT interval. The medication is usually initiated during inpatient hospitalization. The digoxin level must be followed during amiodarone administration because of its impaired excretion and elevated serum level when the two are used together. Generally, the digoxin dose is decreased by half when amiodarone is added. Phenytoin metabolism is also affected, so the dose should be decreased and blood levels followed when amiodarone is started.

Pearls

Marked hypotension and depressed ventricular contractility may occur with the intravenous administration of the medication. Frequent, small bolus doses of intravenous amiodarone are used in pediatric patients due to the risk of leaching of plasticizers from intravenous tubing during slow intravenous amiodarone flow rates. Amiodarone may increase pacing and defibrillation thresholds.

Sotalol

Indications

Sotalol is used for the treatment of life-threatening and refractory atrial and ventricular arrhythmias. Its indications are similar to those for amiodarone, but it has the advantage of a faster onset of action and a shorter duration of activity. Sotalol has the added benefit of decreasing defibrillation and pacing capture thresholds.

Mechanism of Action

Sotalol has nonselective β-blocker effects at low doses, but it has Class III activity at higher doses. As such, sotalol increases cardiac tissue refractoriness and prolongs the action potential duration through effects on the cardiac potassium channel. Sotalol decreases tissue automaticity but has little effect on the phase 0 upstroke and tissue conduction velocity.

Dosage

Sotalol is available only for oral administration in the United States. Usual pediatric doses range from 80 to 160 mg/m^2/day, divided into two or three doses. Neonates and infants seem to metabolize the drug more rapidly, thus requiring the more frequent dosing regimen of three daily doses.

Metabolism and Half-Life

Sotalol is excreted exclusively in the urine. The elimination half-life is 7–12 hours.

Adverse Effects

Side effects include proarrhythmia, including torsades de pointes in 2–4% of adult patients, negative inotropy, bradycardia, and atrioventricular block. Noncardiac side effects include fatigue and gastrointestinal distress.

Monitoring

Levels are not followed, but clinical effects include QT interval prolongation on the electrocardiogram. Other electrocardiographic findings include bradycardia, PR interval prolongation, and atrioventricular block.

Pearls

The commercially available preparation is a racemic mixture of the *d*- and *l*-isomers, resulting in nonselective β-blocking effects. *d*-sotalol was developed for use as an antiarrhythmic agent without β-blocking effects. In the Survival With Oral *d*-sotalol (SWORD) trial, *d*-sotalol was administered to patients with depressed myocardial function after a myocardial infarction to determine whether the pure potassium-channel blocker could reduce mortality risk. The study was terminated after noting that patients treated with *d*-sotalol had increased mortality, presumably due to arrhythmias. Thus, it was concluded that the pure potassium-channel blocker may be associated with increased mortality in high-risk patients, especially those with a history of myocardial infarction.[96] This has resulted in a cautious approach to the drug for pediatric patients, especially those with structural heart disease.

CLASS IV AGENTS

Class IV antiarrhythmics drugs are the calcium channel blockers, specifically verapamil, diltiazem, and nifedipine. Of these, verapamil is used most frequently in pediatric practice for the treatment of arrhythmias, but certain circumstances warrant special attention regarding its use. Diltiazem is frequently used for control of the ventricular rate during an atrial tachycardia by blocking conduction at the atrioventricular node. It is particularly well suited for this indication since it may be administered intravenously with an initial bolus and subsequent infusion that can easily be titrated to effect. The calcium channel blockers are widely used for long-term therapy of pulmonary hypertension. Nifedipine is preferred in those patients since it has little effect on the sinoatrial node, atrioventricular node, and cardiac contractility. Due to its potential for peripheral vasodilation, nifedipine is used for the acute management of hypertension. Nifedipine can be a coronary vasodilator.

Verapamil

Indications

Verapamil is most valuable for the treatment of reentrant supraventricular tachycardias that involve the sinoatrial node or the atrioventricular node. It terminates the atrioventricular reciprocating reentrant tachycardias by interrupting the reentrant circuit in the atrioventricular node. Verapamil can be used for control of the ventricular rate during atrial arrhythmias by decreasing atrioventricular nodal conduction.

Mechanism of Action

Verapamil and the other calcium-channel blockers block the slow inward calcium current in the slow response cells of the sinus node and the atrioventricular node. This cellular activity decreases sinus node automaticity, slows atrioventricular node conduction, and prolongs refractoriness. The calcium-channel blockers have no significant effect on the fast response action potential. Electrocardiographic manifestations of the calcium channel blockers include sinus bradycardia and P-R interval prolongation, without notable changes of the QRS complex and the T wave.

Dosage

Verapamil is available for both intravenous and oral administration. In children greater than 1 year of age, the intravenous dose range is between 0.05 and 0.1 mg/kg/dose and may be repeated after 5 minutes. The maximum single intravenous dose is 5 mg. The oral dose range is 3–6 mg/kg/day divided into three doses. Once or twice daily dosing can be used for the slow-release preparation.

Metabolism and Half-Life

Verapamil is metabolized in the liver. The half-life is 4–7 hours for infants, 2–8 hours for adults, and up to 12 hours during chronic use.

Adverse Effects

Although verapamil is tolerated well in older children, adverse effects include hypotension, sinus bradycardia, atrioventricular block, headache, dizziness, and constipation. Due to the potential negative inotropic effects, which may be synergistic, verapamil should generally not be administered with a β-blocker.

Monitoring

Verapamil serum levels are not routinely assessed. Before the medication is started, the electrocardiogram should be evaluated for Wolff–Parkinson–White syndrome since verapamil may enhance the antegrade conduction properties of the accessory pathway. The electrocardiogram should be followed for excessive P-R interval prolongation or atrioventricular block.

Pearls

Calcium should be available for the treatment of hypotension during the administration of intravenous verapamil. Verapamil should be avoided in children less than 1 year of age due to reports of young infants who have responded to intravenous verapamil with cardiovascular collapse.[97] One suggested mechanism is an increased sensitivity to the cardiac depressant effect of verapamil in the immature animal.[98] Patients with Wolff–Parkinson–White syndrome should not receive chronic verapamil therapy as accessory pathway conduction may be enhanced, whereas atrioventricular nodal conduction may be slowed, particularly during atrial tachycardias.

NON-CLASSIFIED ANTIARRHYTHMICS

Digoxin

Indications

Digoxin is a cardiac glycoside that is useful for the treatment of both arrhythmias and congestive heart failure. Specifically, it is used to treat arrhythmias that occur due to an atrioventricular reciprocating reentrant mechanism by blocking the atrioventricular node and interrupting the circuit. It is also used to achieve ventricular rate control during an atrial tachycardia by blocking the response of the atrioventricular node to the atrial arrhythmia. Due to its ability to decrease automaticity, digoxin may be used for atrial tachycardias, atrial fibrillation, premature atrial complexes, and blocked premature atrial complexes. Digoxin should not be used in patients with Wolff–Parkinson–White syndrome due to its ability to block the atrioventricular node, to shorten the accessory pathway effective refractory period, and, potentially, to enhance antegrade accessory pathway conduction during an atrial tachycardia. Digitalis has been used for the treatment of congestive heart failure for over 200 years, especially in cases of depressed myocardial function. Debate exists regarding whether the same benefit occurs in children with heart failure because of volume overload conditions, such as that seen with a ventricular septal defect.

Mechanism of Action

Digoxin has distinct electrophysiologic effects, along with positive inotropic effects, through a number of complex mechanisms. The most notable cardiac effects of digoxin are decreased automaticity of the sinus node and slowing of conduction in the atrioventricular node. These occur through several pathways of the autonomic nervous system but primarily are in response to an increase in vagal nerve tone and a decrease in sympathetic efferent activity. However, digoxin also has direct cellular effects that seem to vary, depending on plasma levels, patient age, and metabolic conditions. These cellular effects result in changes in the duration of the action potential and refractory periods in all cardiac tissue, including accessory bypass tracts. Toxic concentrations can increase the frequency of spontaneous depolarizations and delayed after-depolarizations, resulting in increased automaticity and triggered arrhythmias. The cellular effects are due to binding of digoxin to sodium-potassium adenosine triphosphatase, which inhibits the sodium pump and ultimately increases intracellular calcium. The inotropic effect of digoxin results in an increase of the force and velocity of cardiac muscle contraction. The increased availability of calcium due to inhibition of the sodium pump results in a more forceful contraction and an increased cardiac output.

Dosage
Digoxin may be administered orally or intravenously for both digitalization and maintenance therapy. Dosage differs between patient age groups and is primarily related to differences in renal excretion. Within a specific age range, individual patients may have very different responses. For the premature infant, who is most sensitive to digoxin, the total oral digitalizing dose is 20 mcg/kg. Term neonates receive 30–40 mcg/kg, infants up to 2 years of age receive 30–50 mcg/kg, and older children usually receive 30 mcg/kg. A standard adult loading dose is 0.75–1.25 mg, divided into two or three doses over 24 hours. Usually, half of the total digitalizing dose is given, followed by two subsequent doses that are one-quarter of the total digitalizing dose at 8 hours and 16 hours after the initial dose. The digitalization may be administered over a shorter or longer period, depending on the clinical situation. Maintenance dosing is initiated 12 hours after the completion of digitalization. The daily maintenance dose is usually one quarter of the loading dose (5–8 mcg/kg/day for premature infants, 10 mcg/kg/day for neonates and older children, and 0.125–0.25 mg/day for adults), and is given as one or two doses. Intravenous dosing is usually 75–80% that of the standard oral dose. Particular caution must be used in dosing digoxin for patients with renal insufficiency as this is the primary method of excretion. In addition, patients with conditions of myocardial ischemia or inflammation, such as those with myocarditis, have an increased sensitivity to digoxin despite serum levels that are in the therapeutic range. If a loading regimen is not used, toxicity may occur later as there is a delay to reaching the ultimate serum steady state concentration of the drug.

Metabolism and Half-Life
Digoxin is the cardiac glycoside preparation used most commonly because of its advantages in bioavailability, absorption, and relatively rapid excretion. The onset of action is 30–120 minutes after an oral dose and 5–30 minutes after an intravenous dose. Digoxin is excreted by the kidney. Half-life varies by age (preterm infants, 60–170 hours; neonates, 40 hours; infants, 20 hours; children, 35 hours). Aside from renal disease, other conditions that affect digoxin metabolism include electrolyte abnormalities and thyroid disease. Digoxin should be used very carefully in the setting of hypokalemia because low extracellular potassium and high intracellular sodium enhance the binding of digoxin to the sodium pump. Hypercalcemia increases digoxin effects, whereas hypocalcemia reduces sensitivity to the drug. Medications can also have significant effects on the plasma digoxin level. Antacids decrease drug absorption, whereas others, such as flecainide, verapamil, and amiodarone, impair elimination. Digoxin is not removed by dialysis or cardiopulmonary bypass.

Adverse Effects
Adverse effects include sinus bradycardia, atrioventricular block, any tachyarrhythmia, nausea, anorexia, somnolence, and vision changes. The noncardiac side effects are nonspecific and are frequently difficult to assess. Therefore, digoxin toxicity is frequently an electrocardiographic diagnosis in children. Digoxin should be avoided or used with caution in patients with atrioventricular block, sinus bradycardia, hypertrophic cardiomyopathy, constrictive pericarditis, Wolff–Parkinson–White syndrome, hypokalemia, hypercalcemia, hypomagnesemia, or renal insufficiency.

Monitoring
Monitoring is important because digoxin has a narrow therapeutic range. The therapeutic plasma level range is 0.5–2.0 ng/mL. Characteristic electrocardiographic findings include sinus bradycardia, PR interval prolongation, shortening of the QT interval, mild depression of the ST segment, and flattening of the T wave. Drug levels are helpful when toxicity is suspected. Toxicity is usually associated with levels greater than 2 ng/mL, but symptoms may not develop in children until higher levels are achieved. Digoxin level accuracy is dependent on the relationship of the time the blood specimen was obtained to the time the dose was given. Blood sampling should occur from 6 hours after an oral dose to just prior to the next dose. Levels drawn too soon after a dose may

appear to be artificially elevated since distribution of the drug is not immediate and a serum steady state has not been achieved. For that reason, serum levels should not be checked until 3–5 days after a loading dose or a change in dose is completed. Serum potassium, magnesium, and calcium levels should be normalized, particularly when patients are also being treated with diuretics. However, potassium supplementation must occur slowly because the inability of the sodium pump to transport potassium intracellularly may result in high serum potassium levels.

Pearls

Digoxin toxicity can result in almost any type of arrhythmia, but the development of arrhythmias is generally a late indicator of toxicity. The electrocardiographic signs of digoxin toxicity are different in children as compared to adults. Infants more frequently present with sinus bradycardia and atrioventricular block. Older children also have bradyarrhythmias, but they can also have atrial and junctional tachyarrhythmias. Pediatric patients, unlike adult patients, rarely develop ventricular tachyarrhythmias. For toxicity, the medication should be discontinued. Serum electrolyte abnormalities should be corrected while continuous monitoring surveys the cardiac rhythm. Atrial and ventricular arrhythmias can be treated with phenytoin or lidocaine. Atropine or a temporary pacemaker can be used to treat bradycardia or atrioventricular block. Digoxin-immune antigen-binding fragments (Fabs) are specific antibodies and may be used to bind digoxin; they may be especially helpful in potentially life-threatening cases of toxicity. Each vial of the antidote is intended to bind 0.5 mg of digoxin. The amount of antidote necessary is based on the body burden of drug, on either the known ingested amount of drug or the serum drug level. Based on the serum digoxin level, the Fab dose is calculated as number of vials = serum level (ng/mL) × body weight (kg) ÷100. Empiric treatment for acute toxicity is 20 vials administered in two divided doses.

Adenosine

Indications

Adenosine is an endogenous purine nucleoside that is useful for terminating supraventricular tachycardia. Because adenosine blocks atrioventricular node conduction, it can be used to help differentiate between an atrioventricular reciprocating reentrant mechanism and automatic, ectopic, or reentrant atrial arrhythmias. It will terminate the atrioventricular reciprocating reentrant circuit by abruptly blocking the atrioventricular node, but the atrial tachycardia will persist with block at the atrioventricular node, resulting in a less than 1:1 ventricular response to the atrial arrhythmia.

Mechanism of Action

Adenosine administered as a large bolus blocks atrioventricular nodal conduction and slows sinoatrial node automaticity. The effects are brief because the drug is rapidly metabolized. Adenosine slows the phase 0 upstroke in atrioventricular nodal tissue. The sinoatrial node and atrial myocytes are affected through stimulation of a specific potassium current channel that results in hyperpolarization, decreased action potential duration, and decreased phase 4 automaticity. There is little effect on ventricular myocardium or accessory pathway tissue. After the characteristic effects on the sinoatrial node and atrioventricular node, adenosine frequently results in a period of sinus tachycardia that is probably due to sympathetic activation or vagal withdrawal.

Dosage

The initial intravenous dose is usually 0.05–0.1 mg/kg. This can be doubled until an effect is seen or to a maximum dose of 0.3 mg/kg. In cases of low cardiac output or in which the medication is administered slowly or peripherally, higher doses may be necessary. If the arrhythmia immediately recurs after a successful termination, the dose may need to be decreased because sympathetic stimulation from the higher dose may provoke premature atrial contractions that act as initiating events. The medication should be rapidly administered and followed with a flush. Due to its rapid metabolism, there is no role for adenosine to be administered orally or as a continuous infusion.

Metabolism and Half-Life

Metabolism is extremely rapid, occurring by deamination or phosphorylation in erythrocytes, endothelial cells, and cardiac myocytes. The half-life is less than 10 seconds, with clinical effects that may last up to 30 seconds.

Adverse Effects

Adverse effects include dyspnea, chest discomfort, headache, and flushing. Bronchospasm can be seen, especially in asthmatics. Long sinus pauses can result and should be anticipated. Transient new arrhythmias can occur at the time of conversion back to sinus rhythm, including complex ventricular ectopy and atrial fibrillation.

Monitoring

An electrocardiographic rhythm strip should be running at the time that the medication is administered. This will help to document sinus rhythm after conversion of the arrhythmia. In addition, information regarding the mechanism of arrhythmia termination and post-conversion arrhythmias can be documented. Resuscitation equipment, including a defibrillator, should be present.

Pearls

There are a few clinical circumstances in which adenosine must be used with extra caution. Dipyridamole is a nucleoside transport blocker that increases the duration and severity of the adenosine effect through activity involving the adenosine specific receptor. Adenosine should be avoided or used with one-fourth of the usual dose in patients who are taking dipyridamole.[99] Caffeine and the methylxanthines cause competitive and reversible antagonism through the specific adenosine receptor, requiring higher doses of adenosine for clinical effect. Orthotopic heart transplant patients have a denervation-induced supersensitivity to adenosine. Therefore, a dose of one-third to one-half of the standard dose is recommended.[100]

DUCTAL MANIPULATORS

Control of patency of the ductus arteriosus is important in certain clinical situations. Indications to maintain patency of the ductus include the cyanotic newborn and the newborn whose systemic circulation is dependent on ductal flow. In contrast, it may be necessary to encourage closure of the structure in a premature infant with lung disease and a left-to-right shunt. Medical manipulation of the ductus became possible in the 1970s with the therapeutic application of prostaglandins.[101] This allowed for stabilization of the newborn with ductal-dependent cardiac lesions prior to surgical repair or palliation. Since then, prostaglandins and indomethacin have become important and common methods of altering the ductal circulation for various derangements of cardiovascular pathophysiology.

Prostaglandin E$_1$

Indications

As a potent vasodilator, particularly of the ductus arteriosus in the fetus and newborn, prostaglandin E$_1$ (PGE$_1$) is indicated for the treatment of ductal-dependent lesions such as cyanotic heart disease with severely limited or no pulmonary blood flow. Specific lesions include tricuspid atresia, pulmonary atresia, and critical pulmonary stenosis. Children with obstruction of systemic blood flow may depend on ductal patency and may benefit from administration of PGE$_1$. Lesions in this category include aortic atresia, critical aortic stenosis, critical coarctation of the aorta, interrupted aortic arch, and hypoplastic left heart syndrome. Children with these lesions present in shock when the ductus arteriosus closes. Patients with transposition of the great arteries benefit from patency of the ductus arteriosus because the pulmonary and systemic circulations are in parallel and the ductus allows for mixing of the two circulations. The resultant improvement

in oxygenation allows for stabilization until a balloon atrial septostomy or a surgical repair can be performed. PGE$_1$ may be effective in newborns up to 1 month of age if ductal closure has not been complete.[102]

Mechanism of Action

PGE$_1$ appears to allow for relaxation of the smooth muscle that lines the ductus arteriosus, although the exact mechanism is not clear. In other tissues, PGE$_1$ has been shown to result in increased levels of nitric oxide and nitric oxide synthase.[103]

Dosage

PGE$_1$ should be administered intravenously initially at a rate of 0.05–0.1 mcg/kg/min. The dose can be doubled every 15–30 minutes, up to a maximum dose of 0.2 mcg/kg/min or until a clinical effect is observed. Once an effective level of the medication is achieved, the rate of the infusion can be titrated down to between 0.01 and 0.04 mcg/kg/min. Studies have shown effective maintenance of ductal patency at doses less than 0.02 mcg/kg/min. The lowest effective dosage should be used, because this decreases the likelihood of side effects, particularly apnea.

Metabolism and Half-Life

PGE$_1$ is primarily metabolized in the lung, and its metabolites are excreted in the urine. The half-life is between 5 and 10 minutes.

Adverse Effects

Adverse effects include respiratory depression and apnea, especially in the smaller infants.[104] Systemic hypotension and bradycardia have also been seen. Fevers are sometimes observed in patients receiving PGE$_1$. PGE$_1$ inhibits platelet aggregation, which may impair clotting. Prolonged use of PGE$_1$ has been associated with gastric outlet obstruction (i.e., pyloric stenosis) and cortical hyperostosis of the long bones.

Monitoring

As with all critically ill patients, vital signs, including pulse oximetry, should be monitored closely in these patients. Arterial blood gas monitoring is particularly useful when attempting to determine if there is adequate pulmonary and systemic blood flow.

Pearls

After initial stabilization, the PGE$_1$ infusion rate can often be weaned to 0.01–0.025 mcg/kg/min. At this level, apnea and the need for endotracheal tube placement are less common. It is recommended that a secure airway be established in newborns receiving PGE$_1$ who require transport to another facility. Finally, there are some situations in which PGE$_1$ therapy cannot help stabilize the infant. For example, a newborn with total anomalous pulmonary venous connection requires surgical repair, and PGE_1 may only increase the pulmonary blood flow, resulting in increased pulmonary edema in the setting of obstructed pulmonary venous return.

Indomethacin

Indications
Indomethacin is indicated in infants, particularly those born prematurely with a patent ductus arteriosus and excessive pulmonary blood flow. Closure of the ductus in premature neonates frequently provides significant benefits to this patient population. In fact, some data suggest that simply the presence of a ductus, without associated hemodynamic sequelae, is indication enough to treat the newborn with indomethacin.[105]

Mechanism of Action
Indomethacin inhibits the activity of cyclooxygenase, thereby decreasing the synthesis of endogenous prostaglandins. In the absence of prostaglandins, smooth muscle within the ductus arteriosus will contract, closing the vessel.

Dosage
Indomethacin should be administered intravenously when treating a patient with a patent ductus arteriosus. Dosing schedules vary, but the intended course of therapy is usually three doses. The medication may be discontinued if the ductus is documented to be closed before completion of the course. If there is a decrease in urinary output, fewer doses may be administered or the time interval between doses may be extended. The initial dose is 0.2 mg/kg, followed by two subsequent doses that vary depending on the postnatal age. If the postnatal age at the time of the first dose is < 48 hours, then the two subsequent doses are 0.1 mg/kg at 12-24-hour intervals; if the postnatal age is 2-7 days, then the two subsequent doses are 0.2 mg/kg at 12-24-hour intervals; if the postnatal age is > 7 days, then the two subsequent doses are 0.25 mg/kg at 12-24-hour intervals. If the ductus arteriosus does not close or if clinical signs reappear after an initially successful first course, then a second course may be repeated at the same doses. Alternative treatment strategies have been used with success, including a more prolonged course of therapy.[106] In general, surgical closure of the patent ductus arteriosus is recommended if there is persistent, uncontrolled congestive heart failure despite medical management that includes indomethacin therapy or if indomethacin is contraindicated.

Metabolism and Half-Life
Indomethacin is metabolized by the liver. The half-life in children under 2 weeks of age is 20 hours, while the half-life in children with a postnatal age greater than 2 weeks is 11 hours.

Adverse Effects
Adverse effects include hypertension, bleeding, edema, thrombocytopenia, oliguria, and renal failure. Indomethacin should be avoided in patients with renal insufficiency, necrotizing enterocolitis, or shock.

Monitoring
The urine output, serum creatinine, platelet count, and blood urea nitrogen should be monitored in children receiving indomethacin. The blood pressure should be followed carefully. Echocardiography is necessary to confirm complete ductal closure.

Pearls
As for all administered medications, the risk-to-benefit ratio of indomethacin therapy must be evaluated. If the medication is deemed too high of a risk in a particular patient, then surgical ligation and division of the ductus arteriosus may be indicated as primary therapy. Prophylactic treatment with indomethacin on the first day of life does not appear to confer any advantage and runs the risk of unnecessary treatment of infants in whom the ductus may close spontaneously.[107]

MAJOR POINTS

- Large pediatric clinical trials are uncommon, resulting in few cardiovascular drugs that are studied and labeled for use in children.
- Recent legislation encourages manufacturers to sponsor pediatric clinical trials for established drugs and requires studies for labeling of new drugs that are considered to have a potentially significant impact in children.
- The current use of cardiovascular drugs in pediatric patients is based on limited published data, anecdotal experience, conventional wisdom, and extrapolation from large adult trials.
- Extrapolation of practice guidelines from adult studies is difficult since the use of identical drugs in pediatric patients is frequently associated with a different efficacy and side effect profile.
- Children often require a higher medication dose per unit of body weight for the same clinical effect, may need more frequent dosing schedules due to their more rapid metabolism and elimination, and may have a different incidence and spectrum of side effects due to variation in their development and physiologic maturity.
- As with prescribing medications in adults, the most important considerations in pediatrics include preexisting diagnoses and comorbidities that may change the intended effects and side effects of the drug, the consequences of the application of any drug

Continued

MAJOR POINTS—CONT'D

in a particular clinical situation, and the interactions between medications.
- Despite the limited quantity of information available regarding the use of cardiovascular drugs in the pediatric population, there exists an abundance of drug classes that may benefit children on a daily basis.

REFERENCES

1. Perkin RM, Levin DL, Webb R, et al: Dobutamine: A hemodynamic evaluation in children with shock. J Pediatr 100: 977-983, 1982.

2. Schranz D, Stopfkuchen H, Jungst BK, et al: Hemodynamic effects of dobutamine in children with cardiovascular failure. Eur J Pediatr 139:4-7, 1982.

3. Barrington K, Chan W: The circulatory effects of epinephrine infusion in the anesthetized piglet. Pediatr Res 33:190-194, 1993.

4. Cutaia M, Porcelli RJ: Pulmonary vascular reactivity after repetitive exposure to selected biogenic amines. J Appl Physiol 55:1868-1876, 1983.

5. Lock JE, Olley PM, Coceani F: Enhanced beta-adrenergic-receptor responsiveness in hypoxic neonatal pulmonary circulation. Am J Physiol 240:H697-H703, 1981.

6. Meadow WL, Rudinsky BF, Strates E: Selective elevation of systemic blood pressure by epinephrine during sepsis-induced pulmonary hypertension in piglets. Pediatr Res 20:872-875, 1986.

7. Brown CG, Martin DR, Pepe PE, et al: A comparison of standard-dose and high-dose epinephrine in cardiac arrest outside the hospital. The Multicenter High-Dose Epinephrine Study Group. N Engl J Med 327:1051-1055, 1992.

8. Goetting MG, Paradis NA: High dose epinephrine in refractory pediatric cardiac arrest. Crit Care Med 17:1258-1262, 1989.

9. Caspi J, Coles JG, Benson LN, et al: Age-related response to epinephrine-induced myocardial stress. Circulation 84:III394-399, 1991.

10. Bartelds B, Gratama JW, Meuzulaar KJ, et al: Comparative effects of isoproterenol and dopamine on myocardial oxygen consumption, blood flow distribution, and total body oxygen consumption in conscious lambs with and without an aortopulmonary left to right shunt. J Am Coll Cardiol 31:473-481, 1998.

11. Nishioka K, Nakanishi T, George BL, Jarmakani JM. The effect of calcium on the inotropy of catecholamine and paired electrical stimulation in the newborn and adult myocardium. J Mol Cell Cardiol 13:511-520, 1981.

12. Stueven HA, Thompson B, Aprahamian C, et al: The effectiveness of calcium chloride in refractory electromechanical dissociation. Ann Emerg Med 14:626-629, 1985.

13. Cardenas-Rivero N, Chernow B, Stoiko MA, et al: Hypocalcemia in critically ill children. J Pediatr 114:946-951, 1989.

14. Broner CW, Stidham GL, Westenkirchner DF, Watson DC. A prospective, randomized, double-blind comparison of calcium chloride and calcium gluconate therapies for hypocalcemia in critically ill children. J Pediatr 117: 986-989, 1990.

15. Odeh M: Tumor necrosis factor-alpha as a myocardial depressant substance. International J Cardiol 42:231-238, 1993.

16. Barton P, Garcia J, Kouatli A, et al: Hemodynamic effects of IV milrinone lactate in pediatric patients with septic shock. Chest 109:1302-1312, 1996.

17. Lawless S, Burckart G, Diven W, et al: Amrinone in neonates and infants after cardiac surgery. Crit Care Med 17:751-754, 1989.

18. Berner M, Jaccard C, Oberhansli I, et al: Hemodynamic effects of amrinone in children after cardiac surgery. Intensive Care Med 16:85-88, 1990.

19. Robinson BW, Gelband H, Mas MS: Selective pulmonary and selective vasodilation effects of amrinone in children: New therapeutic implications. J Am Coll Cardiol 21:1461-1465, 1993.

20. Hoffman TM, Wernovsky G, Atz AM, et al: Efficacy and safety of milrinone in preventing low cardiac output syndrome in infants and children after corrective surgery for congenital heart disease. Circulation 107:996-1002, 2003.

21. Chang AC, Atz AM, Wernovsky G, et al: Milrinone: Systemic and pulmonary hemodynamic effects in neonates after cardiac surgery. Crit Care Med 23:1907-1914, 1995.

22. Beekman RH, Rocchini AP, Dick M Jr, et al: Vasodilator therapy in children: Acute and chronic effects in children with left ventricular dysfunction or mitral regurgitation. Pediatrics 73:43-51, 1984.

23. Dillon TR, Janos GG, Meyer RA, et al: Vasodilator therapy for congestive heart failure. J Pediatr 96:623-629, 1980.

24. Nakano H, Ueda K, Saito A: Acute hemodynamic effects of nitroprusside in children with isolated mitral regurgitation. Am J Cardiol 56:351-355, 1985.

25. Benzing G III, Helmsworth JA, Schrieber JT, et al: Nitroprusside after open-heart surgery. Circulation 54:467-471, 1976.

26. Benzing G III, Helmsworth JA, Schrieber JT, Kaplan S: Nitroprusside and epinephrine for treatment of low output in children after open-heart surgery. Ann Thorac Surg 27:523-528, 1979.

27. Appelbaum A, Blackstone EH, Kouchoukos NT, Kirklin JW: Afterload reduction and cardiac output in infants early after intracardiac surgery. Am J Cardiol 39:445-451, 1977.

28. Fleischmann LE: Management of hypertensive crisis in children. Pediatr Ann 6:410-414, 1977.

29. Gordillo-Paniagua G, Velasquez-Jones L, Martini R, Valdez-Bolanos E: Sodium nitroprusside treatment in severe arterial hypertension in children. J Pediatr 87:799-802, 1975.

30. Will RJ, Walker OM, Traugott RC, Treasure RL: Sodium nitroprusside and propranolol therapy for management for postcoactectomy hypertension. J Thorac Cardiovasc Surg 75:722-724, 1978.

31. Bennett NR, Abbott TR: The use of sodium nitroprusside in children. Anaesthesia 32:456-463, 1977.

32. Moncada S, Palmer RM, Higgs EA: Nitric oxide: Physiology, pathophysiology, and pharmacology. Pharmacol Rev 43:109-142, 1991.

33. Damen J, Hitchcock JF: Reactive pulmonary hypertension after a switch operation. Successful treatment with glyceryl trinitrate. Br Heart J 53:223-225, 1985.

34. Ilbawi MN, Idriss FS, DeLeon SY, et al: Hemodynamic effects of intravenous nitroglycerin in pediatric patients after heart surgery. Circulation 72:II101-II107, 1985.

35. Cohn JN, Archibald DG, Ziesche S, et al: Effect of vasodilator therapy on mortality in chronic congestive heart failure. Results of a Veterans Administration Cooperative Study. N Engl J Med 314:1547-1552, 1986.

36. Edwards BS, Weir EK, Edwards WD, et al: Coexistent pulmonary and portal hypertension: Morphologic and clinical features. J Am Coll Cardiol 10:1233-1238, 1987.

37. Petitpretz P, Brenot F, Azarian R, et al: Pulmonary hypertension in patients with human immunodeficiency virus infection: Comparison with primary pulmonary hypertension. Circulation 89:2722-2727, 1994.

38. Abenhaim L, Moride Y, Brenot F, et al: Appetite-suppressant drugs and the risk of primary pulmonary hypertension. N Engl J Med 335:609-616, 1996.

39. Journois D, Pouard P, Mauriat P, et al: Inhaled nitric oxide as a therapy for pulmonary hypertension after operations for congenital heart defects. J Thorac Cardiovasc Surg 107:1129-1135, 1994.

40. Russell IA, Zwass MS, Fineman JR, et al: The effects of inhaled nitric oxide on postoperative pulmonary hypertension in infants and children undergoing surgical repair of congenital heart disease. Anesth Analg 87:46-51, 1998.

41. Adatia I, Perry S, Landzberg M, et al: Inhaled nitric oxide and hemodynamic evaluation of patients with pulmonary hypertension before transplantation. J Am Coll Cardiol 25:1656-1664, 1995.

42. Schulze-Neick I, Bultmann M, Werner H, et al: Right ventricular function in patients treated with inhaled nitric oxide after cardiac surgery for congenital heart disease in newborns and children. Am J Cardiol 80:360-363, 1997.

43. Frostell C, Fratacci MD, Wain JC, et al: Inhaled nitric oxide. A selective pulmonary vasodilator reversing hypoxic pulmonary vasoconstriction. Circulation 83:2038-2047, 1991.

44. Wessel DL, Adatia I, Thompson JE, Hickey PR: Delivery and monitoring of inhaled nitric oxide in patients with pulmonary hypertension. Crit Care Med 22:930-938, 1994.

45. Laguenie G, Berg A, Saint-Maurice JP, Dinh-Xuan AT: Measurement of nitrogen dioxide formation from nitric oxide by chemiluminescence in ventilated children. Lancet 341:969, 1993.

46. Barst RJ, Rubin LJ, Long WA, et al: A comparison of continuous intravenous epoprostenol (prostacyclin) with conventional therapy for primary pulmonary hypertension. N Engl J Med 334:296-302, 1996.

47. Barst RJ: Vasodilator therapy for primary pulmonary hypertension in children. Circulation 99:1197-1208, 1999.

48. Kermode J, Butt W, Shann F: Comparison between prostaglandin E1 and epoprostenol (prostacyclin) in infants after heart surgery. Br Heart J 66:175-178, 1991.

49. Rubin LJ: Primary pulmonary hypertension. N Engl J Med 336:111-117, 1997.

50. Hoeper MM, Schwarze M, Ehlerding S, et al: Long-term treatment of primary pulmonary hypertension with aerosolized iloprost, a prostacyclin analogue. N Engl J Med 342:1866-1870, 2000.

51. Olschewski H, Ghofrani HA, Schmehl T, et al: Inhaled iloprost to treat severe pulmonary hypertension: An uncontrolled trial. Ann Intern Med 132:435-443, 2000.

52. Channick RN, Simonneau G, Sitbon O, et al: Effects of the dual endothelin-receptor antagonist bosentan in patients with pulmonary hypertension: A randomized placebo-controlled study. Lancet 358:1119-1123, 2001.

53. Galie N, Hinderliter AL, Torbicki A, et al: Effects of the oral endothelin-receptor antagonist bosentan on echocardiographic and Doppler measures in patients with pulmonary arterial hypertension. J Am Coll Cardiol 41:1380-1386, 2003.

54. Barst RJ, Ivy D, Dingemanse J, et al: Pharmacokinetics, safety, and efficacy of bosentan in pediatric patients with pulmonary arterial hypertension. Clin Pharmacol Therap 73:372-382, 2003.

55. Rosenzweig EB, Starc TJ, Chen JM, et al: Intravenous arginine-vasopressin in children with vasodilatory shock after cardiac surgery. Circulation 100(19 suppl):II182-II186, 1999.

56. Heart Failure Society of America: HFSA guidelines for management of patients with heart failure caused by left ventricular systolic dysfunction: Pharmacological approaches. Pharmacotherapy 20:495-522, 2000.

57. Pitt B, Zannad F, Remme WJ: The effect of spironolactone on morbidity and mortality in patients with severe heart failure. N Engl J Med 341:709-717, 1999.

58. Cohn JN, Johnson G, Ziesche S, et al: A comparison of enalapril with hydralazine-isosorbide dinitrate in the treatment of chronic congestive heart failure. N Engl J Med 325:303-310, 1991.

59. The SOLVD Investigators: Effect of enalapril on survival in patients with reduced left ventricular ejection fractions and congestive heart failure. N Engl J Med 313:1617-1620, 1991.

60. Wilson NJS, Dickinson D: Captopril in heart failure secondary to a left to right shunt. Arch Dis Child 63:360-363, 1988.

61. Lewis AB, Chabot M: The effect of treatment with angiotensin-converting enzyme inhibitors on survival of pediatric patients with dilated cardiomyopathy. Pediatr Cardiol 14:9-12, 1993.

62. Pereira CM, Tam YK, Collins-Nakai RL: The pharmacokinetics of captopril in infants with congestive heart failure. Ther Drug Monit 13:209-214, 1991.

63. Fogari R, Zoppi A, Tettamanti F, et al: Effects of nifedipine and indomethacin on cough induced by angiotensin-converting enzyme inhibitors: A double-blind, randomized, cross-over study. J Cardiovasc Pharmacol 19:670-673, 1992.

64. Reisin L, Schneeweiss A: Complete spontaneous remission of cough induced by ACE inhibitors during chronic therapy in hypertensive patients. J Human Hypertens 6:333-335, 1992.

65. The CONSENSUS Trial Study Group: Effects of enalapril on mortality in severe congestive heart failure: Results of the cooperative north Scandinavian enalapril survival study (CONSENSUS). N Engl J Med 316:1429-1435, 1987.

66. The SOLVD Investigators: Effect of enalapril on survival in patients with reduced left ventricular ejection fractions and congestive heart failure. N Engl J Med 325:293-302, 1991.

67. The SOLVD Investigators: Effect of enalapril on mortality and the development of heart failure in asymptomatic patients with reduced left ventricular ejection fractions. N Engl J Med 327:685-691, 1992.

68. Miller K, Atkin B, Rodel PV Jr., Walker JF: Enalapril: A well-tolerated and efficacious agent for the pediatric hypertensive patient. J Cardiovasc Pharmacol 10:S154-S156, 1987.

69. Frenneaux M, Stewart RAH, Newman CMH, Hallidie-Smith KA: Enalapril for severe heart failure in infancy. Arch Dis Child 64:219-223, 1989.

70. Webster MWI, Neutze JM, Calder AL: Acute hemodynamic effects of converting enzyme inhibition in children with intracardiac shunts. Pediatr Cardiol 13:129-135, 1992.

71. Pitt B, Poole-Wilson PA, Segal R, et al: Effect of losartan compared with captopril on mortality in patients with symptomatic heart failure: Randomized trial. The Losartan Heart Failure Survival Study (ELITE II). Lancet 355:1582-1587, 2000.

72. Cohn JN, Tognoni G: Valsartan heart failure trial investigators. A randomized trial of the angiotensin-receptor blocker valsartan in chronic heart failure. N Engl J Med 345:1667-1675, 2001.

73. Pfeffer MA, McMurray JJ, Velazquez EJ, et al: Valsartan in Acute Myocardial Infarction Trial (VALIANT) Investigators. Valsartan, captopril, or both in myocardial infarction complicated by heart failure, left ventricular dysfunction, or both. N Engl J Med 349:1893-1906, 2003.

74. Pfeffer MA, Swedberg K, Granger CB, et al: CHARM Investigators and Committees. Effects of candesartan on mortality and morbidity in patients with chronic heart failure: The CHARM-Overall programme. Lancet 362:759-766, 2003.

75. Wong M, Staszewsky L, Latini R, et al: Val-HeFT Heart Failure Trial Investigators. Valsartan benefits left ventricular structure and function in heart failure. Val-HeFT echocardiographic study. J Am Coll Cardiol 40:970-975, 2002.

76. Cohn JN, Tognoni G: Valsartan Heart Failure Trial Investigators. A randomized trial of the angiotensin-receptor blocker valsartan in chronic heart failure. N Engl J Med 345:1667-1675, 2001.

77. Wyman MG, Slaughter RL, Farolino DA, et al: Multiple bolus technique for lidocaine administration in acute ischemic heart disease. II. Treatment of refractory ventricular arrhythmias and the pharmacokinetic significance of severe left ventricular failure. J Am Coll Cardiol 2:764-769, 1983.

78. Holt DW, Walsh AC, Curry PV, Tynan M: Pediatric use of mexiletine and disopyramide. Br Med J 2:1476-1477, 1979.

79. Echt DS, Liebson PR, Mitchell LB, et al: Mortality and morbidity in patients receiving encainide, flecainide, or placebo. The cardiac arrhythmia suppression trial. N Engl J Med 324:781-788, 1991.

80. Fish FA, Gillette PC, Benson DW Jr: Proarrhythmia, cardiac arrest, and death in young patients receiving encainide and flecainide. The Pediatric Electrophysiology Group: J Am Coll Cardiol 18:356-365, 1991.

81. Perry JC, Garson A Jr: Flecainide acetate for treatment of tachyarrhythmias in children: Review of world literature on efficacy, safety, and dosing. Am Heart J 124:1614-1621, 1992.

82. MERIT-HF Study Group: Effect of metoprolol CR/XL in chronic heart failure: Metoprolol CR/XL Randomized Intervention Trial in Congestive Heart Failure (MERIT-HF). Lancet 353:2001-2007, 1999.

83. Packer M, Coats AJ, Fowler MB, et al: Carvedilol Prospective Randomized Cumulative Survival Study Group. Effect of carvedilol on survival in severe chronic heart failure. N Engl J Med 344:1651-1658, 2001.

84. Smerling A, Gersony WM: Esmolol for severe hypertension following repair of aortic coarctation. Crit Care Med 18:1288-1290, 1990.

85. Vincent RN, Click LA, Williams HM, et al: Esmolol as an adjunct in the treatment of systemic hypertension after operative repair of coarctation of the aorta. Am J Cardiol 65:941-943, 1990.

86. Nussbaum J, Zane EA, Thys DM: Esmolol for the treatment of hypercyanotic spells in infants with tetralogy of Fallot. J Cardiothorac Anesth 3:200-202, 2989.

87. Cuneo BF, Zales VR, Blahunka PC, Benson DW Jr: Pharmacodynamics and pharmacokinetics of esmolol, a short-acting beta-blocking agent, in children. Pediatr Cardiol 15:296-301, 1994.

88. Wiest DB, Garner SS, Uber WE, Sade RM: Esmolol for management of pediatric hypertension after cardiac operations. J Thorac Cardiovasc Surg 115:890-897, 1998.

89. Wiest DB, Trippel DL, Gillette PC, Garner SS: Pharmacokinetics of esmolol in children. Clin Pharmacol Ther 49:618-623, 1991.

90. Trippel DL, Wiest DB, Gillette PC: Cardiovascular and antiarrhythmic effects of esmolol in children. J Pediatr 119:142-147, 1991.

91. Ostman-Smith I, Wettrell G, Riesenfeld T: A cohort study of childhood hypertrophic cardiomyopathy. J Am Coll Cardiol 34:1813-1822, 1999.

92. Perry JC, Fenrich AL, Hulse JE, et al: Pediatric use of intravenous amiodarone: Efficacy and safety in critically ill patients from a multicenter protocol. J Am Coll Cardiol 27:1246-1250, 1996.

93. Kudenchuk PJ, Cobb LA, Copass MK, et al: Amiodarone for resuscitation after out-of-hospital cardiac arrest due to ventricular fibrillation. N Engl J Med 341:871–878, 1999.

94. Dorian P, Cass D, Schwartz B, et al: Amiodarone as compared with lidocaine for shock-resistant ventricular fibrillation. N Engl J Med 346:884–890, 2002.

95. Guiccione P, Paul T, Garson A Jr: Long-term follow-up of amiodarone therapy in the young. J Am Coll Cardiol 15:1118–1124, 1990.

96. Waldo AL, Camm JA, deRuyter H, et al: Effect of *d*-sotalol on mortality in patients with left ventricular dysfunction after recent and remote myocardial infarction. Lancet 348:7–12, 1996.

97. Epstein ML, Kiel EA, Victoria BE: Cardiac decompensation following verapamil therapy in infants with supraventricular tachycardia. Pediatrics 75:737–740, 1985.

98. Gibson R, Driscoll D, Gillette P, et al: The comparative electrophysiologic and hemodynamic effects of verapamil in puppies and adult dogs. Dev Pharmacol Ther 2:104–116, 1981.

99. Watt AH, Bernard MS, Webster J, et al: Intravenous adenosine in the treatment of supraventricular tachycardia: A dose-ranging study and interaction with dipyridamole. Br J Clin Pharmacol 21:227–230, 1986.

100. Ellenbogen KA, Thames MD, DiMarco JP, et al: Electrophysiological effects of adenosine in the transplanted human heart. Evidence of supersensitivity. Circulation 81:821–828, 1990.

101. Lang P, Freed MD, Rosenthal A, et al: The use of prostaglandin E1 in an infant with interruption of the aortic arch. J Pediatr 91:805–807, 1977.

102. Freed MD, Heymann MA, Lewis AB, et al: Prostaglandin E1 in infants with ductus arteriosus-dependent congenital heart disease. Circulation 64:899–905, 1981.

103. Escrig A, Marin R, Mas M: Repeated PGE1 treatment enhances nitric oxide and erection responses to nerve stimulation in the rat penis by upregulating constitutive NOS isoforms. J Urology 162:2205–2210, 1999.

104. Lewis AB, Freed MD, Heymann MA, et al: Side effects of therapy with prostaglandin E1 in infants with critical congenital heart disease. Circulation 64:893–898, 1981.

105. Mahony L, Carnero V, Brett C, et al: Prophylactic indomethacin therapy for patent ductus arteriosus in very-low-birth-weight infants. N Engl J Med 306:506–510, 1982.

106. Seyberth HW, Rascher W, Hackenthal R, Wille L: Effect of prolonged indomethacin therapy on renal function and selected vasoactive hormones in very-low-birth-weight infants with symptomatic patent ductus arteriosus. J Pediatr 103:979–984, 1983.

107. Mahony L, Caldwell RL, Girod DA, et al: Indomethacin therapy on the first day of life in infants with very low birth weight. J Pediatr 106:801–805, 1985.

Surgery for Congenital Heart Disease

BRADLEY S. MARINO

ADAM M. OSTROW

MERYL S. COHEN

Congenital heart disease is the most common anomaly of the newborn, affecting 8/1000 children. Of these, 3 will have critical heart defects that require surgical or catheter-directed intervention within the first 6 months of life.

Since the first cardiac surgeries for structural heart disease, performed in the late 1930s and early 1940s, pediatric cardiac surgery has evolved as a field at a staggering pace. Many contributions have led to this expansion, including the introduction of cardiopulmonary bypass and circulatory arrest to undertake intracardiac repairs, the development of prostaglandin E₁ therapy for ductal-dependent cardiac lesions, innovative operative techniques for cardiac reconstruction, safe cardiac anesthetics, and improving medical and mechanical forms of support for pre- and postoperative management.

In the early era of pediatric cardiac surgery, morbidity and mortality were quite high. Children with critical heart disease underwent palliative procedures that did not correct the defect but rather altered the physiology to sustain life. Today, palliative procedures are still necessary for some lesions, but complex reconstructive surgeries are now possible for neonates and even premature infants with structural defects. Even successful fetal cardiac interventions have been reported.[1] Because cardiac disease is known to progress in utero, it has been postulated that fetal intervention may alter the course of certain disease states; for example, dilation of a severely stenotic aortic valve in utero may prevent the development of hypoplastic left heart syndrome.

Overall, mortality has significantly diminished over the years for almost every cardiac defect. Patients with congenital heart disease are now faced with long-term issues including maintenance of health; neurodevelopmental issues; school, social, and work performance; and pregnancy.

PREOPERATIVE MANAGEMENT OF CONGENITAL HEART DISEASE

By improving hemodynamics and minimizing the sequelae of heart disease such as end-organ damage, preoperative management of the child with critical congenital heart disease has a dramatic impact on overall outcome. Many factors have contributed to the improvement in this management over the last half-century.

Prostaglandin E₁ Therapy

The fetal circulation is uniquely adaptable to most hemodynamic disturbances. In general, the fetus with critical congenital (i.e., single-ventricle) heart disease grows normally and survives to term as a result of this distinctive physiology. In utero, the systemic and pulmonary circulations function in parallel; the placenta acts as the oxygenator, and patency of the ductus venosus, foramen ovale, and ductus arteriosus allows for the oxygen-rich blood to be directed toward the vital organs, namely the heart and brain. In the 1940s, Dr. Helen Taussig recognized that maintenance of the fetal circulation after birth sustained life in infants with cyanotic heart disease. This observation eventually led to a partnership with her surgical colleague, Dr. Alfred Blalock, and the development of a systemic artery to pulmonary artery communication (i.e., an aortopulmonary shunt) that became the surgical equivalent of a patent ductus arteriosus.[2] It was soon learned through animal model studies that the ductus arteriosus remains patent in those receiving intravenous infusion of E-type prostaglandin.[3]

By the late 1970s, prostaglandin E_1 became entrenched as a mainstay of therapy to ensure ductal patency in infants with a variety of cardiac lesions, including those with ductal-dependent pulmonary blood flow (e.g., pulmonary atresia or tricuspid atresia), ductal-dependent systemic blood flow (e.g., critical coarctation of the aorta, critical aortic stenosis, interrupted aortic arch, or hypoplastic left heart syndrome), and transposition of the great arteries. Thus, infants with critical heart defects could be stabilized and could have a more thorough and extensive assessment rather than being urgently ushered to the operative room for emergency palliative procedures. Prostaglandin E_1 continues to play a critical role in the preoperative management of patients with ductal-dependent cardiac lesions.

Noninvasive Imaging

Transthoracic echocardiography, developed in the 1970s and, more recently, cardiac magnetic resonance imaging (MRI) have changed the field of pediatric cardiology. In fact, accurate diagnosis of heart disease by these methods has replaced cardiac catheterization and angiography as the primary diagnostic tools. These imaging modalities provide both anatomic and physiologic information about structural and acquired heart disease. In addition to being noninvasive, echocardiography is portable and is applied in real time, so diagnoses are made as the studies are being performed.

Interventional Cardiac Catheterization

Advances in cardiac catheterization have changed the field from a diagnostic tool to a mode of treatment. Since the first catheter-directed intervention (relief of valvar pulmonary stenosis), interventional cardiac catheterization has improved our ability to stabilize patients with heart disease prior to or to the exclusion of surgical intervention.

In the 1960s, Dr. William Rashkind of The Children's Hospital of Philadelphia introduced a procedure called balloon atrial septostomy to palliate infants with transposition of the great arteries who were markedly cyanotic.[4] In transposition, the systemic and pulmonary circulations are in parallel and mixing between the two is required to oxygenate the systemic arterial blood. The septostomy essentially tears a hole in the atrial septum, thereby allowing mixing at that level. The balloon atrial septostomy, followed by balloon dilation valvuloplasty for pulmonary stenosis, launched the field of pediatric interventional cardiac catheterization.

More recently, interventional catheterization procedures have eliminated the need for some surgical interventions. Devices have been developed that close atrial septal defects, ventricular septal defects, the ductus arteriosus, and collateral vessels. In addition, balloon catheters and intravascular stents similar to those used to open coronary arteries can be used to relieve semilunar valve obstruction, branch pulmonary artery stenosis, and coarctation of the aorta.

Pediatric Cardiac Intensive Care

Pediatric cardiac intensive care has developed into a subspecialty of pediatric cardiology and critical care. Many pediatric institutions have intensive care units that provide care exclusively to children with congenital heart disease. In addition to staffing with highly trained physicians, nurses, and ancillary personnel, advances in management in the intensive care unit include improved ventilator strategies, new pharmacological agents, and mechanical support devices (e.g., extracorporeal membrane oxygenation and ventricular assist devices).

CARDIOPULMONARY BYPASS

The techniques of cardiopulmonary bypass (CPB) and myocardial preservation used in open procedures are critical for an adequate hemodynamic result without permanent secondary organ damage. In CPB, venous blood is siphoned into the venous reservoir of the heart-lung bypass apparatus from a single cannula placed into the right atrium or from two smaller catheters inserted into each vena cava. After traversing a membrane oxygenator, a heat exchanger, a filter, and a roller pump, blood is returned to the patient's ascending aorta through an aortic cannula. Figure 14-1 delineates the path of blood in the cardiopulmonary bypass circuit. The time during which blood is continuously exchanged between the heart–lung apparatus and the patient is referred as the *total bypass time*. The *cross clamp time*

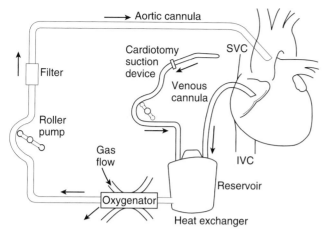

Figure 14-1 Basic components of cardiopulmonary bypass. Venous blood is drained from the heart through a cannula in the right atrium (shown here) or, alternately, bicaval cannulation in the superior vena cava (SVC) and inferior vena cava (IVC). Blood drains by gravity to a venous reservoir and mixes with blood drained from the operative field by cardiotomy suction catheters. After passing through a heat exchanger, the blood is passed through an oxygenator, through a roller pump and a micropore filter, and back to the body through an aortic cannula. (Adapted from Chang AC, Hanley FL, Wernovsky G, Wessel DL: Pediatric Cardiac Intensive Care. Baltimore: Williams & Wilkins, 1998, p 190.)

refers to the time during which the aorta is clamped and the heart is ischemic.

Despite notable and continuing improvements in the technical aspects of CPB, significant morbidity may be associated with its use. During CPB, the blood is exposed to prosthetic material and undergoes sheer stresses. These alterations lead to the activation of neutrophils, platelets, endothelial cells, and the serum proteins that mediate blood clotting, complement fixation, and fibrinolysis.[5] The combined effect of this activation is a generalized inflammatory response, which can result in endothelial cell injury, increased capillary permeability, and tissue edema. CPB can cause increase in total body water, transient myocardial dysfunction, elevated pulmonary vascular resistance, abnormalities of gas exchange, and stress and hormonal responses leading to fluid and electrolyte disturbances. Despite these perturbations, most children who undergo CPB tolerate it well, with few if any significant complications.

Some intraoperative techniques have helped reduce the morbidity associated with CPB, including modified ultrafiltration (MUF). MUF is performed in the immediate post-bypass period. It removes excess water from the patient directly and provides a method of salvaging, from the circuit, red blood cells that may be infused during postoperative convalescence. MUF after cardiac surgery has several beneficial effects, including improved

cardiovascular hemodynamics, decreased pulmonary vascular resistance, cytokine removal and reduction in complement activation, decreased postoperative bleeding, and a decreased need for hemodilution necessitated blood transfusion.

During many cardiac operations, the body temperature is lowered to 18–20°C to decrease tissue oxygen consumption and to protect the heart and other organs. Body temperatures of 20°C or lower are referred to as *deep hypothermia*. As metabolic demands decrease with hypothermia, pump flow can be temporarily reduced to as low as 25–50 mL/kg/min for *low flow bypass,* or the pump can be turned off altogether, causing *circulatory arrest.* At 18°C, circulatory arrest times of less than 45 minutes are generally well tolerated, but the incidence of neurologic sequelae increases in some patients with periods of greater than 60–75 minutes. Most surgeons use a combination of low flow and circulatory arrest to perform complex neonatal heart surgery.

GENERAL CONSIDERATIONS OF PEDIATRIC CARDIAC SURGERY

The field of pediatric cardiac surgery has changed dramatically over the years. In the early era, children were either palliated or they waited for growth prior to surgical intervention. These practices were in part due to the lack of appropriately sized surgical instruments and cannula for cardiopulmonary bypass and also to the uncertainty of how neonates would fare undergoing early open-heart repairs. Critical congenital heart defects that are palliated or uncorrected may cause progressive and irreversible secondary organ damage, principally to the heart, the lungs, and the central nervous system, and may interfere with normal postnatal changes such as myocardial hyperplasia, coronary angiogenesis, and pulmonary vascular and alveolar development.[6,7] In addition to these anatomic and functional sequelae, psychomotor and cognitive abnormalities may be present and may limit the development of the child with palliated or uncorrected critical congenital heart disease.[8,9]

Over the past decade, it has become apparent that the cumulative morbidity and mortality of palliative operations, followed by later repair, is greater than that of early corrective procedures. In the present model, primary reparative surgery in the neonate offers the opportunity to decrease the mortality caused by the primary defect and also to prevent secondary damage to other organ systems.[10] However, as we seek to further reduce morbidity and mortality through refinement of the timing and technique of cardiac surgery and postoperative care, our field continues to evolve.

SURGICAL INTERVENTIONS FOR CONGENITAL HEART DISEASE

TWO-VENTRICLE REPAIRS

Left-to-Right Shunt Lesions

Left-to-right shunts within the cardiovascular system cause undue volume overload to the heart. In many cases, congestive heart failure develops. The metabolic demands of the body are not adequately met because of the excessive volume load, usually in the presence of a normal myocardium. In general, large left-to-right shunts should be addressed prior to 1 year of age (excluding atrial septal defects) because progressive pulmonary vascular disease may develop, significantly increasing the risk of the procedure and affecting long-term outcome.

Atrial Septal Defects

An atrial septal defect (ASD) is a communication between the left atrium and right atrium. There are several anatomic types, including secundum ASDs, ostium primum ASDs, and sinus venosus ASDs. Ostium primum ASDs are a form of atrioventricular canal defect. Sinus venosus ASDs are located at the superior vena cava (SVC) or inferior vena cava (IVC) entries into the right atrium and may have associated partial anomalous pulmonary venous return. Left-to-right shunting at the atrial level results in right atrial and right ventricular volume overload and increased pulmonary blood flow. The degree of left-to-right shunting depends not only on the size of the defect but also on the relative compliance of the ventricles.

Timing of Surgery

The majority of infants and children are asymptomatic despite increased pulmonary blood flow and right ventricular volume overload. Although congestive heart failure (CHF) may occur in the second or third decade of life because of chronic right ventricular volume overload, up to 5% of children with ASD will have symptoms of CHF within the first year of life.[11] Pulmonary hypertension is rare in childhood, but it can occur in up to 13% of unoperated patients with ASD younger than 10 years of age.[12]

Spontaneous closure of small secundum-type ASDs may occur in the first few years of life. Ostium primum and sinus venosus ASDs do not close spontaneously and are addressed surgically. The timing of ASD repair in the asymptomatic infant or child is more controversial. In general, the defect should be repaired when circulatory arrest is not needed and when the likelihood of needing a blood transfusion is low. After 6 months of age, both of these criteria are generally met. In asymptomatic children with suitable small and moderate secundum ASDs, repair is sometimes delayed to allow for either the spontaneous closure of small defects or transcatheter closure, generally undertaken after 2 years of age. This is discussed in Chapter 11.

Method of Repair

Small ASDs, especially secundum-type ASDs, can often be closed directly with sutures. Larger ASDs and most primum ASDs require patch closure, typically with polytetrafluoroethylene (PTFE) (GORE-TEX®) or a small piece of native pericardium. Children with primum ASDs have a common AV valve; the left-sided portion usually has a "cleft," or deficit of tissue, which results in mitral regurgitation. In some cases, mitral valvuloplasty may be required in association with primum ASD closure. Sinus venosus ASDs may require more extensive atrial baffling when right-sided partial anomalous pulmonary venous connection is present.

Follow-Up

Postpericardiotomy syndrome with pericardial effusion is particularly common after all types of ASD repairs. Long-term postoperative problems after secundum ASD repair are extremely uncommon. Transient atrial arrhythmias or sinus node dysfunction occurs in a small percentage of children. Sequelae for primum ASDs are discussed in the section "Common Atrioventricular Canal Defects." Postoperative evaluation should include ruling out superior vena cava and, in the case of sinus venosus type ASDs, right pulmonary vein obstruction. Sinus node dysfunction is not uncommon, and temporary atrial pacing may be necessary.

Ventricular Septal Defects

Ventricular septal defects (VSDs) are categorized anatomically by their location in the ventricular septum (Fig. 14-2). A wide variety of terms are used to classify VSDs. At The Children's Hospital of Philadelphia, the following terms are used: muscular, conoventricular (perimembranous), malalignment, inlet (atrioventricular canal), and conoseptal hypoplasia (supracristal, subpulmonary, infundibular, or outlet). Muscular defects can occur anywhere in the muscular septum. Conoventricular defects are the most common.

Timing of Surgery

Left-to-right shunting at the ventricular level results in left atrial and left ventricular volume overload

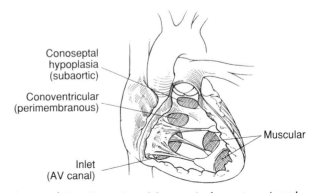

Figure 14-2   Illustration of the ventricular septum viewed from the right ventricle, showing the different types of ventricular septal defect. *AV*, atrioventricular. (Modified from Chang AC, Hanley FL, Wernovsky G, Wessel DL: Pediatric Cardiac Intensive Care. Baltimore: Williams & Wilkins, 1998, p 213.)

and increased pulmonary blood flow. The degree of left-to-right shunting depends not only on the size of the defect but also on the relative resistance between the pulmonary and the systemic circulations. If the VSD is restrictive (i.e., significantly smaller than the aortic root diameter), the degree of shunting is determined by the size of the defect. If the VSD is unrestrictive (i.e., there is no pressure gradient between the left and right ventricles), the degree of left-to-right shunting is determined by the relative resistances between the pulmonary and systemic vascular beds. As the pulmonary vascular resistance falls in the first weeks of life, left-to-right shunting increases and symptoms of congestive heart failure develop.

Spontaneous closure can occur in up to 50% of muscular and conoventricular defects.[13] Malalignment, inlet, and conoseptal hypoplasia VSDs rarely close spontaneously. If the VSD does not close, the clinical spectrum ranges from children with profound CHF and failure to thrive to asymptomatic children who takes subacute bacterial endocarditis prophylaxis when indicated.

The symptomatic child with CHF and failure to thrive is repaired at presentation. Malalignment and inlet VSDs are generally repaired during infancy since these defects are large and will not close spontaneously. If aortic insufficiency develops in a patient with a VSD, surgical closure is generally recommended to minimize the progression of valve insufficiency. Repair may be delayed if a child is asymptomatic, has no pulmonary hypertension, and has a VSD that may spontaneously close. VSD closure by device closure is briefly discussed in Chapter 11.

Method of Repair
Conoventricular, muscular, and inlet VSDs are repaired with a right atriotomy, whereas the conoseptal hypoplasia VSD is repaired with a pulmonary arteriotomy. The malalignment VSD is repaired through either a right atriotomy or a right ventriculotomy. Small VSDs, as well as the extent of larger VSDs, may be difficult to identify due to the trabeculated surface of the interventricular septum on the right ventricle side. As a result, patients are occasionally left with residual VSDs postoperatively.

Like ASDs, small defects can sometimes be directly closed with sutures. Larger defects or multiple defects are usually closed with patches. In some patients with many or complex VSDs, repair may be delayed to allow for growth of the child. Pulmonary artery banding (discussed later in this chapter) is sometimes employed to restrict pulmonary blood flow and to prevent heart failure in these situations. Rarely, a VSD may be so large that there is little ventricular septum. In such cases, the patient is palliated as a single ventricle type lesion.

Follow-Up
Injury to the conduction tissue, most commonly the right bundle branch, is the most common electrophysiologic complication of VSD closure. Right bundle branch block is generally found on an electrocardiogram and has no known significant long-term sequelae. Complete heart block may occur in up to 2% of patients after VSD closure. Temporary atrioventricular pacing is used to treat postoperative heart block. It is prudent to wait at least 7–14 days before implanting a permanent pacemaker as some cases of postoperative heart block will be transient. Despite timely and complete closure, the rare patient will go on to develop pulmonary hypertension for unclear reasons. Patients with trisomy 21 appear to be at increased risk for this late complication.

Patent Ductus Arteriosus
A patent ductus arteriosus (PDA) is a vascular communication between the junction of the main and left pulmonary arteries and the lesser curvature of the descending aorta just distal to the left subclavian artery. Left-to-right shunting at the ductus results in increased pulmonary blood flow and left atrial and left ventricular volume overload. Just as with VSDs, the degree of left-to-right shunting is determined by the size of the communication and the relative resistance between the systemic and pulmonary circulations.

Timing of Surgery
The incidence of PDA is higher in the preterm neonate. Approximately 20% of neonates weighing less than 1750 grams have a PDA.[14] In the preterm infant, treatment for the PDA includes medical management of left ventricular failure, indomethacin or ibuprofen therapy,[15,16] surgical ligation, or a combination thereof. If indomethacin or ibuprofen therapy fails to close the PDA, surgical ligation can be performed with minimal morbidity and mortality.[17] In this population, surgical closure before 10 days of age reduces the duration of ventilatory support and hospital stay and lowers morbidity.[18]

In symptomatic term infants, surgical closure is indicated when congestive heart failure or failure to thrive is present despite maximal medical therapy. Indomethacin is ineffective in term infants and should not be used. An asymptomatic PDA in a term infant is unlikely to close spontaneously after several months of age and should be closed electively to remove the risk of endocarditis. There is controversy as to the management of the incidental finding of a silent ductus, which cannot be appreciated by auscultation. Some clinicians advocate closure of the PDA to remove an undefined risk of endocarditis.

Method of Repair
In the term infant, therapy for the PDA includes medical management of left ventricular volume load, followed by surgical ligation, transcatheter device occlusion, coil embolization, or video-assisted thoracoscopic surgery (VATS).[19] Surgical ligation of the ductus by open thoracotomy or VATS may or may not include division of the ductus (Figs. 14-3 to 14-5). Ligation alone carries a risk of recannulation. In preterm infants, ligation without division of the ductus arteriosus is recommended because the tissues in these patients are very friable and complications may occur.

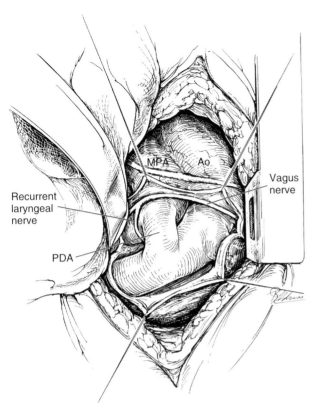

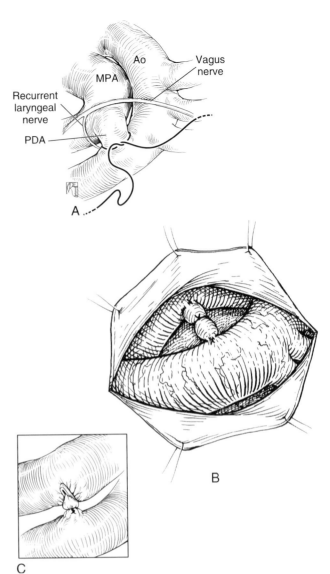

Figure 14-3 Operative exposure of a patent ductus arteriosus through a left thoracotomy. The mediastinal pleura is opened and reflected anteriorly and posteriorly. The vagus nerve and the recurrent laryngeal nerves are identified and preserved by retracting them medially. *Ao*, aorta; *MPA*, main pulmonary artery; *PDA*, patent ductus arteriosus. (From Mavroudis C, Backer CL: Pediatric Cardiac Surgery, 3rd ed. Philadelphia: Mosby, 2003, p 227.)

Figure 14-4 Surgical ligation of patent ductus arteriosus. Cardiopulmonary bypass is not used. The surgical perspective through a left thoracotomy is shown. In premature infants, a single ligature is typically placed using either suture material or metal clips. In children beyond the newborn period, typically three separate surgical ligatures are placed to minimize the chance of recanalization of the ductus. Techniques for ligation include **A,** single suture ligation; **B,** multiple ligation; and **C,** ligation and hemoclip placement of the PDA. Ao, aorta; MPO, main pulmonary artery, PDA, patent ductus arteriosus. (From Mavroudis C, Backer CL: Pediatric Cardiac Surgery, 3rd ed. Philadelphia: Mosby, 2003, p 227; Kouchoukos NT, Blackstone EH, Doty DB, et al:. Kirklin/Barratt-Boyes Cardiac Surgery, 3rd ed. Philadelphia: Churchill Livingstone, 2003, p 937.)

Mediastinal complications include phrenic or recurrent laryngeal nerve injury (i.e., vocal cord paralysis),[21] as well as pneumothorax, hemothorax, and chylothorax. Smaller neonates have a higher risk for these complications.

Closure of PDAs in the cardiac catheterization laboratory by coil embolization or device closure is now common in older children and, to a lesser extent, in term infants. This is discussed in greater detail in Chapter 11.

Follow-Up

In an isolated PDA, no further cardiology follow-up is generally indicated after the last postoperative visit unless there is evidence of recannulation.

Common Atrioventricular Canal Defects

The endocardial cushions form the atrioventricular (AV) valves and the septum of the AV canal. The normal AV canal septum fuses with the lower portion of the atrial septum and the upper portion of the ventricular septum, thereby dividing the canal into two atria and two ventricles. When the endocardial cushions fail to join, a common atrioventricular canal (CAVC) results. The defects found in CAVC include a common AV valve, an ostium primum ASD, and an inlet VSD.

Lesions associated with AV canal defects include patent ductus arteriosus, tetralogy of Fallot, coarctation of the aorta, heterotaxy syndrome, left superior vena cava, or a combination thereof. Common atrioventricular canal accounts for 40% of the congenital heart defects found in children with trisomy 21.

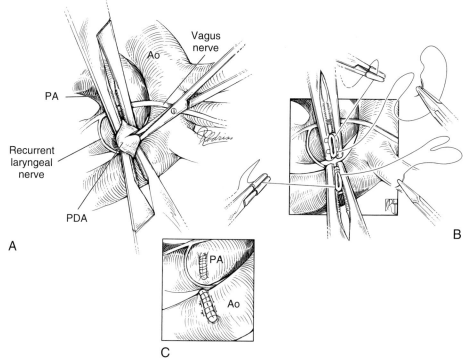

Figure 14-5   Surgical division of patent ductus arteriosus. The surgical perspective through a left thoracotomy is shown. The adventitia underlying the aortic isthmus and ductus arteriosus has been opened and retracted with sutures. **A,** Clamps have been placed across the aortic and pulmonary ends of the ductus arteriosus, and the ductus has been partially divided between the clamps. **B,** The aortic and pulmonary stumps of the ductus are oversewn with a running suture technique. **C,** The clamps are carefully removed and the overlying adventitia is closed. This technique is typically performed in older patients, especially those with anatomic variants that have a large diameter and a short length, and in older patients who have acquired degenerative changes within the ductus arteriosus. Ao, aorta; PA, pulmonary artery; PDA, patent ductus arteriosus. (From Mavroudis C, Backer CL: Pediatric Cardiac Surgery, 3rd ed. Philadelphia: Mosby, 2003, p 229.)

Timing of Surgery

Signs and symptoms depend on the magnitude of the left-to-right shunt and the amount of atrioventricular valve regurgitation. The symptomatic patient should be repaired at less than 6 months, generally at the time of presentation, whereas the asymptomatic child without pulmonary hypertension (i.e., ASD physiology) may undergo elective repair within the first few years of life. Infants with a large VSD component should be repaired by 6 months to decrease the risk of pulmonary artery hypertension and pulmonary vascular obstructive disease.

Method of Repair

The ASD and VSD portions are patched closed by a one- or two-patch technique to divide the common AV valve into a left ventricle (LV) inflow and an RV inflow and to close the septal defects resulting from the endocardial cushion defects (Fig. 14-6). Suture closure of the cleft leaflets of the septated left-sided AV inflow is performed to make the LV inflow as competent as possible.

Follow-Up

These patients have all the potential sequelae of patients with ASD and VSD closures along with some additional risks associated with this particular lesion. Arrhythmias in the postoperative period are common, including sinus node dysfunction and junctional ectopic tachycardia (generally a sign of low cardiac output). Many patients have a right bundle branch block postoperatively. There is also an increased incidence of complete atrioventricular block, which occurs in up to 6% of patients. Ninety-five percent of patients have preoperative left-axis deviation of 0 to −30 degrees on electrocardiogram, and this finding will persist postoperatively. The incidence of immediate postoperative pulmonary hypertension is high and is correlated with older age at operation. These episodes correlate closely with postoperative mortality.[21] There is also evidence that postoperative pulmonary vascular resistance is higher in children with Down syndrome.[22]

Aorticopulmonary Windows

An aorticopulmonary (AP) window is a conotruncal defect that results in a communication between the aorta and the pulmonary artery. The defect may be proximal, midway between the semilunar valves and the pulmonary bifurcation, or it may be distal to the pulmonary bifurcation, resulting in a descending aorta to right

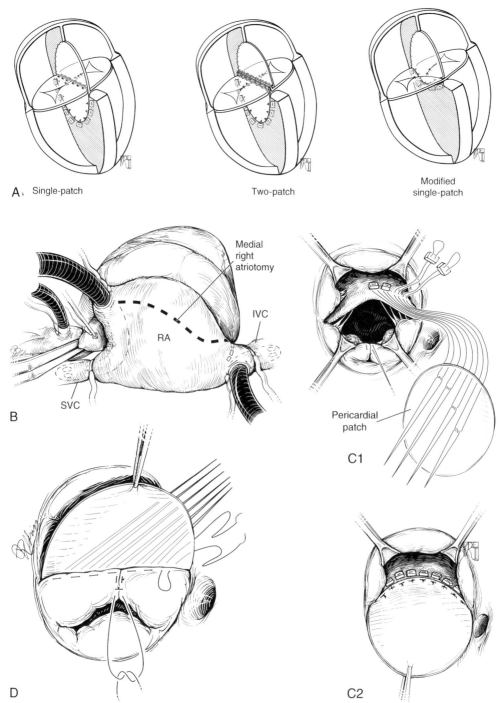

Figure 14-6 Surgical repair of a common atrioventricular (AV) canal defect. **A,** Three-dimensional reconstructions of the three different surgical techniques, single-patch, double-patch, and modified single-patch, are shown; the single-patch technique will be further described here. This repair proceeds using cardiopulmonary bypass and either moderate or deep hypothermia with cardioplegic arrest. **B,** Exposure of the AV canal is achieved through a longitudinal right atriotomy. Thereafter, the bridging leaflets will be divided to create the superior and inferior bridging leaflets. These incisions will parallel the crest of the ventricular septum, dividing the bridging leaflets into the left-ventricular and right-ventricular components. **C,** After division of the bridging leaflets, a patch, typically of pericardium, is placed along the crest of the interventricular septum to obliterate the interventricular communication. **D,** The patch is reflected anteriorly, and a row of horizontal mattress sutures attaches the left AV valve tissue to the appropriate level. The cleft in the new mitral valve becomes apparent and can be closed, as indicated.

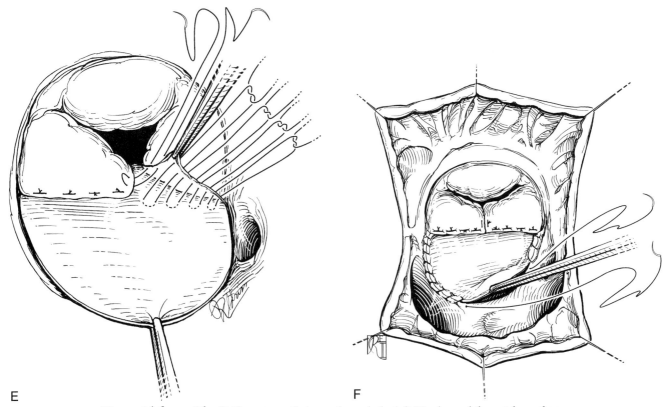

E

F

Figure 14-6, cont'd   E, The sutures that pass through the left AV valve and the patch are then passed through the edge of the right-sided AV valve. These sutures, once tied, anchor the valves to the patch at an appropriate height above the ventricular septum. **F,** The single-patch closure technique is completed by using the pericardial patch to close the atrial septal component of the AV canal with a running suture technique. After completion of the reconstruction, the atrial incision will be closed, and the patient will be weaned from cardiopulmonary bypass. IVC, inferior vena cava; RA, right atrium; SVC, superior vena cava. (From Mavroudis C, Backer CL: Pediatric Cardiac Surgery, 3rd ed. Philadelphia: Mosby, 2003, pp 326–328.)

pulmonary artery window. AP window may be associated with ventricular septal defect, coarctation of the aorta, or interrupted aortic arch.

Timing of Surgery

Left-to-right shunting leads to increased pulmonary blood flow and left atrial and left ventricular volume overload. Neonates with AP window usually present in the first month of life after the pulmonary vascular resistance falls and the pulmonary blood flow increases, resulting in congestive heart failure. These lesions are repaired at the time of diagnosis because of the increased risk for the development of early pulmonary vascular disease. Of note, AP windows can be missed (especially if other lesions are identified) unless very careful transthoracic echocardiography is performed.

Method of Repair

Surgical closure of an AP window is approached through a midline sternotomy. The repair requires incision in the aorta, in the pulmonary artery, or directly into the window (Fig. 14-7). A patch is placed to close the defect, and the incision is closed to incorporate the patch.

Follow-Up

The prognosis for children with AP window is excellent if surgical correction is performed early in life, before irreversible pulmonary vascular changes develop. Residual small windows are possible and branch pulmonary artery stenosis may occur.

Mixing Lesions

Truncus Arteriosus

Truncus arteriosus is a conotruncal defect defined as a single arterial vessel that originates from the heart, overrides the ventricular septum (i.e., the malalignment VSD), and supplies (1) the coronary circulation, (2) the pulmonary arterial circulation, and (3) the systemic circulation. Types I–III are characterized by increasing separation of the right and left pulmonary arteries from the truncus. Type IV includes interruption of the aortic arch, which is found in 18% of patients.[23] Although the truncal valve usually has three leaflets, the number of leaflets may vary anywhere from two to six. The valve is often dysmorphic, and there may be truncal stenosis or

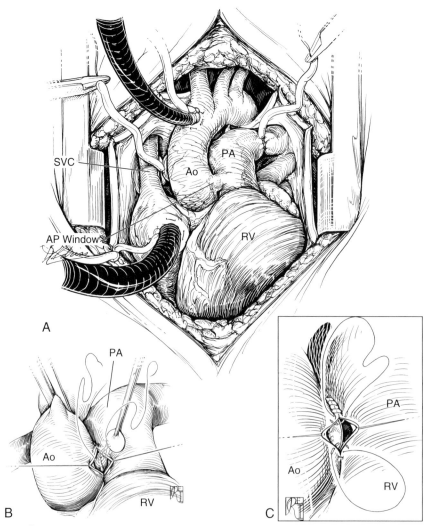

Figure 14-7   Anterior sandwich patch closure of aortopulmonary window. **A,** The aorta is cross-clamped after institution of cardiopulmonary bypass. **B,** The defect is opened anteriorly, and a prosthetic patch is sutured to the superior posterior and inferior rims. **C,** The patch is incorporated in the closure of the anterior incision. *Ao,* Aorta; *AP,* aortopulmonary; *PA,* pulmonary artery; *RV,* right ventricle; *SVC,* superior vena cava. (From Mavroudis C, Backer CL: Pediatric Cardiac Surgery, 3rd ed. Philadelphia: Mosby, 2003 p 357.)

regurgitation. Truncus arteriosus may also be associated with a right-sided aortic arch. Extracardiac anomalies are common (seen in 21–40%) as is 22q11 deletion (seen in 40%).[24]

Timing of Surgery

The initial physiology is that of complete mixing at the ventricular and arterial levels, with blood flow to the systemic and pulmonary circulations determined by pulmonary and systemic vascular resistance. Both right and left ventricles have pressure and volume overload, which can be further increased by the presence of truncal valve stenosis, truncal valve insufficiency, or both. In the absence of pulmonary artery stenosis, the normal fall in pulmonary vascular resistance results in significant left-to-right shunting, pulmonary overcirculation, and symptoms of CHF and failure to thrive within the first few weeks of life.

If left untreated, truncus arteriosus has a mortality rate of 90% by 1 year of age. This is due to the rapid development of pulmonary overcirculation, pulmonary hypertension, and pulmonary vascular obstructive disease, which have been noted as early as 3 months of life. Based on these data, most centers repair infants with truncus arteriosus during the neonatal period.[24]

Method of Repair

Surgical repair includes patch closure of the malalignment VSD to the aorta, removal of the pulmonary arteries from the trunk, and placement of a conduit from the right ventricle to the pulmonary arteries. A valved conduit is often used to minimize pulmonic insufficiency in the perioperative period (Fig. 14-8).

Follow-Up

Postoperative care after truncus arteriosus is challenging due to the risks of pulmonary hypertension and right ventricular dysfunction. Residual VSD and neoaortic valvular regurgitation may occur following truncus arteriosus repair and may ultimately lead to reoperation in the perioperative period or later in life. Over the long term, right ventricular dysfunction may be seen. Complete heart block occurs in 3–5% of patients. Homograft conduits may calcify and do not grow with the patient, leading to conduit replacement in early to late childhood.

Total and Partial Anomalous Pulmonary Venous Connection

Total anomalous pulmonary venous connection (TAPVC) and partial anomalous pulmonary venous connection (PAPVC) are congenital defects in which the pulmonary vein (or veins) drain anomalously into a systemic venous structure rather than into the left atrium. There are four types of TAPVC: supracardiac, cardiac, infracardiac, and mixed type. In the supracardiac and infracardiac types, the pulmonary veins drain to a confluence behind the left atrium and then drain through an anomalous vein into the systemic venous circulation. These are discussed in greater detail in the Chapter 3. In the obstructed form of TAPVC, pulmonary venous blood flow usually is impeded because the distal vessel that connects the veins to the heart is narrowed or atretic. Pulmonary venous hypertension results in pulmonary edema, pulmonary hypertension, and hypoxemia. In unobstructed TAPVC, pulmonary venous return is to the systemic venous circulation, where blood from systemic and venous circulations mix.

PAPVC varies in severity from a single anomalous pulmonary vein to all but one pulmonary vein draining anomalously. Like TAPVC, PAPVC may be obstructed or unobstructed. Scimitar syndrome is a unique form of PAPVC in which only the right pulmonary vein (or veins) drain to the right-sided inferior vena cava in association with right lung sequestration, aortopulmonary collateral to the right lung, and, often, malpositioning of the heart.

Timing of Surgery

In obstructed TAPVC, repair is generally done at the time of presentation, especially when the patient is markedly cyanotic.[26] In unobstructed TAPVC, the child presents later in infancy with CHF. Repair is performed

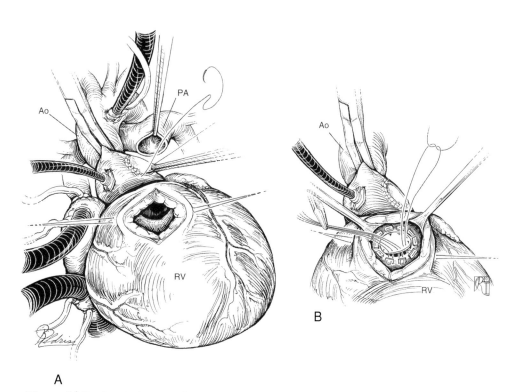

A

B

Figure 14-8 Surgical repair of truncus arteriosus. The procedure utilizes cardiopulmonary bypass with moderate or deep hypothermia and cardioplegic arrest. **A,** The pulmonary artery has been disconnected from the arterial trunk, and the aorta has been reconstructed with a PTFE patch to avoid coronary flow complications. **B,** Transventricular closure of the ventricular septal defect is shown with interrupted pledgeted sutures and a Dacron patch.

Continued

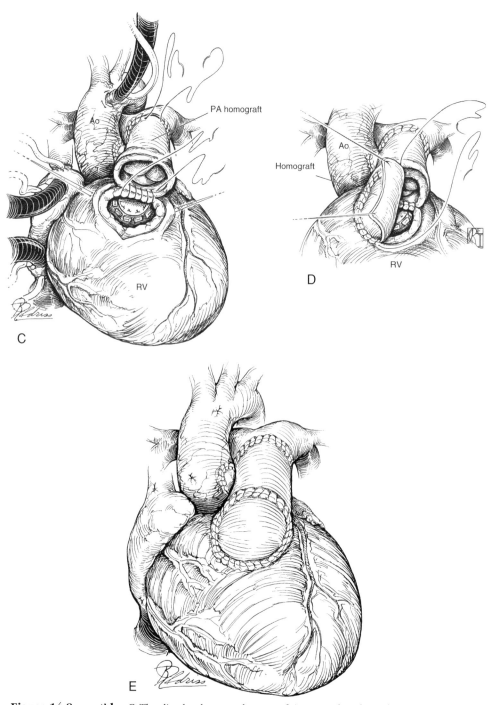

Figure 14-8, cont'd   C, The distal pulmonary homograft is sutured to the pulmonary artery, and the posterior one-third portion of the homograft annulus is sutured directly to the superior rim of the right ventriculotomy. **D,** A homograft hood is sutured to the annulus of the proximal homograft and to the remaining portion of the right ventriculotomy. **E,** Completed homograft hood technique. The homograft hood is used to ensure a generous opening from the right ventricle to the pulmonary artery. *Ao,* Aorta; *PA,* pulmonary artery; *RV,* right ventricle. (From Mavroudis C, Backer CL: Pediatric Cardiac Surgery, 3rd ed. Philadelphia: Mosby, 2003, pp 345–347.)

at that time. The timing of PAPVC repair varies with the severity of the problem. In cases in which the connection is extensive (i.e., two or more pulmonary veins) or the veins are obstructed, repair is usually done at presentation. If a single pulmonary vein drains anomalously and is unobstructed, producing no symptoms or hemodynamic effects, repair may be deferred indefinitely.

Method of Repair

In supracardiac and infracardiac types of TAPVC, the pulmonary venous confluence (where all four pulmonary veins come together) is opened and anastomosed to the left atrium (Fig. 14-9). The vein that connects the pulmonary venous confluence to the heart may or may not be ligated. For cardiac TAPVC, the pulmonary veins are baffled to the left atrium within the heart. Mixed TAPVC is the most technically challenging anatomy for the cardiac surgeon.

Follow-Up

Postoperative care after repair of obstructed TAPVC is challenging due to preoperative respiratory insufficiency and pulmonary arterial hypertension. Persistent pulmonary hypertension in the immediate postoperative period is a significant risk factor for death.[26] Paroxysmal severe pulmonary hypertensive crises have been mini-mized in the postoperative period by the use of neuromuscular blockade and high-dose narcotic infusions for the first few days after surgery. If pulmonary hypertension persists, residual pulmonary venous obstruction must be ruled out either by echocardiography or by cardiac catheterization. Those with unobstructed TAPVC usually have a benign postoperative course. Atrial arrhythmias may occur after repair. There is also a risk of recurrent obstruction at the level of the anastomosis over the long term.

D-Transposition of the Great Arteries

Transposition of the great arteries (TGA) is defined as the aorta arising from the anatomic right ventricle and the pulmonary artery arising from the anatomic left ventricle. D-transposition is the most common form of transposition. In D-transposition, deoxygenated blood from the body is ejected into the aorta and oxygenated blood from the lungs is ejected into the pulmonary artery. Mixing of deoxygenated and oxygenated blood can occur at the atrial (in ASDs) or ventricular (in VSDs) levels, or both, or by a PDA.

Anomalies associated with TGA include VSDs (40%), coronary branching anomalies (33%), aortic arch obstruction (10%), and left ventricular outflow tract

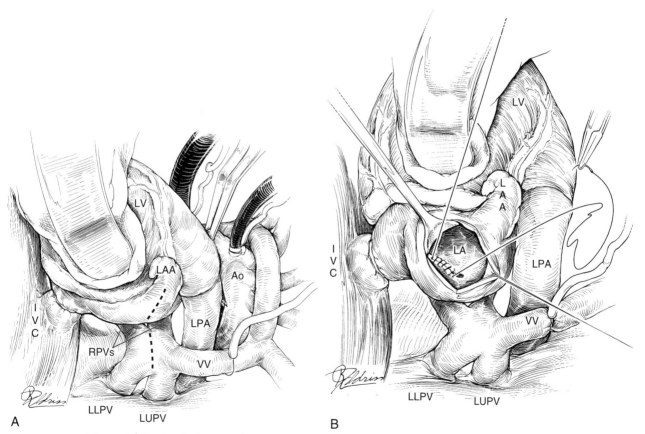

Figure 14-9   Surgical repair of supracardiac TAPVC with a vertical vein (VV) to the left innominate vein. After median sternotomy and institution of cardiopulmonary bypass with moderate or deep hypothermia and cardioplegia arrest, access to the posterior pericardial space is obtained. **A,** The vertical vein is ligated, while care is taken to avoid the left phrenic nerve. **B,** The atrial septal defect is closed through the left atriotomy.

Continued

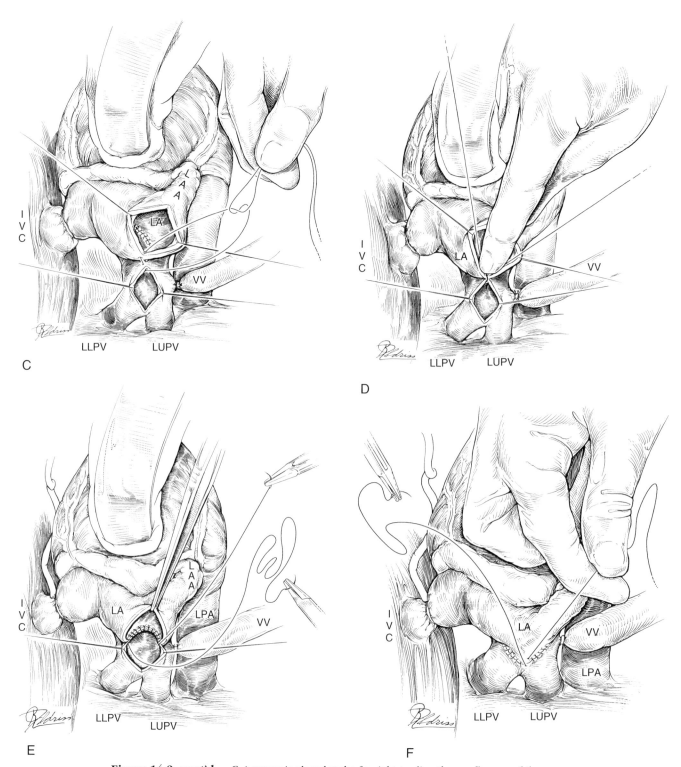

Figure 14-9, cont'd   **C,** A suture is placed at the far right to align the confluence of the pulmonary veins and the left atrium. **D,** The suture is tied, and the knot is left within the cavities. **E,** The anastomosis is performed with running suture technique. The superior and inferior suture lines are alternated to allow the retracted heart to fall back into the pericardial cavity. **F,** The completed anastomosis before the suture is tied. *Ao,* Aorta; *IVC,* inferior vena cava; *LA,* left atrium; *LAA,* left atrial appendage; *LLPV,* left lower pulmonary vein; *LPA,* left pulmonary artery; *LUPV,* left upper pulmonary vein; *LV,* left ventricle; *RPV,* right pulmonary vein, *VV,* vertical vein. (From Mavroudis C, Backer CL: Oper Tech Thorac Cardiovasc Surg 6:12, 2001.)

obstruction (5–10%). Of particular surgical importance are the malalignment type VSDs. Anterior (rightward) displacement of the infundibular septum is associated with crowding of the right ventricular outflow tract (connected to the aorta) with subsequent distal arch obstruction.[27] Conversely, posterior (leftward) displacement of the infundibular septum is associated with varying degrees of left ventricular outflow obstruction including subpulmonary stenosis, pulmonary annulus hypoplasia, or pulmonary valve atresia, or a combination thereof.[28]

Timing of Surgery

Surgery is performed at the time of presentation. Unlike patients with ductal dependent pulmonary or systemic blood flow, many patients with D-TGA cannot be stabilized with prostaglandin E_1 infusion. In TGA with an intact ventricular septum, there is often inadequate mixing at the atrial or ductal level. In such cases, either surgery must be undertaken on an emergent basis or a larger ASD must be created (i.e., atrial septostomy) by transcatheter intervention. The balloon atrial septostomy is discussed in greater detail in Chapter 11.

Method of Repair

Over the years, surgical intervention for TGA has changed dramatically. In the 1960s, the atrial switch became the

first successful procedure for TGA associated with long-term survival. Although the arterial switch was attempted in the same era, mortality for this procedure was extremely high. The trend toward the arterial switch began in the 1980s when surgeons improved the coronary transfer technique.

Atrial inversion procedures (e.g., Mustard and Senning operations) involve baffling the pulmonary venous blood flow to the tricuspid valve (i.e., systemic circulation) and the systemic venous blood flow to the mitral valve (i.e., pulmonary circulation), leaving the right ventricle as the systemic pumping chamber. Although previously the principal surgical procedure for TGA, atrial switch is now reserved for those high-risk patients with significantly abnormal pulmonary valves (i.e., the neo-aortic valve after the arterial switch), challenging coronary artery anatomy, or late diagnosis (greater than a few months of age).

In the present era, children with TGA without right ventricular outflow tract obstruction or left ventricular outflow tract obstruction and suitable coronary artery anatomy undergo an arterial switch operation (ASO). In the ASO, the aorta and the pulmonary artery are transected above their respective semilunar valves and switched with reimplantation of the coronary arteries

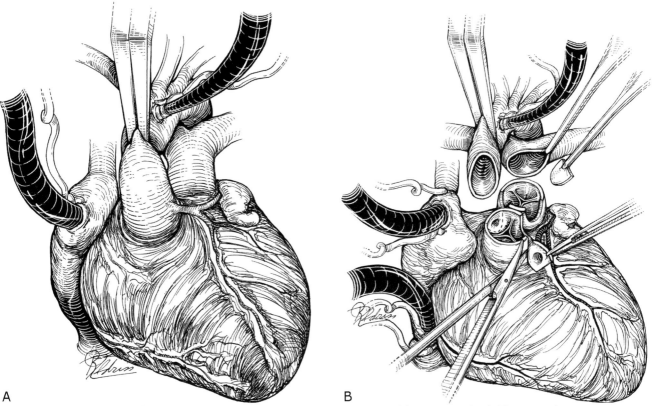

A

B

Figure 14-10 Arterial switch operation for D-transposition of the great arteries. **A,** The external anatomy of transposition of the great arteries is shown, with the anterior and rightward aorta arising from the right ventricle and the posterior and leftward pulmonary artery arising from the left ventricle. In the aorto-uniatrial cardiopulmonary bypass, the aorta is cross-clamped in anticipation of cardioplegia and great vessel transection. **B,** The aorta and pulmonary arteries are transected and the coronary ostia are removed from the native aortic root.

Continued

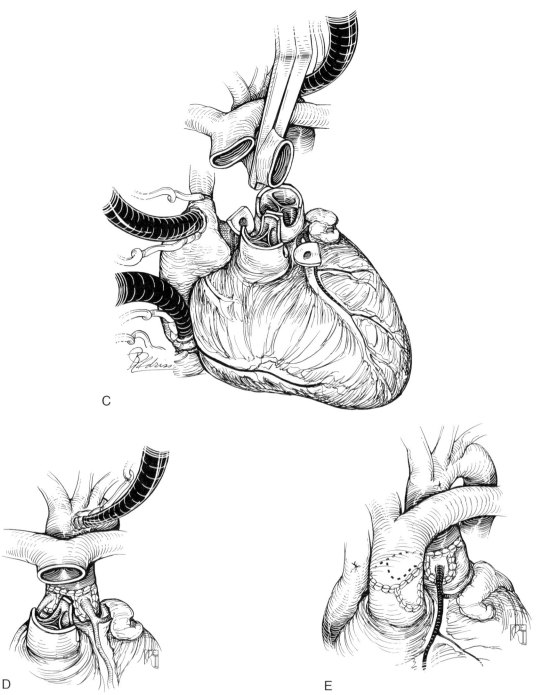

C

D   E

Figure 14-10, cont'd   **C,** The Lecompte maneuver (i.e., positioning of the pulmonary artery anterior to the aorta) is shown. The coronary buttons are mobilized in anticipation of anastomosis to the native pulmonary artery (i.e., the neoaortic root). **D,** The coronary transfer is completed, and the neoaortic root is anastomosed end-to-end to the ascending aorta. Coronary artery reperfusion is established after the cross-clamp is removed. **E,** The coronary explantation sites on the native aorta (i.e., the neopulmonic root) are repaired with a patch, and the pulmonary artery is moved anteriorly and anastomosed to the distal main pulmonary artery. (From Mavroudis C, Backer CL: Pediatric Cardiac Surgery, 3rd ed. Philadelphia: Mosby, 2003, pp 451–456.)

into the neoaorta (Fig. 14-10). Certain types of coronary artery anomalies associated with TGA preclude performing the ASO because of the distance that the coronary arteries would have to be moved. In these cases, more complex surgical solutions are required. The ASO is usually performed in the first few weeks of life. If performed after the pulmonary vascular resistance falls, the left ventricle must be prepared to take on the systemic pressure by banding the pulmonary artery for several weeks.

More complex surgical intervention is required for TGA with malalignment VSD with ventricular outflow tract obstruction. In those with left ventricular outflow tract obstruction and pulmonic stenosis, the Rastelli operation is performed. In this procedure, the proximal main pulmonary artery is divided and oversewn, the left ventricular output is directed to the aorta by placement of a patch from the left ventricle to the aorta, and the right ventricle is connected to the main pulmonary artery by a homograft conduit. The VSD must be adequate in size to permit unobstructed outflow from the left ventricle, necessitating enlargement of the defect by anterior excision of septal muscle in some cases.[29] If right ventricular outflow tract obstruction with aortic stenosis occurs in association with TGA/VSD, the VSD is closed with a patch, the right ventricular outflow is enlarged (in a manner similar to the technique used for tetralogy of Fallot), and the distal arch is repaired.

Follow-Up

Perioperative and long-term follow-up are variable, depending upon the preoperative anatomy and the surgery performed. The long-term consequences of the atrial switch operation have become evident with time. The extensive atrial surgery required for this procedure often results in significant scar tissue and subsequent arrhythmias, including sick sinus syndrome, atrial flutter, and atrial fibrillation. Frequently, a pacemaker is required for sinus node dysfunction and bradyarrhythmias. In addition, because the right ventricle performs as the systemic pumping chamber, right ventricular failure and tricuspid regurgitation are common.

ASO is generally associated with excellent outcome in most surgical centers, and the repair is physiologic, in that the left ventricle pumps to the aorta. In rare cases, myocardial ischemia may occur in the postoperative period, particularly when the coronary arteries come from one orifice (i.e., single coronary) or course in part through the wall of the aorta (i.e., intramural). Long-term issues after ASO include coronary insufficiency (i.e., stenosis after coronary reimplantation), neoaortic (i.e., native pulmonary valve) dilation and regurgitation, and supravalvar pulmonary and aortic stenosis (at the site of the anastomoses). There is a small but real risk of sudden death from coronary ischemia[30] and arrhythmias after the ASO.

After Rastelli repair, right ventricle to pulmonary artery conduit replacement is often required as the patient grows. In some cases, the VSD (i.e., the pathway from the left ventricle to aorta) becomes restrictive and may require revision. Complete heart block can occur.

Congenitally Corrected Transposition of the Great Arteries

In congenitally corrected transposition of the great arteries (L-TGA), the pulmonary artery is connected to the left ventricle and the aorta is connected to the right ventricle. The ventricles are L-looped (i.e., reversed in position). As a result, desaturated blood returns to the right atrium, enters the left ventricle, and is ejected into the pulmonary arteries. Oxygenated blood returns to the left atrium, enters the right ventricle, and then is ejected to the body through the aorta. Thus, the circulation remains in series but the anatomic right ventricle acts as the systemic pumping chamber. Patients with L-TGA may also have ventricular septal defect, Ebstein's anomaly of the left-sided AV valve, pulmonary stenosis, complete heart block, or a combination thereof.

Timing of Surgery

Historically, patients with L-TGA did not have surgery performed unless the pulmonary stenosis or the Ebstein valve needed to be addressed. Today, some L-TGA patients are candidates for a double-switch operation to decrease the risk of right ventricular failure in the long term. The timing of this very complex surgical procedure is variable but is usually delayed until at least 6 months of age.

Method of Repair

The double switch operation is actually a combination of two operations, the ASO and the atrial switch operation (see "D-Transposition of the Great Arteries"). The goal of

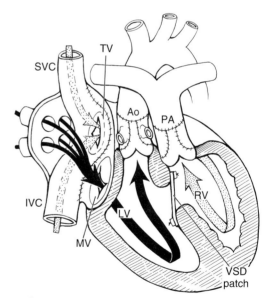

Figure 14-11 Double-switch operation for L-transposition of the great arteries. For patients with congenitally corrected transposition of the great vessels without left ventricular outflow tract obstruction, the arterial-switch operation can be combined with the Senning procedure to achieve atrioventricular and ventricular arterial concordance. Note that a patch closure of a large ventricular septal defect has been performed. *Ao,* Aorta; *IVC,* inferior vena cava; *LV,* left ventricle; *MV,* mitral valve; *PA,* pulmonary artery; *RV,* right ventricle; *SVC,* superior vena cava; *TV,* tricuspid valve. (From Mavroudis C, Backer CL: Pediatric Cardiac Surgery, 3rd ed. Philadelphia: Mosby, 2003, p 488.)

such an endeavor is to restore the left ventricle as the systemic pumping chamber (Fig. 14-11).

Follow-Up

Since this operation is relatively new in the field of congenital heart disease, long-term outcome is not known. Similar issues arise, as discussed, after the atrial switch and ASO. Complete heart block is common.

Left-Sided Obstructive Lesions

Left-sided obstructive lesions present as a spectrum of diseases, ranging from bicuspid aortic valve without stenosis or regurgitation to hypoplastic left heart syndrome. Frequently, multiple levels of obstruction are seen in association with one another, such as aortic stenosis and coarctation of the aorta. Shone's complex is a combination of defects including supravalvar mitral ring (which can cause mitral stenosis), subaortic stenosis, and coarctation of the aorta. Each lesion will be discussed individually; hypoplastic left heart syndrome will be discussed under the section titled "Single-Ventricle Repairs."

Aortic Stenosis

Anatomic abnormalities of the aortic valve may range from a bicuspid aortic valve with little stenosis or regurgitation to a unicommissural, myxomatous, severely obstructive valve with severe left ventricular outflow tract obstruction. Aortic stenosis may occur at the level of the annulus, the supravalvar level (in Williams syndrome), or the subvalvar level. In the most severe cases of aortic stenosis, there is severe dysfunction of the left ventricle, endocardial fibroelastosis (i.e., ischemia of the endocardium), and mitral or left ventricular hypoplasia (or both).[31]

Critical aortic stenosis is defined as severe valvular aortic stenosis with ductal dependent systemic blood flow.

Timing of Surgery

Critical aortic stenosis requires treatment at the time of presentation. Depending on the constellation of associated anomalies and the severity of left ventricular dysfunction, treatment for aortic stenosis may include balloon or surgical valvotomy, Stage I Norwood palliation, a neonatal Ross or Ross–Konno procedure, or cardiac transplantation.[32,33]

Less severe forms of aortic stenosis may be addressed when the gradient across the aortic valve reaches 50 mmHg or when there is evidence of left ventricle dysfunction or other symptomatology such as decreasing exercise tolerance. Isolated, less severe forms of aortic valve lesions may be addressed by balloon dilation valvuloplasty; surgical valvotomy or valvuloplasty; or valve replacement with autograft (i.e., Ross or Ross–Konno procedures), mechanical, homograft, or xenograft valves.

Method of Repair

For isolated aortic stenosis, in which the aortic valve is deemed adequate for a two-ventricle palliation, balloon dilation valvuloplasty is undertaken in the cardiac

catheterization laboratory. This is discussed in greater detail in Chapter 11. Similarly, such valves can be addressed in the operating room by incising the ascending aorta and performing a commissurotomy under direct visualization.

In cases in which there is severe aortic stenosis or aortic valve regurgitation, a Ross or Ross–Konno procedure may be performed. In the Ross procedure, the pulmonic valve is excised and replaced with an RV-to-PA valved homograft conduit (Fig. 14-12). The aortic valve is excised and replaced with the native pulmonary valve (i.e., an autograft). The coronary arteries are excised from the native aorta and reimplanted into the pulmonary autograft. In cases in which there is both aortic valve and subaortic stenosis, the Ross procedure is modified, adding the Konno operation to relieve the subaortic obstruction. In the Konno operation, the interventricular septum is divided and a homograft patch is placed to enlarge the left ventricular outflow tract (Fig. 14-13). The Ross operation is an alternative to prosthetic aortic valve replacement and has the advantages of potential growth of the subaortic area as the patient grows and lack of need for anticoagulation.

Follow-Up

Children with aortic stenosis require close follow-up for evidence of increasing left-sided obstruction, aortic insufficiency, or both. Repeat procedures during the first year of life are required if significant obstruction recurs. Children who have had a Ross or a Ross–Konno procedure must also be followed for evidence of conduit obstruction, coronary artery insufficiency, neoaortic root dilation, and regurgitation. Prosthetic valve replacement is required if the Ross fails, or if the native pulmonary valve is abnormal.

Coarctation of the Aorta

Coarctation of the aorta is defined as a discrete narrowing of the thoracic aorta distal to the left subclavian artery. Coarctation of the aorta typically results in a narrowing of the upper thoracic aorta, caused by posterior infolding or indentation opposite the insertion of the ductus arteriosus. In neonates, coarctation of the aorta is commonly associated with hypoplasia of the transverse aortic arch and ventricular septal defect.[34] Critical coarctation of the aorta (i.e., ductal-dependent systemic blood flow) presents similarly to other critical left-sided obstructive lesions, with cardiovascular collapse and shock after closure of the ductus arteriosus. The clinical presentation of coarctation of the aorta in the neonate varies from profound shock, metabolic acidosis, and end-organ ischemia to slowly progressive CHF. Older children often present with systolic hypertension and a blood pressure gradient from the upper to the lower extremities.

Timing of Surgery

Repair of symptomatic patients is done at the time of presentation. In general, neonates who present with cardiovascular collapse are repaired after stabilization with prostaglandin E_1 and recovery of end-organ function.

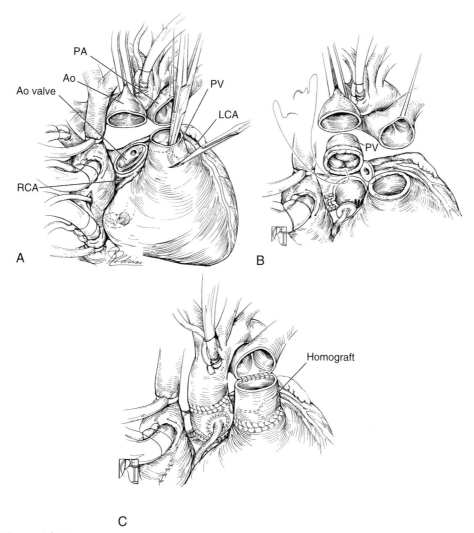

Figure 14-12   Aortic valve replacement with the pulmonary autograft (i.e., Ross procedure).
A, After the institution of a cardiopulmonary bypass with moderate hypothermia and cardioplegic
arrest, the diseased aortic valve is resected and the native pulmonary valve (i.e., the pulmonary
autograft) is harvested from the right ventricular outflow tract. **B,** The two coronary arteries are
removed with a button of sinus of Valsalva tissue. The pulmonary autograft is implanted into the
left ventricular outflow tract, anastomosing the infundibular tissue to the remaining annulus of
the left ventricular outflow tract. **C,** The coronary buttons are reimplanted into the appropriate
sinuses of the autograft, and the autograft is anastomosed into the end of the ascending aorta.
The operation is completed by placing a pulmonary homograft conduit into the right ventricular
outflow tract. *Ao,* Aorta; *LCA,* left coronary artery; *PA,* pulmonary artery; *PV,* pulmonary valve;
RCA, right coronary artery. (From Mavroudis C, Backer CL: Pediatric Cardiac Surgery, 3rd ed.
Philadelphia: Mosby, 2003, pp 544–545.)

Ideally, in asymptomatic patients, repair should be undertaken before 1 year of age. Persistent systemic hypertension is less likely to occur in children repaired before 1
year of age, compared with children repaired after 1 year
of age.[35] The asymptomatic neonate with coarctation is
usually repaired after the first month of life to minimize
the risk of recoarctation. Older children and young
adults are generally repaired at the time of diagnosis.

Method of Repair
Treatment options include percutaneous balloon angioplasty with or without stent placement and surgical

repair. During balloon dilation, there is physical disruption of the intimal and media layers of the aorta. Due to
the nontrivial incidence of aortic aneurysm formation
and recoarctation with primary balloon angioplasty, most
large centers generally manage native coarctation of the
aorta with surgery.[36,37] Surgical options include resection
and end-to-end anastomosis, end-to-side anastomosis, subclavian flap angioplasty, and patch aortoplasty.[38,39]
Figures 14-14 through 14-18 depict the surgical options
for correcting coarctation of the aorta. Repair of coarctation of the aorta is accomplished through a posterolateral

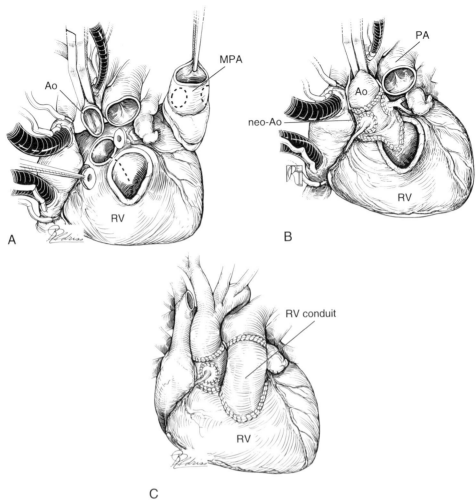

Figure 14-13   Ross–Konno procedure. **A,** The incisions noted for the standard Ross procedure (see Fig. 14-12) are performed; however, the infundibular incision is brought lower onto the free wall of the right ventricle, creating a longer apron of tissue on the anterior component of the circumference of the autograft for the ventriculoseptoplasty part of the operation. The interventricular septal incision (i.e., the Konno procedure) is noted by the dotted line. **B,** The neoaortic left ventricular outflow reconstruction is shown, using the pulmonary autograft extension into the interventricular septum to widen the subvalvar region. This relieves the valvar and subvalvar components of the left ventricular outflow tract obstruction. The coronary reimplantations and the remainder of the aortic reconstruction and the right ventricular outflow tract reconstruction are the same as the standard Ross procedure. **C,** The completed Ross-Konno is shown after placement of the right ventricle-to-pulmonary artery homograft conduit. *Ao,* Aorta; *MPA,* main pulmonary artery; *PA,* pulmonary artery; *RV,* right ventricle. (From Mavroudis C, Backer CL: Pediatric Cardiac Surgery, 3rd ed. Philadelphia: Mosby, 2003, p 547.)

thoracotomy incision. Cardiopulmonary bypass is not necessary in the vast majority of cases.

Follow-Up

The immediate postoperative evaluation should include assessment for residual obstruction, low cardiac output, spinal cord ischemia, and injury to structures adjacent to the aortic arch. Phrenic nerve palsy or paresis can lead to hemidiaphragmatic paralysis, and recurrent laryngeal nerve damage can cause stridor, hoarseness, and aphonia.[40] Disruption of the thoracic duct may result in chylothorax.[41]

Residual or recurrent coarctation (or both) is sometimes observed, particularly in neonates and infants. If residual coarctation occurs with no clinical symptoms, balloon dilation at least 2 months after coarctation repair is recommended. The procedure is delayed for at least 2 months to allow for proper wound healing of the surgically altered aorta. Spinal cord ischemia is a catastrophic complication that occurs in less than 1% of patients after coarctation repair, but it is even rarer in neonates and infants. This complication may be a result of inadequate collateral circulation to the anterior spinal artery.[42]

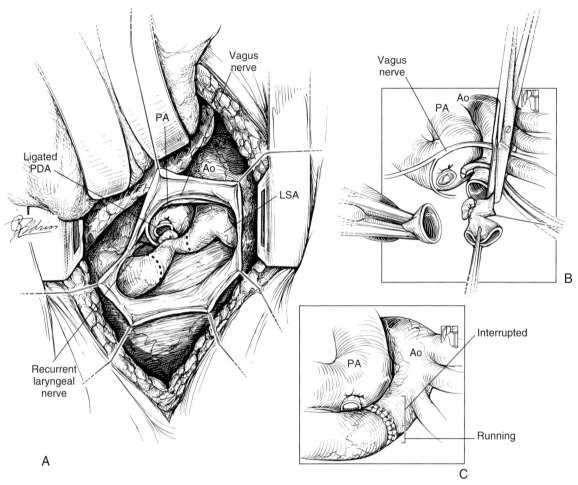

Figure 14-14   End-to-end repair technique. **A,** *Dotted lines* indicate the area to be resected. The PDA has been ligated and divided. **B,** Clamps have been applied, and the coarctation segment is being resected. **C,** An end-to-end anastomosis has been constructed, with running suture for the back wall and interrupted suture anteriorly. *Ao,* Aorta; *LSA,* left subclavian artery; *PA,* pulmonary artery. (From Mavroudis C, Backer CL: Pediatric Cardiac Surgery, 3rd ed. Philadelphia: Mosby, 2003, pp 257–263.)

Interrupted Aortic Arch

Interrupted aortic arch (IAA) results from a disconnection between the ascending and descending aorta and may be subdivided into three types (Fig. 14-19). IAA Type A can be considered an extreme form of coarctation of the aorta. IAA Type B, the most common form of IAA, usually occurs in association with posterior malalignment type VSD and subaortic stenosis. In addition, many patients with IAA Type B have 22q11 deletion (i.e., DiGeorge syndrome or velo-cardio-facial syndrome), especially if the arch is right-sided. IAA type C is extremely rare. IAA may be associated with truncus arteriosus, aorticopulmonary window, double-outlet right ventricle, and single ventricle complexes.

Timing of Surgery

The clinical presentation and preoperative management of IAA is similar to critical coarctation of the aorta. Prostaglandin E_1 (PGE_1) is used to maintain patency of the ductus arteriosus, which provides systemic blood flow to the lower half of the body when aortic interruption is present.

Method of Repair

In most cases, arch reconstruction can be accomplished by end-to-end anastomosis (as in coarctation repair).[43] In some cases, patch augmentation or a conduit may be required to connect the ascending and descending aorta. A VSD (if present) is generally closed with a patch during the same operation. If the left ventricular outflow tract is too small to support the systemic circulation (generally, if it is less than 4 mm in diameter in a neonate), then a Ross–Konno procedure may be indicated (see "Aortic Stenosis").

Follow-Up

The long-term issues associated with the care of patients with interrupted aortic arch are similar to those of coarctation of the aorta. In addition, if the subaortic region is small, subaortic stenosis may

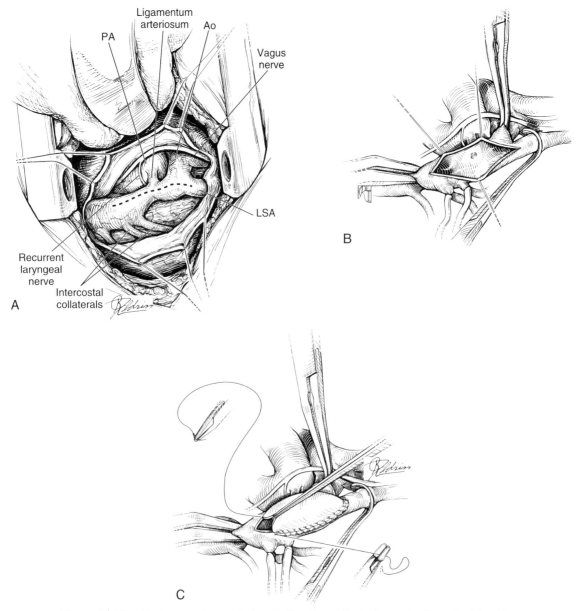

Figure 14-15   Patch aortoplasty technique. **A,** The *dotted line* indicates the line of incision. Note the involuted ligamentum arteriosum and the enlarged intercostals arteries. **B,** Clamps have been applied and the aorta opened laterally opposite to the side of the ligamentum. **C,** A synthetic patch or a pericardial patch is used to augment the hypoplastic area and the coarctation site. *Ao,* Aorta; *LSA,* left subclavian artery; *PA,* pulmonary artery. (From Mavroudis C, Backer CL: Pediatric Cardiac Surgery, 3rd ed. Philadelphia: Mosby, 2003, p 257-263.)

develop over time and may need to be addressed in a subsequent operation.

Mitral Stenosis and Cor Triatriatum
Congenital mitral stenosis in isolation is a rare defect in children and is generally seen in association with other left-sided obstructive lesions. There are two main subtypes: parachute mitral valve, in which the chordae tendinae insert into only one papillary muscle, and mitral valve arcade, in which the mitral valve leaflets insert directly

into the papillary muscles with no chordae. Often, mitral valve hypoplasia is also seen with these disorders. Cor triatriatum is defined as a membranous diaphragm in the left atrium that separates the pulmonary venous return from the mitral valve orifice. For both mitral stenosis and cor triatriatum, pulmonary venous obstruction can cause pulmonary arterial hypertension.

Timing of Surgery
As surgical options for mitral stenosis are limited, repair is reserved for the symptomatic patient or the patient

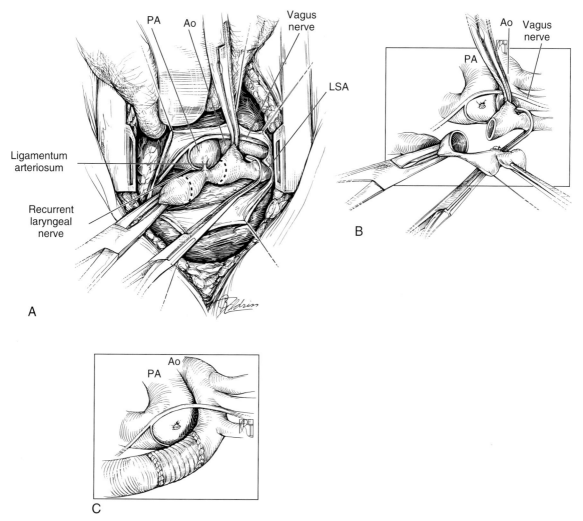

Figure 14-16   Interposition graft technique. **A,** The area to be resected in shown by *dotted lines.* **B,** Clamps have been applied, and the coarctation segment is being resected. **C,** Completed interposition graft. *Ao,* Aorta; *LSA,* left subclavian artery; *PA,* pulmonary artery; *PDA,* patent ductus arteriosus. (Reprinted with permission from Mavroudis C, Backer CL: Pediatric Cardiac Surgery, 3rd ed. Philadelphia: Mosby, 2003, pp 257–263.)

who manifests pulmonary arterial hypertension. Delaying repair is ideal, particularly if mitral valve replacement is considered, because prosthetic mitral valves have not yet been designed for the neonate. Cor triatriatum should be addressed surgically in the symptomatic patient.

Method of Repair

Mitral stenosis is difficult to treat because valvuloplasty often results in either residual mitral obstruction or the development of significant mitral regurgitation. Correction of associated lesions that may increase flow across the mitral valve (i.e., VSDs or PDAs) may lessen the severity of the mitral stenosis, delaying the need for intervention on the valve. If intervention is necessary but the mitral valve is not deemed repairable, mitral valve replace-ment becomes an alternative option. Ideally, mitral valve replacement should be delayed until a child is large enough for the valve to be placed in the annulus. However, if an infant is critically ill, placement of a prosthetic mitral valve in the supra-annular region (within the larger left atrium) is a viable option. Cor triatriatum is surgically repaired by removal of the membrane from the left atrium. This procedure is generally associated with an excellent result.

Follow-Up

Patients who undergo mitral valvuloplasty require close follow-up to assess the mitral valve for restenosis or the development of mitral regurgitation. Mitral valve replacement is generally performed using a prosthetic valve. Lifelong anticoagulation is required to prevent thrombosis. Follow-up echocardiograms are necessary to assess the prosthetic

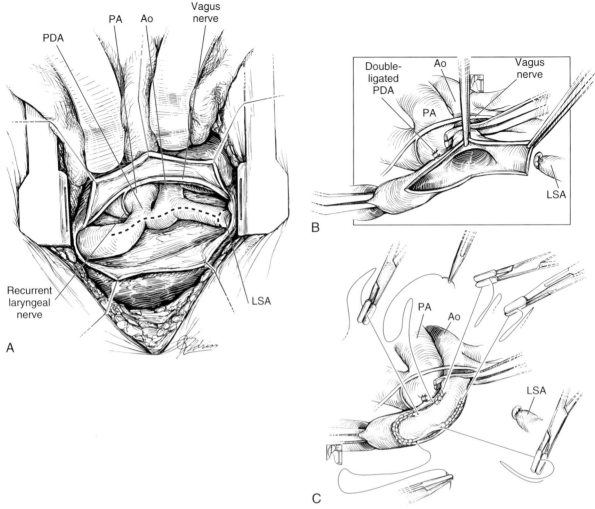

Figure 14-17   Subclavian flap aortoplasty. **A,** The *dotted line* indicates the line of incision. **B,** Clamps are applied, and the left subclavian artery is ligated, opened, and divided. **C,** The left subclavian artery is then turned down as a flap over the coarctation site, carrying the flap as far distal as possible. The ductus arteriosus is ligated and divided. *Ao,* Aorta; *LSA,* left subclavian artery; *PA,* pulmonary artery; *PDA,* patent ductus arteriosus. (From Mavroudis C, Backer CL: Pediatric Cardiac Surgery, 3rd ed. Philadelphia: Mosby, 2003, 257–263.)

valve for perivalvar leak and stenosis of the valve. Indeed, as the child grows, replacement of the mitral prosthesis may be required because the valve becomes relatively stenotic for the patient's increased size. Frequent assessment of anticoagulation is required.

Right-Sided Obstructive Lesions

Right-sided obstructive lesions vary in severity from mild pulmonic stenosis to pulmonary atresia with aortopulmonary collaterals providing pulmonary blood flow. Pulmonary outflow obstruction can be seen in patients with other conotruncal anomalies such as tetralogy of Fallot (TOF), double-outlet right ventricle, or single-ventricle lesions.

Pulmonic Stenosis

Pulmonic valve stenosis is characterized by thickened, doming pulmonary valve leaflets with a hypertrophied right ventricle and a normal tricuspid valve annulus. Critical pulmonic stenosis is defined as severe valvular pulmonic stenosis with duct-dependent pulmonary blood flow.

Timing of Surgery

Critical and symptomatic pulmonic stenosis is addressed at presentation. In asymptomatic older patients, intervention is generally recommended when the right ventricular pressure exceeds 50 mmHg[44] or three-quarters systemic pressure. It is also frequently addressed if the patient is cyanotic or if other lesions, such as a VSD, require intervention.

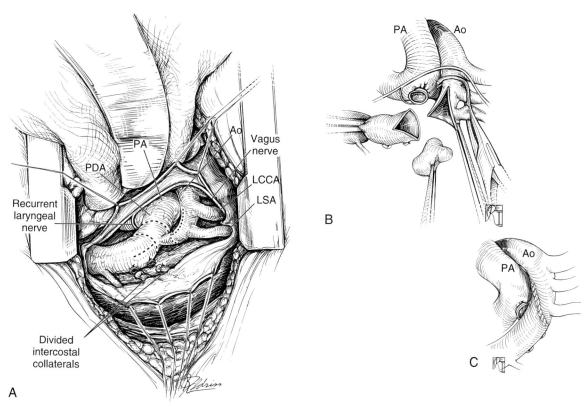

Figure 14-18   Extended end-to-side repair technique. This technique is used when transverse arch hypoplasia is present, typically in the newborn. **A,** The *dotted lines* show the areas to be resected and the incisions to be made on the undersurface of the transverse arch and in the lateral descending aorta. **B,** The ductus has been ligated and divided and the coarctation resected. The proximal clamp is occluding the left carotid and the left subclavian arteries. **C,** Completed oblique anastomosis extends to a point opposite from the left carotid artery, addressing arch hypoplasia. *Ao,* Aorta; *LCCA,* left common carotid artery; *LSA,* left subclavian artery; *PA,* pulmonary artery; *PDA,* patent ductus arteriosus. (From Mavroudis C, Backer CL: Pediatric Cardiac Surgery, 3rd ed. Philadelphia: Mosby, 2003, pp 257–263.)

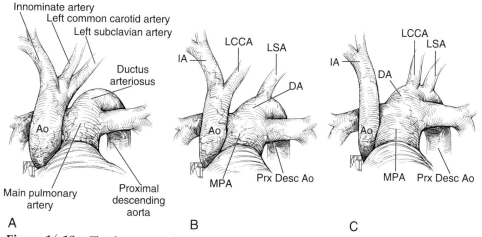

Figure 14-19   The three types of interrupted aortic arch. **A,** In IAA Type A, interruption is distal to the left subclavian artery. **B,** In IAA Type B, interruption occurs between the left subclavian artery and the left carotid artery. **C,** In IAA Type C, the aorta is interrupted between the right innominate artery and the left carotid artery. *Ao,* Aorta; *DA,* ductus arteriosus; *IA,* innominate artery; *LCCA,* left common carotid artery; *LSA,* left subclavian artery; *MPA,* main pulmonary artery; *Prx Des Ao,* proximal descending aorta. (Reprinted with permission from Mavroudis C, Backer CL: Pediatric Cardiac Surgery, 3rd ed. Philadelphia: Mosby, 2003, p 274.)

Method of Repair

Balloon valvuloplasty in the cardiac catheterization laboratory is the initial procedure of choice for valvar pulmonic stenosis. In some patients with a dysplastic pulmonary valve (i.e., Noonan's syndrome) surgical valvotomy may be necessary. After either procedure, a small right-to-left shunt may persist at the atrial level until right ventricular hypertrophy regresses and diastolic compliance of the right ventricle improves. Balloon valvuloplasty of the stenotic pulmonary valve is discussed in greater detail in the Chapter 11.

Follow-Up

Patients must be followed closely for recurrent stenosis of the valve, and they occasionally require reintervention. Pulmonic regurgitation following valvotomy or valvuloplasty is generally well tolerated in the absence of significant tricuspid insufficiency. Patients with severe regurgitation must be assessed frequently for progressive right ventricular dilation or dysfunction.

TOF

Although characterized as having four components (i.e., malalignment VSD, pulmonic stenosis, right ventricular hypertrophy, and overriding aorta), TOF is primarily a single conotruncal defect, namely anterior malalignment of the infundibular septum. This results in a malalignment VSD and a narrowing of the pulmonary outflow tract, a combination that leads to right ventricular hypertrophy (RVH). Furthermore, due to the malalignment VSD, the aorta, although actually in the normal position, appears to be overriding the ventricular septum. The anatomy and physiology of TOF is discussed in greater detail in Chapter 3. There are several variations of TOF, including TOF with pulmonary atresia and TOF with absent pulmonary valve leaflets. TOF with common atrioventricular canal will not be discussed in this chapter.

Typical ToF

Timing of Surgery

Controversy still exists regarding the surgical management of infants with TOF. In asymptomatic children, recommendations for the timing of elective repair have varied from the neonatal period to 1 year of age. For symptomatic patients, (neonates who are progressively cyanotic or have had a hypercyanotic "Tet" spell), a staged repair (i.e., placement of a Blalock–Taussig shunt followed by complete repair later) or early complete repair has been advocated.[45]

Method of Repair

If there is significant pulmonary valve hypoplasia, TOF repair involves using a transannular patch, a procedure that enlarges the right ventricular outflow tract to extend from below the pulmonary valve to the branch pulmonary arteries (Fig. 14-20). The transannular patch results in pulmonary regurgitation, which is generally well tolerated in the young child. Occasionally, if the right ventricular outflow tract is well developed, a transannular patch is not necessary. The malalignment VSD is also closed with a patch.

Follow-Up

In the immediate perioperative period, right-heart diastolic dysfunction can be seen because the right ventricular hypertrophy takes time to regress. In some cases, the dysfunction can be severe and the patient develops symptoms of low cardiac output. Over the long term, patients with TOF must be followed closely for recurrent right ventricular outflow obstruction, right ventricular dilation secondary to pulmonary regurgitation, or both. TOF patients have an increased risk for sudden death from ventricular arrhythmias later in life, which may be related to RV volume overload, residual RV outflow tract obstruction, ventricular scarring, or a combination thereof.

TOF with Pulmonary Atresia

TOF with pulmonary atresia (TOF/PA) has been referred to as PA with ventricular septal defect (PA/VSD). TOF/PA is an extremely heterogeneous defect because of the variability of pulmonary artery architecture. When evaluating the pulmonary arteries, three subgroups of TOF/PA emerge:

1. Confluent "true" pulmonary arteries, normal to slightly small in caliber, perfused by the patent ductus arteriosus
2. Small mediastinal pulmonary arteries and aortopulmonary collateral arteries with multiple segments of lung receiving dual supply
3. Absent or extremely diminutive "true" pulmonary arteries, less than 2 mm, with multiple aortopulmonary collateral arteries (MAPCAs)

Timing of Surgery

In neonates with confluent true pulmonary arteries, prostaglandin E_1 will ensure pulmonary blood flow until either a palliative aortopulmonary shunt or a complete repair can be performed.[46] In rare cases, TOF/PA is not diagnosed until late childhood or adulthood.

Method of Repair

For patients with confluent true pulmonary arteries, a complete repair consists of VSD closure and establishment of unobstructed flow from the right ventricle to the pulmonary arteries, either with a conduit or with a homograft patch (Fig. 14-21). The therapeutic approach to the other two subgroups, in which MAPCAs are a prominent feature, involves establishing forward flow into the true pulmonary arteries, followed by angiography to determine the segments of the lungs that are supplied by the true pulmonary arteries, the MAPCAs alone, or both. Surgical options to establish flow into the true pulmonary arteries include an aortopulmonary shunt, a direct connection of the back of

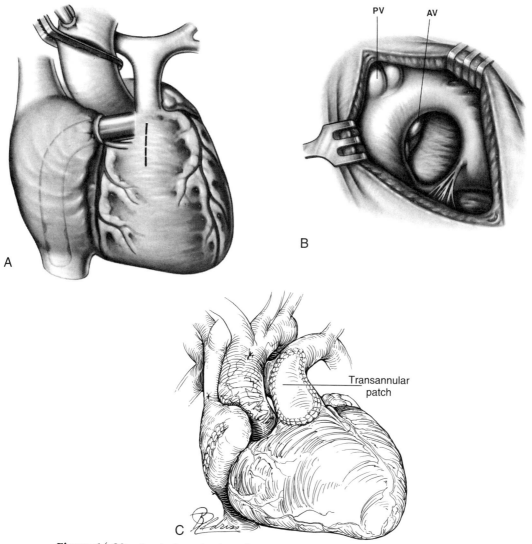

Figure 14-20   Surgical repair of tetralogy of Fallot. **A,** The position of the subvalvar infundibular incision is shown by *dotted lines.* This incision is used when the pulmonary annulus is adequate and a transannular patch is not necessary. When the pulmonary valve annulus is inadequate, a transannular incision is utilized. **B,** A transannular incision is shown, with the edges of the infundibular muscle retracted laterally. The hypoplastic pulmonary valve is revealed along with the malalignment ventricular septal defect. The repair proceeds by resecting the hypertrophied septal and parietal bands of the infundibulum to relieve the infundibular stenosis. The ventricular septal defect is patched, taking care not to injure the overriding aorta beneath the superior aspect of the defect. **C,** A transannular patch is placed to augment the hypoplastic right ventricular outflow tract at the levels of the infundibulum, the valve annulus, and the main pulmonary artery. The patch extends onto the origin of the left pulmonary artery. The proximal extent of the patch on the right ventricular outflow tract should be as short as possible. When a transannular patch is used, postoperative pulmonary insufficiency is almost a certainty. Some surgeons prefer to add a monocusp to the transannular patch to reduce the amount of pulmonary insufficiency in the postoperative period. *PV,* pulmonary valve; *AV,* aortic valve. (**A, B,** From Stark J, De Leval M: Surgery for Congenital Heart Defects, 2nd ed. Philadelphia: W.B. Saunders, 1994, p 409. **C,** From Mavroudis C, Backer CL: Pediatric Cardiac Surgery, 3rd ed. Philadelphia: Mosby, 2003, p 390.)

the aorta to the diminutive central pulmonary arteries, or a right ventricle to pulmonary artery conduit. Segments supplied by MAPCAs may need to be connected (i.e., unifocalized) to the true pulmonary arteries[47] (Fig. 14-22). In theory, this forward flow allows the pulmonary arterial supply to grow as the child grows. Once the cross-sectional area of the pulmonary vascular bed is sufficient to allow a normal cardiac output through the true pulmonary arteries without significantly elevated right ventricular pressure, ventricular septal defect closure is attempted.[48]

Follow-Up

In those patients with TOF and good-sized branch pulmonary arteries, outcome is similar to those with the

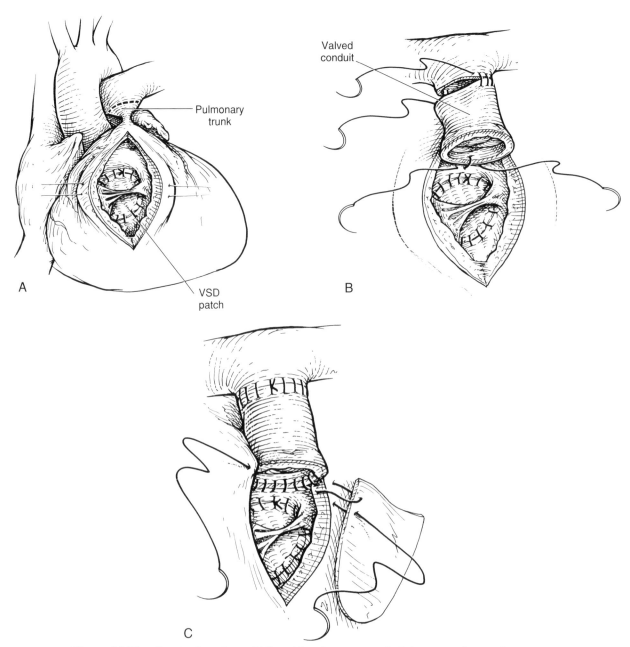

Figure 14-21   Repair of tetralogy of Fallot with pulmonary atresia. Pulmonary valve atresia can take two forms: short segment pulmonary atresia, in which the pulmonary artery is in physical continuity with the infundibulum, or **A,** long-segment pulmonary atresia, in which the pulmonary artery is discontinuous with the heart. Note the incisions in the central main pulmonary artery and in the blind-ended right ventricular infundibulum. **B,** a homograft-valved conduit is anastomosed to the central pulmonary arteries. **C,** The homograft is anastomosed to the infundibulotomy using a proximal hood to augment the anastomoses and to prevent distortion of the valve itself. Tetralogy of Fallot with pulmonary atresia can also be repaired without a valved homograft by using either direct anastomosis of the pulmonary artery to the infundibulum with patch augmentation or a nonvalved conduit. Free pulmonary insufficiency should be expected when a valved conduit is not used. *VSD,* Ventricular septal defect. (From Kouchoukos NT, Blackstone EH, Doty DB, et al: Kirklin/Barratt-Boyes Cardiac Surgery, 3rd ed. Philadelphia: Churchill Livingstone, 2003, p 1029.)

typical form of TOF. In those with diminutive pulmonary arteries, the unifocalized arteries often become stenotic over time; these patients frequently require serial cardiac catheterizations with balloon angioplasty of the affected segments. In general, outcome for the group of TOF patients with MAPCAs is poor over the long term, and there is controversy over whether aggressive intervention is warranted. Right ventricular hypertension with an inadequate pulmonary vascular bed is common.

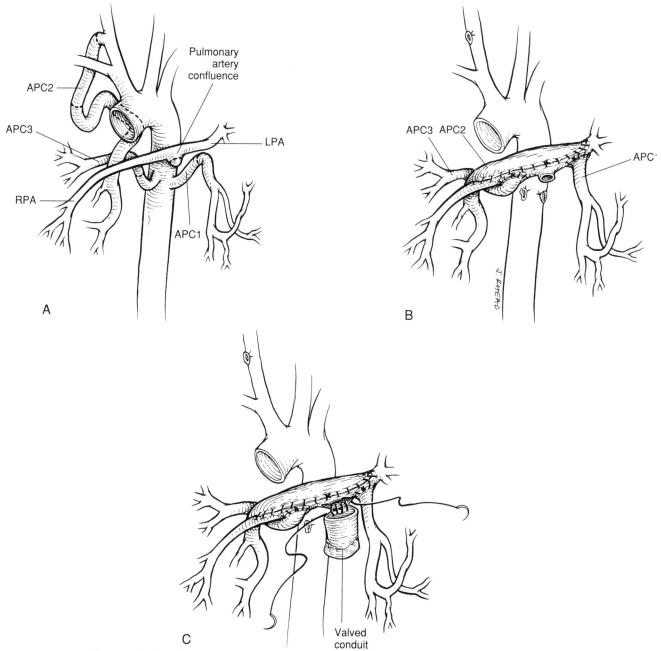

Figure 14-22   Unifocalization of collaterals. **A,** MAPCAs are shown coming off the descending aorta. Small hypoplastic true pulmonary arteries are present. **B,** The MAPCAs are removed from the descending aorta and are brought together with the central pulmonary arteries reconstructed with homograft material. **C,** The reconstructed main pulmonary artery and the branch pulmonary arteries, which may be anastomosed directly to the right ventricle infundibulum or by valved homograft conduit, as shown. *APC,* Aortopulmonary collateral artery; *LPA,* left pulmonary artery; *RPA,* right pulmonary artery. (From Kouchoukos NT, Blackstone EH, Doty DB, et al: Kirklin/Barratt-Boyes Cardiac Surgery, 3rd ed. Philadelphia: Churchill Livingstone, 2003, pp 1025–1027.)

TOF with Absent Pulmonary Valve Syndrome

TOF with absent pulmonary valve (TOF/APV) is a variant of TOF marked by dysgenesis of the pulmonary valve (which is severely malformed and incompetent), annular stenosis, and severe pulmonary regurgitation. Massive enlargement of the branch pulmonary arteries is common due to in utero pulmonary regurgitation. Tracheobronchomalacia is typically present; this airway abnormality is thought to be due to compression from the massive branch pulmonary arteries (Fig. 14-23).

Timing of Surgery
Neonates with TOF/APV typically present soon after birth with severe respiratory distress, cyanosis, and hyperinflation caused by tracheobronchial compression. Repair is usually undertaken in the first days to weeks of life.

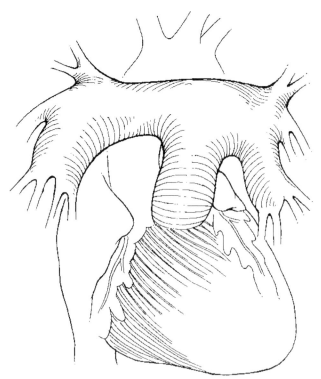

Figure 14-23   External cardiac anatomy of tetralogy of Fallot with absent pulmonary valve. Note the massively dilated main, central, right, and left pulmonary arteries. The aneurysmal changes in the pulmonary arteries may extend into the secondary pulmonary artery branches or even into the distal pulmonary vascular bed. Tracheobronchial obstruction secondary to the massive pulmonary arteries commonly accompanies this lesion. The intracardiac anatomy is similar to that of simple tetralogy of Fallot. (From Chang AC, Hanley FL, Wernovsky G, Wessel DL: Pediatric Cardiac Intensive Care. Baltimore: Williams & Wilkins, 1998, p 263.)

Method of Repair

Repair of this defect includes VSD closure and placement of a monocusp or a valved homograft in the right ventricular outflow tract to minimize pulmonary regurgitation.[49,50] In addition, the large pulmonary arteries are plicated (i.e., made smaller) (Fig. 14-24).

Follow-Up

Despite adequate repair, symptomatic neonates often continue to have airway problems. The clinical spectrum varies from mild bronchospastic disease to ventilatory compromise that requires tracheostomy and chronic mechanical ventilation.

Double-Outlet Right Ventricle

This conotruncal lesion will not be discussed in detail in this chapter because of the variability of the lesion. In double-outlet right ventricle (DORV), both great vessels arise from the anatomic right ventricle and the only outflow from the left ventricle is through the VSD. DORV can mimic TGA/VSD, TOF, or hypoplastic left heart syndrome. The VSD in DORV can be subaortic (similar to TOF), sub-

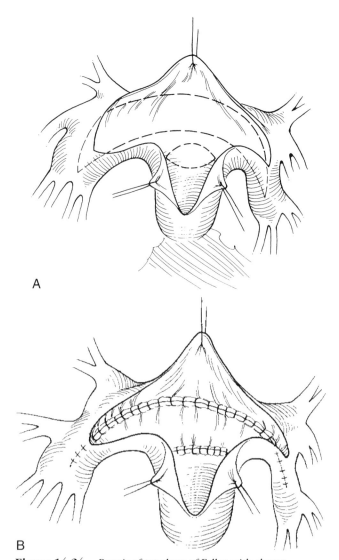

A

B

Figure 14-24   Repair of tetralogy of Fallot with absent pulmonary valve. **A,** The aneurysmal pulmonary arteries are plicated by longitudinal anterior and posterior incisions in the enlarged pulmonary arterial segments. Redundant longitudinal strips of pulmonary artery tissues are removed, and the longitudinal incisions are closed with running suture techniques. **B,** The posterior pulmonary artery plication has been completed. Free pulmonary insufficiency will result if the absent pulmonary valve itself is not addressed. In older infants and children with this syndrome who are stable and asymptomatic at the time of repair, pulmonary insufficiency may be reasonably tolerated. However, in young infants who are unstable with both cardiac and pulmonary involvement, the best results have been achieved by using a monocusp or by placing a valved homograft in the pulmonary position. In all cases, the repair is completed by closing the typical anterior malalignment ventricular septal defect. (From Chang AC, Hanley FL, Wernovsky G, Wessel DL: Pediatric Cardiac Intensive Care. Baltimore: Williams & Wilkins, 1998, p 264.)

pulmonic (similar to TGA), under both great vessels, or not committed to either (i.e., muscular VSD). Surgical treatment depends on many variables, including which outflow tract is obstructed and the location and size of the VSD. Of note, in the TOF type of DORV, outcome is similar to TOF except that those with DORV are more likely to develop subaortic obstruction because muscle (which can hypertrophy) separates the aorta from the left ventricle. Occasionally, DORV subtypes are so complex that separation of the pulmonary and systemic circulations is not possible, and the patient undergoes single ventricle palliation.

Ebstein's Anomaly

Ebstein's anomaly is a rare malformation of the right ventricle and the tricuspid valve. The septal and posterior leaflets of the tricuspid valve are displaced downward with abnormal attachments to the right ventricular wall. The atrialized right ventricle is the proximal inlet portion of the right ventricle that is above the inferiorly displaced tricuspid valve, and the functional right ventricle is the remaining right ventricle that lies distal to the tricuspid valve. The abnormal tricuspid valve is usually regurgitant but may also be stenotic or even imperforate.

Hemodynamic abnormalities are related to the severity of tricuspid regurgitation, the size of the functional right ventricle, and the degree of right-to-left shunting at the atrial level. Ebstein's anomaly can be associated with atrial septal defect, pulmonary outflow obstruction, and L-TGA. In addition, there is an increased incidence of Wolff–Parkinson–White syndrome in patients with Ebstein's anomaly. If there is severe tricuspid regurgitation in utero, massive cardiomegaly, secondary pulmonary hypoplasia, hydrops fetalis, or a combination thereof may result.[51]

Timing of Surgery

Ebstein's anomaly has a clinical spectrum that varies from severe cyanosis and circulatory collapse in the neonate to minimal or no symptoms in the child or adult.[52] Cyanosis is the most common presenting symptom in infancy. Cyanosis without any other symptomatology may be managed conservatively because the hypoxemia may resolve as the pulmonary vascular resistance falls and anterograde pulmonary blood flow increases. Neonates with severe tricuspid regurgitation present at birth with cyanosis, metabolic acidosis, and circulatory collapse. If the heart is massively dilated from right atrial dilatation, pulmonary hypoplasia is common and outcome is poor. The mortality rate is at least 20% when a child with Ebstein's anomaly presents in the neonatal period.[53] In older patients, supraventricular tachydysrhythmias are a significant cause of morbidity. Surgery is reserved for the symptomatic patient with Ebstein's anomaly since repair of the valve is often not possible.

Method of Repair

In the neonate, an additional source of pulmonary blood flow (i.e., an aortopulmonary shunt) may be required if cyanosis is significant. If the tricuspid regurgitation is severe, tricuspid valvuloplasty may be attempted or the tricuspid valve can be oversewn, subsequently necessitating Fontan operation (see Single-

Ventricle Repairs). In older children and adults, right-to-left shunting at the atrial level can often be addressed by surgical or device closure of the atrial septal defect. Occasionally, tricuspid valve repair or replacement (or both) is required.

Follow-Up Mortality remains high for Ebstein's anomaly in association with severe tricuspid regurgitation and pulmonary hypoplasia; in some cases, referral for heart/lung transplant is recommended. For those with less severe forms of the disease, specific postoperative problems include low cardiac output (secondary to diminished forward flow from the right ventricle), residual tricuspid regurgitation, and postoperative dysrhythmias.[54] Complete heart block can occur with tricuspid valve surgery. In long-term follow-up, the function of the tricuspid valve must be observed closely.

Other Lesions

Anomalous Left Coronary Artery from the Pulmonary Artery (ALCAPA) and Other Coronary Artery Anomalies

Normally, the right coronary artery (RCA) arises from the right sinus of Valsalva and the left coronary artery (LCA) arises from the left sinus of Valsalva. The origins and courses of the coronaries can vary widely. There are particular rare anatomic variations of note, including ALCAPA. ALCAPA usually presents with symptoms of heart failure and coronary ischemia (i.e., irritability while feeding) in the 6- to 12-week-old infant (after pulmonary vascular resistance drops). In addition, infants with ALCAPA often have hemodynamically significant mitral regurgitation secondary to ischemia or infarction of the papillary muscles.

Other rare coronary malformations include a coronary that courses between the two great vessels, a high take-off of a coronary artery, and coronary artery fistulae. The LCA coursing between the aorta and the main pulmonary artery may result in compression of the coronary and anginal symptoms or syncope or sudden death during extreme exercise. Unfortunately, patients are commonly completely asymptomatic and the initial presentation can be sudden death. If the origin of a coronary lies significantly above a sinus of Valsalva, an excessive take-off angle, a narrowing of the coronary ostium, or both, may result.

Coronary arterial fistulas can occur from either the RCA or LCA to any chamber of the heart, the coronary sinus, the venae cavae, the pulmonary artery, or the pulmonary veins. Although typically there is a single fistulous connection, there may be multiple ones. In patients with coronary fistulas, presentation in infancy is unusual. Late presentation, even into adulthood, is not uncommon. Typically, patients are asymptomatic and present with a murmur or, less commonly, with heart failure caused by a large left-to-right or a large circular shunt from the fistula. Although there can be coronary insufficiency, it is rare for a patient to present with angina as an isolated symptom.

Timing of Surgery

ALCAPA repair is done at the time of diagnosis. Whether to repair the coronary artery that courses between the aorta and the main pulmonary artery is controversial in an asymptomatic patient because the postoperative risk of sudden death is not known. In general, these coronary anomalies are repaired at the time of diagnosis. Very small fistulous connections will sometimes close spontaneously, and conservative management may be employed. Small coronary arterial fistulas may enlarge over time, and careful follow-up is required. In asymptomatic patients with moderate to large fistulas, elective closure is usually indicated. Symptomatic patients should be addressed at the time of presentation.

Method of Repair

Surgical intervention for ALCAPA generally involves reimplantation of the coronary from the pulmonary artery to the aorta (Fig. 14-25). If the coronary cannot be mobilized, an aortopulmonary window can be created with a

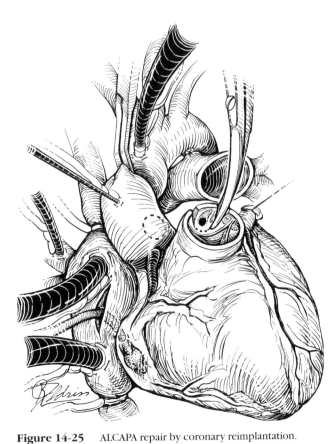

Figure 14-25 ALCAPA repair by coronary reimplantation. After institution of cardiopulmonary bypass and induction of cardioplegia, the pulmonary artery is transected above the sinotubular junction and the anomalous coronary ostium is excised with a generous button of pulmonary artery wall. The circle on the ascending aorta is the proposed site of aortic transfer. (From Mavroudis C, Backer CL: Pediatric Cardiac Surgery, 3rd ed. Philadelphia: Mosby, 2003, p 666.)

baffle within the pulmonary artery, which channels the coronary blood flow to the aorta (i.e., the Takeuchi repair) (Fig. 14-26). The incision in the pulmonary artery is closed with a patch to compensate for the decrease in pulmonary artery size caused by the baffle. Before surgeons became facile at coronary reimplantation, intervention for ALCAPA previously included ligation of the LCA in those with good collateral circulation from the RCA. This practice has been discontinued due to suboptimal outcomes.[55] If mitral regurgitation remains severe, mitral valvuloplasty or mitral valve replacement may be necessary.

In patients who have an anomalous course of a coronary artery between the aorta and the pulmonary artery, the method of repair varies depending on the subtype. If the coronary ostium is normal, reimplantation in a manner similar to that described for ALCAPA may be possible. In other cases, the coronary ostium is slit-like and must be remodeled to prevent compression. Finally, in some patients, bypass grafting may be necessary.

The manner in which coronary arterial fistulas are addressed is dependent upon location. In some patients, the fistula is very distal and the area of myocardium supplied is insignificant. In such patients, the coronary may be ligated proximal to the fistula. In cases in which the fistula opens into an accessible area such as an atrium or the right ventricle, the opening may be sutured closed or patched from within the heart with an atriotomy (or a pulmonary arteriotomy if the connection is to the PA). In selected cases, the coronary arterial segment over the fistula may be opened longitudinally and the fistula oversewn from within the vessel. The overlying coronary artery is then carefully sutured closed. Coil embolization by cardiac catheterization is often possible to address these lesions, avoiding open-heart surgery altogether.

Follow-Up

Coronary insufficiency is the primary concern after any intervention on the coronary arteries. In addition to echocardiography to assess ventricular function, nuclear studies are often indicated as a child grows to assess adequate myocardial perfusion. In some cases, cardiac catheterization is necessary to evaluate the coronary. In those with ALCAPA, long-term follow-up of mitral valve and ventricular function is required.

Vascular Rings and Slings

Vascular rings and slings are abnormalities of the aortic arch and the arch vessels. Presentation can vary widely. Complete vascular rings result from either a double aortic arch, which is most common, or from a variety of vascular malformations which, together with the ligamentum arteriosum or PDA, form a ring around the trachea and esophagus and can result in compression of these structures. The most common vascular ring involving the ductus arteriosus is a right aortic arch with an aberrant left subclavian artery.

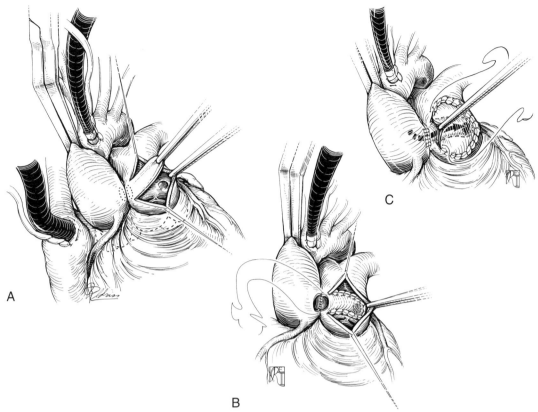

Figure 14-26   ALCAPA repair by Takeuchi repair. **A,** After institution of cardiopulmonary bypass and induction of cardioplegia, a longitudinal incision is made in the main pulmonary artery, and the ostium of the abnormal coronary artery is identified. **B,** Using a punch, a 5-mm opening is made in the aorta on the leftward aspect above the sinotubular junction. A similar opening is made in the pulmonary artery at the same level, and these are anastomosed to create an aortopulmonary window. A segment of 4-mm PTFE graft is opened longitudinally and used to fashion a baffle that directs blood flow from the aortopulmonary window to the anomalous coronary ostium. **C,** After the baffle is completed, the pulmonary arteriotomy is repaired with a patch to avoid creation of supraventricular right ventricular outflow tract obstruction. (From Dodge-Khatami A, Mavroudis C, Backer CL: Anomalous origin of the left coronary artery from the pulmonary artery: Collective review of surgical therapy. Ann Thorac Surg 74:946, 2002.)

A vascular sling occurs when the left pulmonary artery arises posteriorly from the right pulmonary artery and courses around the trachea. This anatomic arrangement can create a sling around the trachea at the level of the right mainstem bronchus and can result in compression of either portion of the airway. Tracheal stenosis can occur.

Timing of Surgery

Complete vascular rings diagnosed in children of less than 6 months of age are typically associated with symptoms of airway obstruction and are corrected at the time of diagnosis. Very mild symptoms in older children may resolve with growth, and elective division may be unnecessary in asymptomatic patients. Patients with left pulmonary artery slings who present with significant respiratory symptoms undergo repair.

Method of Repair

The double aortic arch is treated by ligation and division of the nondominant arch. The remainder of complete vascu-

lar rings are addressed by division of the ligamentum arteriosum or ligation and division of the PDA. Slings without tracheal stenosis can be addressed with a left thoracotomy. If performed through a sternotomy, repair of a sling includes division of the left pulmonary artery (LPA) at its origin and reimplantation into the main pulmonary artery anterior to the trachea. In all patients with significant tracheal stenosis, the trachea is divided, the stenotic segment removed if necessary, and the LPA mobilized to a position posterior to the trachea and then reanastomosed. Primary anastomosis of the trachea is preferred and usually is possible after removal of a stenotic segment.

Follow-Up

After successful correction of vascular rings, cardiology follow-up is not generally required. However, tracheomalacia may remain, and these patients may have long-term issues with airway obstruction. Follow-up after sling repair is required to assess respiratory insufficiency secondary to tracheal abnormalities.

SINGLE-VENTRICLE REPAIRS

A single ventricle is defined as the presence of only one ventricular chamber or a large dominant ventricle associated with a small additional ventricular chamber. Single-ventricle complexes include those with two functioning atrioventricular valves (e.g., a double-inlet left ventricle), a common atrioventricular valve (e.g., an unbalanced atrioventricular canal defect) or one atretic valve (e.g., hypoplastic left heart syndrome or tricuspid atresia), and the great artery anatomy can be extremely variable. Table 14-1 delineates the anatomic variants that result in single-ventricle physiology.

All of these lesions have complete mixing of the systemic and pulmonary venous circulations at the atrial level, the ventricular level, or both. The ventricular output divides between the pulmonary and systemic arterial circuits. Thus, the pulmonary artery and the aortic oxygen saturations are equal, and the ventricular output is the sum of the pulmonary blood flow (Qp) and the systemic blood flow (Qs). The proportion of the ventricular output that goes to the pulmonary or the systemic vascular bed is determined by the relative resistance to flow into both circuits. In most single-ventricle lesions, one of the outflow tracts is obstructed. It is rare to have no outflow obstruction or to have obstruction to both circulations. With pulmonary outflow obstruction, pulmonary blood flow is determined by the degree of subvalvar or valvar pulmonary stenosis, the pulmonary vascular resistance, and the size of the ductus arteriosus. Systemic blood flow in systemic outflow obstruction is determined by the severity of subaortic or aortic outflow obstruction, the systemic vascular resistance, and the size of the ductus arteriosus.

Table 14-1 Anatomic Variations in Single-Ventricle Physiology in the Preoperative and Postoperative States

Anatomy	Complete Intracardiac Mixing	
	Preoperative	Postoperative
VARIATIONS OF SINGLE LEFT VENTRICLE		
Tricuspid valve atresia		
Normally related great arteries	Yes	Yes
Transposed great arteries*	Yes	Yes
Double-inlet left ventricle		
Normally related great arteries	Yes	Yes
Transposed great arteries[a]	Yes[†]	Yes
Malaligned complete atrioventricular canal with hypoplastic right ventricle	Yes	Yes
Pulmonary atresia with intact ventricular septum	Yes	Variable[†]
VARIATIONS OF SINGLE RIGHT VENTRICLE		
Mitral valve atresia		
Hypoplastic left heart syndrome	Yes	Yes
Double-outlet right ventricle	Yes	Yes
Aortic valve atresia		
Hypoplastic left heart syndrome	Yes	Yes
Large ventricular septal defect and normal left ventricular size	Yes	Variable[†]
Malaligned complete atrioventricular canal with hypoplastic left ventricle	Yes	Yes
Heterotaxy syndromes (most forms have pulmonary stenosis or atresia)	Yes	Yes
TWO-VENTRICLE HEARTS WITH POTENTIAL SINGLE-VENTRICLE PHYSIOLOGY		
Tetralogy of Fallot with pulmonary atresia	Yes	Variable[†]
Truncus arteriosus	Yes[‡]	No
Total anomalous pulmonary venous connection	Yes[‡]	No

Adapted from Marino BS, Wernovsky G: Preoperative Care. In Chang AC, Hanley FL, Wernovsky G, Wessel DL (eds): Pediatric Cardiac Intensive Care. Baltimore: Williams & Wilkins, 1998, p 272.
*In tricuspid atresia or double-inlet left ventricle with transposed great arteries ({S,D,D} or {S,L,L}), right ventricular hypoplasia, subaortic obstruction, arch hypoplasia, and coarctation frequently exist.
[†]Single-ventricle physiology will result if a systemic-to-pulmonary artery shunt or a pulmonary artery band is placed. Two-ventricle repairs with normal series circulation or partial repairs with incomplete mixing are possible in certain anatomic types.
[‡]Streaming may result in incomplete mixing.

All newborn procedures for surgical palliation of the single ventricle are performed to achieve the following: (1) unobstructed blood flow from the ventricle to the aorta, (2) limited pulmonary blood flow to minimize the risk of pulmonary artery hypertension and ventricular volume overload, (3) nondistorted branch pulmonary arteries, (4) unrestrictive pulmonary venous return, and (5) minimal AV valve regurgitation. The surgical palliation is variable depending on the single-ventricle anatomy. Preoperative assessment for end-organ dysfunction, genetic syndromes, and additional congenital defects may be required, depending on the cardiac lesion identified and the preoperative condition of the patient. In rare circumstances, pulmonary venous return is obstructed either at the pulmonary veins or at the atrial septum, and emergent surgery or atrial septostomy is required to relieve the obstruction.

Neonatal (Initial) Palliative Procedures

Systemic-to-Pulmonary Artery Shunt
The modified Blalock–Taussig shunt is the palliative procedure most commonly used to augment pulmonary blood flow in single ventricle lesions with pulmonary outflow obstruction and cyanosis. A synthetic tube is placed from the brachiocephalic artery to the pulmonary artery. In situations in which the arch anatomy is abnormal, a central shunt from the ascending aorta to the pulmonary artery may be required. The classic Blalock–Taussig shunt required sacrifice of the subclavian artery and therefore was abandoned. In the past, the Waterston and Potts shunts were used to provide pulmonary blood flow, but they fell out of favor because they were associated with a high risk of pulmonary artery hypertension and distortion of the pulmonary arteries. Figure 14-27 illustrates the classic Blalock–Taussig shunt, the modified Blalock–Taussig shunt, the Glenn shunt, the Waterston shunt, and the Potts shunt.

Pulmonary Artery Banding
In children with a single ventricle in association with unrestricted pulmonary blood flow, congestive heart failure and eventual development of pulmonary vascular disease must be avoided. Therefore, as an initial procedure, a pulmonary artery band is placed around the main pulmonary artery to limit pulmonary blood flow and pressure. This procedure can be performed without cardiopulmonary bypass. The band must be placed in a position that will not distort either the pulmonary arteries or the pulmonary valve (the distortion of which would result in pulmonary insufficiency) (Fig. 14-28).

Pulmonary Artery–to–Aortic Anastomosis (Damus–Kaye–Stansel Procedure)
In order to provide unobstructed flow from the ventricle to the body, a Damus-Kaye-Stansel (DKS) palliation is per-

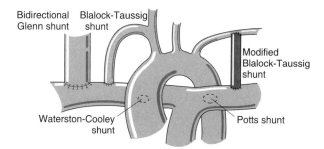

Figure 14-27 Schematic diagram of systemic-to-pulmonary artery shunts. (Modified from Gunn VL, Nechyba C [eds]:The Harriet Lane Handbook, 16th ed. Philadelphia: Mosby, 2002, p 150.)

formed in children with single ventricle in association with subaortic stenosis, with or without distal arch obstruction.[56] The palliation involves amalgamation of the semilunar roots (main pulmonary artery and aorta) to provide unobstructed systemic blood flow, and arch augmentation, if arch obstruction is also present. Neo-aortic (i.e., native pulmonary) valve regurgitation is common after DKS repair, but it is rarely hemodynamically significant.[57]

Norwood Procedure
The Norwood operation is a reconstructive procedure to palliate hearts with a functional single ventricle and aortic atresia or severe aortic hypoplasia; most commonly hypoplastic left heart syndrome.[58] The procedure involves augmentation of the aortic arch with amalgamation of the main pulmonary artery and the ascending aorta to provide unobstructed systemic blood flow and adequate coronary perfusion (Fig. 14-29). An atrial septectomy is performed to assure unobstructed pulmonary venous return, and a modified Blalock–Taussig shunt (MBTS) provides a reliable source of pulmonary blood flow. The Norwood procedure continues to have one of the highest risks of mortality after congenital heart surgery (see "Hypoplastic Left Heart Syndrome").

Norwood with the Sano Modification
In light of the concern for adequate coronary perfusion, a modification of the Norwood has been developed, wherein a small (usually 5-mm) right ventricle-to-pulmonary artery conduit is created, obviating the need for a modified Blalock–Taussig shunt (Fig. 14-30). With a conduit, diastolic blood pressure remains adequate and coronary perfusion is potentially improved. This innovation is quite new, and long-term outcome is completely unknown.

Separation of the Pulmonary and Systemic Circulations

The eventual goal of surgical palliation for single-ventricle lesions is to separate the systemic and pulmonary circulations. Cavopulmonary or atriopulmonary

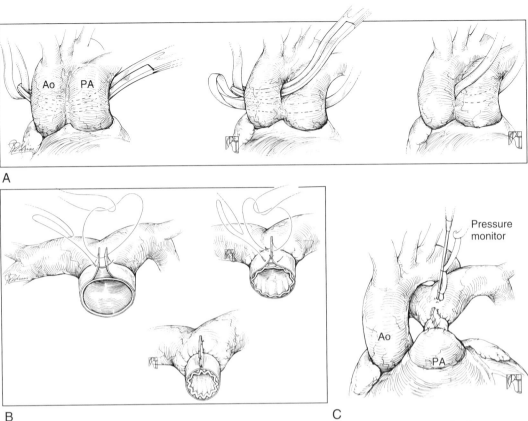

Figure 14-28 Pulmonary artery band placement. **A,** Encircling the pulmonary artery by the subtraction technique. **B,** Suture placement to tighten the band. **C,** Pressure monitor in the distal pulmonary artery to assess band tightness. *Ao,* Aorta; *PA,* pulmonary artery. (From Mavroudis C, Backer CL: Pediatric Cardiac Surgery, 3rd ed. Philadelphia: Mosby, 2003, p 162.)

connections are utilized to divert systemic venous return directly into the pulmonary vascular bed, providing for more effective pulmonary blood flow and reducing the volume load to the single ventricle. Single-ventricle palliations are generally staged to a total cavopulmonary connection (i.e., a modified Fontan operation). Prior to staging with an interim superior cavopulmonary connection, morbidity and mortality were high for single ventricle patients who transitioned directly from their initial palliative procedure to the Fontan operation. Complications included ventricular dysfunction, pleural effusions, low cardiac output, and tachyarrhythmias.

Surgical palliations, in which the single ventricle pumps to both the systemic and the pulmonary circulations, result in increased work for the ventricle, with resultant hypertrophy of the myocardium and increased ventricular mass. The Fontan operation acutely reduces the volume load, but the ventricular hypertrophy takes time to regress; thus, the mass-to-volume ratio is maladaptive and results in increased filling pressures and diastolic dysfunction. By staging to the Fontan with a superior

cavopulmonary connection, many of these hemodynamic alterations are less severe, with significantly lower morbidity and mortality.

Superior Cavopulmonary Connections (Bidirectional Glenn Shunt/Hemi-Fontan)

After the initial palliative procedure, a superior cavopulmonary connection (SCPC) is performed at 4–8 months as an interim procedure prior to the Fontan operation. This operation entails direct connection of the superior vena cava to the right pulmonary artery (i.e., a Glenn shunt) (*see* Fig. 14-31) or the creation of a window between the SVC and the right pulmonary artery along with a patch that prevents the SVC blood from entering the right atrium (i.e., a Hemi-Fontan procedure) (*see* Fig. 14-32) with subsequent takedown of the Blalock–Taussig shunt. In the case in which there is a bilateral SVC, the left SVC is anastomosed to the left pulmonary artery as well. In order to be successful, the pulmonary vascular resistance must fall to a nearly normal level to allow passive flow into the pulmonary arteries.[59]

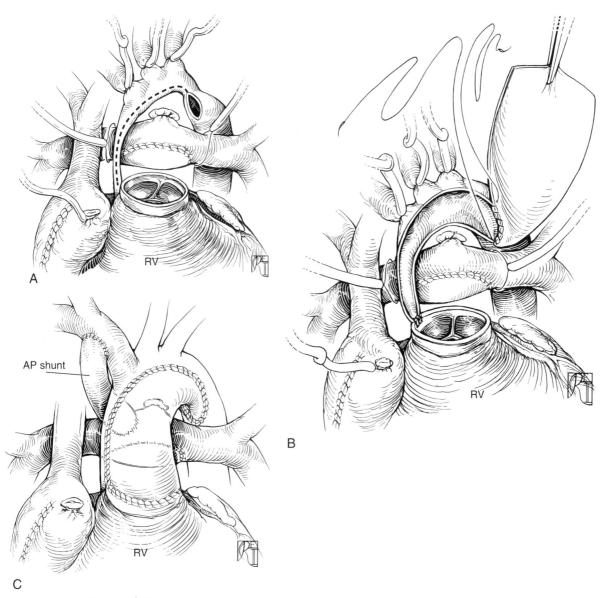

Figure 14-29   Stage I reconstruction for hypoplastic left heart syndrome. The purpose of the Stage I reconstruction for hypoplastic left heart syndrome is to establish unobstructed outflow to the systemic circulation, to balance the systemic and pulmonary circulations. **A,** After establishing circulatory arrest, the main pulmonary artery trunk is divided proximal to the bifurcation, and the ductus is ligated. The remaining ductal tissue is excised completely from the aorta, and the resulting opening is extended both proximally and distally, as shown. **B,** After the hypoplastic aortic arch is opened from the descending aorta retrograde to the level of the aortic valve, the proximal aorta is anastomosed to the adjacent pulmonary artery trunk with interrupted sutures. The proximal transverse descending aortic arch is augmented with a patch of homograft material. **C,** The augmented arch is then connected to the cardiac end of the main pulmonary artery stump. To complete the palliation, an atrial septectomy is performed to ensure unobstructed pulmonary venous outflow; pulmonary blood flow is supplied by a right-sided modified Blalock-Taussig shunt. *AP,* Aortopulmonary; *RV,* right ventricle. (From Mavroudis C, Backer CL: Pediatric Cardiac Surgery, 3rd ed. Philadelphia: Mosby, 2003, pp 564-565.)

In general, the SCPC is well tolerated. Initially, many patients appear to be quite irritable with plethora of the upper half of the body likely secondary to the sudden increase in SVC filling pressure. This headache is treated with pain medication. Pleural effusions can occur in the postoperative period. The oxygen saturation is generally between 75% and 85% after the SCPC.

Fontan Operation

In the modified Fontan operation, the inferior vena cava is connected to the SCPC. There are multiple

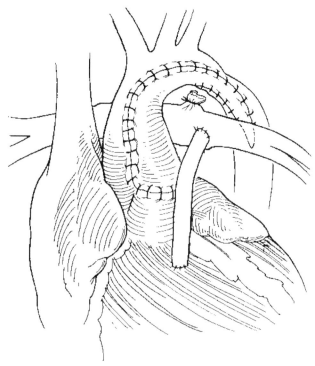

Figure 14-30   Stage I with Sano modification (i.e., 5-mm right ventricle to pulmonary artery shunt). (Adapted from Chang AC, Hanley FL, Wernovsky G, Wessel DL: Pediatric Cardiac Intensive Care. Baltimore: Williams & Wilkins, 1998, p 276.)

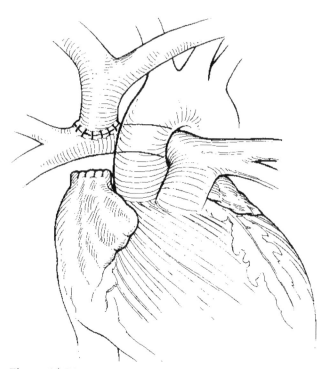

Figure 14-31   Bidirectional Glenn superior cavopulmonary anastomosis. The superior vena cava is transected at the level of the right pulmonary artery, the cardiac end is oversewn, and the cephalad portion of the superior vena cava is anastomosed end-to-side into the proximal right pulmonary artery. (From Chang AC, Hanley FL, Wernovsky G, Wessel DL: Pediatric Cardiac Intensive Care. Baltimore: Williams & Wilkins, 1998, p 278.)

technical modifications of the Fontan operation[60] that have been developed over the past three decades. In most centers, one of two methods is presently used, either the lateral tunnel Fontan (an intra-atrial baffle from the inferior to the superior vena cava) or the extra cardiac conduit (a GORE-TEX® tube connection between the venae cavae).[61] Many centers perform a fenestration in the Fontan baffle to help augment cardiac output during the postoperative period. The Fontan operation is generally performed 12–24 months after the SCPC. In some cases, the procedure is delayed if the patient has adequate oxygen saturation levels (i.e., 87–90%) or if hemodynamic abnormalities are found on echocardiography or cardiac catheterization.

Risk factors for poor outcome after the modified Fontan operation include ventricular hypertrophy,[62] elevated pulmonary vascular resistance,[63] pulmonary artery distortion,[64] atrioventricular valve regurgitation,[65] and ventricular dysfunction. Improved patient selection, surgical technique, and postoperative management have reduced the operative mortality to less than 5% in most centers.[66] The long-term outcomes, however, remain unknown.[67]

Patients who have had the Fontan operation require close follow-up for the remainder of their lives. Long-term follow-up issues include neurodevelopmental outcome, altered cardiovascular mechanics, diminished exercise capacity, arrhythmias, somatic growth retardation, neoaortic insufficiency, and thrombotic complications. Bradyarrhythmias and tachyarrhythmias are common after Fontan, and pacemaker placement or radiofrequency ablation may be required. An idiopathic form of protein-losing enteropathy (PLE) develops in approximately 5–10% of Fontan patients. This disease is characterized by chronic diarrhea with fecal protein loss, leading to loss of vascular oncotic pressure and the subsequent development of peripheral edema, ascites, and pleural or pericardial effusions. Patients often become immunocompromised from a loss of immunoglobulins. The etiology of PLE in Fontan patients remains unknown. Although there are a variety of treatments that achieved limited success in selected cases, many patients are refractory to all therapies; mortality is high, with only 50% survival at 5 years from the time of initial diagnosis.

Common Lesions Receiving Single-Ventricle Palliation

A wide variety of complex lesions can result in the common endpoint of the Fontan procedure. The three most common lesions in this category are described below, with other selected lesions listed in Table 14-1.

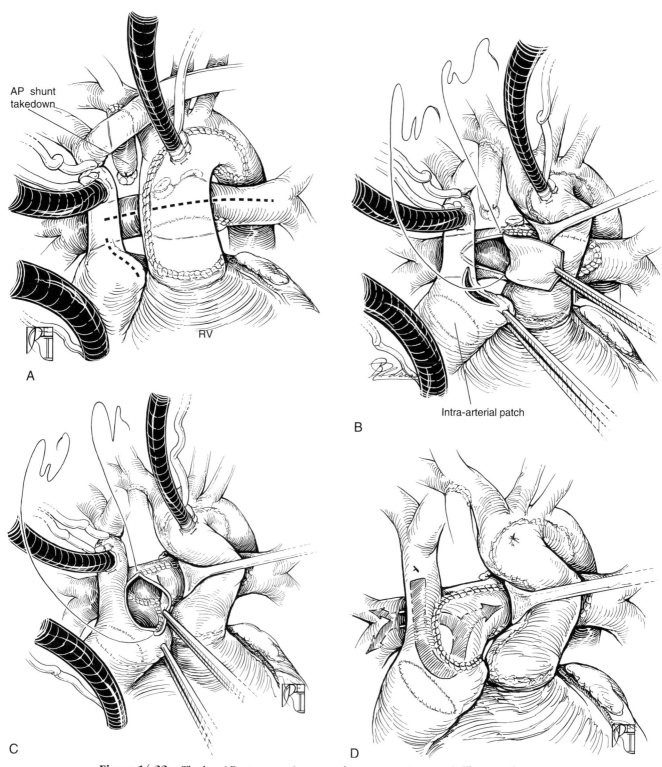

Figure 14-32   The hemi-Fontan superior cavopulmonary anastomoses. **A,** The central pulmonary arteries are opened widely, and an incision is made in the base of the right atrial appendage. The systemic-to-pulmonary artery shunt has been ligated. **B,** An intraarterial patch is placed at the junction of the superior vena cava and the right atrium. Additionally, a patch of homograft material is used to augment the left pulmonary artery. **C,** The posterior aspect of the right atriotomy is anastomosed to the inferior wall of the right pulmonary artery. The homograft patch is then used to roof the cavopulmonary connection. **D,** The final appearance of the hemi-Fontan connection is shown. The patch used to separate the superior vena cava to pulmonary artery connection from the heart is shown within the right atrium; it prevents superior vena cava return from entering the right atrium. At the time of the Fontan procedure, the atrial patch is removed from within the right atrium, leaving a wide connection from the inferior vena cava into the pulmonary arteries. *AP,* Aortopulmonary; *RV,* right ventricle. (From Mavroudis C, Backer CL: Pediatric Cardiac Surgery, 3rd ed. Philadelphia: Mosby, 2003, pp 567–568.)

Hypoplastic Left Heart Syndrome

Hypoplastic left heart syndrome (HLHS) is defined as a cardiac lesion with hypoplasia or atresia of the mitral and aortic valves in association with a left ventricular chamber that is either absent or too small to support the systemic circulation. In the most severe cases, the aortic valve is atretic with a markedly hypoplastic ascending aorta (1 mm in diameter) and retrograde perfusion of the coronaries from the patent ductus arteriosus. The Norwood and Sano procedures are the initial palliative surgeries for this lesion. HLHS poses a significant challenge to the cardiac surgeon and the pediatric cardiologist. Despite significant strides in technique, the incidence of sudden death after the Norwood procedure remains problematic. In some cases, residual hemodynamic abnormalities such as ventricular dysfunction, significant tricuspid regurgitation, and distal arch obstruction portend poor outcome. However, the etiology often remains unclear. Coronary insufficiency and low cardiac reserve are likely to play a role. The long-term outcome for HLHS remains unknown as well. The oldest HLHS survivors at present are in their early 20s and had surgery in a different era than those undergoing intervention today. The durability of the right ventricle, the tricuspid valve, and the pulmonary valve in the systemic circuit remains in question.

A subset of patients with HLHS at particularly high risk for poor outcome despite any intervention include those patients with either an intact atrial septum or an inadequate atrial communication. Intact atrial septum in association with mitral atresia results in significant pulmonary venous obstruction with subsequent development of pulmonary arterial hypertension and vascular disease. Even after the atrial-level obstruction is relieved, either by balloon septostomy or by surgical septectomy, the pulmonary arterial hypertension often remains, making the patient a poor candidate for Norwood palliation. In some cases, heart and lung transplantation is recommended.

Tricuspid Atresia

Absence of the tricuspid valve is often associated with right ventricular hypoplasia. In most cases, a VSD is present. If the VSD is large, the pulmonary outflow may not be obstructed. Depending on the severity of obstruction at the level of the pulmonary outflow, a patient with tricuspid atresia may require a pulmonary artery band (for excessive pulmonary blood flow), a modified Blalock–Taussig shunt (for insufficient pulmonary blood flow), or no surgical intervention (for adequate but not excessive pulmonary blood flow). Tricuspid atresia can also be associated with transposition of the great arteries, pulmonary atresia, or both. Patients with tricuspid atresia were the first survivors of the Fontan operation.

Pulmonary Atresia with Intact Ventricular Septum

Pulmonary atresia with intact ventricular septum (PA/IVS) is defined as atresia of the pulmonary valve with no associated VSD and variable hypoplasia of the right ventricle and tricuspid valve. The main pulmonary artery is usually present and of normal size, and the pulmonary blood flow is supplied by a patent ductus arteriosus. The tricuspid valve may be stenotic, regurgitant, or both. Coronary-to-right-ventricle fistulous communications are common in children with PA/IVS, especially those who have a small hypertensive right ventricle with a small tricuspid valve annulus.[68] A right ventricular-dependent coronary circulation exists when some of the myocardium is perfused only from the high-pressure right ventricle rather than antegrade from the aorta. The presence of right ventricular-dependent coronaries has an important impact on possible surgical management strategies and is associated with a high mortality.[69] In these cases, decompression of the right ventricle (by establishing a communication with the pulmonary artery) results in almost certain death from coronary insufficiency. Thus, almost all patients with PA/IVS undergo cardiac catheterization prior to any surgical procedure to identify the coronary perfusion pattern.

In those PA/IVS patients with an adequately sized tricuspid valve and right ventricle (and normal coronary perfusion), a right ventricle-to-pulmonary artery connection is performed to establish antegrade flow through the right heart. In some cases, a modified Blalock–Taussig shunt is also necessary to provide additional pulmonary blood flow. Right ventricular hypertrophy typically regresses over time with improved right ventricular compliance and increased right ventricular contribution to pulmonary blood flow. By 6 months to 1 year, the shunt is usually taken down surgically or coil occluded in the catheterization laboratory.

In cases with a diminutive right ventricle, right ventricular dependent coronaries, or both, staged single ventricle repair is preferred, with a modified Blalock–Taussig shunt as the initial procedure. Some centers prefer cardiac transplantation to staged palliation when coronary perfusion is right ventricle-dependent.

CARDIAC TRANSPLANTATION

Cardiac transplantation is a viable option for children with end-stage cardiac failure or inoperable congenital heart lesions. Congenital heart disease is the most common indication for heart transplant in children less than 1 year of age. In some institutions, cardiac transplant is the primary treatment for infants with HLHS. Transplantation is considered for patients with cardiomyopathy. Overall, actuarial survival after cardiac transplant appears to be steadily improving, with 75% of children transplanted between 1998 and 2001 and just under 60% of children transplanted between 1993 and 1997 presently alive.[70]

Cardiac transplantation is not the perfect solution for patients with cardiac disease. Although the heart becomes structurally normal, the patient is faced with new long-term problems that are difficult to manage. In addition, there is a significant shortage of donor hearts available for infants and children, limiting the transplant option for many patients. The short- and long-term issues surrounding cardiac transplantation are extraordinarily complex. In general, a pediatric cardiologist with a specialty in transplantation becomes involved in virtually all aspects of a patient's care. Management is complicated by the increased risk for infection associated with immunosuppression. Furthermore, long-term immunosuppression places patients at risk for a form of cancer called post-transplant lymphoproliferative disease. Long-term issues for all cardiac transplant patients include surveillance for rejection episodes and assessment for coronary allograft vasculopathy (an accelerated coronary artery disease that develops after cardiac transplantation). Systemic hypertension is common in this population and often requires treatment.

CONCLUSION

Surgery for congenital heart disease has seen extraordinary growth and progress over the last half century. At present, the overwhelming majority of cardiac lesions can be addressed surgically with good outcomes. Children with complex congenital heart disease are living into adulthood, being employed and having families. At present, congenital heart disease can be identified in utero as early as 14 weeks' gestation. Current challenges in the field of pediatric cardiac surgery include improving methods of cardioprotection and neuroprotection and developing smaller ventricular assist devices for neonates. Innovative treatment approaches are also in development, including gene therapy, fetal cardiac intervention, creation of human tissue valves, and prosthetic hearts. These exciting developments will only enhance the field of pediatric cardiac surgery and will enable us to better care for our patient population.

MAJOR POINTS

- Congenital heart disease is the most common congenital malformation in humans.
- The Blalock–Taussig shunt is the first major development in the field of pediatric cardiac surgery; it allows for a reliable source of pulmonary blood flow in children with severe pulmonary stenosis or pulmonary atresia.

MAJOR POINTS—CONT'D

- Prostaglandin E_1, which entered the clinical realm in the late 1970s, changed the course of management of children with critical congenital heart disease by providing blood flow through the ductus arteriosus for pulmonary blood flow (for treating pulmonary atresia) or systemic blood flow (for treating hypoplastic left heart syndrome or critical coarctation of the aorta).
- Transthoracic echocardiography and cardiac MRI provide noninvasive, accurate diagnostic information so that most patients do not require cardiac catheterization prior to surgical intervention.
- Interventional cardiac catheterization provides a method of repairing certain cardiac lesions (e.g., atrial septal defects and valvar aortic and pulmonary stenosis) without surgical intervention and also is used frequently to address residual lesions after surgical repair (e.g., residual coarctation of the aorta and residual branch pulmonary stenosis).
- Dr. William Rashkind, the father of pediatric interventional catheterization, developed the live-saving balloon atrial septostomy, in which an atrial communication is made with a balloon catheter to allow mixing of oxygenated and deoxygenated blood in transposition of the great arteries and similar lesions.
- Cardiopulmonary bypass and circulatory arrest are methods used to perform complex intracardiac repairs; despite innovations in these techniques, morbidity continues to be associated with their use.
- Many congenital heart defects (e.g., atrial septal defect, ventricular septal defect, and patent ductus arteriosus) can have complete repairs with little if any residual sequelae.
- Complete repair is not available for more complex cardiac lesions; therefore, palliative procedures, which can have significant residual sequelae, are performed.
- The arterial switch operation for transposition of the great arteries provides a more anatomic repair with fewer complications than the previous atrial switch operation, in which the right ventricle remained the systemic ventricle.
- The Norwood procedure for hypoplastic left heart syndrome, developed in 1980 by Dr. William Norwood and still performed today, successfully palliates children with a previously uniformly fatal cardiac defect.
- The Fontan operation for single-ventricle lesions provides passive flow of all systemic venous return to the pulmonary arteries with no pumping chamber; over the long term, this procedure is associated with significant morbidity, including atrial arrhythmias, pleural effusions, protein-losing enteropathy, and heart failure.
- Cardiac transplantation is a viable option for children with end-stage cardiac failure or inoperable congenital heart lesions, with 75% 5-year survival.

REFERENCES

1. Tworetzky W, Marshall AC: Balloon valvuloplasty for congenital heart disease in the fetus. Clin Perinatol 30(3):541-550, 2003.

2. Blalock A, Taussig HB: The surgical treatment of malformations of the heart in which there is pulmonary stenosis or pulmonary atresia. J Am Med Assoc 128:189-192, 1945.

3. Heymann MA, Rudolph AM: Ductus arteriosus dilatation by prostaglandin E$_1$ in infants with pulmonary atresia. Pediatrics 59:325-329, 1973.

4. Rashkind WJ, Miller WW: Creation of an atrial septal defect without thoracotomy: A palliative approach to complete transposition of the great arteries. J Am Med Assoc 196:991-992, 1966.

5. Kirklin JK, Westaby S, Blackstone EH, et al: Complement and damaging effects of cardiopulmonary bypass. J Thorac Cardiovasc Surg 98:1100, 1989.

6. Rabinovitch M, Herrera-Deleon V, Castaneda AR, Reid LM: Growth and development of the pulmonary vascular bed in patients with tetralogy of Fallot, with or without pulmonary atresia. Circulation 64:1234-1249, 1981.

7. Flanagan MF, Fujii AM, Colan SD, et al: Myocardial angiogenesis and coronary perfusion in left ventricular pressure-overload hypertrophy in the young lamb: Evidence for inhibition with chronic protamine administration. Circ Res 68:1458-1470, 1991.

8. Wernovsky G, Stiles KM, Gauvreau K, et al: Cognitive development after the Fontan operation. Circulation 102:883-889, 2000.

9. Bellinger DC, Wypij D, duPlessis AJ, et al: Neurodevelopmental status at eight years in children with dextrotransposition of the great arteries: The Boston Circulatory Arrest Trial. J Thorac Cardiovasc Surg 126:1385-1396, 2003.

10. Castaneda AR, Mayer JE, Jr, Jonas RA, et al: The neonate with critical congenital heart disease: Repair—a surgical challenge. J Thorac Cardiovasc Surg 98:869-875, 1989.

11. Hunt CE, Lucas RV: Symptomatic atrial septal defect in infancy. Circulation 47:1042-1048, 1973.

12. Cherian G, Uthaman CB, Durairaj M, et al: Pulmonary hypertension in isolated secundum atrial septal defect: High frequency in young patients. Am Heart J 105:952-957, 1983.

13. Moe DG, Guntheroth WG: Spontaneous closure of uncomplicated ventricular septal defect. Am J Cardiol 60:674-678, 1987.

14. Gersony WM, Peckham GJ, Ellison RC, et al: Effects of indomethacin in premature infants with patent ductus arteriosus: Results of a national collaborative study. J Pediatr 102:895-906, 1983.

15. Heymann MA, Rudolph AM, Silverman NH: Closure of the ductus arteriosus in premature infants by inhibition of prostaglandin synthesis. N Engl J Med 295:530-538, 1976.

16. Van Overmeire B, Follens T, Hartmann S, et al: Treatment of patent ductus arteriosus with ibuprofen. Arch Dis Child Fetal Neonatal Ed 76:F179-184, 1997.

17. Wagner HR, Ellison RC, Zierler S, et al: Surgical closure of patent ductus arteriosus in 268 preterm infants. J Thorac Cardiovasc Surg 87:870-875, 1984.

18. Cotton RB, Stahlman MT, Berder HW, et al: Randomized trial of early closure of symptomatic patent ductus arteriosus in small preterm infants. J Pediatr 93:647-651, 1978.

19. Laborde F, Noirhomme P, Karam J, et al: A new video-assisted thoracoscopic surgical technique for interruption of patent ductus arteriosus in infants and children. J Thorac Cardiovasc Surg 105:278-280, 1993.

20. Fan LL, Campbell DN, Clarke DR, et al: Paralyzed left vocal cord associated with ligation of the patent ductus arteriosus. J Thorac Cardiovasc Surg 98:611-613, 1989.

21. Pozzi M, Remig J, Fimmers R, et al: Atrioventricular septal defect: Analysis of short-and mid-term results. J Thorac Cardiovasc Surg 101:138-142, 1991.

22. Morris CD, Magilke D, Reller M: Down syndrome affects results of surgical correction of complete atrioventricular canal. Pediatr Cardiol 13:80-84, 1992.

23. McElhinney DB, Driscoll DA, Emanuel BS, Goldmuntz E: Chromosome 22q11 deletion in patients with truncus arteriosus. Pediatr Cardiol 24(6):569-573, 2003.

24. Bove EL, Lupinetti FM, Pridjian AK, et al: Results of a policy of primary repair of truncus arteriosus in the neonate. J Thorac Cardiovasc Surg 105:1057-1065, 1993.

25. Sano S, Brawn WJ, Mee RBB: Total anomalous pulmonary venous drainage. J Thorac Cardiovasc Surg 97:886-892, 1989.

26. Lincoln CR, Rigby ML, Mercanti C, et al: Surgical risk factors in total anomalous pulmonary venous connection. Am J Cardiol 61:608-611, 1988.

27. Moene RJ, Oppenheimer-Dekker A, Bartelings MM: Anatomic obstruction of the right ventricular outflow tract in transposition of the great arteries. Am J Cardiol 51:1701-1704, 1983.

28. Kurosawa H, Van Mierop LHS: Surgical anatomy of the infundibular septum in transposition of the great arteries with ventricular septal defect. J Thorac Cardiovasc Surg 91:123-132, 1986.

29. Rastelli GC, McGoon DC, Wallace RB: Anatomic correction of transposition of the great arteries with ventricular septal defect and subpulmonary stenosis. J Thorac Cardiovasc Surg 58:545-552, 1969.

30. Pasquali SK, Hasselblad V, Li JS, et al: Coronary artery pattern and outcome of arterial switch operation for transposition of the great arteries: A meta-analysis. Circulation 106(20):2575-2580, 2002.

31. Sharland GR, Chita SK, Fagg NLK, et al: Left ventricular dysfunction in the fetus: Relation to aortic valve anomalies and endocardial fibroelastosis. Br heart J 66:419-424, 1991.

32. Rychik J, Murdison KA, Chin AJ, et al: Surgical management of severe aortic outflow obstruction in lesions other than the hypoplastic left heart syndrome: Use of the pulmonary artery to aortic anastomosis. J Am Coll Cardiol 18:809-816, 1991.

33. Van Son JA, Falk V, Mohr FW, et al: Ross–Konno operation with resection of endocardial fibroelastosis for critical aortic stenosis with borderline-sized left ventricle in neonates. Ann Thorac Surg 63:112–116, 1997.

34. Pellegrino A, Deverall PB, Anderson RH, et al: Aortic coarctation in the first three months of life: An anatomopathological study with respect to treatment. J Thorac Cardiovasc Surg 89:121–126, 1985.

35. Ohye RG, Bove EL: Current Topics in Congenital Heart Surgery. In Allen HD, Gutgesell HP, Clark EB, Driscoll DJ (eds): Moss and Adams' Heart Disease in Infants, Children, and Adolescents: Including the Fetus and Young Adult, 6th ed. Philadelphia: Lippincott Williams & Wilkins, 2001; pp 382–394.

36. DeLezo JS, Fernandez R, Sancho M, et al: Percutaneous transluminal angioplasty for isthmus coarctation in infancy. Am J Cardiol 54:1147–1149, 1984.

37. Brandt B, Marvin WJ, Rose EF, et al: Surgical treatment of coarctation of the aorta after balloon angioplasty. J Thorac Cardiovasc Surg 94:715–719, 1987.

38. Cobanoglu A Teply TF, Grunkemeier GL, et al: Coarctation of the aorta in patients younger than 3 months. J Thorac Cardiovasc Surg 89:128–135, 1985.

39. Clarkson PM, Brandt PWT, Barratt-Boyes BG, et al. Prosthetic repair of coarctation of the aorta with particular reference to Dacron onlay patch grafts and late aneurysm formation. Am J Cardiol 56:342–346, 1985.

40. Trinquet F, Vouhe PR, Vernant F, et al: Coarctation of the aorta in infants: Which operation? Ann Thorac Surg 45:186–191, 1988.

41. Park JK, Dell RB, Ellis K, Gersony WM: Surgical management of the infant with coarctation of the aorta and ventricular septal defect. J Am Coll Cardiol 20:176–180, 1992.

42. Brewer LA, Fosburg RG, Mulder GA, et al: Spinal cord complications following surgery for coarctation of the aorta: A study of 66 cases. J Thorac Cardiovasc Surg 64:368–381, 1972.

43. Sell JE, Jonas RA, Mayer JE, et al: The results of a surgical program for interrupted aortic arch. J Thorac Cardiovasc Surg 96:864–877, 1988.

44. Hayes CJ, Gersony WM, Driscoll DJ, et al: Second natural history study of congenital heart defects: Results of treatment of patients with pulmonary valvar stenosis. Circulation 87(2 Suppl):28–37, 1993.

45. Perryman RA, Jaquiss RDB: Tetralogy of Fallot. In Kaiser LR, Kron IL, Spray TL (eds): Mastery of Cardiothoracic Surgery. Philadelphia: Lippincott-Raven, 1998; pp 831–838.

46. Hennein H, Mosca R, Urcelay G, et al: Intermediate results after complete repair of tetralogy of Fallot in neonates. J Thorac Cardiovasc Surg 109:332–344, 1995.

47. Reddy VM, Liddicoat JR, Hanley FL: Midline one-stage complete unifocalization and repair of pulmonary atresia with ventricular septal defect and major aortopulmonary collaterals. J Thorac Cardiovasc Surg 109:832–845, 1995.

48. Shimazaki Y, Lio M, Nakano S, et al: Pulmonary artery morphology and hemodynamics in pulmonic valve atresia with ventricular septal defect before and after repair. Am J Cardiol 67:744–748, 1991.

49. Snir E, de Leval M, Elliot M, et al: Current surgical technique to repair Fallot's tetralogy with absent pulmonary valve syndrome. Ann Thorac Surg 51:979–982, 1991.

50. Watterson K, Malm T, Karl T, Mee R: Absent pulmonary valve syndrome: Operation in infants with airway obstruction. Ann Thorac Surg 54:1116–1119, 1992.

51. Lang D, Obenhoffer R, Cook A, et al: Pathologic spectrum of malformations of the tricuspid valve in prenatal and neonatal life. J Am Coll Cardiol 17:1161–1167, 1991.

52. Celermajer DS, Bull C, Till JA, et al: Ebstein's anomaly: Presentation and outcome from fetus to adult. J Am Coll Cardiol 23:170–176, 1994.

53. Celermajer DS, Cullen S, Sullivan ID, et al: Outcome in neonates with Ebstein's anomaly. J Am Coll Cardiol 19:1041–1046, 1992.

54. Danielson GK, Furster V: Surgical repair of Ebstein's anomaly. Ann Surg 196:499–506, 1982.

55. Gaynor JW: Coronary Artery Anomalies in Children. In Kaiser LR, Kron IL, Spray TL (eds): Mastery of Cardiothoracic Surgery. Philadelphia: Lippincott-Raven, 1998; pp 880–893.

56. Gates R, Laks H, Elami A, et al: Damus-Stansel-Kaye procedure: Current indications and results. Ann Thorac Surg 56:111–119, 1993.

57. Van Son JAM, Reddy VM, Haas GS, Hanley FL. Modified surgical techniques for relief of aortic obstruction in [S,L,L] hearts with rudimentary right ventricle and restrictive bulboventricular foramen. J Thorac Cardiovasc Surg 110:909–915, 1995.

58. Jacobs M, Rychik J, Murphy J, et al: Results of Norwood's operation of lesions other than hypoplastic heart syndrome. J Thorac Cardiovasc Surg 110:1555–1562, 1995.

59. Chang AC, Hanley FL, Wernovsky G, et al: Early bidirectional cavopulmonary shunt in young infants: Postoperative course and early results. Circulation 88:149–158, 1993.

60. Fontan F, Baudet E: Surgical repair of tricuspid atresia. Thorax 26:240–248, 1971.

61. Laschinger JC, Redmond JM, Cameron DE, et al: Inter-mediate results of the extracardiac Fontan procedure. Ann Thorac Surg 62:1261–1267, 1996.

62. Cohen AJ, Cleveland DC, Dyck J, et al: Results of the Fontan procedure for patients with univentricular heart. Ann Thorac Surg 52:1266–1271, 1991.

63. Knott-Craig C, Danielson G, Schaff H, et al: The modified Fontan operation: An analysis of risk factors for early postoperative death or takedown in 702 consecutive patients from one institution. J Thorac Cardiovasc Surg 109:1237–1243, 1995.

64. Senzaki H, Isoda T, Ishizawa A, Hishi T: Reconsideration of criteria for the Fontan operation: Influence of pulmonary artery size on postoperative hemodynamics of the Fontan operation. Circulation 89:1196–1202, 1994.

65. Imai Y, Takanashi Y, Hoshino S, et al: Modified Fontan procedure in 99 cases of atrioventricular valve regurgitation. J Thorac Cardiovasc Surg 113:262-269, 1997.

66. Gentles TL, Mayer JE Jr., Gauvreau K, et al: Fontan operation in 500 consecutive patients: Factors influencing early and late outcome. J Thorac Cardiovasc Surg 114:376-391, 1997.

67. Fontan F, Kirklin JW, Fernandez G, et al: Outcome after a "perfect" Fontan operation. Circulation 81:1520-1536, 1990.

68. Hanley FL, Sade RM, Blacksone EH, et al: Outcomes in neonatal pulmonary atresia with intact ventricular septum: A multi-institutional study. J Thorac Cardiovasc Surg 105:406-427, 1993.

69. Giglia TM, Mandell VS, Connor AR, et al: Diagnosis and management of right ventricular-dependent coronary circulation in pulmonic atresia with intact ventricular septum. Circulation 86:1516-1628, 1992.

70. Boucek MM, Edwards LB, Keck BM, et al: The Registry of the International Society for Heart and Lung Transplantation: Sixth Official Pediatric Report, 2003. J Heart Lung Transplant 22(6):636-652, 2003.

CHAPTER 15

Special Considerations in Children and Young Adults with Heart Disease

BERNARD J. CLARK III

A continuing goal of pediatric cardiology has been and should be to maximize the quality of life of each child with heart disease. Achieving this goal requires an understanding of the impact of pediatric heart disease on the activities and events of everyday life. When possible, we should encourage normalcy; when we cannot, we should understand how to maximize these children's quality of life.

How are infants, children, and young adults with congenital or acquired heart disease different from children without heart disease? How different are these children from others with reference to activities of daily living, participation in school gym or organized sports, taking common medications, and the application of common preventive health measures such as immunizations and preventive dental care? At what points in their lives does the presence of heart disease impact their activity? As these children become adults, what is the expected quality of life, and what might be their limitations? When can a woman with heart disease expect to have a successful pregnancy?

The purpose of this chapter is to consider these issues in the infant, child, adolescent, and young adult with mild to moderate structural heart disease, repaired structural heart disease, or chronic cardiac conditions, including cardiac arrhythmias and myocardial dysfunction.

Cardiac diagnosis and age generally determine the impact of heart disease on a child's life. The impact can be dynamic, changing over time as the cardiac condition may evolve for both unrepaired and repaired structural congenital heart disease. Mild aortic valve disease, for example, may become more significant with age. The toddler with mild aortic stenosis may grow to become the adolescent with moderate to severe aortic stenosis. In children with repaired or palliated cardiac disease, we are continuing to learn the late medical complications seen following repair of congenital heart disease. Cardiac follow-up and anticipatory guidance for these children is partially dictated by these potential complications.

Equally important, activity level and its resultant demands on the cardiovascular system change with age from infancy to adolescence. Consequently, activities permitted at 6 years of age may not be possible or advisable during adolescence; participatory guidance by caregivers is a continuous process.

The American Heart Association estimates that there are 1 million people in the United States with congenital heart disease.[1-3] By comparison, there are approximately 250,000 survivors of childhood cancer.[4] Because of the advances in treatment over the past 20 years, the vast majority of these children are under the age of 18. Each year, 35,000 children are born in the United States with congenital heart disease.[5] Current survival for infants and children following treatment for congenital heart disease, including surgery, is excellent, and the large majority of these infants currently being born with congenital heart disease will live to adulthood. The number of infants, children, adolescents, and adults with congenital heart disease can be expected to grow both absolutely and relatively to the total population of children in the United States in the coming decades.

THE INFANT WITH UNREPAIRED MILD CONGENITAL HEART DISEASE

Nearly 20% of the cases of congenital heart disease are due to a small ventricular septal defect or another form of minor acyanotic congenital heart disease (*see* Box 15-1). The large majority of these infants are diagnosed within the first month of life by virtue of a murmur; once diagnosed, they are followed clinically with the expectation that they will not have cardiac symptoms. A restrictive, small ventricular septal defect (VSD) usually becomes smaller, and, in a high percentage of patients, the VSD will close by 2–3 years of age. Infants with mild heart disease will be identified in the first 6 months of life, generally by the presence of a murmur. In such a child, there need be little difference in the health care provided from normal pediatric care. Immunizations are given as recommended for the normal infant. Diet does not require alteration, and normal weight gain can be expected. The child with mild acyanotic congenital heart disease receives routine pediatric care and intermittent follow-up with a pediatric cardiologist. In patients with a moderate VSD, a failure to gain weight may be a criterion for having the defect surgically closed.

THE INFANT WITH PALLIATED OR UNREPAIRED CONGENITAL HEART DISEASE

Approximately 3/1000 live births result in a newborn with critical cardiac disease that requires early surgical intervention within the first 30 days of life. Many of these children undergo reparative surgery. After recovery from surgery, they can be expected to resume normal infant development

Box 15-1   Asymptomatic Congenital Heart Disease

ASYMPTOMATIC UNREPAIRED CONGENITAL HEART DISEASE IN INFANCY

Mild to moderate pulmonary stenosis
Restrictive VSD
ASD
Small patent ductus arteriosus
Bicuspid aortic valve without stenosis

ASYMPTOMATIC REPAIRED CONGENITAL HEART DISEASE WITHOUT CARDIOVASCULAR RESIDUA

Repaired coarctation of the aorta
Repaired tetralogy of Fallot
Repaired VSD
Arterial switch procedure for D-transposition of the great vessels

and growth. This is the case for both simple cardiac malformations such as coarctation of the aorta and for more complex lesions such as transposition of the great vessels. Once these infants have undergone surgical repair and have recovered, general pediatric care is not different from that of the infant or child without heart disease with respect to nutrition, immunizations, and treatment of infections.

There is a significant proportion of infants with critical heart disease who will have only palliative surgery in infancy and, after surgery, will continue to be cyanotic and have abnormalities of circulation. Most of these infants will have only a single ventricle, with pulmonary blood flow supplied by a systemic to pulmonary artery shunt. Under these conditions, cardiac output to the systemic circulation and the pulmonary circulation is supplied by the single pumping ventricle, representing a sustained increased workload for the heart. These infants are at risk for decreased growth rate secondary to several factors, including decreased nutritional intake, increased metabolic demand, and increased circulating catecholamines that oppose insulin, a principal growth hormone in infancy.[6-9] In addition, these infants can develop evidence of heart failure, requiring medication, and they can exhibit an increased rate of respiratory infections and are at risk for sudden death.[10-12] Despite the nearly five-fold improvement in outcome after infant cardiac surgery over the past 15 years, infants with palliated complex heart disease remain at risk for significant morbidity after surgery. These infants are at increased risk for infections and require close follow-up with special attention to nutrition and cardiovascular well-being.

Nutritional needs of infants with palliated congenital heart disease are increased to approximately 140–150 kcal/kg/day.[13-15] To achieve this, a formula with increased caloric density may be required. This can be achieved by the addition of specific carbohydrate or fat supplements to the existing formula or by the mixing of powdered formula with less water to achieve a formula with 24–27 kcal/oz. In addition, many of these infants have delayed development of normal suck and swallow reflexes possibly related to the delay of normal feeding immediately after birth because of their heart disease and the surgery performed. As many as 20% of infants undergoing early palliative surgery will require nasogastric feeds in the first months of life. If possible, these should be bolus feedings to mimic normal feeding patterns. Simultaneously, these infants can benefit from infant feeding stimulation protocols to develop suck and swallowing skills.[16-19]

Immunizations are given per normal routine to infants and children with mild, repaired, or palliated congenital heart disease. In addition, because of the increased morbidity associated with respiratory syncytial viral (RSV) infections in children with palliated congenital heart disease, it is now recommended that these infants receive a course of Synagis, a monoclonal antibody manufactured using recombinant DNA technology and effective in the prevention of RSV infections. This treatment has been recommended for monthly dosage in premature infants or in those with residual bronchopulmonary dysplasia during the season most likely to result in RSV infections (September–March). Box 15-2 shows the current recommendations in infants with congenital heart disease. The decision to use palivizumab

---

Box 15-2   Current Recommendations for Use of Palivizumab (Synagis)

Infants less than 2 years of age with chronic lung disease who have required medical therapy in the last 6 months

Infants born at 32 weeks gestation or earlier

Infants and children 24 months of age and younger with hemodynamically significant cyanotic and acyanotic congenital heart disease

---

Box 15-3   Responsibilities of Care Team for Infants with Complex Palliated Congenital Heart Disease

Nutritional and feeding teams
(Generally not available in the community and are set up at the tertiary center)
   Calorie counts
   Nutritional supplements
   Feeding-stimulation protocols
Physical therapists
(May be available in the community)
   Growth and development
   Physical therapy
   Infant stimulation
Social workers
   Medical insurance
   Appointments and follow-up
   Parent and family education
Visiting nurses
   Medical checkups
   Family education
Pediatricians
   General medical care
   Anticipatory guidance
   Growth
   Immunizations
   Synagis
Cardiologists
   Cardiac care and appointments
   Medications
   Interaction of cardiac performance and growth
   Planning for future procedures

(Synagis) in infants with mild acyanotic congenital heart disease should be made based on the prenatal history of the infant and the state of the congenital heart disease.[20-23]

Patients with staged palliative surgery for complex congenital heart disease discharged from the hospital are at risk for sudden changes in cardiovascular stability. Patients with systemic-to-pulmonary artery shunts can develop sudden changes in the distribution of systemic and pulmonary blood flow, leading to cyanosis or decreased systemic perfusion. Consequently, some cardiac centers have developed a close follow-up protocol in which the families are discharged to home after surgery with a baby weight scale and a pulse oximeter. Families are instructed to track weekly weights and saturations; if deviations from expected values are found, the infant is hospitalized for observation. The use of such a protocol has been shown to substantially decrease incidence of out-of-hospital cardiovascular collapse and death.[24] Box 15-3 presents an outline for a coordinated care team for infants with complex congenital heart disease.

A SPECIAL CASE: THE INFANT AFTER HEART TRANSPLANT

For a small number of infants with complex heart disease, palliative or reparative surgery is not possible; these infants can be listed for heart transplantation. Although orthotopic heart transplant restores the cardiac circulation to normal, these infants do have special needs similar to those of the infant with palliated critical heart disease, discussed previously. In addition, these infants are immunologically compromised because of the multiple antirejection medications that they are taking and are at risk for more serious symptoms during otherwise routine pediatric infections. Nutrition and growth are critically important because these infants will often wait several months to undergo transplant and, they will do so with abnormal cardiac function, which will impair growth. After transplant, infants cannot receive attenuated live virus immunizations. This prevents them from receiving the measles-mumps-rubella (MMR) immunization. However, they can and should receive the diphtheria-pertussis-tetanus (DPT), *Haemophilus influenzae* type B (HIB), hepatitis B, and inactivated polio vaccines. In addition, they should receive an influenza immunization yearly. Parents and families require extensive education regarding each of these components of care in the infant after transplant. Table 15-1 lists appropriate immunizations for children with a heart transplant and for their family members.[22] After transplantation, resume immunization schedule once on maintenance immunosuppressant therapy or 6 months after a rejection episode. Patients under evaluation or newly listed should be given MMR and Varivax beginning at 9 months of

Table 15-1	Recommendations Regarding Immunizations for Heart Transplant Recipients and Their Siblings	
VACCINE	**RECIPIENT**	**SIBLING(S)**
DTP/DT	Yes	Yes
FluMist (for influenza)	No	No
Hepatitis A*	Yes	Yes
Hepatitis B	Yes	Yes
Hib	Yes	Yes
Influenza (non-live injection)	Yes	Yes
IPV	Yes	Yes
MMR	No	Yes
Neisseria meningitidis	Yes	Yes
Oral polio	No	No
Prevnar or Pneumovax	Yes	Yes
Synagis	Yes	Yes
Varivax (for chickenpox)	No	Yes

DT, Diphtheria-tetanus; *DTP*, diphtheria-tetanus-pertussis; *IVP*, inactive poliomyelitis vaccine; *MMR*, measles-mumps-rubella.
*Administered to patients residing in Alaska, Arizona, California, Idaho, Nevada, New Mexico, Oregon, South Dakota, Utah, and Washington.

age. Patients listed in the hospital can safely receive the MMR and Varivax vaccines while hospitalized.

TRAVEL AND THE CHILD WITH HEART DISEASE

Good anticipatory guidance will often allow children with heart disease to enjoy traveling for vacation. Several issues need to be addressed. First is the mode of travel. With the exception of children with significant cyanosis, air travel does not pose particular problems. For children with residual cyanosis, it needs to be recognized that the cabin pressure aboard most planes is equal to that at 10,000 feet and can result in a lower oxygen saturation in the patient. As such, the infant with cyanosis may benefit from the addition of oxygen on a plane trip. This can be done successfully but requires significant planning on the part of the family. Some smaller planes are not equipped or are restricted from having pressurized oxygen on board. Children with pacemakers should show the airport secuity personnel their pacemaker identification card and be allowed to bypass metal detectors or electromagnetic devices.

It is important that families carry sufficient medications for the duration of the trip, since obtaining medication away from home, out of state, or out of country can be difficult. In addition, the family should carry a medical history, including current condition and medications, in the case of emergency care. The medical history should provide information for the possible adjustment of medication dosage, if appropriate, related to time zone changes. Finally, consideration should be given to the type of activity that the family and child will experience. Some limitations may be advised

regarding the amount or type of exercise required to participate in the planned activities.

A common question is that of participation on different amusement park rides. Many rides stipulate that persons with a cardiac condition are restricted. This may or may not apply to the child with heart disease. Children with significant arrhythmias or those at risk for loss of consciousness with sudden changes in position should be restricted from some rides that could produce significant physical and emotional stress. This is especially true of children with arrhythmias triggered by increased catecholamine activity and children with moderate to severe pulmonary hypertension.

EXERCISE AND THE CHILD AND ADOLESCENT WITH HEART DISEASE

Activities that encourage aerobic exercise are healthy for all children, including those with heart disease. The current epidemic of childhood obesity is, to some extent, the result of a decrease in the daily activity levels of children today. Exercise, including competitive exercise, generally can be encouraged in all but a minority of children with heart disease.

Appropriate detailed guidelines are required in counseling the family and the child with heart disease with regard to exercise. Several factors need to be considered. The first consideration is the cardiac diagnosis and the cardiovascular condition of the child. Most patients with repaired congenital heart disease without significant residual anatomic or functional abnormalities can participate in unrestricted exercise. On the other hand, many children have significant residual defects that need to be considered when exercise is suggested. A second consideration is whether the specific form of exercise can be associated with sufficient cardiac stress to promote a sudden loss in cardiac function, such as an exercise-induced ventricular arrhythmia or coronary ischemia, resulting in sudden cardiac death. A final consideration is whether the type of exercise carries with it a risk of bodily injury if there were to be a cardiovascular event resulting in dizziness or loss of consciousness during exercise.

Most exercise can be classified according the type and intensity of activity and, in sports, whether there is risk of bodily injury, as from collision. With respect to the type of activity, there are two broad categories, divided by the expected cardiovascular response. Dynamic or isotonic exercise is defined as exercise that requires repetitive rhythmic contraction of muscles groups and is associated with an increase in heart rate and cardiac stroke volume. Systolic blood pressure is increased, but overall peripheral vascular resistance is decreased. Running would be considered a dynamic exercise. Static or isometric exercise is associated primarily with a significant increase in blood pressure and peripheral resistance with relatively little increase in heart rate or stroke volume. Activities such as heavy weight lifting or competitive wrestling would be considered high static activities.

Each form of exercise has both static and dynamic components.[24] Bike riding on level ground is primarily dynamic, but riding during hill climbing would be increasingly static, depending on the slope of the hill. Primarily, dynamic exercise results in an increase in volume load, whereas static exercise results in a pressure load on the heart. Both forms of exercise increase myocardial oxygen demand and are associated with an increased myocardial contractility and circulating catecholamines.

Table 15-2 outlines common recreational and competitive activities, categorized by the type of exercise involved. Each sport has both dynamic and static components. Columns A–C present increasing levels of dynamic exercise, and rows I-III present increasing levels of static exercise.[24]

One can separate exercise into recreational and competitive. Competitive exercise includes regular competition by an individual or an organized team against others, and it stresses the importance of individual performance to achieve success, or to win. Competitive sports require some form of recurrent ongoing training or practice. In addition, competitive sports are very different from recreational sports in that they do not provide an environment in which a participant can easily withdraw from activity. This last factor is particularly important in assessing the activity permissible for the older school age child and adolescent. In the height of competition, it may be difficult for an adolescent to differentiate cardiac symptoms such as tachycardia, shortness of breath, or chest pain from anxiety or the stress of competition. Finally, pediatric cardiologists need to consider the impact of restricting activity on the quality of life of the

Table 15-2   Classification of Sports

		A. Low Dynamic (<40% Max O_2)	Increasing Dynamic Component → B. Moderate Dynamic (40 – 70% Max O_2)	C. High Dynamic (>70% Max O_2)
Increasing Static Component ↓	1. Low Static (<20% MVC)	Billiards Bowling Cricket Curling Golf Riflery	Baseball/Softball* Fencing Table tennis Volleyball	Badminton Cross-country skiing (classic technique) Field hockey* Orienteering Race walking Racquetball/Squash Long-distance running Soccer* Tennis
	2. Moderate Static (20 – 50% MVC)	Archery Auto racing*† Diving*† Equestrian*† Motorcycling*†	American football Field events (jumping) Figure skating* Rodeoing*† Rugby* Running (sprint) Surfing*† Synchronized swimming†	Basketball* Ice hockey* Cross-country skiing (skating technique) Lacrosse* Running (middle-distance) Swimming Team handball
	3. High Static (>50% MVC)	Bobsledding/Luge *† Field events (throwing) Gymnastics*† Martial arts Sailing Sport climbing*† Water-skiing*† Weight lifting*† Windsurfing*†	Body building† Downhill skiing*† Skateboarding*† Snowboarding*† Wrestling*	Boxing* Canoeing/kayaking Cycling*† Decathlon Rowing Speed-skating*† Triathlon*†

The classification is based on peak static and dynamic components achieved during competition. It should be noted, however, that higher values may be reached during competition. It should be noted, however, that higher values may be reached during training. The increasing dynamic component is defined in terms of the estimated percent of maximal oxygen uptake (Max O_2) achieved and results in an increasing cardiac output. The increasing static component is related to the estimated percent of maximal voluntary contraction (MVC) reached and results in an increasing blood pressure load. The lowest total cardiovascular demands (cardiac output and blood pressure) are shown in the upper left corner and the highest in the lower right corner.

Adapted from Mitchell JH, et al: Classification of sports. J Am Coll Cardiol 45(8):1364-1366, 2005.

*Danger of bodily collision.

†Increased risk if syncope occurs.

child with heart disease. Modifications of activity may allow sports participation in many children with heart disease. This may include the choice of lower impact or less stressful sports (such as baseball or golf), a less physically competitive position (such as goalie, as opposed to forward, when playing soccer), or a limited time in the game (such as 5 minutes instead of an entire quarter).

At present, there are no evidence-based recommendations regarding suggested levels of recreational or competitive activity for children with heart disease. In 1994, the 26th Bethesda Conference attempted to provide "prudent consensus recommendations regarding the eligibility of athletes with an identified cardiovascular abnormality for competition in a sport."[25-28] In doing so, the authors recognized that there were little prospective data on which to base guidelines and that extrapolation of the guidelines to recreational activities would be difficult. Nonetheless, the conference, in addition to developing a severity index of activities, shown in Table 15-2, developed guidelines for structural heart disease, either repaired or unrepaired; several are highlighted below. Finally, the conference concluded that the recommendations should not be regarded as absolutely restrictive but, alternatively, as a vehicle offering physicians a better understanding of when they may wish to justify selective deviations from the guidelines. In the end, the most prudent anticipatory guidance must be made based on multiple factors, with full disclosure to the family and the child or adolescent.

The Child with Repaired Congenital Heart Disease

Children with repaired structural heart disease and little residual disease can generally participate in most recreational and competitive sports. This includes patients who have undergone repair of acyanotic heart disease, including patent ductus arteriosus, atrial septal defect (ASD), and VSD, without evidence of residual defects or pulmonary hypertension. In addition, it includes select patients with successfully repaired complex heart disease, including tetralogy of Fallot, transposition of the great vessels, and total anomalous pulmonary venous connection.

Special consideration should be given to children who have undergone a successful Fontan procedure. These children have decreased exercise tolerance because of the inability to appropriately augment stroke volume during exercise; they are not likely to achieve a high competitive level. In the absence of residual lesions, significant cyanosis, or significant arrhythmias, children with a Fontan procedure should be allowed to participate in some high dynamic sports. Individual evaluation and exercise testing should precede any such participation. In consideration of the fact that they only have a single ventricle, some cardiologists would suggest these children's restriction from high static activities because of their propensity to develop ventricular hypertrophy and diastolic dysfunction.

An additional special case is the older child after an arterial switch procedure for transposition of the great vessels. It has been suggested that these children should undergo an evaluation to determine if coronary insufficiency develops during exercise, because movement of the coronary button from the aortic root to the pulmonary (i.e., neoaortic) root is part of this surgical procedure. Small case series have found a small incidence of silent coronary insufficiency after repair of transposition of the great vessels. If suspected from echocardiographic studies, such children should undergo formalized exercise tress testing with radionuclide imaging or stress echocardiography to determine whether there is exercise-induced coronary insufficiency.

Left-Sided Obstructive Lesions

Patients with unrepaired left-sided obstructions, including mild subaortic stenosis, mild aortic valve stenosis, or coarctation of the aorta with a small pressure gradient, participate in many competitive sports, but they should be restricted from high static exercise. Patients with severe aortic stenosis, defined as a peak instantaneous gradient greater than 50 mmHg measured at cardiac catheterization or a mean gradient greater than 40 mmHg measured by echocardiography, should be restricted from all competitive sports. Evaluation of the child with aortic stenosis can include the use of exercise testing to look for arrhythmias or electrocardiographic changes suggesting cardiac ischemia during exercise.

After surgery for left-sided obstructive lesions, participation in sports is guided by the degree of residual obstruction, with the exception of continued restriction from high static exercise. Weight lifting is very popular currently, and often cardiologists are asked if the child with a mild left-sided obstruction can participate in a weight-lifting program. An easy guide to this is to explain the impact of high static exercise on the cardiovascular system and to recommend a maximal weight limitation that is below the child's actual weight or less than 50–75 lb. This weight should be light enough to allow at least 15 repetitions of an individual weight protocol. This provides some assurance that the child will not be doing high static exercise.

Pulmonary Hypertension

Patients with pulmonary hypertension require restriction from most competitive sports, especially patients with Eisenmenger's syndrome These children have significant right-to-left shunting, are cyanotic, and become more cyanotic with the fall in peripheral vascular resistance during exercise. Included in patients with pulmonary hypertension are children with complex forms of tetralogy of Fallot with residual peripheral pulmonary artery stenosis and elevated pulmonary vascular resistance, resulting in elevated right ventricular systolic pressure.

These children should be restricted from moderate and high dynamic exercise and all but mild static exercise because of the risk of arrhythmias, which can occur with increased catecholamine release, and the further increase in right ventricular pressure during exercise.

Other Considerations

Other special considerations with reference to exercise and competitive sports exist in patients with atrial and ventricular arrhythmias. In general, patients with supraventricular tachycardia without atrial flutter and well-controlled on medication, as well as patients with isolated premature atrial contractions, can participate in competitive sports without restriction. Atrial flutter is an uncommon form of arrhythmia in children without structural heart disease. Children with atrial flutter have the potential to have 1:1 atrial-to-ventricular conduction and a very fast ventricular response rate. Children with known atrial flutter should be exercised to determine the ventricular response to exercise. Children with Wolff–Parkinson–White (WPW) syndrome can usually participate in competitive sports if their SVT is controlled; these patients should undergo evaluation, including a 24-hour Holter monitor and exercise testing prior to participation. Patients with WPW and atrial flutter or fibrillation should be restricted from competitive exercise because of the potential for rapid atrioventricular conduction and ventricular fibrillation. In the current era, catheter ablation is recommended for these individuals. Children with WPW who have undergone successful catheter ablation can participate in competitive sports without restriction.[28]

Patients with structural heart disease and ventricular ectopy should be evaluated as to the severity of their heart disease and the association between exercise and their arrhythmia profile. Patients with isolated premature ventricular contractions (PVCs) in the absence of structural heart disease who do not require medications can participate in sports without restriction if the PVCs suppress, do not increase, or become more complex with exercise. Because of the risk of sudden death, children with long QT syndrome often are restricted from all competitive sports. Finally, children with Marfan syndrome should be restricted from sports because of the risks of significant contact injury and progression of aortic dilation or aortic rupture.

SUBACUTE BACTERIAL ENDOCARDITIS PROPHYLAXIS

Subacute bacterial endocarditis (SBE) or infective endocarditis is an indolent bacterial infection in the heart, often caused by the introduction of bacteria into the bloodstream at the time of a nonsterile surgical or medical procedure. In patients with congenital heart disease, abnormal patterns of blood flow, left-to-right intraventricular shunts, and areas of valvular stenosis or insufficiency can give rise to turbulent flow of blood, which enhances the likelihood of sequestration of bacteria in the endocardium of the heart or heart valves. To prevent this from occurring, patients with congenital heart disease are given oral or intravenous antibiotics prior to undergoing a procedure that may lead to bacteremia. The most common of these procedures in children are dental cleaning and the filling of dental caries. Others include tonsillectomy and adenoidectomy, placement of myringotomy tubes, endoscopy or similar gastrointestinal diagnostic procedures, and procedures requiring manipulation of the urogenital tract such as a voiding cystourethrogram in a child following recurrent urinary tract infections. Eye surgery to correct strabismus does not require preoperative antibiotics.

Special cases for school-age children are orthodontic procedures, including the wearing of braces and other orthodontic appliances. These children have frequent visits to the dentist for the adjustment of braces and orthodontic appliances. It is recommended that bacterial prophylaxis be used for application of the braces. Once appliances are in place and visits are confined to checking the integrity of the braces or minor wire corrections, prophylaxis is not necessary. If visits include the removal of appliances or the application of new appliances, prophylaxis should again be used.

The current American Heart Association recommendations for the use of antibiotics for endocarditis prophylaxis have largely been derived from empiric data and clinical experience. Recommendations are determined by the type of congenital heart disease and the specific procedure.

Patients at highest risk are those with left-sided valve disease, those with aortic or mitral valve replacement, and children with cyanotic heart disease and systemic-to-pulmonary artery shunts. Boxes 15-4 and 15-5 list recommendations for prophylaxis for children with heart disease, as well as the procedures that currently do and not require prophylaxis. Table 15-3 lists the various regimens required for patients. These will depend on weight, the procedure, the current use of antibiotics, and the patient's diagnosis.[30]

Although SBE prophylaxis has been recommended in various forms for some time, the guidelines are derived from empiric data and recently have been challenged by those concerned about the overuse of antibiotics in general and the development of resistant strains of bacteria. It has been suggested that insufficient evidence exists regarding the efficacy of antibiotic prophylaxis, particularly after dental

Box 15-4   Cardiac Conditions Associated With Endocarditis

ENDOCARDITIS PROPHYLAXIS RECOMMENDED
High-risk category

Prosthetic cardiac valves, including bioprosthetic and
   homograft valves
Previous bacterial endocarditis
Complex cyanotic congenital heart disease (e.g., single
   ventricle states, transposition of the great arteries, and
   tetralogy of Fallot)
Surgically constructed systemic to pulmonary shunts or
   conduits

Moderate-risk category

Most other congenital cardiac malformations (other than
   above and below)
Acquired valvar dysfunction (e.g., rheumatic heart disease)
Hypertrophic cardiomyopathy

Mitral valve prolapse with valvar regurgitation, thickened
   leaflets, or both

ENDOCARDITIS PROPHYLAXIS NOT RECOMMENDED
**Negligible-risk category (i.e., no greater risk than the
general population)**

Physiologic, functional, or innocent heart murmurs
Isolated secundum ASD
Surgical repair of ASD, VSD, or patent ductus arteriosus
   (without residua beyond 6 months)
Previous coronary artery bypass graft surgery
Mitral valve prolapse without valvar regurgitation
Previous Kawasaki disease without valvar dysfunction
Previous rheumatic fever without valvar dysfunction
Cardiac pacemakers (intravascular and epicardial) and
   implanted defibrillators*

Adapted from Dajani AS, Taubert KA, Wilson W, et al: JAMA 277: 1794–1801, 1997.
*Prophylaxis is recommended for high-risk patients; it is optional for medium-risk patients.
ASD, Atrial septal defect; *VSD,* ventricular septal defect.

Box 15-5   Dental Procedures and Endocarditis Prophylaxis

**DENTAL PROCEDURES—ENDOCARDITIS PROPHYLAXIS
RECOMMENDED***

Dental extractions
Periodontal procedures including surgery, scaling and root
   planing, probing, and recall maintenance
Dental implant placement and reimplantation of avulsed teeth
Endodontic (root canal) instrumentation or surgery only
   beyond the apex
Subgingival placement of antibiotic fibers or strips
Initial placement of orthodontic bands but not brackets
Intraligamentary local anesthetic injections
Prophylactic cleaning of teeth or implants where bleeding
   is anticipated

**DENTAL PROCEDURES—ENDOCARDITIS PROPHYLAXIS NOT
RECOMMENDED**

Fluoride treatments
Taking of oral radiographs
Orthodontic appliance adjustment
Shedding of primary teeth
Oral impressions

**OTHER PROCEDURES—ENDOCARDITIS PROPHYLAXIS
RECOMMENDED**

Respiratory tract
   Tonsillectomy and/or adenoidectomy
   Surgical operations that involve respiratory mucosa
   Bronchoscopy with a rigid bronchoscope
Gastrointestinal
   Sclerotherapy for esophageal varices
   Esophageal stricture dilation
   Endoscopic retrograde cholangiography with biliary
      obstruction

   Biliary tract surgery
   Surgical operations that involve intestinal mucosa
Genitourinary tract
   Prostatic surgery
   Cystoscopy
   Urethral dilation

**OTHER PROCEDURES—ENDOCARDITIS PROPHYLAXIS NOT
RECOMMENDED**

Respiratory tract
   Endotracheal intubation
   Bronchoscopy with a flexible bronchoscope, with or
      without biopsy
   Tympanostomy tube insertion
Gastrointestinal tract
   Transesophageal echocardiography†
   Endoscopy with or without gastrointestinal biopsy†
Genitourinary tract
   Vaginal hysterectomy†
   Vaginal delivery†
   Cesarean section
In uninfected tissue:
   Urethral catheterization
   Uterine dilatation and curettage
   Therapeutic abortion
   Sterilization procedures
   Insertion or removal of intrauterine devices
Other
   Cardiac catheterization, including balloon angioplasty
   Implanted cardiac pacemakers, implanted defibrillators,
      and coronary stents
   Incision or biopsy of surgically scrubbed skin
   Circumcision

Adapted from Dajani AS, Taubert KA, Wilson W, et al: JAMA 277: 1794–1801, 1997.
*Prophylaxis is recommended for patients with high- and moderate-risk cardiac conditions.
†Prophylaxis is recommended for high-risk patients; it is optional for medium-risk patients.

Table 15-3   Prophylactic Regimens

PROPHYLACTIC REGIMENTS FOR DENTAL, ORAL, RESPIRATORY TRACT, OR ESOPHAGEAL PROCEDURES

Situation	Agent	Regimen
Standard general prophylaxis	Amoxicillin	Adults: 2.0 gm; children: 50 mg/kg; orally 1 hour before procedure
Unable to take oral medications	Ampicillin	Adults: 2.0 gm; children: 50 mg/kg; IM or IV within 30 minutes before procedure
Allergic to penicillin	Clindamycin *or*	Adults: 600 mg; children: 20 mg/kg; orally 1 hour before procedure
	Cephalexin† *or* cefadroxil† *or*	Adults: 2.0 gm; children; 50 mg/kg; orally 1 hour before procedure
	Azithromycin or clarithromycin	Adults: 500 mg; children: 15 mg/kg; orally 1 hour before procedure
Allergic to penicillin and unable to take oral medications	Clindamycin *or*	Adults: 600 mg; children: 20 mg/kg; IV within 30 minutes before procedure
	Cefazolin†	Adults: 1.0 g; children: 25 mg/kg; IM or IV within 30 minutes before procedure

PROPHYLACTIC REGIMENS FOR GENITOURINARY/GASTROINTESTINAL (EXCLUDING ESOPHAGEAL) PROCEDURES

Situation	Agents*	Regimen‡
High-risk patients	Ampicillin plus gentamicin	Adults: ampicillin, 2.0 gm IM or IV, plus gentamicin, 1.5 mg/kg (not to exceed 120 mg) within 30 min of starting procedure; 6 hours later, ampicillin, 1 gm IM/IV, *or* amoxicillin, 1 gm orally Children: ampicillin, 50 mg/kg IM or IV (not to exceed 2.0 gm), plus gentamicin, 1.5 mg/kg, within 30 minutes of starting the procedure; 6 hours later, ampicillin, 25 mg/kg IM/IV, *or* amoxicillin, 25 mg/kg orally
High-risk patients allergic to ampicillin or amoxicillin	Vancomycin plus gentamicin	Adults: vancomycin, 1.0 gm IV over 1–2 hours, plus gentamicin, 1.5 mg/kg IV/IM (not to exceed 120 mg); complete injection/infusion within 30 minutes of starting procedure Children: vancomycin, 20 mg/kg IV over 1–2 hours, plus gentamicin, 1.5 mg/kg IV/IM; complete injection/infusion within 30 minutes of starting procedure
Moderate-risk patients	Amoxicillin or ampicillin	Adults: amoxicillin, 2.0 gm orally 1 hour before procedure, or ampicillin, 2.0 gm IM/IV within 30 minutes of starting procedure Children: amoxicillin, 50 mg/kg orally 1 hour before procedure, or ampicillin, 50 mg/kg IM/IV within 30 minutes of starting procedure
Moderate-risk patients allergic to ampicillin/amoxicillin	Vancomycin	Adults: 1.0 gm IV over 1–2 hours; complete infusion within 30 minutes of starting procedure Children: 20 mg/kg IV over 1–2 hours; complete infusion within 30 minutes of starting procedure

IM, Intramuscularly; *IV,* intravenously.
*Total children's dose should not exceed adult dose.
†Cephalosporins should not be used in individuals with immediate-type hypersensitivity reaction (i.e., urticaria, angioedema, or anaphylaxis) to penicillins.
‡No second dose of vancomycin or gentamicin is recommended.

procedures. New recommendations are under consideration by the American Heart Association. Studies have suggested that the chance of contracting bacterial endocarditis after a dental procedure is sufficiently small to warrant eliminating the use of antibiotic prophylaxis for certain groups of patients.[31,32] At present, however, the recommendations of the American Heart Association continue to suggest bacterial prophylaxis in patients with existent or repaired congenital heart disease, with the exceptions of mild pulmonary stenosis, suture repaired ASD, and repaired patient ductus arteriosus.

MEDICATION RESTRICTIONS

Patients with arrhythmias should be restricted from medications that may provoke their arrhythmia. Cold medications that contain ephedrine or pseudoephedrine

---

Box 15-6 Medication for Symptomatic Treatment of Respiratory Infections in Children with Arrhythmias

ANTIHISTAMINES:

Chlorpheniramine
Promethazine
Diphenhydramine
Loratadine
Fexofenadine (Allegra)
Cetirizine (Zyrtec)

COUGH SUPPRESSANTS:

Guaifenesin ± dextromethorphan
Promethazine with codeine

NO DECONGESTANTS INCLUDING NASAL SPRAYS WITH STIMULANTS

No phenylephrine or oxymetazoline

---

should not be used in patients with supraventricular tachycardia or ventricular tachycardia. Box 15-6 lists cold medications (primarily antihistamines) that can be used instead.

Careful consideration should be given to the patient with attention-deficit hyperactivity disorder (ADHD). Medications for treatment of this disorder are often sympathomimetics and, as such, could cause an increase in the frequency of arrhythmia. However, they are commonly very effective in treating ADHD and often can be the difference between a productive school experience and academic failure. Thus, in spite of the potential effect of these medications on the frequency of arrhythmias, they should not be withheld in the child with ADHD and arrhythmias. The medication for ADHD should be started and the patient monitored for a change in the frequency of arrhythmia. The choice of medication for ADHD can occasionally be guided by the history of arrhythmias.

In contrast, several psychotropic medications cause a prolongation of the corrected QT (QTc) interval, and their clinical risk benefit should be carefully considered in the child with symptomatic ventricular ectopy or long QT syndrome. If used in children with long QT syndrome, frequent electrocardiograms (ECGs) and Holter monitoring should be used once a child is at a steady medication state to determine if there is any change in the rhythm or QTc interval. Administration

of a medication to a child with suspected or diagnosed long QT syndrome should only be undertaken after consultation with a pediatric cardiologist.

PREGNANCY AND HEART DISEASE

With the increased success of reparative surgical techniques and improved survival, there are an increasing number of young women of childbearing age who have undergone reparative and palliative surgery for congenital heart disease. For the majority of these women, pregnancy can have a favorable maternal, as well as fetal, outcome. Despite this, pregnancy in a woman with all but the simplest heart diseases, such as mild pulmonary valve stenosis or mitral valve prolapse, should be considered high-risk, demanding careful coordination between the obstetrician and the cardiologist. In general, treatment of existent congenital heart disease amenable to correction should be done prior to planned pregnancy. In women with repaired congenital heart disease and residual defects not requiring correction, increased symptoms secondary to the cardiovascular stress of pregnancy may be experienced.

During pregnancy, hormone-mediated increases in circulating blood volume, red cell mass, and resting heart rate lead to an increased cardiac stroke volume and cardiac output that peaks in the second trimester and remains elevated until after delivery. In addition, elevated gestational hormone levels, as well as circulating vasoactive metabolites such as prostaglandins and the low resistance circulation of the placenta, contribute to a lowering of peripheral vascular resistance and blood pressure. Labor and delivery can present considerable stress to the cardiovascular system, resulting from anxiety, pain, uterine contraction, and blood loss. After delivery, cardiac output is further augmented by the decompression of the inferior vena cava and the increased blood volume resulting from the contraction of the uterus. These cardiovascular changes resolve within 2 weeks after delivery.[33]

Previously, pregnancy in the woman with unrepaired or repaired complex heart disease was felt to carry very significant risks by virtue of the physiologic demands of pregnancy on the cardiovascular system. The first early studies suggested that the underlying cardiovascular function was the largest single determinant of outcome; women with cyanosis and arterial saturations, less than 85% tended to have small (for gestational age) infants. There were high rates of morbidity and mortality for both mothers and fetuses when pregnancy was complicated by pulmonary hypertension and Eisenmenger's syndrome. These early findings have subsequently been supported by recent multicenter studies.[34,35]

Maternal cardiac status during pregnancy can be stratified according to the type of cardiac disease and state of the cardiac function (Box 15-7). Patients with repaired congenital heart disease or minor acyanotic forms of heart disease should remain largely symptom-free from a cardiac standpoint throughout pregnancy. Even patients with complex but repaired heart disease, such as tetralogy of Fallot, with good biventricular function may have minimal cardiac risk during pregnancy. Women with residual cardiac disease, such as a moderate to large left-to-right shunt, mitral or aortic stenosis, or a moderate cardiac dysfunction, may have the onset of new cardiac symptoms, including heart failure, pulmonary edema, or arrhythmias, that may require close cardiac follow-up and treatment. Women at high cardiac risk during pregnancy

include women with decreased cardiac function and New York Heart Association (NYHA) Class III or IV symptoms, severe aortic stenosis, moderate to severe pulmonary hypertension, Marfan syndrome and aortic root involvement, and Eisenmenger's syndrome. In women who have severe pulmonary hypertension, either primary or secondary, mortality can be high. Women with Marfan syndrome and an aortic root diameter of greater than 40 mm are at significant risk of aortic dissection during pregnancy. In women with high-risk heart disease, planned pregnancy should be discouraged and termination of the pregnancy should be strongly considered if the risk to the mother's life is known to be increased.

Women with palliated heart disease and cyanosis, although largely asymptomatic prior to pregnancy, have a high rate of cardiac complications during pregnancy, and there is a significant incidence of fetal complications, however. Women with cyanosis and right-to-left shunts may become more cyanotic during pregnancy because of the associated fall in peripheral vascular resistance. Maternal complications include significant exercise intolerance consistent with NYHA Class III symptoms, heart failure, arrhythmias, stroke, and death. Cyanosis has a significant impact on the fetus as well. Pregnancy associated with cyanosis results in high rates of prematurity (37%), low birth weight (40%), and early fetal demise (40%). These complications are more common in women with arterial oxygen saturations of less than 85%.[36] The Fontan operation eliminates cyanosis in congenital cardiac disease with a single ventricle but does so at the expense of limiting the ability to increase cardiac output. Pregnancy in the woman with a Fontan procedure can be successful, but cardiac complications, including arrhythmias and peripheral edema, are significant, and the risk to the fetus is high, including first trimester miscarriage in 30–40%.

Women who have had mitral or aortic valve replacement pose additional management issues during pregnancy because of the need for adequate anticoagulation. Although warfarin is often considered more effective as an anticoagulant and is better accepted by patients, compared with subcutaneous heparin, it carries risk to the fetus in early pregnancy during organ development, and there is a risk to the fetus for intracranial bleeding throughout pregnancy, particularly during vaginal delivery unless the drug has been stopped at least 2 weeks prior to delivery. Recent recommendations for anticoagulation during pregnancy include low-dose warfarin and aspirin either throughout pregnancy or with the use of subcutaneous heparin during the peak risk period of warfarin embryopathy, weeks 6–12 of gestation.[37]

A multidisciplinary team combining specialists in congenital cardiology and high-risk obstetrics should undertake management of the planned pregnancy in

---

Box 15-7   Maternal Cardiac Status and Risk of Cardiac Complications During Pregnancy

LOW RISK

Small left-to-right shunts, ASD, small VSD, or small PDA
Repaired lesions without residual cardiac dysfunction
Isolated mitral valve prolapse without significant regurgitation
Bicuspid aortic valve without stenosis
Mild to moderate pulmonic stenosis
Valvar regurgitation with normal systolic ventricular function

INTERMEDIATE RISK

Unrepaired or palliated cyanotic congenital heart disease
Large left-to-right shunts
Uncorrected coarctation of the aorta
Mitral or aortic stenosis
Mechanical prosthetic valves
Severe pulmonic stenosis
Moderate to severe systemic ventricular dysfunction
History of peripartum cardiomyopathy with no residual ventricular dysfunction

HIGH RISK

New York Heart Association Class III or IV symptoms
Severe pulmonary hypertension
Marfan syndrome with aortic root dilation or aortic or mitral valve involvement
Severe aortic stenosis
History of peripartum cardiomyopathy with residual ventricular dysfunction

From Siu SC, Colman JM: Heart disease and pregnancy. Heart 85(6):710–715, 2001.

women with heart disease (Box 15-8). Women should receive detailed counseling regarding the maternal and fetal risks of pregnancy, tailored to the expectant mother's cardiac diagnosis and condition. Detailed plans for treatment of potential cardiac complications should be developed. A genetic counselor should be part of the multidisciplinary team and should discuss the potential risk of congenital cardiac disease occurring in the fetus. The presence of congenital heart disease in an expectant mother or a first-degree relative increases the risk to the fetus by a factor of 10, from 0.6% in the general population to 4-6% in an at-risk fetus. Counseling may require genetic testing to determine whether the mother has a known genetic marker for heart disease, such as a microdeletion of chromosome 22, associated with conotruncal cardiac defects, because, if found, it would increase the risk of occurrence to 50%.

Vaginal delivery is recommended in women at term with heart disease, with labor usually carried out in the lateral decubitus position. Caesarean section should be considered only for obstetric indications, with the exception of Marfan syndrome with dilated aortic root or in the patient in whom heparin has not been instituted at least 2 weeks prior to labor. In certain cases, intra-arterial blood pressure monitoring can be useful in patients who would suffer deleterious effects with a sudden drop in blood pressure, such as the woman with significant aortic stenosis.

Box 15-8   Management Strategy for Pregnancy Complicated by Maternal Heart Disease

ALL PATIENTS

Define cardiac lesion and any anatomic residual abnormalities

Assess cardiac functional status

Determine predictors of risk

Eliminate teratogens

Arrange genetic counseling

Consider referral to a regional high-risk obstetric center

Assess need for endocarditis prophylaxis

INTERMEDIATE- AND HIGH-RISK PATIENTS

Refer to regional center for high-risk pregnancy

Consider antepartum interventions to reduce maternal risks

Engage a multidisciplinary team

Develop and disseminate detailed management plan

Anticipate vaginal delivery in almost all cases unless there are obstetrical contraindications

Consider early epidural anesthesia

Modify labor and delivery to reduce cardiac work

Plan postpartum monitoring, potentially in a coronary or intensive care unit setting

Adapted from Siu SC, Colman JM: Heart disease and pregnancy. Heart 85(6):710-715, 2001.

MAJOR POINTS

- Medical and surgical treatment of infants and children has improved dramatically in the past 15 years, and an ever-increasing number of these children are experiencing near-normal levels of activities of daily living as they grow to adulthood.
- Early care of the infant after cardiac surgery is directed toward promoting appropriate growth and development. In the most complicated infants, this is accomplished best with the help of a multidisciplinary team.
- Anticipatory guidance regarding activities of daily living is an important component of care for school-aged children with congenital heart disease for the primary care provider and the pediatric cardiologist. Areas of education and decision-making include use of immunizations, prevention of bacterial endocarditis, and guidance regarding level of physical activity and participation in competitive sports.
- Sports and competitive physical activity are important to the successful physical and emotional growth of children. Children with congenital heart disease should be offered options regarding participation in sports based on their cardiac diagnosis and condition and the expected effect of a specific activity on the cardiovascular system.
- Certain cardiac conditions, especially those with arrhythmias, require careful monitoring of prescription medications.
- Young women of childbearing age with congenital heart disease can often carry a fetus to successful delivery; this area of medicine, however, requires careful prepregnancy patient education, patient monitoring during pregnancy, and a trained team of caregivers, including obstetricians trained in the management of high-risk pregnancies.

REFERENCES

1. Hoffman JIE: Incidence, Prevalence, and Inheritance of Congenital Heart Disease. In Moller JH, Hoffman JIE (eds): Pediatric Cardiovascular Disease. New York, Churchill Livingstone, 2000, pp 257-262.

2. Mitchell SC, Korones SB, Berendes HW: Congenital heart disease in 56,109 births: Incidence and natural history. Circulation 43(3):323-332, 1971.

3. Green A: Outcomes of congenital heart disease: A review. Pediatr Nurs 30(4):280-284, 2004.

4. Bleyer WA: The impact of childhood cancer on the United States and the world. CA Cancer J Clin 40(6):355-367, 1990.

5. Hoffman JIE: Congenital heart disease: Incidence and inheritance. Pediatr Clin North Am. 37:25-43, 1990.

6. Mitchell IM, Davies PS, Day JM, et al: Energy expenditure in children with congenital heart disease, before and after cardiac surgery. J Thorac Cardiovasc Surg 107(2):374-380, 1994.

7. Barton JS, Hindmarsh PC, Scrimgeour CM, et al: Energy expenditure in congenital heart disease. Arch Dis Child 70(1):5-9, 1994.

8. Day RW, Denton DM, Jackson WD: Growth of children with a functionally single ventricle following palliation at moderately increased altitude. Cardiol Young 10(3):193-200, 2000.

9. Avitzur Y, Singer P, Dagan O, et al: Resting energy expenditure in children with cyanotic and noncyanotic congenital heart disease before and after open heart surgery. JPEN J Parenter Enteral Nutr 27(1):47-51, 2003.

10. Buchhorn R, Hammersen A, Bartmus D, Bursch J: The pathogenesis of heart failure in infants with congenital heart disease. Cardiol Young 11(5):498-504, 2001.

11. Ross RD: Medical management of chronic heart failure in children. Am J Cardiovasc Drugs 1(1):37-44, 2001.

12. Mahle WT, Spray TL, Gaynor JW, Clark BJ: Unexpected death after reconstructive surgery for hypoplastic left heart syndrome. Ann Thorac Surg 71(1):61-65, 2001.

13. Smith P: Primary care in children with congenital heart disease. J Pediatr Nurs 16(5):308-319, 2001.

14. Leitch CA: Growth, nutrition and energy expenditure in pediatric heart failure. Prog Pediatr Cardiol 11(3):195-202, 2000.

15. Leitch CA, Karn CA, Peppard RJ, et al: Increased energy expenditure in infants with cyanotic congenital heart disease. J Pediatr 133(6):755-760, 1998.

16. Forchielli ML, McColl R, Walker WA, Lo C: Children with congenital heart disease: A nutrition challenge. Nutr Rev 52(10):348-353, 1994.

17. Jackson M, Poskitt EM: The effects of high-energy feeding on energy balance and growth in infants with congenital heart disease and failure to thrive. Br J Nutr 65(2), 1991.

18. Imms C. Feeding the infant with congenital heart disease: An occupational performance challenge. Am J Occup Ther. 2001 May-Jun;55(3):277-84.

19. van der Kuip M, Hoos MB, Forget PP, et al: Energy expenditure in infants with congenital heart disease, including a meta-analysis. Acta Paediatr 92(8):921-917, 2003.

20. Tulloh R, Marsh M, Blackburn M, et al: Working Group of the British Pediatric Cardiac Association. Recommendations for the use of palivizumab as prophylaxis against respiratory syncytial virus in infants with congenital cardiac disease. Cardiol Young 13(5):420-423, 2003.

21. Feltes TF, Cabalka AK, Meissner HC, et al: Cardiac Synagis Study Group. Palivizumab prophylaxis reduces hospitalization due to respiratory syncytial virus in young children with hemodynamically significant congenital heart disease. J Pediatr 143(4):532-540, 2003.

22. Pickering LK (ed): Red Book 2003 Report of the committee on infectious diseases, 26th ed. Elk Grove Village, IL: American Academy of Pediatrics, 2003.

23. American Academy of Pediatrics Committee on Infectious Diseases and Committee on Fetus and Newborn. Revised indications for the use of palivizumab and respiratory syncytial virus immune globulin intravenous for the prevention of respiratory syncytial virus infections. Pediatrics 112(6 Pt 1):1442-1446, 2003.

24. Ghanayem NS, Cava JR, Jaquiss RD, Tweddell JS: Home monitoring of infants after stage one palliation for hypoplastic left heart syndrome. Semin Thorac Cardiovasc Surg Pediatr Card Surg Annu 7:32-38, 2004.

25. Mitchell JH, Haskell WL, Raven PB: Classification of sports. J Am Coll Cardiol 24(4):864-866, 1994.

26. Graham TP Jr, Bricker JT, James FW, Strong WB: Twenty-sixth Bethesda conference: Recommendations for determining eligibility for competition in athletes with cardiovascular abnormalities. Task Force 1: Congenital heart disease. J Am Coll Cardiol 24(4):867-873, 1994.

27. Cheitlin MD, Douglas PS, Parmley WW: Twenty-sixth Bethesda conference: Recommendations for determining eligibility for competition in athletes with cardiovascular abnormalities. Task Force 2: Acquired valvular heart disease. J Am Coll Cardiol 24(4):874-880, 1994.

28. Maron BJ, Isner JM, McKenna WJ: Twenty-sixth Bethesda conference: Recommendations for determining eligibility for competition in athletes with cardiovascular abnormalities. Task Force 3: Hypertrophic cardiomyopathy, myocarditis and other myopericardial diseases and mitral valve prolapse. J Am Coll Cardiol 24(4):880-885, 1994.

29. Zipes DP, Garson A Jr: Twenty-sixth Bethesda conference: Recommendations for determining eligibility for competition in athletes with cardiovascular abnormalities. Task Force 6: Arrhythmias. J Am Coll Cardiol 24(4):892-899, 1994.

30. Dajani AS, Taubert KA, Wilson W, et al: Prevention of bacterial endocarditis: Recommendations by the American Heart Association. Clin Infect Dis 25(6):1448-1458, 1997.

31. Gewitz MH: Prevention of bacterial endocarditis. Curr Opin Pediatr 9(5):518-522, 1997.

32. Cabell CH, Abrutyn E, Karchmer AW: Cardiology patient page. Bacterial endocarditis: The disease, treatment, and prevention. Circulation 107(20):e185-187, 2003.

33. Siu SC, Colman JM: Heart disease and pregnancy. Heart 85(6):710-715, 2001.

34. Siu SC, Sermer M, Harrison DA, et al: Risk and predictors for pregnancy-related complications in women with heart disease. Circulation 96(9):2789-2794, 1997.

35. Siu SC, Sermer M, Colman JM, et al: Cardiac Disease in Pregnancy (CARPREG) Investigators. Prospective multicenter study of pregnancy outcomes in women with heart disease. Circulation 104(5):515-521, 2001.

36. Siu SC, Colman JM, Sorensen S, et al: Adverse neonatal and cardiac outcomes are more common in pregnant women with cardiac disease. Circulation 105(18):2179-2184, 2002.

37. Oron G, Hirsch R, Ben-Haroush A, et al: Pregnancy outcome in women with heart disease undergoing induction of labour. BJOG 111(7):669-675, 2004.

CHAPTER 16

Preventive Cardiology

FRAZ A. ISMAT

RICHARD M. DONNER

It is most unusual for pediatricians to study risk factors that produce a disease responsible for virtually no morbidity or mortality during the first two decades of life. Coronary artery disease (CAD) is surely the exception because it is the single largest cause of death in the United States, affecting 7–10% of the population, and because it may burden the taxpayer with $75 billion per year in direct and indirect costs. Compared with other commonly addressed issues in pediatric cardiology, prevention of CAD may have a greater positive impact on the lives of more patients than any other aspect of the field.

There is a growing body of evidence suggesting that the CAD process begins in childhood. Current algorithms suggest that this process is multifactorial, requiring identification and examination of multiple possible risk factors, each of which may have complex relationships with CAD and among themselves. A number of these risk factors have already been identified in the adult population and have been studied in some detail. Whether any or all of these factors should be identified and addressed during childhood is a difficult subject with no definitive answer, but it is a subject that must be explored. Risk factors for other cardiovascular diseases such as peripheral vascular disease, renal vascular disease, and stroke are less well correlated with these disease processes and will not be speculated on here.

THE THROMBOTIC MODEL

CAD has been defined in adults for more than half a century. Much of this investigative work has centered on the critical event of coronary artery thrombosis leading to acute myocardial infarction. Current models of the process leading to thrombosis have shifted away from the traditional concept implicating the chronic, most severely narrowed segments of coronary artery to the notion of a smaller vulnerable plaque, characterized by an accumulation of lipids, T-lymphocytes, macrophages, and smooth muscle cells that become activated in response to inflammatory triggers. This concept explains, in part, why some interventions that reduce lipid content or address the inflammatory sequence result in a significant decrease in the risk for serious coronary events in the absence of any easily recognizable change in coronary artery pathology. This observation holds even with the use of intravascular ultrasound to detect alterations in plaque size and morphology that are transparent to coronary angiography. Secondary prevention studies demonstrating a more favorable effect of lipid lowering than for percutaneous coronary angioplasty are also consistent with this hypothesis.

Among the components of the coronary artery thrombosis model, the endothelium is crucial and participates in the initial phase. With the description of acetylcholine-induced conversion of L-arginine to nitric oxide (NO) by NO synthase, a number of targets for previously known risk factors were identified. Hypercholesterolemia is a potent cause of endothelial dysfunction through detrimental effects on the production and availability of NO. Endothelial dysfunction associated with hypercholesterolemia is described in a wide variety of situations, including familial hypercholesterolemia in childhood. Hypertension decreases production of NO, availability of NO, or both, and it increases medial smooth muscle mass, with all of these effects promoting vasoconstriction. Smoking causes endothelial dysfunction by a variety of mechanisms. The hyperglycemia of diabetes has a direct, destructive effect on the endothelial cell membrane in addition to causing the release of prostanoids that facilitate platelet aggregation. The prothrombotic effect of homocysteine may be related to diminished endothelial-related vasodilatation. Finally, age-related changes in the NO pathway may contribute to acceleration of atherosclerosis later in life.

Endothelial injury and dysfunction are recognized as the major triggers for subsequent inflammation. Endothelial cell adhesion molecules appear as a consequence of injury and permit migration of macrophages and T-lymphocytes into the arterial wall. In the presence of low-density lipoprotein cholesterol (LDLC), particularly the highly oxidized forms of cholesterol mentioned below, these inflammatory cells become foam cells and coalesce into structures that are referred to as "fatty streaks." Cytokines and growth factors are released, and these advance the inflammatory process and initiate the production of smooth muscle cells, forming the initial plaque. A collection of enzymes, the metalloproteinases, causes remodeling of the arterial wall, sometimes increasing the effective arterial lumen. A necrotic fibrous cap, consisting of many of the inflammatory components, eventually forms with the capability of rupture in the presence of abnormal flow dynamics and shear forces. Interest in measuring general markers of inflammation, such as high-sensitivity C-reactive protein (hs-CRP), as a clinical tool for diagnosis and assessing prognosis has recently intensified despite recent caution regarding its usefulness as a screening tool. Increased interest in infectious agents, particularly *Chlamydia pneumoniae,* has generated debate regarding the use of macrolide antibiotics following myocardial infarction.

The universal presence of free radicals such as hydrogen peroxide and the hydroxyl group contributes to coronary artery thrombosis by participating in the process of oxidative stress. Oxidized LDLC is not well bound to hepatic LDL receptors (LDL-Rs) and, through additional oxidative processes, is more available for foam cell formation.

Antioxidants such as amlodipine reduce oxidative stress by several mechanisms. Studies have shown clinical reduction of major cardiac events for some of these compounds.

RISK FACTORS IN THE ADULT POPULATION

Dyslipidemia

Among the clinical risk factors contributing to coronary artery thrombosis, dyslipidemia figures most prominently in adults. Although lipid metabolism is an extremely complex subject, it is not necessary to explore its full scope to gain a useful understanding of dyslipidemia states. Figure 16-1 illustrates the more important pathways and relationships in a simplified format. Because the risk for CAD depends on the cholesterol and triglyceride content of individual lipoproteins, the standard fasting lipid profile (with some elective components), illustrated in Table 16-1, has become commonplace.

The relationship between total serum cholesterol and coronary artery disease was initially described by two major studies, the Framingham Study[1] and the Multiple Risk Factor Intervention Trial (MRFIT). The authors of both studies found a direct, continuous relationship between total cholesterol and serious coronary events such as acute myocardial infarction. This relationship is commonly known as the "cholesterol hypothesis." Similar results were obtained over a wide range of studies and methods. Based upon this evidence, the National Cholesterol Education Program (NCEP) Expert Panel has issued three reports detailing the detection, evaluation, and treatment of hypercholesterolemia in adults. The most recent of these, the Adult Treatment Panel III (ATP III),[2] accounts for the more current models of coronary thrombosis, including a better understanding of and appreciation for the antioxidant effects of some standard lipid-lowering medications and their effects on certain lipid subfractions. The potential benefits of this approach, in addition to documented poor compliance with previous guidelines by both patients and physicians, led ATP III to adopt more stringent guidelines addressing elevations of LDLC. The guidelines are established according to three categories of risk rather than an individual's LDLC. These are (A) existing coronary artery disease and its equivalents (i.e., other atherosclerotic disease or diabetes mellitus), (B) the presence of two or more risk factors plus an assessment of 10-year risk, and (C) the presence of no risk factors or only one risk factor. The goal for category A is LDLC < 100 mg/dL; for category B, LDLC < 130 mg/day; and for category C, LDLC < 160 mg/dL. However, within each category are subcategories that modify the recommendation and define the timing of intervention. Two major studies published in early 2004 suggest that reduction of LDLC

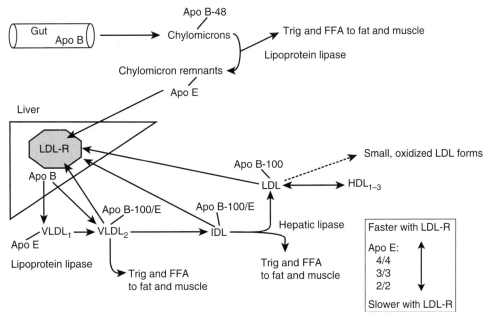

Figure 16-1   Simplified lipid scheme. Lipoproteins are complex particles that consist of a core of lipids (i.e., triglycerides and cholesterol esters in varying types and amounts, depending on the type) surrounded by a layer of phospholipids and apoproteins. Lipids are transported to various locations in the body by the movement of these different lipoproteins. Apolipoprotein B (APOB), present in the liver and the gut wall, is the precursor of most lipoproteins. The chylomicron, a lipoprotein containing apoprotein B-48 (APOB-48), carries dietary cholesterol and triglycerides to the liver after some triglycerides and free fatty acids are split off to fat and muscle by lipoprotein lipase (LpL). In the fasting state, hepatocytes express APOB fully as APOB-100 and add cholesterol and triglycerides to make the large very low density lipoprotein $VLDL_2$, which also expresses apolipoprotein E (APOE). Another hepatocyte product, $VLDL_1$, only expresses APOE. In the plasma, $VLDL_2$ loses some triglycerides and free fatty acids by LpL and is reduced in size to intermediate density lipoprotein (IDL). Through hepatic lipase and the loss of additional lipids to fat and muscle, IDL is reduced further in size to low-density lipoprotein (LDL). LDL may be reduced further in size by oxidation to form a number of smaller lipoproteins that are significantly altered and that participate in the atherogenic process. High density lipoprotein (HDL) consists of three subsets and exists in equilibrium with LDL. An important property of HDL is its scavenger function—its ability to remove lipids from other lipoproteins and to transport them to the liver. The hepatic LDL receptor (LDL-R), required for entry of lipids into the hepatocyte, recognizes only lipoproteins expressing APOB. Lipoproteins also expressing APOE compete with LDL for LDL-R according to the APOE phenotype, the 4/4 phenotype combining more readily, thereby slowing clearance of LDL from the plasma. *Apo B*, Apolipoprotein B; *Apo B-48*, apoprotein B-48; *Apo B-100*, apoprotein B-100; *Apo E*, apolipoprotein E; *FFA*, free fatty acid; *IDL*, intermediate density lipoprotein; *LDL-R*, low-density lipoprotein receptor; *Trig*, triglycerides; *VLDL*, very low density lipoprotein.

Table 16-1   Suggested Components of the Fasting Lipid Profile

Lipid Fraction	Description	Laboratory Method	FLP Component Type
Total cholesterol (TC)	Cholesterol content of all lipoproteins	Measured	Standard
HDL-c	Cholesterol content of HDL	Measured	Standard
Triglycerides	Triglyceride content of all lipoproteins	Measured	Standard
LDL cholesterol (LDLC)	Cholesterol content of LDL	Calculated when triglycerides < 400 mg/dL: LDLC = TC − [HDL-C + (triglycerides / 5)] When triglycerides > 400 mg/dL, use ultracentrifugation	Standard
Apolipoprotein B (APOB)	Total APOB: a rough measure of the total number of lipoprotein particles	Measured	Elective
Lipoprotein (a)	Total lipoprotein (a)	Measured	Elective
Homocysteine (nonlipid)	Homocysteine	Measured	Elective

to values below these goals might achieve a further reduction of morbidity and mortality.

NCEP ATP III guidelines focus on the major risk, assumed to have no specific underlying etiology, posed by LDLC elevation in the general population. However, the report does recognize a relatively small population that presents with recurring patterns of lipid and lipoprotein elevations of significant degree. These adults are assumed to represent genetic abnormalities of lipoprotein metabolism. In most (but not all) cases, the genetic abnormality confers some risk for serious CAD. Because values for cholesterol and triglycerides are usually much higher than in the general population at risk, recommendations regarding timing of intervention, drug therapy, and lifestyle issues are considered separately. As discussed later in this chapter, the recognition and significance of mild or moderate LDLC elevations during the first two decades of life is poorly developed. Therefore, it is the child with genetic disease who most often presents for evaluation.

Hypertension

The Sixth Report of the Joint National Committee on the Prevention, Detection, Evaluation, and Treatment of High Blood Pressure (JNC VI, 1997), reexamined a large number of adult studies and meta-analyses. The report reaffirmed the link between hypertension and coronary artery disease in adults. It pointed out that reduction in the incidence of coronary disease had occurred after successful institution of previous treatment guidelines, but that the rate of decrease was again slowing. Like the NCEP ATP III guidelines, recommendations for treatment were individualized according to risk group.

Metabolic Syndrome

Metabolic syndrome is a grouping of CAD risk factors that are related clinically and are associated with a two- to five-fold increased risk of CAD. The well-recognized components, characteristics of which are listed in Table 16-2, are dyslipidemia, diabetes, insulin resistance, obesity, hypertension, and a procoagulant state. All components may not be present simultaneously. It is generally agreed that insulin resistance of peripheral tissues (particularly muscle) probably represents the closest approximation to a fundamental etiology present at this time. The impaired glucose tolerance and hyperglycemia that follow lead to CAD through a variety of mechanisms including direct effect on the endothelial cell and glycation of lipoproteins, which increases their susceptibility to oxidation.

The diagnosis is generally made on easily available clinical and laboratory findings. ATP III suggests that at least three of the following five criteria be present: obesity

Table 16-2	**Components of Metabolic Syndrome**
Component	**Characteristics**
Dyslipidemia	Elevated VLDL triglycerides, low HDL-C, and normal total LDLC, with increased percentage of small, dense LDLC
Diabetes mellitus	May be type 1 but usually type 2. Risk for CAD may more than double and is a function of the degree of hyperglycemia and impaired glucose tolerance.
Insulin resistance	Hyperinsulinemia is probably the final common pathway.
Obesity	Usually central with increased waist-to-hip ratio
Hypertension	Mechanism in type 1 diabetes may be nephropathy, but hypertension is also present in type 2 diabetes
Procoagulant state	Increased platelet aggregation and increased fibrinogen

with an elevated waist circumference (males > 40 inches, females > 35 inches), triglycerides $\geq$ 150 mg/dL, HDL-c (high-density lipoprotein-cholesterol) < 40 mg/dL in males and < 50 mg/dL in females, blood pressure $\geq$ 130/85, and fasting glucose $\geq$ 110 mg/dL. Treatment is directed primarily at the insulin resistance and can therefore be ineffective if the totality of the syndrome is not recognized. Effective treatment for insulin resistance is primarily weight loss and exercise. Drug treatment of the dyslipidemia and hypertension is also beneficial. In adults, drug therapy is used routinely to increase insulin release from the pancreas. The glitazones are a newer class of agents that increase sensitivity to insulin by decreasing the release of mediators of insulin resistance from adipose tissue.

Obesity

The percentage of adults defined as obese has grown rapidly in the past 25 years, reaching nearly 70% in 2002 with an increasing upward trend. Obesity in adults probably raises the risk of CAD through the factors associated with metabolic syndrome and insulin resistance. Another pathway may be through hypertension and its effect on left ventricular mass, systolic and diastolic function, and arrhythmias. Other organ systems that may suffer directly or indirectly from obesity include the pulmonary, skeletal, and endocrine systems. The presence of an independent effect on general health is not certain, although overall mortality and the risk for other systemic disease such as some cancers is also increased.

The Third National Health and Nutritional Examination Surveys (NHANES III) defines obesity in terms of the ratio of mass (kg) to square of the height (m), otherwise known as the body mass index (BMI). Obesity is present when BMI is > 27.8 kg/m² in men and > 27.3 kg/m² in women. Recognizing that the risk for nonfatal CAD-related events may increase when one is overweight but not obese, NIH clinical guidelines define an individual as "overweight" at a BMI from 25–29.9 kg/m² and obese at a BMI of 30 kg/m² or greater.

These definitions may not take into account the more benign effect of increased lean body mass (e.g., acquired through isometric exercise), and a number of studies have shown that central obesity, as defined by the waist-to-hip ratio or the waist circumference (males > 102 cm, females > 88 cm), is more closely associated with the development of CAD. There is ample evidence that CAD risk varies with ethnicity and lifestyle for a given BMI. Treatment of obesity in adults has been exceedingly difficult with very high failure rates. Most methods utilize some form of behavior modification combined with regular aerobic and isometric exercise.

Smoking

Tobacco use raises the risk for CAD through a number of mechanisms. Nicotine increases catecholamine-induced vasoconstriction and increased blood pressure, along with increased heart rate. Together, these increase myocardial oxygen demand. Carbon monoxide acts directly on hemoglobin to decrease oxygen carrying capacity. The result is myocardial ischemia. Additional effects of smoking include endothelial dysfunction from decreased NO availability, increased platelet aggregation, a hypercoagulable state, and increased LDLC. These effects are both acute and chronic.

There is much epidemiologic evidence demonstrating increased morbidity and mortality from CAD in both male and female smokers. The risks of suffering most (but not all) CAD-related events are proportional to the cumulative exposure to tobacco, whether acquired by heavy smoking over a brief period of time or by occasional tobacco exposure over many years. Once CAD becomes manifest, continued exposure to tobacco increases risk disproportionately. Similar findings exist for passive exposure to cigarette smoke, although the magnitude of the effect is smaller. The mechanisms are thought to be identical to those in smokers, and risk increases in a dose-dependent fashion.

There are many studies demonstrating the tremendous benefit of smoking cessation in terms of CAD risk reduction. Physician and other professional input and encouragement are identified as strong components of success. However, more than half of all individuals who diminish or eliminate their tobacco exposure eventually return to prior levels. Smokers who have achieved some level of cessation, as well as those who have not yet contemplated doing so, may benefit from a number of aids including nicotine-replacement products administered by the oral, skin patch, or inhalation route. Bupropion, an antidepressant that functions by inhibiting norepinephrine and dopamine uptake, has also been an effective tool.

Hyperhomocystinemia

High plasma levels of homocysteine are associated with a number of disease states, including CAD. The mechanism is primarily related to endothelial cell damage and dysfunction, but adverse effects on platelet function, clotting factors, and smooth muscle function have also been described. A plasma homocysteine level greater than 15 µmol/L is shown in several studies to be an independent risk for events such as myocardial infarction. Levels at the upper end of this normal range have also been identified as risk factors for CAD. Elevated plasma homocysteine may result from absence of a key enzyme such as cystathionine β-synthase, the cause of homocystinuria or other rare enzyme abnormalities.

In many others, however, alteration of cofactors such as vitamins B_6 and B_{12} and folic acid in the homocysteine-methionine cycle may be implicated. These include age-associated deficiencies, deficiencies associated with some chronic diseases such as chronic renal disease, and agents like methotrexate or estrogen, which contain compounds that disturb the metabolism of vitamins B_6 and B_{12}. Treatment of hyperhomocystinemia has centered on supplementation with folic acid along with vitamins B_6 and B_{12} if levels of the latter are found to be low. The generally accepted dose of folic acid for adults is 0.4 mg/day. The efficacy of this approach for diminishing the risk of CAD has not been proven conclusively.

RISK FACTORS IN THE PEDIATRIC POPULATION

Evidence has accumulated showing that some risk factors leading to CAD in adulthood are operative during the first two decades of life. The relationships among these risk factors are certainly complex and may not be fully understood. Still other factors remain to be identified. There has been considerable debate as to whether any or all of the possible risk factors warrant attention from the pediatric healthcare system. Although much data remain to be collected, most authors and consensus reports identify the following risk factors in childhood as worthy of study: dyslipidemia, hypertension, obesity or sedentary lifestyle, and smoking. Others, such as hyperhomocystinemia, are currently under study and may join the list in the near future.

Childhood risk factors for CAD may be addressed by two methodologies. The first is to target all children by incorporating recommended strategies into the current healthcare process—a population-based approach. Examples might be to discuss general and specific nutrition guidelines or to recommend age-specific forms of physical activity at the time of the well-child visit.

The second methodology—an individual approach—is to utilize a screening algorithm to identify individuals with risk factors that may then be targeted by specific therapies. This approach, for example, might attempt to identify a strong family history of CAD that would lead to laboratory testing and treatment if guidelines are exceeded. Various combinations of these methodologies have also been proposed and, in practice, the pediatrician often selects one as more appropriate for a given family or population in his or her practice.

Dyslipidemia

Normal Values

In 1980, the Lipid Research Clinics Program Prevalence Study published plasma lipid and lipoprotein levels for Caucasian and African Americans by age and sex. These data greatly improved our understanding of the distribution of lipid values in children and formed the basis for screening algorithms and treatment recommendations. Subsequent studies during the 1980s, particularly the Bogalusa Heart Study, further defined the significance of these normal ranges by examining selected portions of the U.S. population and comparing them with similar data from diverse cultures throughout the world. New analyses suggest that other factors such as pubertal status may further modify our ability to discriminate normal from abnormal and to identify those children truly at risk.

Systematic Approach

Physicians involved in the care of children with dyslipidemia need to consider a systematic approach to the subject that not only defines a comprehensive clinical pathway but also allows incorporation of new guidelines, diagnostic tools, and innovative treatments. An example is the following three-step approach in which *risk assessment* identifies subjects in whom a *diagnostic algorithm* is initiated, sometimes leading to *treatment options*:

Risk assessment is the identification of individuals or segments of the population who qualify for diagnosis and possible therapy of their dyslipidemia. Unlike the adult population, for whom an individual screening process is recommended, children may benefit from both population-based and individual approaches.

The *diagnostic algorithm* identifies an etiology for the dyslipidemia that refines knowledge of outcome and inheritance patterns, establishes realistic treatment goals, and insures that correct and efficient therapy is initiated without undo experimentation or delay. The

importance of such an algorithm in adult medicine is diminished in favor of universal treatment options that are invoked to meet specific lipid target values regardless of etiology.

Treatment options for children are generally based on those available for adults. The caution with which they are recommended for pediatric use needs to be balanced with any new information suggesting that early intervention modifies the course of CAD in the adult.

Risk Assessment

Data from many studies throughout the adult cardiovascular literature demonstrate a clear relationship between the risk of CAD and certain forms of morbidity and mortality in the fifth, sixth, and seventh decades to various dyslipidemias encountered during early adult life. No such relationship exists for the pediatric patient because, with few exceptions, there is no morbidity or mortality encountered during childhood from dyslipidemia. The rationale for concern, then, is founded upon the notion that dyslipidemia encountered during the childhood years will *track* into the early adult years and will then be subject to the relationship between early adult dyslipidemia and later adverse coronary artery events.

The existence of tracking was hotly debated during the 1980s, and it was argued by some that there was little rationale for addressing pediatric dyslipidemia. There is now sufficient evidence to support the concept of tracking, although it is unlikely that a definitive longitudinal study over many years will ever be performed. Short- and medium-term data from the Muscatine study were acquired by examining lipid values at ages 8–18 and again at ages 20–25 or 26–30. There was impressive tracking of the upper quartiles and quintiles into early adulthood, resulting in a greater than 50% chance that these individuals will maintain their abnormal lipid profiles as young adults. Data from the Bogalusa Heart Study, interpreted by many authors, show convincing evidence that pathologic findings in young adults correlate with abnormal lipoprotein profiles in children and particularly with the presence of multiple risk factors, including hypertension and smoking. Primary genetic disease, first identified in childhood, would be expected to promote the morbidity and mortality that are found in adults with these diseases. Finally, the link between childhood distributions of lipids and adult risk for CAD is illustrated by certain homogenous populations that exhibit increased CAD as adults when subject to Westernization of their dietary habits during childhood.

Most children will appear in a lipid specialist's office for one of two reasons. The first is anxiety within the child's family regarding an unexpected death (usually of a parent) from CAD or multiple family members being treated for CAD. The second is the finding of abnormal lipid values identified by laboratory testing obtained for some other indication. Unfortunately, neither of these is often driven by population- or individual-oriented guidelines; consequently, there is a large at-risk pediatric population that is excluded from the screening process. Despite strong support for the existence of tracking, there has not yet been a consensus recommendation for universal laboratory screening of children, which is part of an individual-based approach that exists for the adult. Instead, an individual approach to identify high-risk individuals and families, together with some population-based recommendations and definitions of acceptable, borderline, and elevated lipid values, has been advocated by a number of individuals and consensus groups. These include The National Cholesterol Education Program Expert Panel on Blood Cholesterol Levels in Children and Adolescents,[3] the American Heart Association,[4] and the Council on Cardiovascular Disease in the Young of the American Heart Association.[5] These recommendations for screening and intervention are mostly consistent among expert groups and are summarized in Table 16-3. Since these guidelines were established, more recent findings argue for their revision. Findings that normal lipid values in preteens and teenagers are affected by puberty and hormonal changes diminish

the usefulness of single cutoff values for all children and may exclude some teenagers from receiving proper therapy. The growing experience with the safety of diet and drug therapy at younger ages and evidence that behavior modification during childhood may lead to favorably altered lipid profiles as an adult also argue for revision of the guidelines.

There is generally agreement that population-based initiatives and dyslipidemia screening fall within the responsibility of the pediatrician or primary care physician. The decision to proceed with diagnosis and to initiate therapy is now the responsibility of a variety of individuals, including the pediatrician, the pediatric cardiologist, the pediatric gastroenterologist, and the lipid specialist. In our experience, many pediatricians feel uncomfortable with the diagnostic algorithm and with the mechanics of diet and drug therapy. We hope that this trend will be reversed by incorporating the basic principles of dyslipidemia risk assessment, diagnosis, and treatment into both the pediatric training core curriculum and postgraduate education.

Diagnostic Algorithm

Pediatric patients with dyslipidemia may be conveniently placed into one of three categories: primary genetic disease, secondary dyslipidemia, and unclassified dyslipidemia. Examples of each are given in Box 16-1. It is likely that the distribution of children within these

Table 16-3 Composite Recommendations for Dyslipidemia Screening and Intervention

Population-Based Recommendations	Individual High-Risk Assessment From History	Individual High-Risk Assessment From Lipid Profile
Avoid excess simple carbohydrates (sugar)	Family history of premature CAD in first degree relatives < age 55	Acceptable: Total cholesterol < 170 mg/dL*
Total fat should remain between 20% and 30% of total calories	and/or	LDL cholesterol < 110 mg/dL
Limit saturated fats to < 10% of total calories	Parents with total cholesterol > 240 mg/dL and/or	HDL cholesterol > 35 mg/dL
Limit trans fatty acids†	Presence of other childhood risk factors§ and/or	Triglycerides ≤ 150 mg/dL
Limit cholesterol to < 300 mg/day	Family history is unknown	Borderline: Total cholesterol 170–199 mg/dL
		LDL cholesterol 110–129 mg/dL
Encourage fruits and vegetables, whole-grain foods, and fiber‡		Elevated: Total cholesterol ≥ 200 mg/dL*
		LDL cholesterol ≥ 130 mg/dL
		HDL cholesterol ≤ 35 mg/dL
		Triglycerides > 150 mg/dL
Action: Apply to all children > 2 years old at times of health checkups and, where appropriate, at times of illness	**Action**: Perform serial laboratory screening	**Action**: Begin therapy for individuals in the elevated group

* For total cholesterol, 170 mg/dL and 200 mg/dL are approximately the 75th and 95th percentiles, respectively.
† American Heart Association Guidelines.
‡ American Heart Association Council on Cardiovascular Disease in the Young: 5 or more daily servings of fruits and vegetables, 6–11 daily servings of whole-grain foods and fiber equal to (years of age + 5) gm/day.
§ Obesity, diabetes, hypertension, smoking.

Box 16-1 Categories of Pediatric Dyslipidemia

PRIMARY GENETIC DISEASE

Familial hypercholesterolemia
Familial defective APOB-100
Autosomal recessive hypercholesterolemia
Familial combined hyperlipidemia
Familial hypertriglyceridemia
Lipoprotein lipase deficiency
Small, dense LDL syndromes
Abnormalities of APOA-1 with diminished HDL
Elevated lipoprotein (a)

SECONDARY DYSLIPIDEMIA

Metabolic syndrome, diabetes mellitus, and insulin
  resistance
Nephrotic syndrome
Chronic renal disease
Hypothyroidism
Drug therapies
Obesity

UNCLASSIFIED DYSLIPIDEMIA

Dyslipidemia that does not fit a pattern characteristic of
  one of the known genetic diseases
Dyslipidemia that may be polygenic in origin

three categories will resemble, but not be identical, to that found in adults since the expression of some primary genetic dyslipidemias and secondary dyslipidemias may be delayed until the third decade or later. It is likely that the pediatric distribution will account for a similar, corresponding proportion of morbidity and mortality during adulthood. For example, familial combined hyperlipidemia, first identified in a childhood cohort, may account for up to 20% of premature CAD in that same cohort after reaching the fourth and fifth decades. As laboratory techniques become more available, small, dense LDL syndromes first identified in childhood may account for even more morbidity and mortality during early adulthood. Appropriate treatment of children identified with dyslipidemia might therefore diminish overall morbidity and mortality and change the spectrum of adult coronary artery disease.

Whether dyslipidemia is identified by parental involvement, by routine laboratory studies, or through the mechanisms in Table 16-3, efforts should be made to place the abnormality into one of the three major categories. Treatment for adult dyslipidemia is often selected only by the established lipoprotein pattern, ignoring its origin. Although this often leads to the correct treatment pathway, a great deal of information is lost to the patient and physician by this approach. For example,

treatment of a mild LDLC elevation with appropriate diet or drug therapy, or both, at 10 years of age, without identifying a history for familial combined hyperlipidemia in first-degree relatives, will deprive the patient of the correct diagnosis, namely, a knowledge of the serious morbidity and mortality that is part of the disease, and subsequently may delay proper diet and drug therapy. It is essential that an attempt be made to identify a specific diagnosis, whether primary genetic disease or secondary dyslipidemia, before placing the dyslipidemia into the unclassified category. It has been our experience that more then 80% of patients referred to us with dyslipidemia present with characteristics attributable to one of the known genetic syndromes. This may be due, in part, to the natural selection bias that occurs when primary care physicians choose to refer those children with only the most abnormal fasting lipid profile or family history, both of which are likely to be related to a primary genetic abnormality. It is quite possible that a higher percentage of polygenic and unclassified dyslipidemia exists in the general pediatric population.

Figure 16-2 illustrates the process of establishing a specific diagnosis. This is achieved by matching the observed fasting lipid profile with one or more primary genetic, secondary, or unclassified disorders. Care must be taken to obtain one or, preferably, several lipid profiles (Table 16-1) under conditions of a fairly uniform diet and a stable BMI. Knowledge of the lipoprotein pattern is useful and sometimes essential, but for most common disorders, the lipid elevations (i.e., cholesterol, triglycerides, or both) are sufficient. In situations in which several abnormalities match the abnormal lipid pattern or an abnormality may present with more than one lipid pattern, examinations of the family history and lipid profiles of key members are used to identify the diagnosis. It is often helpful to utilize a family history form, on which lipid profiles and clinical data may be assembled prior to the office visit.

Characteristics of Some Primary Genetic Dyslipidemias

Familial hypercholesterolemia is notable for an early clinical presentation of atherosclerotic cardiovascular disease and occurs with a prevalence of about 1/500 people across most populations. It is inherited in an autosomal-dominant pattern, mapping to chromosome 19 (p13.2–p13.1). Hundreds of different mutations have been noted, including point mutations, deletions, and gene rearrangements, leading to a variety of abnormalities. The primary defect is in the LDL receptor (Fig. 16-1), either through a reduced number of receptors or through reduced receptor activity. With this condition, there is a reduction in hepatic clearance of intermediate density lipoprotein (IDL) and LDL, as well as hepatic overproduction of LDL. As expected, the same lipoprotein pattern is seen in children and the affected parent.

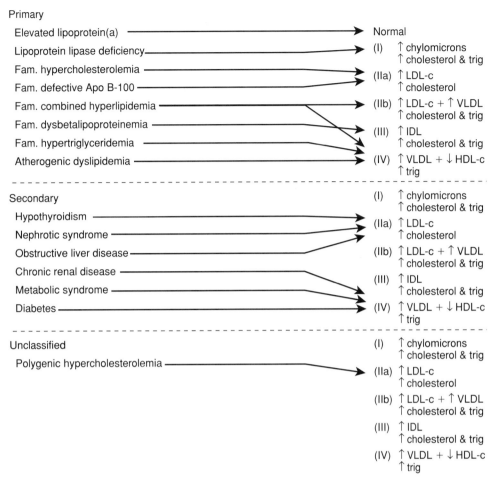

Figure 16-2   Relationship of primary genetic, secondary, and unclassified dyslipidemias to common abnormal lipid patterns (i.e., the Fredrickson classification). This figure is meant to serve as a rough guide for matching specific elevations of lipoproteins and lipids to known primary genetic, secondary, and unclassified dyslipidemias. The Fredrickson classification of abnormal fasting serum lipids was one of the earlier described, and it has maintained its usefulness among specialists. This is the case despite the more recent understanding that multiple diseases may be responsible for each class of abnormality, and that single diseases may present as more than one type of dyslipidemia, as is illustrated here.

Naturally, there is a much more severe presentation in the homozygous state, in which both alleles of the LDL receptor gene are abnormal, usually in different ways. In this extremely rare condition of homozygous dysfunction of the LDL receptor (occurring at a frequency of approximately 1/1,000,000 individuals), cholesterol levels > 2000 mg/dL may be seen, as may cardiac events in the first decade of life. Typically, men with heterozygous disease present with myocardial infarction or other cardiac events in the fourth decade, with women presenting with similar problems a decade later. Other clinical findings include a significant fraction of patients with tendinous xanthoma or arcus corneae, although these signs tend to be seen in adulthood. Among adolescents, up to 10% may have tendinous xanthomas. Laboratory studies show severely elevated total cholesterol (250–450 mg/dL) and LDLC (180–300 mg/dL). It should be noted that

these extremely high values may fall by 20% or more during adolescence before rising again, sometimes obscuring the diagnosis. There are no consistent changes in HDL-C, and triglycerides and apolipoprotein B (APOB) are normal. Treatment is directed at agents that decrease the hepatocellular concentration of saturated fats and cholesterol, both of which, in excess, further diminish the activity of LDL receptors. Alone, diet is seldom effective. Treatment for homozygous disease is extremely difficult and includes plasmapheresis, liver or heart-liver transplantation, gene therapy trials, and various enzyme infusions.

More recently, children have been described with lipid profiles similar to those seen in familial hypercholesterolemia, but with normal parental lipoprotein profiles. Affected patients had total cholesterols of 500–650 mg/dL, with LDLC at 350–550 mg/dL. Analysis of LDL receptors usually demonstrates normal or slightly decreased function. In this autosomal recessive disease, mapped to chromosome 1, abnormally encoded proteins lead to dysfunction of the LDL receptor, resulting in a pattern of disease usually seen in familial hypercholesterolemia.

In *familial defective APOB-100*, disease mutations in the gene on chromosome 2 at 2p24 may result in the inability of the APOB-100 ligand on LDL to properly interact with the LDL receptor, thus impairing the ability of LDL to bind to the LDL receptor. This ultimately leads to reduced plasma LDL clearance and elevated LDL levels. The defect is inherited in an autosomal dominant fashion and is seen in approximately 1 in 600–1000, with about 5% mimicking familial hypercholesterolemia and the remainder demonstrating a slightly lower LDLC, usually 210–280 mg/dL. Premature atherosclerotic vascular disease may be seen in these individuals. Rarely, elevated triglycerides (1500–2000 mg/dL) and pancreatitis appear due to similar impairment of VLDL clearance (Fig. 16-1).

Familial combined hyperlipidemia, the most common inherited disorder of lipid metabolism (with a prevalence of 1/50) was first described by Goldstein and associates in 1973 and is notable for a particularly complex pattern of serum lipid abnormalities. The disease may account for as much as 10–20% of premature CAD. It is inherited in an autosomal dominant manner, with appearance of cardiovascular disease in the fourth and fifth decades in men and in the fifth decade in women. Xanthomas are not present. Half of patients and affected family members present with Fredrickson type IIb lipid profiles (Fig. 16-2) with elevations of LDLC (130–180 mg/dL) and moderate elevations of triglycerides (150–300 mg/dL). The other half present with a type IV pattern, with elevated very low density lipoprotein (VLDL) triglycerides (200–400 mg/dL) and APOB (140–250 mg/dL). HDL-C may be normal or low. Although obesity and diabetes may be associated with this disease, many individuals have a normal BMI. The precise genetic defect is not known, but multiple genes on chromosomes 1 and 11 may result in overproduction of APOB by the liver. Treatments target available triglycerides through weight control and carbohydrate restriction. Additional strategies reduce hepatic production of APOB (e.g., niacin) and increase catabolism of VLDL (e.g., fibric acid derivatives and statins).

Familial hypertriglyceridemia has a prevalence of approximately 1 in 300 individuals, and inheritance is autosomal dominant. Cardiovascular disease presents in the fourth or fifth decade in men and in the fifth decade in women, with earlier appearance of CAD in the setting of obesity. No single genetic locus has been identified, but recent analysis of Mexican-American families has shown linkage of triglyceride level with sites on chromosomes 6, 7, and 15. Familial hypertriglyceridemia pres-

ents with the Fredrickson type IV lipid profile (Fig. 16-2), notable for elevation of VLDL triglycerides (325–600 mg/dL) and low HDL-C levels. APOB is elevated (140–250 mg/dL). LDLC may be low. In younger individuals, there may be only modest increases in triglycerides (100–200 mg/dL). Xanthomas are not seen. The most striking feature of this abnormality is the occasional sudden increase of triglycerides to 1000–4000 mg/dL, sometimes accompanied by pancreatitis. This phenomenon is thought to be related to the use of alcohol, contraceptives, and steroids or the simultaneous presence of hypothyroidism. Components of metabolic syndrome may also be present. As in familial combined hyperlipidemia, treatment is oriented toward control of triglycerides with weight reduction (when possible) through carbohydrate restriction and with niacin, fibric acid derivatives, and statins.

Lipoprotein lipase deficiency is a rare disease, most notable for severe chylomicronemia, eruptive xanthomas, lipemia retinalis, hepatosplenomegaly, and pancreatitis. The serum lipid pattern is type I (Figs. 16-1 and 16-2). Classical presentation in infancy is that of creamy blood seen during a routine fasting phlebotomy. If not diagnosed early, pancreatitis may begin in the first few years of life. The elevations of triglycerides may be in the thousands of mg/dL, and not uncommonly they are in the tens of thousands. The gene for lipoprotein lipase has been mapped to chromosome 8q22. Dozens of different mutations have been found. A familial loss of serum lipoprotein lipase or, more rarely, an apoprotein (C-II) is responsible for this disease. The inheritance is autosomal recessive and occurs with a frequency of approximately 1/100,000. Heterozygous deficiency is seen in 3–7% of Caucasians and is largely clinically silent, but it may have findings of mild disease manifested by slightly elevated triglycerides and reduced levels of HDL-C. Except for the occurrence of pancreatitis with severe elevation of triglycerides (> 1000 mg/dL), there is no known association with CAD in these individuals. Lipoprotein lipase activity may be determined through the intravenous injection of heparin (60 u/kg), which releases the enzyme from the endothelial surface. Restriction of dietary fat (e.g., with the use of medium-chain triglycerides that are not transported by chylomicrons) can reduce the severity of the triglyceridemia and can help prevent the complications of the disease.

Familial dysbetalipoproteinemia (i.e., broad β disease) is a relatively rare autosomal recessive condition with a prevalence of 1/5000. The usual lipid pattern is type III, marked by an accumulation of IDL and chylomicron remnants due to diminished VLDL catabolism (Figs. 16-1 and 16-2). The disease results, in part, from the presence of two alleles of apolipoprotein E_2 (APOE$_2$) associated with diminished binding of VLDL to hepatic receptors. Clinically, there is an increased incidence of

CAD beginning in the third and forth decade. Most notable are the unique eruptive xanthomas and planar xanthomas that may occur in teens but are more common in early adulthood.

Small, dense LDL syndromes include a number of genetic abnormalities such as hyperapobetalipoproteinemia and LDL subclass pattern B, as well as acquired syndromes due to oxidative stress. These syndromes are part of the triad characterized by small LDL particles, elevated VLDL triglycerides, and low HDL-C, often referred to as atherogenic dyslipidemia. The acquired forms of atherogenic dyslipidemia constitute the majority of findings in diabetes and metabolic syndrome. All feature normal or only mildly altered lipid profiles in most relatives but are associated with significantly increased prevalence of CAD after the third decade. At the present time, routine, inexpensive detection of small, dense LDL particles is not available in all laboratories. Treatment is usually directed at lowering triglycerides and addressing any LDLC increase that may be present.

Elevated lipoprotein A levels may represent an independent risk factor for CAD. The mechanism is unknown, but many isoforms of lipoprotein A resemble units of the clotting cascade, particularly plasminogen. This suggests a role for increased thrombosis, diminished thrombolysis, or both. Measurement is difficult, and treatment is limited to the mild lowering effect of nicotinic acid, although there is no universal recommendation to begin treatment unless it accompanies another genetic dyslipidemia.

Familial hypoalphalipoproteinemia and abnormalities of apolipoprotein A-1 (APOA-1) are identified by a low level of HDL (35 mg/dL) in the absence of other lipoprotein abnormalities. In this autosomal dominant condition associated with early-onset CAD, APOA-1 levels are low (Table 16-4). Coronary and cerebrovascular disease often presents as early as the fourth decade.

Characteristics of Some Secondary Dyslipidemias
Although the majority of children who are brought to a lipid specialist have an identifiable primary genetic disease, there are a significant number who have other conditions that secondarily cause abnormalities of blood lipids.

Type 1 (juvenile or insulin-deficient) and type 2 (adult-onset or insulin resistant) *diabetes mellitus* have both been shown to express atherogenic dyslipidemia with elevations of VLDL triglycerides and a reduction of HDL-C, particularly in the setting of poor glucose control (Fig. 16-2). In some, there may be a mild elevation of LDLC. In adults, these have been shown to improve with tighter glycemic control. Because diabetes is a major risk factor for CAD, there has been a special effort to manage lipids aggressively in adults with this disease. Despite the lack of clearly demonstrable findings showing an elevated risk for the development of CAD in children and adolescents with diabetes, a similarly aggressive approach would seem appropriate for this population. Of particular concern is the growing prevalence of type 2 diabetes in association with obesity and metabolic syndrome.

Metabolic syndrome, like type 2 diabetes, appears to be increasing in the pediatric population. The lipid profile of atherogenic dyslipidemia (Fig. 16-2) generally shows elevations of VLDL triglycerides and low HDL-C. Unlike isolated diabetes, LDLC is usually normal. There are also relationships with overall obesity, body composition (adiposity), and the distribution of fat. Abdominal fat is associated with larger elevations of triglyceride and circulating insulin levels. For children, efforts are made to improve glycemic control, to stabilize or eliminate obesity, and to monitor and treat hypertension when appropriate.

In *hypothyroidism,* elevations of LDL and VLDL lead to modest increases of both cholesterol and triglycerides. Fortunately, pharmacologic correction of hypothyroidism normalizes these abnormalities. Interestingly, HDL cholesterol is also often elevated in the setting of hypothyroidism.

The *nephrotic syndrome,* marked by proteinuria, hypoalbuminemia, and hypercholesterolemia, is a classic cause of secondary dyslipidemia. The most marked abnormality is elevation of LDLC, thought to occur as a result of hepatic overproduction of LDL and VLDL in response to the hypoalbuminemia. This may be the result of a general overproduction of proteins by the liver; it is not due to a specific effect on apolipoprotein synthesis. Overproduction of cholesterol in the liver also leads to down-regulation of the LDL receptors, resulting in diminished LDL clearance. In severe, prolonged cases of the nephrotic syndrome, triglycerides may also be elevated due to the elevated production of VLDL and to their reduced peripheral lipolysis. With treatment of the underlying disease, the lipoprotein abnormalities generally resolve. Due to the (largely) short periods of elevated serum lipids in these patients, the long-term effect on the risk of developing CAD is unknown. Chronic renal insufficiency, however, has a significant association with cardiovascular disease with low HDL-C and elevated triglycerides.

In *obstructive liver disease,* LDLC is usually elevated. This is related to a number of factors including dysfunction

Table 16-4 Low Cut-Off Levels for APOA-I	
Class	**APOA-1 level**
Boys	110 mg/dL
Girls	120 mg/dL
Adult males	90 mg/dL
Adult females	105 mg/dL

or reduced numbers of LDL receptor sites and an inability to excrete cholesterol in bile acids.

Characteristics of Unclassified Dyslipidemias
Polygenic hypercholesterolemia is the most common unclassified dyslipidemia in our lipid specialty practice, accounting for about one-fourth of all patients referred. It is characterized by mild to moderate elevations of LDLC, ranging from 135 to 200 mg/dL, with total cholesterol at 220–280 mg/dL. Triglycerides, HDL-C, and APOB are usually normal. Prevalence is approximately 1/20–1/100, with a similar distribution of these lipid values and clinical CAD on both sides of the family. There are no cutaneous manifestations of hyperlipidemia. The diagnosis can be vague, especially when total cholesterol and LDLC are at the upper end of the range and overlap some criteria for familial hypercholesterolemia and familial defective APOB. In these cases, the absence of autosomal dominant inheritance usually identifies the disease. The etiology is related to multiple gene effects, probably including variations of APOE. Treatment depends on the magnitude of the LDLC elevation, generally adhering to consensus guidelines (Table 16-3). A progressive approach, beginning with diet therapy, is usually successful, but, in some instances, bile acid sequestrants or, very rarely, statins are required.

On occasion, close inspection of laboratory profiles and family history will fail to reveal the etiology of a mild or moderate hyperlipidemia. For example, a child may present with a typical picture for familial combined hyperlipidemia, but there will be no similar lipid profiles or evidence for clinical cardiovascular disease in either side of the family. It is always helpful to assume the most likely possibility and to counsel the family that further data may establish the diagnosis. For at least some period of time, however, the hyperlipidemia will remain unclassified and the therapeutic approach will be to single out and to address the individual lipid abnormalities.

Treatment Options

The rationale for treatment of children with dyslipidemia is unclear. Diet-related behavioral modification that persists into adulthood will certainly be more successful if begun during the childhood years. Whether drug intervention must begin during childhood or would be equally effective when initiated as a young adult is unknown. The Bogalusa Heart Study has identified the presence of vascular lesions in the first decade, but their significance in terms of reversibility and link to morbidity and mortality is uncertain. These questions must be answered satisfactorily in order to formulate future recommendations.

Diet and drug therapies for hyperlipidemia are often effective for specific lipid elevations, regardless of their origin. For instance, cholesterol-lowering agents will usually reduce serum cholesterol, whether it is related to familial hypercholesterolemia or is a product of poly-genic origin. Refinements of drug use, such as timing and dosage, may improve the response significantly for individuals with specific dyslipidemias. Current NCEP recommendations specify the use of drug treatment in children 10 years of age or older, but it is likely that this age limitation will be reduced in the near future. Recommendations for specific drugs from manufacturers are likely to remain conservative. Although the reduction of lipid values to normal is desirable, this is often not possible, especially in children with some primary genetic diseases. More modest goals of partial reductions have become accepted and must be balanced against potential physical and emotional effects of the treatment.

Hypercholesterolemia
With few exceptions, diet therapy is the initial treatment of children with hypercholesterolemia of any cause. The goal is to reduce saturated fat and cholesterol in the hepatocyte with the intention of promoting LDL receptor production. Because saturated fat comes principally from the diet, the strategy is often effective for mild elevations of cholesterol. Reductions of hepatic cholesterol are not as easily achieved because cholesterol is mostly synthesized in the liver. Population-wide recommendations for reducing LDLC in individuals over 2 years of age with borderline elevations of cholesterol (110–129 mg/dL) begin with the Step 1 diet (Table 16-5). If normalization of LDLC (< 100 mg/dL) is not achieved with the Step 1 diet over a 3–6 month period, the Step 2 diet is recommended. Greater restrictions on fat and cholesterol intake in the Step 2 diet may require the supervision of a dietitian. In both diets, the recommended number of total calories from fat is to be the

Table 16-5	1991 NCEP Dietary Guidelines (with total calories to achieve and maintain ideal body weight)	
Nutrient	**Step 1 Diet**	**Step 2 Diet**
Total fat calories (% total calories)	< 30%	< 30%
Saturated fat calories (% total calories)	< 10%	< 7%
Polyunsaturated fat calories (% total calories)	≤ 10%	≤ 10%
Monounsaturated fat calories (% total calories)	10–15%	10–15%
Carbohydrate calories (% total calories)	50–60%	50–60%
Protein calories (% total calories)	10–20%	10–20%
Cholesterol*	< 300 mg/day	< 200 mg/day

*This maximum value is indexed to 100 mg per 1000 calories consumed for younger children.

average percentage over a few days, rather than a day-by-day or meal-by-meal total. Additionally, the American Academy of Pediatrics recommends a minimum percentage of 20% of calories from fat. In children with borderline elevation of cholesterol, the Step 1 diet results in a 3–10% reduction of LDLC. An additional 4–14% LDLC reduction may be seen with the Step 2 diet. For elevations of LDLC in the abnormal range (≥ 130 mg/dL), a smaller reduction can be expected with little or no reduction demonstrated for individuals who have large elevations of LDLC that are characteristic of familial hypercholesterolemia. In most cases, dietary intervention has little effect on HDL-C. The effectiveness of diet therapy is enhanced by addressing other factors such as smoking and obesity. The latter may require some restrictions of total calories and a prescription for regular physical exercise.

The primary lipid-lowering agents recommended for pediatric hypercholesterolemia are bile acid sequestrants such as cholestyramine and colestipol. Their mechanism of action is to bind intestinal bile acids, removing them from the enterohepatic circulation and reducing hepatic cholesterol, thereby increasing the production of LDL receptors. The starting dose is usually 4 gm (i.e., 1 packet or 1 scoop) of cholestyramine or 5 gm of colestipol administered daily, 30–60 minutes before the largest meal of the day (usually dinner), with additional doses given before another meal if necessary and tolerated. Some children may become more accustomed to the gritty taste of the powder by initiating therapy with a smaller dose. The maximum dose is 16–20 gm/day. The powder is often mixed in a citrus juice, but it can be combined with almost anything. Side effects such as nausea, constipation, and bloating are frequent but are usually minor and well tolerated. Malabsorption of the fat-soluble vitamins A, E, D, and K, along with folate and iron, usually requires that these supplements be administered daily, usually in the form of an over-the-counter preparation. Hepatic function should also be monitored periodically. Bile acid sequestrants may lower total and LDL cholesterol up to 50 and 40 mg/dL, respectively, when used in children with LDLC > 130 mg/dL.

The 3-hydroxy-3-methylglutaryl coenzyme A (HMG CoA) reductase inhibitors (i.e., statins) inhibit the rate-limiting step in endogenous cholesterol production. In a mechanism similar to that seen in sequestrant therapy, the lowering of intrahepatic cholesterol levels enhances the production of LDL receptors. Use in children is currently limited to those with genetic disorders associated with extremely high LDLC, such as familial hypercholesterolemia, and to children in whom dietary therapy and sequestrants are unsuccessful. However, marked reduction in total cholesterol and LDLC (35–40% in some studies) may be achieved. In addition, elevations of HDL-C of up to 20% may also occur. Rarely, statins are combined with a bile acid sequestrant to yield reductions of total cholesterol in excess of 50%. Initial statin doses are usually quite low (e.g., 5 mg of pravastatin or simvastatin once per day) and are increased only after repeating the fasting lipid profile. In most cases, the objective is to achieve a reasonable reduction of LDLC that is not necessarily within the normal range.

Much concern has been generated regarding the adverse effects of statins. Hepatic transaminase elevation is seen in few children and is almost always reversible with discontinuation of the drug. Usually, restarting it after a number of weeks does not reproduce the effect. Myositis with renal failure related to myoglobinuria is a potentially serious complication that must be considered. Cataract formation is described in adults but is not a feature of statin use in children. Hepatic function tests and creatine phosphokinase (CPK) are usually monitored a few weeks after initiating therapy and periodically thereafter. An elevation of CPK is an absolute indication to discontinue the medication. At the present time, there are no generally accepted guidelines specifying who may prescribe statins. It is not our policy to limit their use to lipid specialists, but some institutions utilize this restriction.

Cholesterol-absorption blockers such as ezetimibe are a new class of agents that also reduce the enterohepatic reabsorption of cholesterol. In adults, ezetimibe is used principally with the statins to provide an additional 15–25% reduction of LDLC. Some data suggest that monotherapy is effective but yields smaller reductions. Ezetimibe is not related to abnormalities of hepatic function, and it does not cause CPK elevation or malabsorption of fat soluble vitamins, making it attractive for study in children. Its availability may be affected by coadministration of bile acid sequestrants.

Hypertriglyceridemia

Hypertriglyceridemia usually responds to diet therapy. Reduction of total carbohydrates, the substrate for triglyceride formation, may be possible in many children who also have elevated BMI. Often, a small weight loss will result in a very significant reduction of triglycerides. Some (but not all) statins have a measurable triglyceride-lowering effect. Niacin (i.e, nicotinic acid) is thought to decrease the production of APOB and has been used successfully in children. The dose ranges from 0.5 to 3 gm/day and is usually limited by marked side effects of flushing, itching, abdominal pain, and headaches. These may be limited by the coadministration of low-dose aspirin or the use of the niacin substitute inositol hexaniacinate. Additional concerns are hyperuricemia and hepatic toxicity, which require periodic laboratory testing. Fibric acid derivatives such as gemfibrozil (600–1200 mg/day) have been used in adults to lower triglycerides, but little experience has been accumulated in children. Adverse effects such as myositis and gallstones are not uncommon and must be watched for closely, especially when used with HMG CoA reductase inhibitors. The use of these drugs should also be restricted to lipid specialists.

Hyperchylomicronemia

The hypertriglyceridemia of hyperchylomicronemia responds well to restriction of dietary fat. Often, medium-chain triglycerides may be substituted to provide sufficient calories in younger individuals. Such intervention may be needed to prevent the occurrence of pancreatitis in some individuals with lipoprotein lipase deficiency.

Mixed Lipid Elevations

The approach to mixed lipid elevations such as the type IIb pattern (Fig. 16-2) found in familial combined hyperlipidemia is to target the most abnormal elevation as an initial step. Often, success in lowering triglycerides will result in a decrease of LDLC, probably related to a reduction of total lipoprotein particles. Treatment of elevated LDLC with statins usually has a beneficial effect on triglycerides. Occasionally, combined drug therapy is required, but this approach should be used cautiously.

Other Therapies

In the most seriously affected individuals, such as those with homozygous familial hypercholesterolemia, diet and medication may not have any impact on LDLC. Other methods of treatment in these circumstances include liver transplantation (i.e., transplantation of LDL receptors) and plasmapheresis or LDL apheresis to remove LDLC from the serum. Experimental approaches with gene therapy have been explored for these severely affected patients.

Hypertension

Technique and Normal Values

The measurement of blood pressure by sphygmomanometer is recommended to be part of the routine annual examination of children over 3 years of age conducted by primary care providers. Utilization of a properly sized cuff is important for an accurate reading. A bladder width of approximately 40% of the arm circumference should be selected, with a bladder length that encircles 80–100% of the circumference, as shown in Figure 16-3. This usually results in the cuff covering two-thirds to three-quarters of the arm, a useful approximation for the practitioner. Readings should be obtained with the child seated in a calm, quiet setting with the arm outstretched and the cubital fossa at the level of the heart. The systolic and diastolic values for all ages are those at the onset (K_1) and loss (K_5) of the Korotkoff tapping sounds. In young children in whom K_5 reaches 0, the diastolic pressure cannot be measured, but this is sufficient to exclude diastolic hypertension. Normal blood pressure is defined as being below the 90th percentile. Values from the 90th to just below the 95th percentile are considered borderline, and those at or above the 95th percentile for systolic or diastolic readings on three separate occasions, separated by weeks or months, are defined as hypertensive. Values at or above the 99th percentile represent significant elevations that require additional diagnostic testing and, possibly, more aggressive therapy. A table of normal values for height percentile, based upon the use of K_1 and K_5 obtained by manual cuff blood pressure determinations, was published in 1996 in the Update on the Task Force Report (1987) on High Blood Pressure in Children and Adolescents,[6] but it was recently revised to include the 50th and 99th percentiles (Tables 16-6 and 16-7). As of press time, a new Task Force Report from NHLBI is expected soon.

The use of automated oscillometric devices for blood pressure measurement in children has gained wide popularity. These devices measure the heart rate and the systolic and mean arterial pressures from which a diastolic pressure is calculated. They are extremely useful, especially when repeated measurements are necessary. Caution is advised in their use, and the preferred method of blood pressure determination remains the manual cuff, since normal values have been determined using the manual cuff.

Distribution of Hypertension in Pediatrics

Essential hypertension is the most common form of pediatric hypertension encountered. In most cases, it remains a diagnosis of exclusion, supported by a family history of high blood pressure. It is often chronic, and it is not usually associated with any symptoms; presentation is usually at an older age. Secondary causes of hypertension are listed in Box 16-2. The younger the child and the more severe the elevation of blood pressure, the more likely that the cause of the blood pressure elevation is secondary and identifiable.

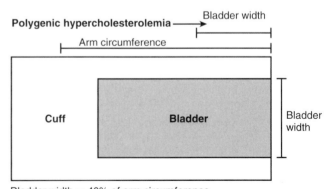

Bladder width = 40% of arm circumference
Bladder length = 80–100% of arm circumference

Figure 16-3 A cuff is selected based on the arm circumference and the width of the bladder.

Table 16-6   Blood Pressure Levels for Girls by Age and Height Percentile

Age (Years)	BP Percentile	Systolic BP (mmHg) Percentile of Height							Diastolic BP (mmHg) Percentile of Height						
		5th	10th	25th	50th	75th	90th	95th	5th	10th	25th	50th	75th	90th	95th
1	50th	83	84	85	86	88	89	90	38	39	39	40	41	41	42
	90th	97	97	98	100	101	102	103	52	53	53	54	55	55	56
	95th	100	101	102	104	105	106	107	56	57	57	58	59	59	60
	99th	108	108	109	111	112	113	114	64	64	65	65	66	67	67
2	50th	85	85	87	88	89	91	91	43	44	44	45	46	46	47
	90th	98	99	100	101	103	104	105	57	58	58	59	60	61	61
	95th	102	103	104	105	107	108	109	61	62	62	63	64	65	65
	99th	109	110	111	112	114	115	116	69	69	70	70	71	72	72
3	50th	86	87	88	89	91	92	93	47	48	48	49	50	50	51
	90th	100	100	102	103	104	106	106	61	62	62	63	64	64	65
	95th	104	104	105	107	108	109	110	65	66	66	67	68	68	69
	99th	111	111	113	114	115	116	117	73	73	74	74	75	76	76
4	50th	88	88	90	91	92	94	94	50	50	51	52	52	53	54
	90th	101	102	103	104	106	107	108	64	64	65	66	67	67	68
	95th	105	106	107	108	110	111	112	68	68	69	70	71	71	72
	99th	112	113	114	115	117	118	119	76	76	76	77	78	79	79
5	50th	89	90	91	93	94	95	96	52	53	53	54	55	55	56
	90th	103	103	105	106	107	109	109	66	67	67	68	69	69	70
	95th	107	107	108	110	111	112	113	70	71	71	72	73	73	74
	99th	114	114	116	117	118	120	120	78	78	79	79	80	81	81
6	50th	91	92	93	94	96	97	98	54	54	55	56	56	57	58
	90th	104	105	106	108	109	110	111	68	68	69	70	70	71	72
	95th	108	109	110	111	113	114	115	72	72	73	74	74	75	76
	99th	115	116	117	119	120	121	122	80	80	80	81	82	83	83
7	50th	93	93	95	96	97	99	99	55	56	56	57	58	58	59
	90th	106	107	108	109	111	112	113	69	70	70	71	72	72	73
	95th	110	111	112	113	115	116	116	73	74	74	75	76	76	77
	99th	117	118	119	120	122	123	124	81	81	82	82	83	84	84
8	50th	95	95	96	98	99	100	101	57	57	57	58	59	60	60
	90th	108	109	110	111	113	114	114	71	71	71	72	73	74	74
	95th	112	112	114	115	116	118	118	75	75	75	76	77	78	78
	99th	119	120	121	122	123	125	125	82	82	83	83	84	85	86
9	50th	96	97	98	100	101	102	103	58	58	58	59	60	61	61
	90th	110	110	112	113	114	116	116	72	72	72	73	74	75	75
	95th	114	114	115	117	118	119	120	76	76	76	77	78	79	79
	99th	121	121	123	124	125	127	127	83	83	84	84	85	86	87
10	50th	98	99	100	102	103	104	105	59	59	59	60	61	62	62
	90th	112	112	114	115	116	118	118	73	73	73	74	75	76	76
	95th	116	116	117	119	120	121	122	77	77	77	78	79	80	80
	99th	123	123	125	126	127	129	129	84	84	85	86	86	87	88
11	50th	100	101	102	103	105	106	107	60	60	60	61	62	63	63
	90th	114	114	116	117	118	119	120	74	74	74	75	76	77	77
	95th	118	118	119	121	122	123	124	78	78	78	79	80	81	81
	99th	125	125	126	128	129	130	131	85	85	86	87	87	88	89
12	50th	102	103	104	105	107	108	109	61	61	61	62	63	64	64
	90th	116	116	117	119	120	121	122	75	75	75	76	77	78	78
	95th	119	120	121	123	124	125	126	79	79	79	80	81	82	82
	99th	127	127	128	130	131	132	133	86	86	87	88	88	89	90
13	50th	104	105	106	107	109	110	110	62	62	62	63	64	65	65
	90th	117	118	119	121	122	123	124	76	76	76	77	78	79	79
	95th	121	122	123	124	126	127	128	80	80	80	81	82	83	83
	99th	128	129	130	132	133	134	135	87	87	88	89	89	90	91
14	50th	106	106	107	109	110	111	112	63	63	63	64	65	66	66
	90th	119	120	121	122	124	125	125	77	77	77	78	79	80	80
	95th	123	123	125	126	127	129	129	81	81	81	82	83	84	84
	99th	130	131	132	133	135	136	136	88	88	89	90	90	91	92

Table 16-6   Blood Pressure Levels for Girls by Age and Height Percentile—cont'd

Age (Years)	BP Percentile	Systolic BP (mmHg) Percentile of Height							Diastolic BP (mmHg) Percentile of Height						
		5th	10th	25th	50th	75th	90th	95th	5th	10th	25th	50th	75th	90th	95th
15	50th	107	108	109	110	111	113	113	64	64	64	65	66	67	67
	90th	120	121	122	123	125	126	127	78	78	78	79	80	81	81
	95th	124	125	126	127	129	130	131	82	82	82	83	84	85	85
	99th	131	132	133	134	136	137	138	89	89	90	91	91	92	93
16	50th	108	108	110	111	112	114	114	64	64	65	66	66	67	68
	90th	121	122	123	124	126	127	128	78	78	79	80	81	81	82
	95th	125	126	127	128	130	131	132	82	82	83	84	85	85	86
	99th	132	133	134	135	137	138	139	90	90	90	91	92	93	93
17	50th	108	109	110	111	113	114	115	64	65	65	66	67	67	68
	90th	122	122	123	125	126	127	128	78	79	79	80	81	81	82
	95th	125	126	127	129	130	131	132	82	83	83	84	85	85	86
	99th	133	133	134	136	137	138	139	90	90	91	91	92	93	93

BP, blood pressure.
The 90th percentile is 1.28 standard deviations (SD), 95th percentile is 1.645 SD, and the 99th percentile is 2.326 SD over the mean.

Table 16-7   Blood Pressure Levels for Boys by Age and Height Percentile

Age (Years)	BP Percentile	Systolic BP (mmHg) Percentile of Height							Diastolic BP (mmHg) Percentile of Height						
		5th	10th	25th	50th	75th	90th	95th	5th	10th	25th	50th	75th	90th	95th
1	50th	80	81	83	85	87	88	89	34	35	36	37	38	39	39
	90th	94	95	97	99	100	102	103	49	50	51	52	53	53	54
	95th	98	99	101	103	104	106	106	54	54	55	56	57	58	58
	99th	105	106	108	110	112	113	114	61	62	63	64	65	66	66
2	50th	84	85	87	88	90	92	92	39	40	41	42	43	44	44
	90th	97	99	100	102	104	105	106	54	55	56	57	58	58	59
	95th	101	102	104	106	108	109	110	59	59	60	61	62	63	63
	99th	109	110	111	113	115	117	117	66	67	68	69	70	71	71
3	50th	86	87	89	91	93	94	95	44	44	45	46	47	48	48
	90th	100	101	103	105	107	108	109	59	59	60	61	62	63	63
	95th	104	105	107	109	110	112	113	63	63	64	65	66	67	67
	99th	111	112	114	116	118	119	120	71	71	72	73	74	75	75
4	50th	88	89	91	93	95	96	97	47	48	49	50	51	51	52
	90th	102	103	105	107	109	110	111	62	63	64	65	66	66	67
	95th	106	107	109	111	112	114	115	66	67	68	69	70	71	71
	99th	113	114	116	118	120	121	122	74	75	76	77	78	78	79
5	50th	90	91	93	95	96	98	98	50	51	52	53	54	55	55
	90th	104	105	106	108	110	111	112	65	66	67	68	69	69	70
	95th	108	109	110	112	114	115	116	69	70	71	72	73	74	74
	99th	115	116	118	120	121	123	123	77	78	79	80	81	81	82
6	50th	91	92	94	96	98	99	100	53	53	54	55	56	57	57
	90th	105	106	108	110	111	113	113	68	68	69	70	71	72	72
	95th	109	110	112	114	115	117	117	72	72	73	74	75	76	76
	99th	116	117	119	121	123	124	125	80	80	81	82	83	84	84
7	50th	92	94	95	97	99	100	101	55	55	56	57	58	59	59
	90th	106	107	109	111	113	114	115	70	70	71	72	73	74	74
	95th	110	111	113	115	117	118	119	74	74	75	76	77	78	78
	99th	117	118	120	122	124	125	126	82	82	83	84	85	86	86

Continued

Table 16-7   Blood Pressure Levels for Boys by Age and Height Percentile—cont'd

Age (Years)	BP Percentile	Systolic BP (mmHg) Percentile of Height							Diastolic BP (mmHg) Percentile of Height						
		5th	10th	25th	50th	75th	90th	95th	5th	10th	25th	50th	75th	90th	95th
8	50th	94	95	97	99	100	102	102	56	57	58	59	60	60	61
	90th	107	109	110	112	114	115	116	71	72	72	73	74	75	76
	95th	111	112	114	116	118	119	120	75	76	77	78	79	79	80
	99th	119	120	122	123	125	127	127	83	84	85	86	87	87	88
9	50th	95	96	98	100	102	103	104	57	58	59	60	61	61	62
	90th	109	110	112	114	115	117	118	72	73	74	75	76	76	77
	95th	113	114	116	118	119	121	121	76	77	78	79	80	81	81
	99th	120	121	123	125	127	128	129	84	85	86	87	88	88	89
10	50th	97	98	100	102	103	105	106	58	59	60	61	61	62	63
	90th	111	112	114	115	117	119	119	73	73	74	75	76	77	78
	95th	115	116	117	119	121	122	123	77	78	79	80	81	81	82
	99th	122	123	125	127	128	130	130	85	86	86	88	88	89	90
11	50th	99	100	102	104	105	107	107	59	59	60	61	62	63	63
	90th	113	114	115	117	119	120	121	74	74	75	76	77	78	78
	95th	117	118	119	121	123	124	125	78	78	79	80	81	82	82
	99th	124	125	127	129	130	132	132	86	86	87	88	89	90	90
12	50th	101	102	104	106	108	109	110	59	60	61	62	63	63	64
	90th	115	116	118	120	121	123	123	74	75	75	76	77	78	79
	95th	119	120	122	123	125	127	127	78	79	80	81	82	82	83
	99th	126	127	129	131	133	134	135	86	87	88	89	90	90	91
13	50th	104	105	106	108	110	111	112	60	60	61	62	63	64	64
	90th	117	118	120	122	124	125	126	75	75	76	77	78	79	79
	95th	121	122	124	126	128	129	130	79	79	80	81	82	83	83
	99th	128	130	131	133	135	136	137	87	87	88	89	90	91	91
14	50th	106	107	109	111	113	114	115	60	61	62	63	64	65	65
	90th	120	121	123	125	126	128	128	75	76	77	78	79	79	80
	95th	124	125	127	128	130	132	132	80	80	81	82	83	84	84
	99th	131	132	134	136	138	139	140	87	88	89	90	91	92	92
15	50th	109	110	112	113	115	117	117	61	62	63	64	65	66	66
	90th	122	124	125	127	129	130	131	76	77	78	79	80	80	81
	95th	126	127	129	131	133	134	135	81	81	82	83	84	85	85
	99th	134	135	136	138	140	142	142	88	89	90	91	92	93	93
16	50th	111	112	114	116	118	119	120	63	63	64	65	66	67	67
	90th	125	126	128	130	131	133	134	78	78	79	80	81	82	82
	95th	129	130	132	134	135	137	137	82	83	83	84	85	86	87
	99th	136	137	139	141	143	144	145	90	90	91	92	93	94	94
17	50th	114	115	116	118	120	121	122	65	66	66	67	68	69	70
	90th	127	128	130	132	134	135	136	80	80	81	82	83	84	84
	95th	131	132	134	136	138	139	140	84	85	86	87	87	88	89
	99th	139	140	141	143	145	146	147	92	93	93	94	95	96	97

BP, blood pressure.
The 90th Percentile is 1.28 SD, 95th Percentile is 1.645 SD, and the 99th Percentile is 2.36 SD over the mean.

Secondary causes of hypertension are also more often associated with symptoms such as headaches, epistaxis, altered mental status, anorexia, polydipsia, and polyuria.

Rationale for Hypertension Screening
In a manner similar to dyslipidemia, adult CAD and heart failure from myocardial disease are linked to childhood hypertension through tracking. Subtle defects including increased left ventricular mass, diastolic dysfunction, and some structural changes in coronary vasculature have been described, but, with the exception of acutely and severely elevate blood pressure, clinical cardiovascular disease from hypertension is rarely observed. Tracking of high blood pressure is difficult to demonstrate from youth to adulthood, but the Bogalusa

Box 16-2 Secondary Causes of Hypertension

RENAL

Glomerulonephritis and other renal parenchymal
  disease
Renal artery stenosis
Renal vein thrombosis
Tumors (i.e, neuroblastoma and Wilms' tumor)

ENDOCRINE

Steroid hormone abnormalities (i.e., Cushing's
  syndrome, CAH, and primary hyperaldosteronism)
Pheochromocytoma
Hyperthyroidism
Hypercalcemia

CARDIOVASCULAR

Coarctation of the aorta
Diastolic runoff lesions (i.e., PDA, aortic regurgitation,
  and AV malformation)

MEDICATIONS

Steroids (i.e., glucocorticoids and anabolic steroids)
Immunosuppresants (i.e., cyclosporine and tacrolimus)

OTHER CAUSES

Takayasu's arteritis
Klippel-Trenaunay-Weber syndrome
Williams syndrome

Heart Study has shown some evidence for this. For children between 2 and 14 years of age in the upper quartile of systolic and diastolic blood pressure on three occasions, 68% remained in the upper quartile for systolic pressure and 62% for diastolic pressure 9 years after the initial blood pressure determination. The role of exercise stress testing for determining the likelihood of future hypertension is well established in adults but is less clear in children.

Investigation and Treatment

Investigation of hypertension should be tailored to the age and likelihood that a cause will be found. A thorough history and physical exam are essential at all ages, but laboratory testing is usually more extensive in younger children. Children with blood pressure between the 90th and 95th percentile should have repeated blood pressure screening. Children with blood pressure at or just above the 95th percentile should have a urinalysis, blood urea nitrogen and creatinine determinations, and a fasting lipid profile. For children with significant elevations (i.e., 99th percentile or above), laboratory testing should be directed toward establishing a secondary etiology.

Therapy for hypertension is both pharmacologic and nonpharmacologic. Nonpharmacologic therapy is recommended for some children at < 90th percentile with other risk factors (e.g., diabetes or hyperlipidemia), for children at ≥ 90th percentile and < 95th percentile, and for some children at ≥ 95th percentile as initial therapy. Pharmacologic therapy is indicated in those children ≥ 95th percentile who fail nonpharmacologic initial therapy and in all other children ≥ 95th percentile. Using this algorithm, drug therapy will be appropriate for about 1–2% of all children.

If appropriate in a given situation, weight reduction is the mainstay of nonpharmacologic therapy. Because normal and abnormal blood pressures are both related to body size, a reduction of body weight will almost always have a measurable effect. In addition, weight reduction decreases the effect of dietary salt on blood pressure and may reduce other risk factors such as triglycerides and the triglyceride/HDL-C ratio. The effect of exercise on blood pressure is controversial when used alone, but, when combined with weight loss, blood pressure falls more rapidly and farther than with weight loss alone. This is especially true after puberty.

The evidence that salt restriction is beneficial for treatment of hypertension in adults is strong. A similar benefit is presumed for children but has not been entirely verified. It has been suggested by the Task Force Report on High Blood Pressure in Children and Adolescents that sodium intake be restricted to 85–100 mEq/day (i.e., 5–6 gm sodium chloride) for all children with blood pressure consistently above the 90th percentile.

Pharmacologic therapy for childhood hypertension follows the adult recommendations closely. Angiotensin-converting enzyme (ACE) inhibitors (e.g., captopril, enalapril, and lisinopril), angiotensin receptor blockers (ARBs) (e.g., losartan), and calcium channel blockers (e.g., nifedipine, diltiazem, and amlodipine) have been the mainstay of chronic therapy for many years. Each is used at the lowest effective dose. Diuretics have been used for many years, and there is recent evidence in adults that chronic diuretic therapy may have a better long-term outcome, especially when compared with calcium channel blockers. Thus, thiazide diuretics such as chlorothiazide, both alone and in combination with spironolactone, often are recommended as initial antihypertensive therapy.

Obesity

Several studies conducted during the past 10 years have demonstrated a rather rapid increase in the prevalence of childhood obesity. In 2003, approximately 15% of children at all ages met criteria for obesity. This increase affects all segments of the pediatric population but is more marked among African-American (particularly female) and Hispanic children.

Definition and Characteristics

A quantitative assessment of the degree of excess adipose tissue in children is hindered by a number of factors including the effects of puberty and the increased lean body mass produced by adolescent isometric training. Nevertheless, the BMI may serve as a useful tool to evaluate children for obesity and to identify the need for intervention. Figures 16-4 and 16-5 give BMI standards for children; these standards have recently been published by the Centers for Disease Control and Prevention.[7] Obesity is generally defined as a BMI at or greater than the 95th percentile. Selection of children at risk may also be enhanced by utilizing measures of local fat distribution such as skin fold thickness, but these techniques are more subject to inexperience and observer error and are time-consuming. Therefore, it may not be practical to incorporate them into general pediatric practice.

Many studies in both adults and adolescents have shown a variety of relationships among obesity, insulin resistance, and other components of metabolic syndrome. For example, insulin resistance may predate significant obesity, but treatment of obesity is observed to decrease insulin resistance. Altered lipid profiles and the early appearance of vascular lesions may be related to the dyslipidemia of insulin resistance or directly to increased intake of both fats and carbohydrates that promotes obesity. There is ample evidence to suggest a strong genetic influence in the development of obesity. The association of parental obesity with childhood obesity is particularly strong. The prevalence of obesity appears to be modified significantly by a number of environmental factors including climate, socioeconomic status, season of the year in which the study is conducted, urban vs. rural residence, and size of the family. Tracking of obesity from early childhood through adolescence to adulthood has been well documented.

Investigation and Treatment

It has been suggested that individuals with BMI at the 85th percentile with complications of obesity such as insulin resistance, hypertension, and obesity-related sleep and orthopedic disorders, as well as individuals at the 95th percentile without these complications, may benefit from evaluation and intervention.[8] Causes of secondary obesity must be eliminated. These include genetic disorders, of which Prader-Willi syndrome is the most common; endocrine abnormalities such as

hypothyroidism; Cushing's syndrome and polycystic ovary syndrome; and psychological disorders such as bulimia in either the child or other members of the family. A complete investigation should include a fasting lipoprotein profile, serial blood pressure measurements, and a fasting glucose and insulin determination. When endocrine or genetic abnormalities are suggested, consultations with appropriate subspecialists are indicated.

Principles of treatment have been reviewed by a number of authors and consensus groups.[5,8-10] These are also divided into population-based recommendations and those targeted toward the individual who is determined to be at risk. Box 16-3 summarizes these recommendations.

Smoking

The finding in adults that risk for CAD is related to the product of tobacco in both dose and exposure time gives tremendous support for addressing this subject in children. Twenty percent of teens have smoked on a daily basis for some period of time, and increasing numbers of children have begun smoking at the beginning of the second decade. The problem is already widespread and demands both prevention and cessation efforts. Younger children and preteens generally acquire risk factors through secondhand exposure, although emulation of parent habits accounts for some in the 8- to 12-year-old group. During the teen years, peer pressure and social conformity are the most important incentives to smoke. In a manner similar to the adult experience, formal programs initiated and maintained by professionals, parents, and institutions have the most positive effect on prevention and cessation. Recommendations for population-based prevention and individual-oriented cessation efforts are summarized in Box 16-4.

Hyperhomocystinemia

Children with metabolic defects such as cystathionine β-synthase deficiency, the cause of homocystinuria, are at risk for developing premature CAD in addition to other serious abnormalities. It is well known that children with chronic renal disease, children with Down syndrome, and some children with leukemia or sickle cell disease manifest elevated levels of homocysteine. There is legitimate concern that these individuals may incur a higher risk for CAD. In the general pediatric population, it is not known whether higher levels of homocysteine track into adulthood and confer the same risk for CAD described in adults. Studies disagree on a relationship between homocysteine level and a family history of early clinical CAD. Most studies find mean homocysteine

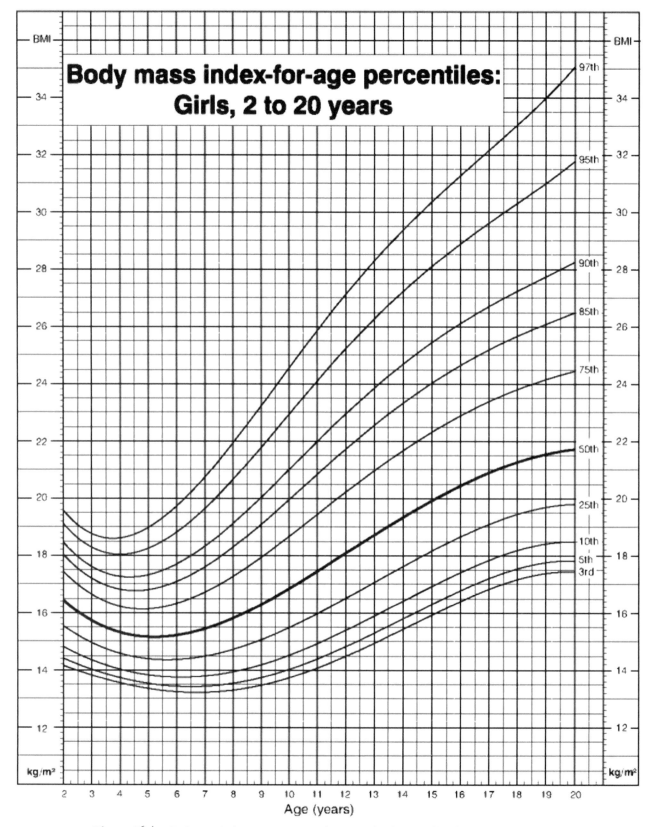

Figure 16-4   Body mass index nomograms. Body mass index for age tables for girls 2–20 years of age. Data from the Centers for Disease Control and Prevention growth chart revision, 2000.

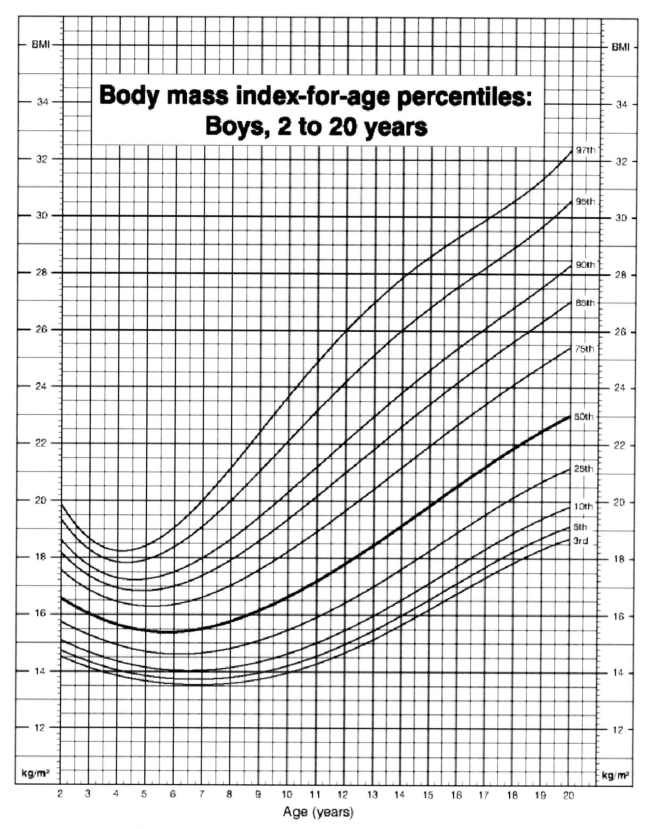

Figure 16-5   Body mass index nomograms. Body mass index for age tables for boys 2–20 years of age. Data from the Centers for Disease Control and Prevention growth chart revision, 2000.

Box 16-3 Population-Based and Individual Recommendations for Treatment of Obesity

POPULATION-BASED RECOMMENDATIONS

- Maintain normal growth patterns and plot BMI at regular visits.
- Encourage moderate aerobic activity for 30 minutes per day.
- Discourage sedentary behavior (e.g., watching TV and playing video games).
- Insert manual activities in the daily routine (e.g., walking up steps and walking to school).
- Encourage the AHA Step 1 diet.
- Advocate for healthy school meal preparation.
- Advocate for community recreational programs.
- Educate families about the seriousness and growing prevalence of obesity and its complications.

INDIVIDUALS AT RISK

- Address obesity early.
- Set realistic goals—the first approach should be maintenance of weight to permit BMI to decrease with growth.
- When a goal of weight loss is accepted by the child and family, institute a program that is based on a calculated balance between energy intake and expenditure. Use a dietitian whenever possible.
- Avoid rapid weight changes to minimize stigmatization, systemic complaints, and eating disorders.
- Review progress at frequent visits.
- Include the entire family in the program and target parents if appropriate.
- When rapid weight loss is required by complications of obesity, utilize an obesity specialist who will evaluate the need for medication or surgery.
- Remember that insufficient data have been collected regarding the efficacy and safety of commercial weight-loss programs.

Box 16-4 Recommendations for Population-Based Prevention and Individual-Oriented Cessation of Smoking

POPULATION-BASED PREVENTION

- Include questions about tobacco use in routine exams beginning at age 8–10. Discuss the harmful short- and long-term effects, the need to resist peer pressure and to substitute other behaviors, the addictive nature of smoking, and the negative role of advertising.
- Inquire about tobacco use by parents at every visit and discuss the effects of secondhand smoke and the increased probability of children smoking from the age of 10.
- Lobby for smoke-free environments in locations where children may assemble.

CESSATION IN INDIVIDUALS

- Assess the child's individual environment and dependence and select a date-oriented quitting program or one that allows for gradual reduction of tobacco exposure with an open-ended plan for quitting entirely.
- Discuss with parents the need to eliminate smoking in the home and to provide support for the child through the difficult period of quitting.
- Discuss with parents the need to maintain a tobacco-free environment and to continue support after smoking is eliminated in the child.
- Consider the use of tobacco substitution products if counseling, encouragement, and behavior modification fail.

---

levels in children to be approximately 5 μmol/L. These are considerably lower than those in adults, but as many as 5% of children have levels comparable to those associated with clinical CAD in adults (i.e., > 9 μmol/L). In the second decade of life, boys have higher levels than girls. The distribution of homocysteine differs among populations and seems to be inversely related to vitamin B6, vitamin B12, and folic acid levels.

At the present time, there is not nearly enough evidence to screen children for hyperhomocystinemia unless there is a family history for this abnormality or a strong family history for CAD in the presence of a normal fasting lipid profile (see Fig. 16-2). Likewise, there is no rationale to begin vitamin supplementation in children with homocysteine levels considerably above the mean unless it is associated with a metabolic defect known to increase the risk of CAD in adults. However, children with levels above the mean should probably have serial levels performed at appropriate intervals.

MAJOR POINTS

- CAD and the thrombotic process begin in childhood.
- CAD is promoted by a number of risk factors that are related in a complex manner. These include dyslipidemia, diabetes, hypertension, obesity, smoking, and hyperhomocystinemia.
- The systematic approach to pediatric dyslipidemia begins with *risk assessment* and progresses through a *diagnostic algorithm* to *treatment options*. This approach is supported by the high probability that lipid values during childhood track into adulthood.
- Essential hypertension is often chronic and mild with onset during mid to late adolescence. Hypertension from secondary causes is more severe and begins earlier.
- Childhood obesity is increasing rapidly. It is strongly associated with insulin resistance.
- Morbidity from smoking is related to its high prevalence among teens and preteens as well as to the effects of secondhand exposure.
- Hyperhomocystinemia in children is a theoretical risk factor for adult CAD.

REFERENCES

1. Kannel WB, Castelli WP, Gordon T, McNamara PM: Serum cholesterol, lipoproteins, and the risk of coronary heart disease. The Framingham study. Ann Intern Med 74:1-12, 1971.

2. Third Report of the National Cholesterol Education Program (NCEP) Expert Panel on Detection, Evaluation, and Treatment of High Blood Cholesterol in Adults (Adult Treatment Panel III) final report. Circulation 106:3143-3421, 2002.

3. American Academy of Pediatrics. National Cholesterol Education Program: Report of the Expert Panel on Blood Cholesterol Levels in Children and Adolescents. Pediatrics 89:525-584, 1992.

4. Kavey RE, Daniels SR, Lauer RM, et al: American Heart Association guidelines for primary prevention of atherosclerotic cardiovascular disease beginning in childhood. Circulation 107:1562-1566, 2003.

5. Williams CL, Hayman LL, Daniels SR, et al: Cardiovascular health in childhood: A statement for health professionals from the Committee on Atherosclerosis, Hypertension, and Obesity in the Young (AHOY) of the Council on Cardiovascular Disease in the Young, American Heart Association. Circulation 106:143-160, 2002.

6. Faulkner B, Daniels SR, Loggie JMH, et al: Update on the 1987 Task Force Report on High Blood Pressure in Children and Adolescents: A Working Group Report from the National High Blood Pressure Education Program. Pediatrics 98:649-658, 1996.

7. Centers for Disease Control: Centers for Disease Control and Prevention 2000 Growth Chart Revisions. CDC publication, 2000. Available at www.cdc.gov/growthcharts.

8. Barlow SE, Dietz WH: Obesity evaluation and treatment: Expert Committee recommendations. The Maternal and Child Health Bureau, Health Resources and Services Administration and the Department of Health and Human Services. Pediatrics 102:E29, 1998.

9. Gidding SS, Leibel DR, Daniels S, et al: Understanding obesity in youth. A statement for healthcare professionals from the Committee on Atherosclerosis and Hypertension in the Young of the Council on Cardiovascular Disease in the Young and the Nutrition Committee, American Heart Association, Writing Group. Circulation 94:3383-3387, 2003.

10. Steinberger J, Daniels, SR: Obesity, insulin resistance, diabetes, and cardiovascular risk in children: An American Heart Association scientific statement from the Atherosclerosis, Hypertension, and Obesity in the Young Committee (Council on Cardiovascular Disease in the Young) and the Diabetes Committee (Council on Nutrition, Physical Activity, and Metabolism). Circulation 107:1448-1453, 2003.

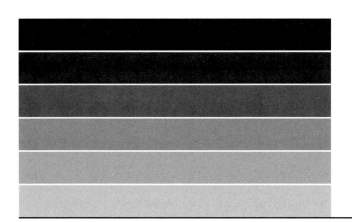

Index